T0327545

Infectious Diseases of Wild Birds

Infectious Diseases of Wild Birds

Edited by Nancy J. Thomas
D. Bruce Hunter
Carter T. Atkinson

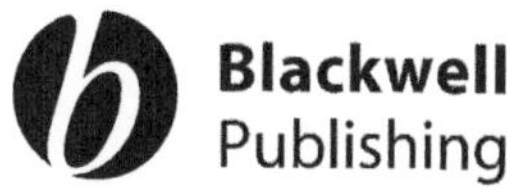

Nancy J. Thomas, DVM, MS, Diplomate, American College of Veterinary Pathologists, is an endangered species specialist for the U.S. Geological Survey, National Wildlife Health Center. She has more than 20 years of experience in diagnostic pathology and research on wild bird diseases.

D. Bruce Hunter DVM, MSC. is a professor in the Department of Pathobiology, Ontario Veterinary College, University of Guelph. His specialty encompasses avian, fur-bearing, and wildlife pathology and ecosystem health. His research interests have included infectious diseases of commercial poultry, West Nile Virus in owls, and diseases of mink.

Carter T. Atkinson, Ph.D., is a research microbiologist with the U.S. Geological Survey, Pacific Island Ecosystems Research Center. His research focuses on protozoan parasites of vertebrates, particularly birds, with a recent emphasis on the effects of introduced avian malaria on Hawaiian forest birds.

Blackwell Publishing Professional
2121 State Avenue, Ames, Iowa 50014, USA

Orders: 1-800-862-6657
Office: 1-515-292-0140
Fax: 1-515-292-3348
Web site: www.blackwellprofessional.com

Blackwell Publishing Ltd
9600 Garsington Road, Oxford OX4 2DQ, UK
Tel.: +44 (0)1865 776868

Blackwell Publishing Asia
550 Swanston Street, Carlton, Victoria 3053, Australia
Tel.: +61 (0)3 8359 1011

Library of Congress Cataloging-in-Publication Data
Infectious diseases of wild birds / edited by Nancy J. Thomas, D. Bruce Hunter, Carter T. Atkinson.
p. cm.
Includes bibliographical references and index.
ISBN-13: 978-0-8138-2812-1 (alk. paper)
ISBN-10: 0-8138-2812-0 (alk. paper)
1. Birds—Infections. 2. Wildlife diseases.
3. Communicable diseases in animals.
I. Thomas, Nancy J. (Nancy Jeanne), 1948–. II. Hunter, D. Bruce III. Atkinson, Carter T.
SF994.I54 2007
636.5'08969—dc22

2006021665

The last digit is the print number: 9 8 7 6 5 4 3

Contents

Preface

At its inception, this book was a revision of *Infectious and Parasitic Diseases of Wild Birds,* edited by John W. Davis, Roy C. Anderson, Lars Karstad, and Daniel O. Trainer and published by the Iowa State University Press in 1971. Advances in the field and the volume of resulting material led us to expand the original work and necessitated launching this work as a new volume solely devoted to infectious diseases of wild, free-living birds. Nevertheless, this book is patterned after the original volume that has been the mainstay of wild bird disease study, despite its dated condition. This book is planned as a companion to *Infectious Diseases of Wild Mammals,* 3rd Edition, edited by Elizabeth S. Williams and Ian K. Barker, and *Parasitic Diseases of Wild Mammals,* 2nd Edition, edited by William M. Samuel, Margo J. Pybus, and A. Alan Kocan (Iowa State University Press). We gratefully acknowledge our colleagues who established such excellent models for us to follow.

This book focuses on diseases affecting free-living wild birds and the agents that cause them. Relevant information and examples are drawn from captive birds or poultry in order to fill in gaps in data or to provide lessons for managers of captive-rearing programs, as captive reintroduction programs are becoming increasingly important for supplementing wild populations of threatened and endangered species. Biologists and wildlife managers, wildlife and veterinary students, professionals in the fields of animal health and wildlife disease, and evolutionary biologists with interests in disease ecology should all find this book to be a valuable reference. The chapters cover classical waterfowl diseases, such as avian cholera, botulism, and poultry disease agents that have taken on new dimensions in wild birds (Newcastle disease, mycoplasmosis, and duck plague). New diseases (circoviral, papilloma and polyomaviral diseases) have risen since the original volume in 1971, and some older diseases, such as avian influenza, have acquired global significance in new zoonotic forms. Included among the chapters are disease agents that are less significant to wild bird health but are important to human health, in which wild birds play an important role in the epizootiologic cycle (certain arboviruses and *Borrelias*).

The chapter authors were selected for their expertise and familiarity with the agents, disease processes, and effects on wild bird populations. This book is the cumulative product of their considerable knowledge and experience. Each chapter provides a classical description of the history, disease, and causative agent, but the authors were also challenged to provide perspectives on the significance of the disease to wild birds and to document population impacts, an aspect that is particularly difficult to quantify in the wild. Chapters concentrate more on the disease processes, recognition, and epizootiologic factors than on treatment. Authors were encouraged to identify unresolved questions and to provide balanced reviews of controversies. It is inevitable that rapid advances in knowledge and the fast pace of environmental changes in today's world will quickly render some aspects of this book outdated, but the authors' treatments of rapidly evolving diseases like avian influenza and West Nile virus are "state of the art" at this time. The authority for avian nomenclature, both scientific and English names, was the American Ornithologists' Union *Checklist of North American Birds,* 7th Edition (http://www.aou.org/checklist/), supplemented for any unlisted species, by James F. Clements' *Birds of the World: A Checklist* (Ibis Publishing Company, 2000). Because many unpublished data on wild bird diseases have been compiled in laboratory and diagnostic files, citations of unpublished data were allowed for repositories of large, permanent, accessible institutions, such as the Canadian Cooperative Wildlife Health Centre, USGS National Wildlife Health Center, and Southeastern Cooperative Wildlife Disease Study.

Grateful acknowledgement goes to Donald J. Forrester, University of Florida, the Iowa State University Press, who guided this project through its initial stages, and to Blackwell Publishing, who took it over and shepherded it through to completion. We also thank Daina Hunter for her significant contribution in the technical editing of this book. We acknowledge the support of the U.S. Geological Survey, Wildlife and Terrestrial Resources Program and the University of Guelph. This book is dedicated to the Wildlife Disease Association, whose members initiated the revision of this book series and who continue to provide the backbone of growing knowledge in the field of wildlife disease. Royalties that accrue from sales of this book will be provided to the Wildlife Disease Association.

Nancy J. Thomas
D. Bruce Hunter
Carter T. Atkinson

Contributors

Arthur A. Andersen
National Animal Disease Center
Agricultural Research Service
U.S. Department of Agriculture
Ames, Iowa, U.S.A.

Trent K. Bollinger
Canadian Cooperative Wildlife Health Centre
Western College of Veterinary Medicine
Department of Veterinary Pathology
University of Saskatchewan
Saskatoon, Saskatchewan, Canada

Richard G. Botzler
Department of Wildlife
Humboldt State University
Arcata, California, U.S.A.

Kathryn A. Converse
U.S. Geological Survey
National Wildlife Health Center
Madison, Wisconsin U.S.A.

Todd Cornish
Wyoming State Veterinary Diagnostic Laboratory
Department of Veterinary Science
University of Wyoming
Laramie, Wyoming, U.S.A.

Pierre-Yves Daoust
Canadian Cooperative Wildlife Health Centre
Department of Pathology and Microbiology
Atlantic Veterinary College
University of Prince Edward Island
Charlottetown, Prince Edward Island, Canada

Douglas E. Docherty
U.S. Geological Survey
National Wildlife Health Center
Madison, Wisconsin, U.S.A.

Mark L. Drew
Idaho Department of Fish and Game
Wildlife Health Laboratory
Caldwell, Idaho, U.S.A.

John R. Fischer
Southeastern Cooperative Wildlife Disease Study, and
Department of Population Health
College of Veterinary Medicine
The University of Georgia
Athens, Georgia, U.S.A.

Scott D. Fitzgerald
Department of Pathobiology and Diagnostic
Investigation
College of Veterinary Medicine
Michigan State University
Lansing, Michigan, U.S.A.

Leanne J. Flewelling
Fish and Wildlife Research Institute
Florida Fish and Wildlife Conservation Commission
St. Petersburg, Florida, U.S.A.

Donald J. Forrester
Department of Infectious Diseases and Pathology
College of Veterinary Medicine
University of Florida
Gainesville, Florida, U.S.A.

J. Christian Franson
U.S. Geological Survey
National Wildlife Health Center
Madison, Wisconsin U.S.A.

Richard E. Gough
Avian Virology
Veterinary Laboratories Agency (Weybridge)
New Haw, Addlestone, Surrey, United Kingdom

Wallace R. Hansen
U.S. Geological Survey
National Wildlife Health Center
Madison, Wisconsin, U.S.A.

Robert A. Heckert
U.S. Department of Agriculture
Agricultural Research Service
Animal Health National Program
Beltsville, Maryland, U.S.A.

Tuula Hollmén
Alaska SeaLife Center, and
University of Alaska Fairbanks
School of Fisheries and Ocean Sciences
Seward, Alaska, U.S.A.

D. Bruce Hunter
Department of Pathobiology
Ontario Veterinary College
University of Guelph
Guelph, Ontario, Canada

Erhard F. Kaleta
Klinik für Vögel, Reptilien, Amphibien und Fische
Justus-Liebig-Universität Giessen
Giessen, Germany

Jan H. Landsberg
Fish and Wildlife Research Institute
Florida Fish and Wildlife Conservation Commission
St. Petersburg, Florida, U.S.A.

Frederick A. Leighton
Canadian Cooperative Wildlife Health Centre
Department of Veterinary Pathology
Western College of Veterinary Medicine
University of Saskatchewan
Saskatoon, Saskatchewan, Canada

Page Luttrell
Southeastern Cooperative Wildlife Disease Study, and
Department of Population Health
College of Veterinary Medicine
The University of Georgia
Athens, Georgia, U.S.A.

Robert G. McLean
U.S. Department of Agriculture
Animal and Plant Health Inspection Service-Wildlife Services
National Wildlife Research Center
Fort Collins, Colorado, U.S.A.

Torsten Mörner
Department of Wildlife, Fish and Environment
National Veterinary Institute
Uppsala, Sweden

Eva Nagy
Department of Pathobiology
Ontario Veterinary College
University of Guelph
Guelph, Ontario, Canada

Björn Olsen
Department of Infectious Diseases
Umeå University
Umeå, Sweden and
Biology and Environmental Sciences
Institute for Zoonotic Ecology and Epidemiology
Kalmar University
Kalmar, Sweden

Jean Paré
Animal Health Centre
Toronto Zoo
Scarborough, Ontario, Canada

David N. Phalen
Wildlife Health and Conservation Centre
Camden, New South Wales, Australia

John F. Prescott
Department of Pathobiology
Ontario Veterinary College
University of Guelph
Guelph, Ontario, Canada

Charlotte F. Quist
Wildlife Health Associates, Inc.
Dillon, Montana, U.S.A.

Charles van Riper III
U.S. Geological Survey
Southwest Biological Science Center
Sonoran Desert Field Station
The University of Arizona
Tucson, Arizona, U.S.A.

Nadia Robert
Center for Fish and Wildlife Health
Institute for Animal Pathology
University of Berne
Berne, Switzerland

Tonie E. Rocke
U.S. Geological Survey
National Wildlife Health Center
Madison, Wisconsin, U.S.A.

Michael D. Samuel
U.S. Geological Survey (USGS)
National Wildlife Health Center, and
USGS-Wisconsin Cooperative Wildlife Research Center
University of Wisconsin
Madison, Wisconsin, U.S.A.

Richard D. Slemons
Department of Veterinary Preventive Medicine
College of Veterinary Medicine
The Ohio State University
Columbus, Ohio, U.S.A.

David E. Stallknecht
Southeastern Cooperative Wildlife Disease
Study, and Department of Population Health
College of Veterinary Medicine
The University of Georgia
Athens, Georgia, U.S.A.

Sonya R. Ubico
Atitlan Green and Wild
Fort Collins, Colorado, U.S.A.

Gabriel A. Vargo
College of Marine Science
University of South Florida
St. Petersburg, Florida, U.S.A.

Faith E. Wiley
Department of Forestry and Natural Resources
Clemson University
Clemson, South Carolina, U.S.A.

Gary A. Wobeser
Canadian Cooperative Wildlife Health Centre
Department of Veterinary Pathology
Western College of Veterinary Medicine
University of Saskatchewan
Saskatoon, Saskatchewan, Canada

Mark J. Wolcott
Field Operations and Training Branch, and
Special Pathogens Branch
U.S. Army Medical Research Institute of Infectious Diseases
Fort Detrick, Maryland, U.S.A.

Roger D. Wyatt
Department of Poultry Science
University of Georgia
Athens, Georgia, U.S.A.

Section 1: Viral Diseases

1
Newcastle Disease and Related Avian Paramyxoviruses

Frederick A. Leighton and Robert A. Heckert

INTRODUCTION

Several related paramyxoviruses infect and cause disease in wild and domestic birds. Of these, avian paramyxovirus type 1 (APMV-1), also known as Newcastle Disease virus, is the best studied. Much less is known about the other eight avian paramyxoviruses (APMV-2 to APMV-9). This chapter is concerned primarily with APMV-1 and the disease it causes: Newcastle Disease (ND). However, some information on the other avian paramyxoviruses also is provided.

Newcastle Disease virus is widespread among several different taxonomic groups of wild birds, and appears capable of infecting all species of birds and some other vertebrates, including humans. ND has caused substantial mortality in free-ranging populations of Double-crested Cormorants (*Phalacrocorax auritus*) and Rock Pigeons (*Columba livia*), and among psittacine birds and other tropical species captured and shipped internationally in the pet bird trade. All of these species have been sources of infection for domestic poultry. ND is one of the most economically important diseases of domestic poultry world-wide. Newcastle Disease and Avian Influenza are the only two diseases of birds included by the World Organization for Animal Health (formerly OIE) among the 15 infectious diseases deemed most economically important to international trade in animals and animal products (World Organization for Animal Health 2004). There are many strains of ND virus, and they vary greatly in their capacity to cause disease in different bird species. Infection may be entirely unapparent or may result in disease that can range from mild to rapidly fatal. Thus, the term "Newcastle Disease virus," in its various contexts, refers to a complex of many virus strains, global in distribution, that infect a wide range of avian hosts and that manifest themselves very differently in different settings.

SYNONYMS

APMV-1:Newcastle Disease, pseudo-fowl pest, pseudovogel-pest, atypische gefugelpest, pseudo-poultry plague, avian pest, avian distemper, Ranikhet disease, Tetelo disease, Korean fowl plague, avian pneumoencephalitis
APMV-2: Yucaipa virus
APMV-5: Kunitachi virus

In general, the terms "Newcastle Disease virus" and "Avian Paramyxovirus Type 1" (APMV-1) are synonyms. However, this broad application of the name "Newcastle Disease" has proved to be problematic for government regulatory veterinary agencies that seek to regulate only those particular strains of the virus that cause significant disease in commercial poultry. Thus, in the context of international trade in poultry and poultry products, the names "Newcastle Disease" and "Newcastle Disease virus" are reserved exclusively for strains of APMV-1 that are highly pathogenic for domestic chickens. Scientists who do not work within this regulatory framework do not often adhere to this restricted use of the name "Newcastle Disease," and more often use the terms APMV-1 and ND virus synonymously.

In the past, diseases in birds caused by avian paramyxoviruses other than APMV-1 also may have been called "Newcastle Disease." As of this writing, nine different avian paramyxoviruses are now recognized. Virological techniques to distinguish some of these viruses from APMV-1 have been available for a relatively short period of time. Thus, some reports in the literature of ND virus may have been of diseases and viruses that were not ND (Kaleta and Baldauf 1988; Alexander 2000a).

HISTORY

The earliest record of Newcastle Disease virus in wild birds may be from 1897 in Great Cormorants

(*Phalacrocorax carbo*) and European Shags (*Phalacrocorax aristotelis*) in Scotland (MacPherson 1956; Kuiken 1999). This inference is made from a poem in Scottish Gaelic, *Call nan cearc* ("The Loss of the Hens") that recounts a die-off of domestic chickens that was strikingly similar to an epidemic of ND that occurred in the same coastal locations in Scotland and in Ireland in 1949–1951. The source of infection for the hens in the 1949–1951 epizootic was determined to be the two cormorant species, which regularly were hunted for food and from which offal was fed to chickens. In the 1949–1951 outbreak, ND virus was isolated from European Shags and also from a Northern Gannet (*Morus bassanus*), and one Great Cormorant was found with a high serological titre to ND virus, indicating recent infection (Wilson 1950; Blaxland 1951; MacPherson 1956). In this mid-century outbreak, there was no evidence that the cormorants suffered disease because of their infection, but lesions that might have been due to ND were observed in the gannet. Whether the ND virus in this outbreak originated from infected domestic poultry carried to wild bird populations by scavenging gulls or was enzootic in the wild seabird populations themselves has been discussed but not resolved (Kuiken 1999; MacPherson 1956). About 20% of Great Cormorants sampled in eastern France from 1997 to 1999 were serologically positive to one or more strains of ND virus (Artois et al. 2002).

From the 1950s onward, numerous serological surveys of free-ranging and captive wild birds were undertaken, some accompanied by attempts at virus isolation. Results of these surveys showed that exposure to ND viruses was widespread, particularly among free-living waterfowl. Published reports of infection of wild birds with ND virus were compiled by Palmer and Trainer (1971) and Kaleta and Baldauf (1988), the latter recording infection in 241 different species of birds encompassing 27 taxonomic Orders. Several strains of the virus were isolated from wild waterfowl; these were of very low virulence to poultry and did not appear to cause disease in the source species (Palmer and Trainer 1971; Vickers and Hanson 1982; Vickers and Hanson 1980; Alexander 1988b; Kaleta and Baldauf 1988; Stallknecht et al. 1991). Nonetheless, from circumstantial evidence it has been inferred that wild waterfowl may have been responsible for spread of a strain of ND virus highly pathogenic to chickens across Europe in 1996–1997 (Alexander et al. 1998).

An epizootic of ND emerged in Rock Pigeons in Europe in the 1980s (Vindevogel and Duchatel 1988). The disease was recognized and followed primarily in domestic racing pigeons (domesticated Rock Pigeons). Its occurrence in wild populations is not well documented. The epizootic may have begun in the Middle East in the 1970s and spread westward and then around the world. The strain of ND virus responsible for this epizootic is distinguishable from other strains by antigenic and molecular criteria, and generally is at least moderately pathogenic in chickens. The virus infected Rock Pigeons inhabiting grain storage facilities in England and was spread to commercial poultry when virus from the pigeons was incorporated into poultry feeds made from contaminated grains (Alexander et al. 1984; Alexander et al. 1985).

Epizootic ND with high rates of morbidity and mortality was observed in young-of-the-year (YOY) Double-crested Cormorants in Canada in 1990 and subsequently recurred both in Canada and the United States throughout that decade (Wobeser et al. 1993; Kuiken et al. 1998b; Kuiken 1999). This is the only wild bird species in which large-scale mortality from ND has been recognized; reported mortality has ranged from <1% to 92% of YOY per affected colony. ND virus also was isolated from one American White Pelican (*Pelecanus erythrorhynchos*), one Caspian Tern (*Sterna caspia*) and one Ring-billed Gull (*Larus delawarensis*) during these epizootics. A single strain of ND virus was isolated consistently from these outbreaks and was highly pathogenic for chickens. This same strain of ND virus spread from wild cormorants to one commercial turkey flock in the United States in 1992 (Heckert et al. 1996).

In domestic poultry, Newcastle Disease was first recognized in the mid-1920s more or less simultaneously at locations that are currently within India, Sri Lanka, Indonesia, Korea, Japan and England. The name of the disease derives from the description of the outbreak in 1926 at Newcastle-Upon-Tyne, England, by T.M. Doyle (Doyle 1927). Three possible explanations for the emergence of these ND virus strains highly pathogenic to chickens have been advanced: 1) that these ND virus strains existed historically in domestic chickens in southeast Asia, and that ND emerged as a major international disease of poultry when large-scale commercial poultry farming and rapid international trade developed in the first half of the twentieth century; 2) that these strains of ND viruses were enzootic among wild birds in tropical rain forests and spread to poultry when human settlement intruded into their natural habitat; and 3) that these strains of ND viruses arose directly by mutation from the many strains of low pathogenicity to chickens found in wild birds. Alexander (2000a) considered the first explanation likely, the second unlikely, and the third at least possible.

The first world-wide occurrence of ND in poultry lasted from the mid-1920s to the early 1960s. A second world-wide epizootic in poultry occurred from 1969 to 1973, and a regional epizootic occurred in Western Europe throughout the 1990s.

Avian Paramyxovirus serotypes 2 to 9 were described in domestic or wild birds between 1956 and 1978, as indicated in Table 1.1. None of these viruses has been recognized to cause disease in free-living wild birds, but all are assumed to persist in wild bird populations. APMV serotypes 2, 3, 6, and 7 have produced disease in domestic poultry (Alexander 2000).

DISTRIBUTION

ND viruses are worldwide in distribution, but detailed knowledge of the distribution of the many different strains of the virus in different host species is fragmentary and incomplete. Natural migration in many groups of wild birds and translocation by humans of wild and domestic birds or bird products occur on so rapid and global a scale that any strain of ND virus has the potential to infect wild or domestic birds in all parts of the planet. Any attempt to define the geographic distribution of ND viruses at one point in time would be radically out of date in a very short while. Antibodies to ND virus have been detected in Antarctic penguins and arctic-nesting geese (Morgan and Westbury 1981; Bradshaw and Trainer 1966). Small poultry flocks in southeast Asia, Central America, parts of South America, and perhaps parts of Africa probably are the principal reservoirs of ND virus strains highly pathogenic to chickens (Alexander 2000a). Double-crested Cormorants, which range across the full width of North America and from the Canadian boreal forest south to Mexico, and Rock Pigeons world-wide appear to maintain within their populations virus strains pathogenic both to themselves and to other species, including domestic poultry. Too little is known about the other avian paramyxoviruses to make an accurate statement about their geographic distributions.

HOST RANGE

All species of birds probably can be infected with one or more of the strains of ND virus. Most infections are asymptomatic and do not result in disease. Infection

Table 1.1. Avian paramyxovirus serotypes.

Prototype virus	Common hosts	Other hosts	Related diseases in Poultry
PMV-1 (Newcastle disease virus)	Many different avian species	—	Spectrum of disease
PMV-2/chicken/California/ Yucaipa/56	turkeys, passerines	chickens, psittacines, rails	Respiratory disease, egg production losses, serious if complicated
PMV-3/turkey/Wisconsin/68	turkeys only	none	egg production losses, respiratory disease
PMV-3/parakeet/Netherlands/ 449/75	psittacines, passerines	none	No infections known
PMV-4/duck/Hong Kong/D3/75	ducks	geese	Inapparent infections in commercial ducks
PMV-5/budgerigar/Japan/ Kunitachi/75	Budgerigars	lorikeets	No infections known
PMV-6/duck/Hong Kong/199/77	ducks	geese, turkeys, rails	Inapparent in ducks and geese, respiratory disease and egg losses in turkeys
PMV-7/dove/Tennessee/4/75	pigeons, doves	turkeys, ostriches	No infections known
PMV-8/goose/Delaware/1053/75	ducks, geese	—	No infections known
PMV-9/duck/New York/22/78	ducks	—	Inapparent infections in commercial ducks

Source: Alexander, D. J. 1997 (with permission).

with ND virus has been reported in more than 241 different avian species (Kaleta and Baldauf 1988; Wobeser et al. 1993; Bailey et al. 1996; Alexander 2000b).

The other eight avian paramyxoviruses are not nearly as well studied as is ND virus (APMV-1), and the full range of hosts that each infects remains to be determined (Table 1.1).

ETIOLOGY

The causative agent of Newcastle Disease (ND) is avian paramyxovirus serotype 1 (APMV-1), classified as belonging to the Order *Mononegavirales,* Family *Paramyxoviridae,* Subfamily *Paramyxovirinae,* Genus *Rubulavirus* (Rima et al. 1995). The virus contains a linear, noninfectious, negative sense, ssRNA genome of 15–16 kb in size with a Mr of $3.5–5 \times 10^6$ that codes for six proteins, including an RNA directed RNA polymerase (L), hemagglutinin-neuraminidase (HN) protein, fusion (F) protein, matrix (M) protein, phosphoprotein (P), and nucleoprotein (N) (de Leeuw and Peeters 1999). The virions are approximately 150 nm or more in diameter, pleomorphic, with a lipid envelope surrounding a helical nucleocapsid. Embedded in the lipid envelope are the HN and F proteins, which form the surface spikes. The virus is sensitive to lipid solvents, unstable at very high or low pH, and shows heat lability, especially above 40°C (Beard et al. 1984).

EPIZOOTIOLOGY

ND virus is readily transmitted among susceptible birds. Virus can be shed by infected birds in feces, body fluids, and eggs, and potentially is present in all tissues, including meat and viscera. The virus can survive for long periods of time outside living hosts, and transmission via contamination of inanimate objects is likely.

Most infections in wild birds appear to cause little or no disease but result both in a detectable immune response and a period of virus replication and shedding by the infected bird. Cormorants shed virus for 21–32 days after experimental infection (MacPherson 1956; Kuiken et al. 1998a). Such experimental results, and the many isolations of ND viruses from apparently healthy birds, indicate that long periods of virus shedding, and thus of potential transmission of the virus to other birds, is usual in infections with ND virus. As noted in the historical account (above), among wild bird populations, Double-crested Cormorants and Rock Pigeons appear to maintain virus strains pathogenic to themselves and to other species, while wild waterfowl (ducks and geese) appear to maintain virus strains generally of low virulence to themselves and to other species.

The virus is relatively stable in nature, remaining infective for weeks at low temperatures and surviving for several hours over a wide pH range. Protected by associated organic matter, it can survive for days in litter, water, soil, carcasses, eggs, and feathers. Virus remained infectious on feather down for 123 days at a temperature of 20°C to 30°C, 255 days when temperatures varied from 11°C to 36°C, and for 538 days at 3°C to 6°C. The virus survived pH extremes of pH 3 and pH 11 for up to one week. It remained infectious in meat and bone for six months at 1°C (Olesiuk 1951; Moses et al. 1947).

Infected Rock Pigeons are reported to shed virus starting two days after infection and to continue shedding for about two weeks. Virus persisted in the intestine for up to three weeks after infection and in the brain for up to five weeks after infection. Rock Pigeons were considered no longer potential sources of infection for other birds six weeks after they became ill with ND. However, infectious virus may persist in pigeon feces for more than six months under natural conditions. In domestic flocks of Rock Pigeons, new cases of clinical ND ceased to appear about five weeks after infection first reached the flock (Kaleta and Baldauf 1988).

Epizootic ND in wild birds has been documented in only two settings: Double-crested Cormorants in North America and Rock Pigeons, initially in the Middle East, Africa, and Europe, and then North America, Japan, and worldwide. Epizootic ND occurred in Rock Pigeons in southern Europe in the early 1980s, preceded by occurrences in the Middle East and Africa, and spread north and west across Europe. The virus was translocated to North America and to Asia by unknown means in the 1980s (Vindevogel and Duchatel 1988; Johnston and Key 1992; Barton et al. 1992). Although documented primarily as a disease of domestic Rock Pigeons (racing pigeons), wild and feral birds were affected as well. Among naive domestic Rock Pigeons, morbidity rates have been reported to range from 30% to 70%, with many affected birds recovering from the disease and mortality seldom exceeding 10%. Morbidity and mortality rates have not been estimated in wild Rock Pigeons, but it is likely that morbidity rates equivalent to those reported in domestic birds would result in much higher mortality rates in wild Rock Pigeons, which must feed themselves, avoid predators, and maintain their balance on roosts. Newcastle Disease first affected free-living urban Rock Pigeons in Saskatoon, Saskatchewan, Canada in the summer of 1990, and this epizootic may be typical of epizootics elsewhere. Initially, ND produced highly visible mortality. There was a slow but steady rain of affected birds from their roosting areas under the city's bridges into the South Saskatchewan

River below that could be witnessed any day during the summer and early fall of 1990. Dead birds accumulated in such quantities around other urban roosts that special collection and disposal were undertaken. Many birds were submitted to the local veterinary college for diagnosis. Within two years, however, such highly visible mortality had ended, although the virus persisted in the pigeon population. A single strain of ND virus was responsible for this world-wide epizootic among Rock Pigeons (Alexander et al. 1985; Pearson et al. 1987). Thus, there appears to be a stable relationship between this strain of ND virus and Rock Pigeon populations in many parts of the world.

Mortality of young-of-the-year (YOY) cormorants caused by ND was first recognized in North America in Saskatchewan in 1990 and subsequently was recognized at various locations in 1992, 1995, 1996, 1997, 1999, 2001, and 2003 (F.A. Leighton, unpublished data; Wobeser et al. 1993; Kuiken 1999; Meteyer et al. 1997). At one breeding colony in Saskatchewan, monitored regularly for epidemic disease, ND occurred at two-year intervals in 1995, 1997, 1999, 2001, and 2003. A single strain of virus was the cause of all of these occurrences of ND. Thus, there may be a stable relationship between this ND virus strain and Double-crested Cormorants. Antibodies to APMV-1 (virus strain not determined) were found in 26% to 56% of migratory Double-crested Cormorants sampled in winter in the southern United States from 1997 to 1999, and in 78% of eggs laid by the nonmigratory Florida subspecies in 1998–1999 (Farley et al. 2001). It is most likely that ND is enzootic in Double-crested Cormorant populations, with periodic epizootic occurrence among YOY. Morbidity rates among cormorants are not known. Rough estimates of mortality rates among YOY have ranged from less than 1% to 92%. A mortality rate within the range of 32% to 64% was estimated in one intensively studied outbreak (Kuiken 1999). ND virus in cormorants is more pathogenic to young birds than to older birds. This also is the case in poultry (Kuiken et al. 1998a; Alexander 1997). An ND virus isolated from an epizootic that killed at least 32% of YOY cormorants on their breeding colony produced minimal disease or none at all when previously unexposed, hand-reared birds from the same colony in the same year were infected at 16 weeks of age. The birds on the colony had been exposed to natural infection at about six weeks of age. The many outbreaks in Double-crested Cormorants have caused mortality and clinical disease exclusively in YOY birds (Meteyer et al. 1997; Kuiken 1999).

Major outbreaks of ND in poultry in the early 1970s were traced to imported infected psittacine birds, and ND virus strains highly pathogenic for chickens have frequently been isolated from dead, sick, or asymptomatic psittacines and other species imported into various countries in the pet bird trade (Clavijo et al. 2000; Ashton 1984; Walker et al. 1973). Because of this, it has been assumed that wild populations of these species, particularly psittacines, are reservoirs for these ND virus strains so highly pathogenic to chickens. All evidence to date indicates that this is a false assumption. Pathogenic ND viruses have not been found in wild populations of these species, whereas highly pathogenic ND viruses continue to be found in rural poultry flocks in many tropical areas. It is probable that tropical wild birds captured for the pet bird trade are placed in contact with small rural flocks of domestic chickens during transportation, marketing, and in holding facilities, and that the captured birds become infected with ND viruses only after capture (Johnson et al. 1986; Goodman and Hanson 1988; Kaleta and Baldauf 1988).

CLINICAL SIGNS

In both Rock Pigeons and Double-crested Cormorants, the signs most characteristic of ND are manifestations of central nervous system dysfunction associated with infection and inflammation of the brain and spinal cord (Kaleta and Baldauf 1988; Barton et al. 1992; Kuiken et al. 1998b). Affected birds may have uncoordinated gait and movements, abnormal positioning of the head and neck, poor balance, and unilateral or bilateral partial or complete paralysis of legs and wings (Figure 1.1). Similar clinical signs in Double-crested Cormorants are described in detail by Kuiken et al. 1998b. Among cormorants, paralysis of legs and wings appears to persist as a permanent debility in many birds that survive acute ND (Figure 1.1). Birds with unilateral wing paralysis thrash across the water with their one functional wing acting like a paddle wheel. They are able to dive but not to fly. Although unilateral wing dysfunction can have many causes, observation of numbers of birds exhibiting such single-wing attempts to fly can be taken as good evidence of a current or recent epizootic of ND in cormorants. In epizootic years, cormorants with such paralysed wings remain on colony lakes after the rest of the birds have departed on southward migration, and can be seen on these lakes until freeze-up in late fall. Live birds falling from their roosts is one manifestation of clinical ND in Rock Pigeons.

Clinical signs associated with dysfunction of the central nervous system are not always evident in cormorants and pigeons with ND. Many affected birds are systemically ill and show only general weakness and prostration. Diarrhea, sometimes with hemorrhage, is a usual feature of ND in Rock Pigeons and is the classical clinical sign of highly pathogenic (visceral, velogenic) ND in domestic chickens (Vindevogel and

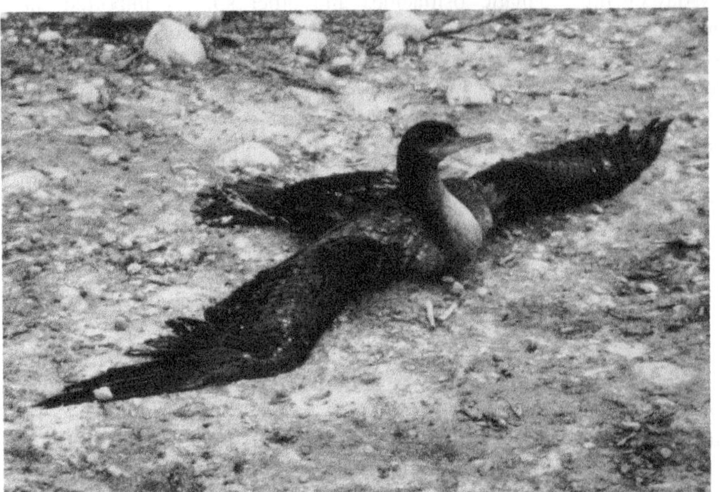
A

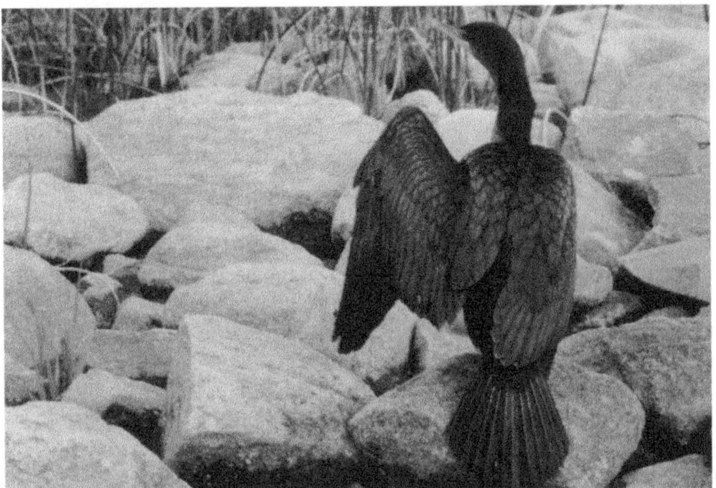
B

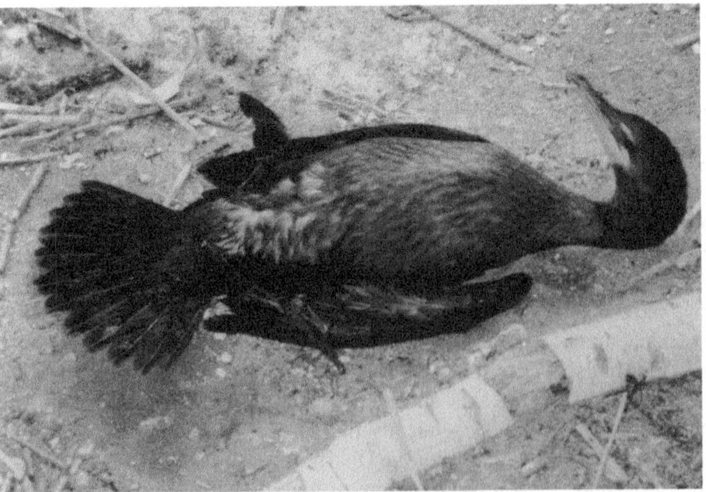
C

Figure 1.1. Clinical signs of Newcastle Disease in Double-crested Cormorants. A. Bilateral leg paralysis. The cormorant is trying to move forward by use of its wings pivoted against the ground. B. Unilateral wing paralysis. The normal wing is spread and the affected wing is held close to the body. C. Loss of balance. The cormorant has fallen on its back and has difficulty in righting itself (From Kuiken 1999, used with permission).

Duchatel 1988; Barton et al. 1992). For all species of birds, ND must be considered as one potential cause of any clinical disease that includes bloody diarrhea, signs of central nervous system dysfunction, or general prostration.

PATHOGENESIS

The pathogenicity of ND virus varies greatly with the strain of virus and the species of host bird. Nearly all research on the pathogenesis of ND virus infection has been done with domestic chickens, thus most of the information presented here is derived from experimental infections in chickens.

The period between infection and the appearance of clinical disease usually is two to six days, but can be up to 15 to 21 days. An outbreak in chickens may be so severe that almost all of an affected flock dies within 72 hours without prior noticeable signs, often causing a suspicion of poisoning.

The primary determinant of virulence of ND viruses in chickens is the amino acid composition of the fusion (F) protein on the virus surface and its effect on the ability of host cell enzymes to cleave this protein. During infection with ND virus, it is necessary for the precursor protein, F0, to be cleaved to proteins F1 and F2 in order for further steps in the process of virus infection to occur. This cleavage of F0 is mediated by host cell proteases, which recognize a specific motif of amino acids at the F protein cleavage site. For example, in chickens it was found that if the cleavage motif contained several basic amino acids, the cleavage and subsequent virus replication could occur in most cells throughout the body, whereas if the cleavage motif contained few or no basic amino acids, cleavage could be mediated only by enzymes found in the respiratory or intestinal tracts, thus confining virus infection to these sites (Nagai et al. 1976; Alexander 2001; Aldous et al. 2001). Mutational changes in this cleavage site, resulting in the addition of basic amino acids, has led to changes in viruses from low virulence to high, as seen in ND outbreaks in Ireland in 1990 and in Australia in 1998–2000 (Collins et al. 1998; Westbury 2001). The marked variation in pathogenicity of ND virus strains in different species and ages of birds may have a similar basis in the interaction between the amino acid structure of virus surface proteins and host enzyme locations and configurations.

PATHOLOGY

Newcastle Disease viruses typically cause lesions in one or more of four organs or body systems: central nervous system, kidney, alimentary tract, and respiratory system.

ND viruses pathogenic to wild bird species appear most often to affect the central nervous system and kidney, or to cause generalized, rapidly fatal disease accompanied by few recognizable gross or histological lesions. In both Double-crested Cormorants and Rock Pigeons, pathological changes often are restricted to the central nervous system and kidney and are evident only microscopically (Kuiken et al. 1999; Meteyer et al. 1997; Wobeser et al. 1993; Kaleta and Baldauf 1988; Barton et al. 1992). Histological lesions in the central nervous system have consisted of nonsuppurative inflammation in the brain and cord, sometimes including the meninges, with cuffs of lymphocytes around blood vessels and with associated gliosis, necrosis of neurons, and swelling of endothelial cells. These lesions occurred most regularly in the brain stem and cerebellum in cormorants but also were evident elsewhere. Nonsuppurative nephritis, consisting of multiple small areas of infiltration of the renal parenchyma with lymphocytes and plasma cells, also has been a regular feature of infection with ND virus in cormorants and pigeons. Small foci of necrosis of renal tubule cells have been observed in association with the inflammatory cells. Focal nonsuppurative pancreatitis has been noted in infected Rock Pigeons. These lesions are particularly well illustrated in Barton et al.(1992) and Kuiken et al. (1999).

Kaleta and Baldauf (1988) tabulated reported clinical signs and lesions from published accounts of ND virus infection in 222 different species of birds infected either naturally or experimentally with ND viruses. The birds in their survey either had no lesions at all or had combinations of lesions in the alimentary, central nervous, and respiratory systems. Because many of the reports did not include microscopic evaluation of tissues, many of the birds said to have clinical signs of central nervous dysfunction but no lesions probably also had encephalomyelitis. This tabulation and the abundant literature about ND in domestic poultry demonstrate that ND viruses can cause a wide range of lesions in any particular species of bird, and further, that none of these lesions is uniquely attributable to ND.

The pathology of ND is well known and well described in domestic chickens and turkeys (Alexander 1997). Highly pathogenic strains of NDV usually cause severe hemorrhage and necrosis of the alimentary tract. Strains of lesser virulence for chickens often affect both the respiratory and central nervous systems. In the respiratory system, lesions typically include hemorrhage and necrosis of the mucosa of trachea and bronchi, sometimes accompanied by pneumonia due to secondary bacterial infection of the lung. Conjunctivitis and rhinitis also may result from these infections. Lesions in the central nervous system are evident only microscopically and consist of a nonsuppurative encephalomyelitis.

DIAGNOSIS

Neither clinical signs nor *post mortem* lesions alone are a reliable basis for diagnosis of ND. Confirmation requires identification and pathotyping of the virus, demonstration of viral genetic material within lesions, or a significant rise in antibody titre between acute and convalescent sera coinciding with a disease outbreak.

When there is suspicion of ND, it is usual to attempt virus isolation from recently dead or moribund birds. Samples from dead birds should include trachea or tracheal swabs and samples of lung, kidney, intestine (including contents), spleen, brain, liver, and heart. Tissue samples may be collected separately or as a pool, but the intestinal samples should be packaged separately. Where possible, a separate set of tissues also should be collected in 10% neutral-buffered formalin for histopathology. Samples from live birds should include tracheal swabs and cloacal swabs visibly coated with fecal material. Small birds may be harmed by swabbing; therefore the collection of freshly voided feces can serve as an adequate alternative. For transportation of samples, it is recommended that appropriate virus transport media be used (Alexander 2004), and if there is a delay longer than 72 hr in getting samples to a diagnostic laboratory, they should be frozen.

Although routine virus isolation procedures in chicken embryos for NDV are generally adequate (Alexander 2004), some highly pathogenic strains of ND virus have failed to cause hemagglutination after isolation in embryonated eggs and were detected only by use of an indirect immunoperoxidase assay. For example, 19 of 21 viruses isolated from epizootic ND in Double-crested Cormorants rapidly killed the chicken embryos used for primary isolation but failed to show hemagglutination with the standard screening test (Kuiken et al. 1999). Such failure of hemagglutination may have been due to the highly pathogenic virus killing the chicken embryos before sufficient virus replication had occurred to produce a high concentration of virus in the allantoic fluid tested by hemagglutination. Alternatively, this virus strain may lack hemagglutinating properties.

After an ND virus has been isolated, its virulence in domestic chickens is assessed by an established procedure of experimental infections, referred to as pathogenicity testing. In many countries, it is a legal requirement that identification of an ND virus be communicated to national veterinary authorities and tested by those authorities for pathogenicity in chickens. Although several potential *in vitro* tests for establishing virulence are being investigated by various groups around the world, at present the assessment of pathogenicity is based on one or more of the following *in vivo* tests (Alexander 2004):

a. Mean death time in eggs: The mean death time (MDT) is the mean time in hours for the minimum lethal dose to kill chicken embryos. The MDT has been used to classify ND virus strains as highly pathogenic (taking less than 60 hours to kill); moderately pathogenic (taking between 60 and 90 hours to kill); and weakly pathogenic (taking more than 90 hours to kill).
b. Intracerebral pathogenicity index: The intracerebral pathogenicity index (ICPI) is a weighted score of clinical signs after intracerebral injection of the virus into each of 10 ND-free day-old chickens. The most virulent viruses will give indices that approach the maximum score of 2.0, whereas strains with low pathogenicity will give values close to 0.0.
c. Intravenous pathogenicity index: The intravenous pathogenicity index (IVPI) is a weighted score of clinical signs after intravenous injection of the virus into 10 six-week-old ND-free chickens. Low pathogenic strains and some moderately pathogenic strains will have IVPI values of 0.0, whereas the indices for virulent strains will approach 3.0.

Based upon these tests, strains of ND virus were classically grouped into three pathotypes: velogenic (highly virulent), mesogenic (moderately virulent), and lentogenic (low virulence) (Table 1.2). In addition, the velogenic viruses have also been further subclassified based on the organ most severely affected in the experimentally-infected chickens: viscerotropic for the intestinal tract, neurotropic for the central nervous system. In the regulation of international trade in domestic poultry and poultry products, the name "Newcastle Disease virus" now is applied exclusively to ND strains that are highly pathogenic (velogenic) for chickens.

Mouse monoclonal antibodies (MAbs) directed against strains of ND virus have been used in HI tests to allow rapid identification of ND viruses without the possible cross-reactions with other APMV serotypes that may occur with polyclonal sera. MAbs have been produced that give reactions in HI tests that are specific for particular strains or variant ND virus isolates. Panels of MAbs have been used to establish antigenic profiles of ND virus isolates. This has proven to be a valuable method for grouping and differentiating isolates of ND virus and has been particularly valuable in understanding the epizootiology of outbreaks (Alexander et al. 1997).

Table 1.2. Examples of pathogenicity indices obtained for strains of Newcastle disease virus.

Virus strain	Pathotype	ICPI[a]	IVPI[b]	MDT[c]
Ulster 2C	Lentogenic	0.0	0.0	>150
Queensland V4	Lentogenic	0.0	0.0	>150
Hitchner B1	Lentogenic	0.2	0.0	120
F	Lentogenic	0.25	0.0	119
La Sota	Lentogenic	0.4	0.0	103
H	Mesogenic	1.2	0.0	48
Mukteswar	Mesogenic	1.4	0.0	46
Roakin	Mesogenic	1.45	0.0	68
Beaudette C	Mesogenic	1.6	1.45	62
GB Texas	Velogenic	1.75	2.7	55
NY Parrot 70181 1972	Velogenic	1.8	2.6	51
Italian	Velogenic	1.85	2.8	50
Milano	Velogenic	1.9	2.8	50
Herts 33/56	Velogenic	2.0	2.7	48
Cormorant/Quebec-Canada/457/75	Velogenic	1.72	2.20	ND
Gull/Saskatchewan-Canada/1477/90	Velogenic	1.51	1.93	ND
Pelican/Saskatchewan-Canada/1478/90	Velogenic	1.65	1.98	ND

Sources: Alexander 1997; Heckert et al. 1996.
Note:
[a]Intracerebral Pathogenicity Index – see text
[b]Intravenous Pathogenicity Index – see text
[c]Mean Death Time – see text
ND = Not determined

In addition to the traditional tests described previously, molecular biology has provided new methods for the detection of the ND virus genome (Aldous et al. 2001). Detection of ND virus by the reverse transcriptase polymerase chain reaction (RT-PCR) assay was first described in 1991 and has been further developed and applied to diagnosis, as reviewed by Aldous and co-authors (Jestin and Jestin 1991; Aldous et al. 2001). Kho showed that RT-PCR was more sensitive than conventional virus isolation, and it has been used to detect ND virus genome in a wide variety of tissues (Kho et al. 2000; Gohm et al. 2000; Wise et al. 2004). RT-PCR not only has been used to detect the presence of ND virus in samples but also has become an integral part in pathotyping; sequence analysis of the F gene cleavage site can provide important information regarding the potential pathogenicity of ND strains (as described previously under pathogenesis).

Newcastle Disease virus or its genome also can be identified in formalin-fixed, paraffin-embedded tissue sections. In fixed tissues from infected chickens, viral RNA was detected in multiple tissues, most prominently in macrophages associated with lymphoid tissue (Brown et al. 1999). With immunohistochemistry applied to paraffin-embedded sections from infected cormorants, Kuiken demonstrated ND virus particularly in the nervous system and kidney (Kuiken et al. 1999).

SEROLOGICAL DIAGNOSIS

Although the presence of anti-ND virus antibodies in the serum provides no information regarding the strain of ND virus to which the bird was exposed, there may be value in knowing that infection with some strain of ND virus has occurred in wild bird species or populations. Newcastle Disease virus antibodies have been detected by a wide variety of serological tests including single radial immunodiffusion, single radial hemolysis, agar gel immunodiffusion, virus neutralization in chick embryos, plaque neutralization, hemagglutination inhibition (HI), enzyme-linked immunosorbent assay (ELISA), and blocking ELISA (Chu et al. 1982; Hari Babu 1986; Gelb and Cianci 1987; Beard 1980; Beard and Hanson 1984; Czifra and Nilsson 1996). Of these assays, the most widely used is HI and ELISA (Allan and Gough 1974; Beard and Wilkes 1985; Brugh et al. 1978; Adair et al. 1989; Miers et al. 1983; Rivetz et al. 1985; Snyder et al. 1983; Wilson et al. 1984).

A variety of commercial ELISA kits are available and are based on several different strategies for the detection of ND virus antibodies, including indirect, sandwich, and blocking or competitive tests using monoclonal antibodies. Usually such tests have been evaluated and validated by the manufacturer, and it is therefore important that the instructions specified for their use be followed carefully. The ELISA lends itself well to screening large numbers of sera, and the results correlate well with those of HI (Adair et al. 1989; Brown et al. 1990; Cvelic-Cabrilo et al. 1992). The blocking ELISA may be most useful when testing sera from a wide variety of bird species. Although more sera are probably tested by ELISA than by HI, the HI test is still the most widely used test internationally due to its simplicity and ease in interpretation. Chicken sera rarely give nonspecific positive reactions in this test, and pretreatment of the sera is unnecessary. Sera from species other than chickens may sometimes cause agglutination of chicken red blood cells (CRBC), so this property should first be determined and then removed by absorption of the serum with CRBC.

HI titers may be regarded as being positive if there is inhibition of hemagglutination at an initial serum dilution of 1:16 or more against 4 HA units of antigen. Some laboratories prefer to use 8 HA units in HI tests. This is permissible, but it affects the interpretation of results such that a positive titer becomes 1:8 or more. Hemagglutination inhibition also has been used to detect antibodies to ND virus in egg yolk in epidemiological monitoring of exposure to the virus (Kuiken et al. 1998b; Farley et al. 2001).

IMMUNITY

Most if not all avian species will produce an immune response upon exposure to ND virus (Kaleta and Baldauf 1988; Alexander 2004; Sousa et al. 1999; Kuiken et al. 1998a). In commercial poultry, this response has been shown to be both humoral (antibody) and cellular (cell mediated). The initial immune response to infection with ND virus is cell mediated and may be detectable as early as two to three days after infection with live vaccine strains (Ghumman and Bankowski 1976; Timms and Alexander 1977). The importance of cell-mediated immunity is still unclear. One study showed that it contributed to protection but in itself was insufficient to provide complete protection (Reynolds and Maraqa 2000a).

When chickens and some other species have been exposed to ND virus, antibodies generally were detectable in the serum within 6 to 10 days. Antibodies against the HN and F proteins are neutralizing antibodies (Russell 1988; Reynolds and Maraqa 2000b). The amount of antibody produced is dependent upon the infecting strain and generally peaks at approximately three to four weeks post infection. As determined by HI, antibodies can persist for as long as one year after infection (Allan and Gough 1974). Secreted antibodies, in particular from the Harderian gland near the eye, are important in providing upper respiratory tract protection in chickens (Holmes 1979a; Holmes 1979b; Parry and Aitken 1977). These antibodies have been shown to be primarily of the IgM and IgA class (Russell 1993; Russell and Ezeifeka 1995).

Antibody titers in experimentally infected cormorants reached a maximum 21 days after infection and were still detectable 70 days after infection when the experiment ended. From the steady rate of decline in titer following the peak, it was predicted that titers would have become undetectable about 126 days after infection (Kuiken et al. 1998a). It is not known when such birds might become susceptible to re-infection or how long virus would be shed from re-infected birds.

PUBLIC HEALTH CONCERNS

Newcastle Disease virus is a human pathogen of minor importance. The Advisory Committee on Dangerous Pathogens of the United Kingdom has assigned ND virus to Hazard Group 2, each member of which is defined as "a biological agent that can cause human disease and may be a hazard to employees; it is unlikely to spread to the community" (Alexander 2000a). Persons most likely to become infected are those who handle infected birds, such as farmers and pigeon fanciers, veterinary health care workers, including those who vaccinate birds on poultry farms, abattoir workers, and personnel of diagnostic laboratories. There are no records of human infections acquired from consumption of infected eggs or meat. Avirulent virus strains used in live vaccines and field strains pathogenic for birds appear to be equally pathogenic for people. Human disease caused by ND virus has been reviewed by M.I. Khan (1994). The common result of ND virus infection in humans is conjunctivitis, which may be severe but is of only a few days duration and without residual effect once resolved, unless complicated by secondary pathogens. Nothing is known of the potential of other avian paramyxoviruses to cause disease in people.

DOMESTIC AND CAPTIVE ANIMAL HEALTH CONCERNS

Newcastle Disease is one of the most important diseases of poultry around the world. Historically, epizootic ND has caused high mortality and massive expenditures on eradication in developed countries (Walker et al. 1973; Alexander 1988a). Vaccination and biosecurity measures required because of ND virus are a constant cost to industrial poultry production. However, the most important economic impact of ND may be on small poultry flocks in Asia, Africa, Central America, and parts of South America because of the major significance of these flocks to local economies and nutrition, and because of the regular high mortality caused by ND in these settings (Alexander 2000a). For example, in Nepal it has been estimated that as many as 90% of chickens in small village flocks die each year from ND. Small rural flocks are the most likely source for infections in birds that enter the pet bird trade.

In addition to effects on traditional domestic species, Newcastle Disease has been a cause of economic loss in captive ratites and domestic pigeons and is a constant hazard to zoos and wild animal rehabilitation facilities, which can suffer losses of birds to disease and, potentially, depopulation orders imposed on healthy specimens that were exposed to ND virus by infected birds brought into these facilities for medical care. Captive breeding programs for endangered bird species experience similar risks (Kaleta and Baldauf 1988; Vindevogel and Duchatel 1988; Bailey et al. 1996).

Strains of ND virus highly pathogenic to domestic poultry are enzootic in free-living populations of Double-crested Cormorants and Rock Pigeons, and both species have been sources of infection for commercial poultry flocks (Alexander et al. 1984; Heckert et al. 1996). Alexander and others (1998) considered it likely that wild ducks, geese, and swans carried strains of ND virus pathogenic to poultry among sites of outbreaks in commercial poultry in Europe in 1997.

WILDLIFE POPULATION IMPACTS AND MANAGEMENT IMPLICATIONS

Few data are available to evaluate the potential effect of ND on wild bird populations. In Double-crested Cormorants, ND appears to cause high mortality, but only among young-of-the-year. Such mortality in the prefledging period, even if it occurs frequently and recurrently, may have little or no impact on overall population size or structure (Kuiken 1999). Population effects of ND in wild Rock Pigeons have not been studied. There may be an indirect negative impact of ND on populations of tropical birds that are popular in the pet bird trade. Stringent import regulations for such birds, imposed to prevent importation of ND viruses, probably are one stimulus for illegal trading practices, which often result in high mortality rates from diseases and handling. This may result in additional captures of wild birds and further reductions in wild populations.

Wildlife managers should be aware that strains of ND highly pathogenic to domestic poultry are enzootic in Double-crested Cormorants and Rock Pigeons but, as far as is currently known, only in these species. Other species of wild birds also are capable of carrying such pathogenic strains of ND for short periods of time. Where vaccination of poultry against ND is not routinely carried out, prevention of ND in poultry requires nonporous physical barriers between domestic and wild birds to ensure that transmission of ND viruses (and several other important pathogens) does not occur. Wherever possible, wildlife managers should work with local poultry enterprises to reduce the risk of having ND enter these premises from wild bird sources and the risk of wild birds becoming exposed to ND virus strains present in poultry.

TREATMENT AND CONTROL

There is no treatment for ND. Vaccination with both live and killed vaccines is used in domestic birds as an adjunct to biosecurity procedures, which are the primary means of prevention of ND in the commercial poultry industry (Alexander 2000a). Vaccination may be an effective method of ND prevention in gallinaceous species in rare or endangered species recovery programs, but is not a practical solution for wild bird populations. ND virus may be eliminated by pasteurization of table eggs and egg products for 4.5 minutes at 64°C; rendering for several minutes at 100°C; processing of meat for 30 minutes at 30°C or one minute at 80°C. The rate at which the virus is destroyed depends on the strain of virus, the quantity of virus, the time of treatment and the media in which the treatment occurs (Beard and Hanson 1984). In the commercial poultry industry of most developed countries, outbreaks of ND trigger "stamping-out," or eradication, responses whereby all infected and potential contact birds are killed, there is sanitary disposal of all carcasses and bird products, and affected premises are disinfected and left without birds for a period of time.

ACKNOWLEDGEMENTS

Thijs Kuiken and Gary Wobeser contributed substantially to the authors' understanding of ND through discussion, collaborative research and review.

UNPUBLISHED DATA

F. A. Leighton, Canadian Cooperative Wildlife Health Centre, Saskatoon, Saskatchewan, Canada.

LITERATURE CITED

Adair, B.M., M.S. McNulty, D. Todd, T.J. Connor, and K. Burns. 1989. Quantitative estimation of Newcastle disease virus antibody levels in chickens and turkeys by ELISA. *Avian Pathology* 18:175–192.

Aldous, E.W., M.S. Collins, A. McGoldrick, and D.J. Alexander. 2001. Rapid pathotyping of Newcastle disease virus (NDV) using fluorogenic probes in a PCR assay. *Veterinary Microbiology* 80:201–212.

Alexander, D.J. 1988a. Historical aspects. In *Newcastle Disease,* 1st Ed., D.J. Alexander (ed.). Kluwer Academic Publishers, Boston, MA, U.S.A., pp.—.

Alexander, D.J. 1988b. Newcastle disease Virus—An Avian Paramyxovirus. In *Newcastle Disease,* 1st Ed. D.J. Alexander (ed.). Kluwer Academic Publishers, Boston, MA, U.S.A., pp. 11–22.

Alexander, D.J. 1997. Newcastle disease and other avian *Paramyxoviridae* infections. In *Diseases of Poultry,* 10th Ed., B. W. Calnek (ed.). Iowa State University Press, Ames, IA, U.S.A., pp. 541–569.

Alexander, D.J. 2000a. Newcastle disease and other avian paramyxoviruses. *Revue Scientifique et Technique de l'Office International des Epizooties* 19:443–462.

Alexander, D.J. 2000b. Newcastle disease in ostriches (*Struthio camelus*)—a review. *Avian Pathology* 29:95–100.

Alexander, D.J. 2001. Gordon Memorial Lecture: Newcastle disease. *British Poultry Science* 42:5–22.

Alexander, D.J. 2004. Newcastle disease. In *Manual of Standards for Diagnostic Tests and Vaccines for Terrestrial Animals (mammals, birds and bees),* 5th Ed. World Organization for Animal Health (OIE), Paris, France, pp. 270–282.

Alexander, D.J., R.J. Manvell, J.P. Lowings, K.M. Frost, M.S. Collins, P.H. Russell, and J.E. Smith. 1997. Antigenic diversity and similarities detected in avian paramyxovirus type 1 (Newcastle disease virus) isolates using monoclonal antibodies. *Avian Pathology* 26:399–419.

Alexander, D.J., H.T. Morris, W.J. Pollitt, C.E. Sharpe, R.L. Eckford, R.M.Q. Sainsbury, L.M. Mansley, R.E. Gough, and G. Parsons. 1998. Newcastle disease outbreaks in domestic fowl and turkeys in Great Britain during 1997. *Veterinary Record* 143:209–212.

Alexander, D.J., G. Parsons, and R. Marshall. 1984. Infection of fowls with Newcastle disease virus by food contaminated with pigeon faeces. *Veterinary Record* 115:601–602.

Alexander, D.J., G.W.C. Wilson, P.H. Russell, S.A. Lister, and G. Parsons. 1985. Newcastle disease outbreaks in fowl in Great Britain during 1984. *Veterinary Record* 117:429–434.

Allan, W.H., and R.E. Gough. 1974. A standard hemagglutination inhibition test for Newcastle disease (1). A comparison of macro and micro methods. *Veterinary Record* 95:120–123.

Artois, M., R. Manvell, E. Fromont, and J-B. Schweyer. 2002. Serosurvey for Newcastle disease and avian influenza A virus antibodies in great cormorants from France. *Journal of Wildlife Diseases* 38:169–171.

Ashton, W.L. G. 1984. The risks and problems connected with the import and export of captive birds. *British Veterinary Journal* 140:317–327.

Bailey, T.A., P.K. Nicholls, J.H. Samour, J. Naldo, U. Wernery, and J. C. Howlett. 1996. Postmortem findings in bustards in the United Arab Emirates. *Avian Diseases* 40:296–305.

Barton, J.T., A.A. Bickford, G.L. Cooper, B.R. Charlton, and C.J. Cardona. 1992. Avian paramyxovirus Type 1 infections in racing pigeons in California. 1. Clinical Signs, Pathology, and Serology. *Avian Diseases* 36: 463–468.

Beard, C.W. 1980. Serologic procedures. In *Isolation and Identification of Avian Pathogens,* S.B. Hitchner, C.H. Domermuth, H.G. Purchase, and J.E. Williams (eds.). *American Association of Avian Pathologists,* Kennet Square, PA, U.S.A., pp. 129–135.

Beard, C.W. and R.P. Hanson. 1984. Newcastle disease. In *Diseases of Poultry,* 8th Ed., M.S. Hofstad, H.J. Barnes, B.W. Calnek, W.M. Reid, and H.W. Yoder (eds.). Iowa State University Press, Ames, IA, U.S.A., pp. 452–470.

Beard, C.W. and W.J. Wilkes. 1985. A comparison of Newcastle disease hemagglutination-inhibition test results from diagnostic laboratories in the south eastern United States. *Avian Diseases* 29:1048–1056.

Blaxland, J.D. 1951. Newcastle disease in shags and cormorants and its significance as a factor in the spread of this disease among domestic poultry. *Veterinary Record* 63:731–733.

Bradshaw, J.E. and D.O. Trainer. 1966. Some infectious diseases of waterfowl in the Mississippi. *Journal of Wildlife Management* 30:570–576.

Brown, C., D.J. King, and B.S. Seal. 1999. Pathogenesis of Newcastle disease in chickens experimentally infected with viruses of different virulence. *Veterinary Pathology* 36:125–132.

Brown, J., R.S. Resurreccion, and T.G. Dickson. 1990. The relationship between the hemagglutination-inhibition test and enzyme-linked immunosorbent assay for detection of antibody to Newcastle disease. *Avian Diseases* 34:585–587.

Brugh, M. Jr., C.W. Beard, and W.J. Wilkes. 1978. The influence of test conditions on Newcastle disease hemagglutination-inhibition titres. *Avian Diseases* 22:320–328.

Chu, H.P., G. Snell, D.J. Alexander, and G.C. Schild. 1982. A single radial immunodiffusion test for antibodies to Newcastle disease virus. *Avian Pathology* 11:227–234.

Clavijo, A., Y. Robinson, T. Booth, and F. Munroe. 2000. Velogenic Newcastle disease in imported caged birds. *Canadian Veterinary Journal* 41:404–408.

Collins, M.S., S. Franklin, I. Strong, G. Meulemans, and D.J. Alexander. 1998. Antigenic and phylogenetic studies on a variant Newcastle disease virus using anti-fusion protein monoclonal antibodies and partial sequencing of the fusion protein gene. *Avian Pathology* 27:90–97.

Cvelic-Cabrilo, V.,H. Mazija, Z. Bidin, and W.L. Ragland. 1992. Correlation of hemagglutination-inhibition and enzyme-linked immunosorbent assays for antibodies to Newcastle disease virus. *Avian Pathology* 21: 509–512.

Czifra, G., and M. Nilsson. 1996. Detection of PMV-1 specific antibodies with a monoclonal antibody blocking enzyme-linked immunosorbent assay. *Avian Pathology* 25:691–703.

De Leeuw, O., and B. Peeters. 1999. Complete nucleotide sequence of Newcastle disease virus: evidence for the existence of a new genus within the subfamily Paramyxovirinae. *Journal of General Virology* 80:131–136.

Doyle, T.M. 1927. A hitherto unrecorded disease of fowls due to a filtre-passing virus. *Journal of Comparative Pathology and Therapeutics* 40:144.

Farley, J.M., S.H. Romero, M.G. Spalding, M.L. Avery, and D.J. Forrester. 2001. Newcastle disease in double-crested cormorants in Alabama, Florida and Mississippi. *Journal of Wildlife Diseases* 37:808–812.

Gelb, J. Jr., and C.G. Cianci. 1987. Detergent-treated Newcastle disease viruses as an agar gel precipitin test antigen. *Poultry Science* 66:845–853.

Ghumman, J.S., and R.A. Bankowski. 1976. *In vitro* DNA synthesis in lymphocytes from turkeys vaccinated with LaSota, TC, and inactivated Newcastle disease vaccines. *Avian Diseases* 20:18–31.

Gohm, D.S., B. Thus, and M.A. Hofmann. 2000. Detection of Newcastle disease virus in organs and faeces of experimentally infected chickens using RT-PCR. *Avian Pathology* 29:143–152.

Goodman, B.B. and R.P. Hanson. 1988. Isolation of avian paramyxovirus-2 from domestic and wild birds in Costa Rica. *Avian Diseases* 32:713–717.

Hari Babu, Y. 1986. The use of a single radial haemolysis technique for the measurement of antibodies to Newcastle disease virus. *Indian Veterinary Journal* 63:982–984.

Heckert, R.A., M.S. Collins, R.J. Manvell, I. Strong, J.E. Pearson, and D.J. Alexander. 1996. Comparison of Newcastle Disease viruses isolated from cormorants in Canada and the U.S.A. in 1975, 1990 and 1992. *Canadian Journal of Veterinary Research* 60:50–54.

Holmes, H.C. 1979a. Resistance of the respiratory tract of the chicken to Newcastle disease virus infection following vaccination: the effect of passively acquired antibody on its development. *Journal of Comparative Pathology* 89:11–19.

Holmes, H.C. 1979b. Virus-neutralizing antibody in sera and secretions of the upper and lower respiratory tract of chickens inoculated with live and inactivated Newcastle disease virus. *Journal of Comparative Pathology* 89:21–29.

Jestin, V., and A. Jestin. 1991. Detection of Newcastle disease virus RNA in infected allantoic fluids by in vitro enzymatic amplification (PCR). *Archives of Virology* 118:151–161.

Johnson, D.C., C.E. Couvillion, and J.E. Pearson. 1986. Failure to demonstrate viscerotropic velogenic Newcastle disease in psittacine birds in the Republic of the Philippines. *Avian Diseases* 30:813–815.

Johnston, K.M. and D.W. Key. 1992. Paramyxovirus-1 in feral pigeons (*Columba livia*) in Ontario. *Canadian Veterinary Journal* 33:796–800.

Kaleta, E.F. and C. Baldauf. 1988. Newcastle disease in Free-Living and Pet Birds. In *Newcastle Disease,* 1st Ed. D.J. Alexander (ed.). Kluwer Academic Publishers, Boston, MA, pp. 197–246.

Khan, M.I. 1994. Newcastle Disease. In *Handbook of Zoonoses, Section B: Viral Diseases,* 2nd. Ed., G.W. Beran (ed.). CRC Press, United States, pp. 473–481.

Kho, C.L., M.L. Mohd-Azmi, S.S. Arshad, and K. Yusoff. 2000. Performance of an RT-nested PCR ELISA for detection of Newcastle disease virus. *Journal of Virological Methods* 86:71–83.

Kuiken, T. 1999. Review of Newcastle Disease in Cormorants: *Waterbirds* 22:333–347.

Kuiken, T., R.A. Heckert, J. Riva, F.A. Leighton, and G. Wobeser. 1998a. Excretion of pathogenic Newcastle disease virus by double-crested cormorants (*Phalacrocorax auritus*) in absence of mortality or clinical signs of disease. *Avian Pathology* 27:541–546.

Kuiken, T., F.A. Leighton, G. Wobeser, K.L. Danesik, J. Riva, and R.A. Heckert. 1998b. An epidemic of Newcastle disease in Double-Crested Cormorants from Saskatchewan. *Journal of Wildlife Diseases* 34: 457–471.

Kuiken, T., G. Wobeser, F.A. Leighton, D.M. Haines, B. Chelack, J.B. Bogdan, L. Hassard, R.A. Heckert, and J. Riva. 1999. Pathology of Newcastle Disease in Double-Crested Cormorants from Saskatchewan, with comparison of diagnostic methods. *Journal of Wildlife Diseases* 35:8–23.

MacPherson, L.W. 1956. Some observations on the epizootiology of Newcastle disease. *Canadian Journal of Comparative Medicine* 10:55–168.

Meteyer, C.U., D.E. Docherty, L.C. Glaser, J.C. Franson, D.A. Senne, and R. Duncan. 1997. Diagnostic findings in the 1992 epornitic of neurotropic velogenic Newcastle disease in Double-crested Cormorants from the upper midwestern United States. *Avian Diseases* 41:171–180.

Miers, L.A., R.A. Bankowski, and Y.C. Zee. 1983. Optimizing the enzyme-linked immunosorbent assay for evaluating the immunity of chickens to Newcastle disease. *Avian Diseases* 27:1112–1125.

Morgan, I.R., and H.A. Westbury. 1981. Virological studies of Adelie penguins (*Pygoscelis adeliae*) in Antarctica. *Avian Diseases* 25:1019–1026.

Moses, H.E., C.A. Brandly, and E.E. Jones. 1947. The pH stability of viruses of Newcastle disease and fowl plague. *Science* 105:477–479.

Nagai, Y., H.D. Klenk, and R. Rott. 1976. Proteolytic cleavage of the viral glycoproteins and its significance for the virulence of Newcastle disease virus. *Virology* 72:494–508.

Olesiuk, O.M. 1951. Influence of environmental factors on viability of Newcastle disease virus. *American Journal of Veterinary Research* 12:152–155.

Palmer, S.F., and D.O. Trainer. 1971. Newcastle Disease. In *Infectious and Parasitic Diseases of Wild Birds,* 1st ed., J.W. Davis, R.C. Anderson, L. Karstad, and D.O. Trainer (eds.). The Iowa State University Press, Ames, IA, U.S.A., pp. 3–16.

Parry, S.H., and I.D. Aitken. 1977. Local immunity in the respiratory tract of the chicken. II. The secretory immune response to Newcastle disease virus and the role of IgA. *Veterinary Microbiology* 2:143–165.

Pearson, J.E., D.A. Senne, D.J. Alexander, W.D. Taylor, L.A. Peterson, and P.H. Russell. 1987. Characterization of Newcastle disease virus (avian paramyxovirus-1) isolated from pigeons. *Avian Diseases* 31:105–111.

Reynolds, D.L., and A.D. Maraqa. 2000a. Protective immunity against Newcastle disease: the role of cell-mediated immunity. *Avian Diseases* 44:145–154.

Reynolds, D.L., and A.D. Maraqa. 2000b. Protective immunity against Newcastle disease: the role of antibodies specific to Newcastle disease polypeptides. *Avian Diseases* 44:138–144.

Rima, B., D.J. Alexander, M.A. Billeter, P.L. Collins, D.W. Kingsbury, M.A. Lipkind, Y. Nagai, C. Orvell, C.R. Pringle, and V. ter Meulen. 1995. Paramyxoviridae. In *Virus Taxonomy: Sixth Report of the International Committee on Taxonomy of Viruses,* F.A. Murphy, C.M. Fauquet, D.H.L. Bishop, S.A. Ghabrial, A.W. Jarvis, G.P. Martelli, M.A. Mayo, and M.D. Summer (eds.). Vienna: Springer-Verlag, Austria, pp. 268–274.

Rivetz, B., W. Weisman, M. Ritterband, F. Fish, and M. Herzberg. 1985. Evaluation of a novel rapid kit for the visual detection of Newcastle disease antibodies. *Avian Diseases* 29:929–942.

Russell, P.H. 1988. Monoclonal antibodies in research, diagnosis and epizootiology of Newcastle disease. In *Newcastle Disease,* 1st Ed., D.J. Alexander (ed.). Kluwer Academic Publishers, Boston, MA, U.S.A., pp. 131–146.

Russell, P.H. 1993. Newcastle disease virus: virus replication in the harderian gland stimulates lacrimal IgA; the yolk sac provides early lacrimal IgG. *Veterinary Immunology and Immunopathology* 37:151–163.

Russell, P.H., and G.O. Ezeifeka. 1995. The Hitchner B1 strain of Newcastle disease virus induces high levels of IgA, IgG and IgM in newly hatched chicks. *Vaccine* 13:61–66.

Snyder, D.B., W.W. Marquart, E.T. Mallinson, and E. Russek. 1983. Rapid serological profiling by enzyme-linked immunosorbent assay. I. Measurement of antibody activity titre against Newcastle disease virus in a single serum dilution. *Avian Diseases* 27:161–170.

Sousa, R.L., T.C. Cardoso, A.C. Paulillo, H.J. Montassier, and A. A. Pinto. 1999. Antibody response to Newcastle disease vaccination in a flock of young partridges (*Rhynchotus rufescens*). *Journal of Zoo and Wildlife Medicine* 30:459–461.

Stallknecht, D.E., D.A. Senne, P.J. Zwank, S.M. Shane, and M.T. Kearney. 1991. Avian paramyxoviruses from migrating and resident ducks in coastal Louisiana. *Journal of Wildlife Diseases* 27:123–128.

Timms, L. and D.J. Alexander. 1977. Cell-mediated immune response of chickens to Newcastle disease vaccines. *Avian Pathology* 6:51–59.

Vickers, M.L. and R.P. Hanson. 1980. Experimental infection and serologic survey for selected paramyxoviruses in red-winged blackbirds (Agelaius phoeniceus). *Journal of Wildlife Diseases* 16:125–130.

Vickers, M.L. and R.P. Hanson. 1982. Newcastle disease virus in waterfowl in Wisconsin. *Journal of Wildlife Diseases* 18:149–158.

Vindevogel, H. and J.P. Duchatel. 1988. Panzootic Newcastle Disease Virus in Pigeons. In *Newcastle Disease,* 1st Ed., D.J. Alexander (ed.). Kluwer Academic Publishers, Boston, MA, U.S.A., pp. 184–196.

Walker, J.W., B.R. Heron, and M.A. Mixson. 1973. Exotic Newcastle disease eradication program in the United States. *Avian Diseases* 17:486–503.

Westbury, H. 2001. Newcastle disease virus: an evolving pathogen. *Avian Pathology* 30:5–11.

Wilson, J.E. 1950. Newcastle disease in a Gannet (*Sula bassana). Veterinary Record* 62:33–34.

Wilson, R.A., C. Perotta Jr., and R.J. Eckroade. 1984. An enzyme-linked immunosorbent assay that measures protective antibody levels to Newcastle disease virus in chickens. *Avian Diseases* 28:1079–1085.

Wise M.G., D.L. Suarez, B.S. Seal, J.C. Pedersen, D.A. Senne, D.J. King, D.R. Kapczynski, and E. Spackman. 2004. Development of a real-time reverse-transcription PCR for detection of Newcastle disease virus RNA in clinical samples. *Journal of Clinical Microbiology* 42:329–338.

Wobeser, G., F.A. Leighton, R. Norman, D.J. Myers, D. Onderka, M.J. Pybus, J.L. Neufeld, G.A. Fox, and D.J. Alexander. 1993. Newcastle disease in wild water birds in western Canada, 1990. *Canadian Veterinary Journal* 34:353–359.

World Organization for Animal Health (OIE). 2004. *International Animal Health Code: mammals, birds and bees.* Paris: World Organization for Animal Health.

2
Arboviruses in Birds

Robert G. McLean and Sonya R. Ubico

INTRODUCTION

Arboviruses (arthropod-borne viruses) are a diverse group of viruses representing 12 different virus families that affect vertebrates and are biologically transmitted by arthropod vectors including different species of mosquitoes, ticks, sand flies (*Phlebotomidae*), or biting midges (*Culicoides, Ceratopogonidae*) in which they multiply. The wide variety of disease patterns caused by arboviruses depends upon the type of virus and hosts involved and includes sub-clinical, acute, chronic progressive disease, and mortality. Overt infections consist of systemic, encephalitic, or hemorrhagic syndromes, and the severity of disease may not be identical in the different host species affected.

The International Catalogue of Arboviruses (Karabatsos 1985) lists 504 registered arboviruses isolated worldwide; but for practical reasons, it also lists certain other viruses of vertebrates that are not vector borne. Calisher and Karabatsos (1988) updated and reviewed the taxonomic relationships of 655 registered and unregistered arboviruses. The most recent reviews for many of the arboviruses are in a five-volume series titled *The Arboviruses: Epidemiology and Ecology* (Monath 1988). Approximately 77 of the arboviruses have been isolated from birds and have been placed taxonomically in five of the 13 virus families listed: Bunyaviridae, Flaviviridae, Rhabdoviridae, Reoviridae, and Togaviridae. A small number of viruses (13) isolated from birds have not been taxonomically classified. Antibodies against additional viruses have been detected in birds, but their role in natural transmission cycles may be incidental or is unknown. Most avian arboviruses have evolved with their hosts and generally do not cause morbidity or mortality in the natural avian hosts.

HISTORY

Arboviruses have undoubtedly existed for many centuries throughout the world in natural transmission cycles, in habitats where wild vertebrates and arthropod vectors coexisted. Human and equine cases during prior centuries were likely sparse and went unnoticed or undetected because human populations were more widely dispersed and their living environments were not highly developed. As humans began to concentrate in urban-suburban centers and develop irrigation projects that favored certain vertebrate host and mosquito vector populations, transmission of arboviruses to humans and their associated domestic animals became more frequent. At the same time, humans were encroaching more into undeveloped areas with natural foci of transmission of arboviruses, increasing their exposure to new pathogens. The advancements in medicine and science in the twentieth century also led to the discovery of the causative agents of diseases. Arboviruses were first isolated in 1901 (Karabatsos 1985), and birds were first implicated in transmission cycles of arboviruses in 1938 (Tenbroeck 1938). Arboviruses were originally named according to the illness that they cause, for example, yellow fever and equine encephalitis; however, it became necessary to add a geographic connotation to differentiate viruses, for example, western equine encephalitis (WEE) from eastern equine encephalitis (EEE) viruses. Arboviruses have also been named after the place from where they were first isolated, for example, West Nile (WN) and St. Louis encephalitis (SLE).

ETIOLOGY, HOST RANGE, AND DISTRIBUTION

Flaviviridae

The 70 viruses in the genus *Flavivirus,* Flaviviridae, are single-stranded RNA viruses composed of three structural proteins containing antigens that react in a variety of serological tests with extensive cross-reactivity, suggesting a high degree of similarity among the viruses. The flaviviruses are subdivided taxonomically into six complexes or serogroups for the vector-associated viruses, two complexes for the vector-unassociated viruses, and 19 viruses that have not been assigned to any antigenic complex (Calisher and Karabatsos 1988).

About 16 flaviviruses have been isolated from birds from the vector-associated and unassigned groups. These include seven in the Japanese Encephalitis (JE) serocomplex, four in the Russian Spring-Summer Encephalitis (RSSE) complex, one each in the Ntaya (Israel turkey meningoencephalitis, IT) and Uganda S complexes, and three in the ungrouped viruses. Birds are important natural hosts for a more limited number of flaviviruses including some of major public health and domestic animal health importance, and only these viruses are discussed separately. Five of the viruses in the JE antigenic complex and an ungrouped virus (Rocio) cause central nervous system infections in humans; at least three viruses cause clinical disease in domestic animals (WN virus in the JE complex, Louping Ill [LI] in the RSSE complex, and IT); and two cause morbidity and mortality in wild birds (WN and LI). Every continent has one or more mosquito-borne flaviviruses of birds that cause significant human disease.

The JE virus serocomplex is a group of closely related flaviviruses (Mackenzie et al. 2002) that include JE virus in SE Asia and recently in Australia; Murray Valley encephalitis (MVE) virus in Australia; SLE virus in North America (NA) and South America (SA); WN virus in Africa, Middle East, Europe, western Asia and recently in NA; and Kunjin (KUN) virus in Australia.

Japanese Encephalitis Virus

Japanese encephalitis (JE) is a common but serious human disease in 16 countries of eastern and southern Asia. The virus was first isolated from a fatal encephalitis case in Japan in 1935 and has caused severe epidemics of more than 6,000 cases in Japan in 1924, 5,548 cases in Korea in 1949, 40,000 cases in China in 1966, 2,000–5,000 cases in Thailand in the 1960s, and more than 6,000 cases in northeastern India in 1978 (Burke and Leake 1988; Endy and Nisalak 2002). It is estimated that approximately 50,000 cases occur annually in this region. Severe clinical disease and death from JE is age related, with most cases occurring in the very young and elderly. Even though all domestic animals can be infected, few develop clinical signs of illness. Nevertheless, fatal encephalitis has been reported in horses, and abortion and fetal loss may occur in infected pigs. Significant disease in wildlife from JE infection is not known to occur.

Japanese encephalitis virus is maintained in enzootic transmission cycles in rural areas of SE Asia by rice field breeding mosquitoes (mostly *Culex tritaeniorhynchus*), water birds, and/or domestic pigs. Pigs are one of the primary amplifying hosts and probably the major determinant of human epidemic activity. Young pigs become intensely infected, develop up to nearly 100% antibody prevalences, and develop viremias capable of infecting mosquitoes. There is high population turnover of pigs, producing a regular supply of susceptible animals (Burke and Leake 1988). Widespread use of vaccines has reduced the risk to humans in these intense epizootic areas in Japan. Water birds, particularly ardeid species (herons), are also primary amplifying hosts and frequently cohabit the irrigated rice fields with the pigs and rice workers. A wide variety of wild vertebrates is infected, but the primary host species for virus maintenance appears to be the Black-crowned Night Heron (*Nycticorax nycticorax*). However, other ardeid species, some passerine species, as well as a few other nonpasserine species have been implicated in various studies. Only selected species of herons and egrets and one passerine species have been shown to be competent hosts to infect mosquitoes. Black-crowned Night Heron, Chinese Pond-Heron (*Ardeola bacchus*), Little Egrets (*Egretta garzetta*), Intermediate or Plumed Egrets (*Egretta intermedia*), Cattle Egrets (*Bubulcus ibis*), and European Starlings (*Sturnus vulgaris*) readily produced viremias sufficient to experimentally infect the primary mosquito vector (Buescher et al. 1959; Soman et al. 1977).

Japanese encephalitis virus was introduced to a new continent at the Torres Strait Islands off the northern coast of Australia, and the first recognized outbreak occurred in 1995 (Hanna et al. 1996). By 1998, JE virus reached mainland Australia as detected by antibody in sentinel and domestic pigs and by the diagnosis of a human case on the Cape York Peninsula (Hanna et al. 1999). Viremic migratory birds may have been responsible for the introduction of JE virus to Australia from the New Guinea mainland (Hanna et al. 1996).

St. Louis Encephalitis

St. Louis encephalitis (SLE) virus (*Flavivirus*) is one of the arboviruses of birds that produces significant disease in humans. It is estimated that more than 10,000 human clinical cases and 1,000 fatalities have occurred in NA since the virus was first identified in 1937 (Chamberlain 1980). St. Louis encephalitis virus was first found infecting vertebrate animals during an investigation of a human epidemic in Washington, U.S.A. in 1940 (Hammon and Howitt 1942). The virus occurs in a discontinuous distribution from Canada in North America to Argentina in South America. Human cases have been reported in every state in the continental U.S.A. except in New England and South Carolina. There have been periodic human outbreaks mostly in urban centers in the midwestern states, Texas, and Florida (Tsai and Mitchell 1988). The virus most likely existed in nearly silent transmission cycles for a long time and became evident only as birds became more closely associated with increasing human population concentrations and their urban environments and in intense agricultural settings during the twentieth century. Even though SLE causes clinical disease in humans, it does not cause disease in any other vertebrate host species and does not cause viremias in horses. Humans and horses are dead-end hosts for the virus and thus do not contribute to additional transmission. Throughout the range of SLE, birds are the natural hosts except for a few species of rodents, bats, and other mammals in specialized circumstances/settings (McLean and Bowen 1980; Spence 1980; Ubico and McLean 1995). Reviews of the epidemiology and ecology (Monath 1980; Tsai and Mitchell 1988) and vertebrate hosts of SLE (McLean and Bowen 1980) provide extensive background information.

In humans, the incubation period is estimated at 4 to 21 days, and infection causes a wide spectrum of response, from asymptomatic to severe clinical disease and death. However, less than 1% of human SLE infections develop clinical symptoms. Clinical disease includes mild symptoms with slight fever; a febrile syndrome usually with fever and intense headaches lasting several days, followed by complete recovery; and aseptic meningitis with a sudden onset of fever and stiffness of the neck but without neurologic dysfunctions. The most severe syndrome is encephalitis that begins suddenly with fever and one or more signs of brain inflammation (confusion, delirium, lethargy, paresis, and convulsions). This last syndrome occurs more frequently in elderly persons, and the majority of deaths occurs in persons over 50 years old, among whom the case fatality rate can be as high as 30% or more.

The basic transmission cycle of SLE virus involves wild birds and ornithophilic mosquitoes. A number of avian species have been identified as the primary hosts and a few species of culicine mosquitoes as the principal vectors in North America (McLean and Bowen 1980; Mitchell et al. 1980). Regional differences of preferred avian host and mosquito vector species have resulted in varying transmission patterns in the U.S.A. In the western U.S.A., SLE virus is transmitted in a wild bird-*Cx. tarsalis* mosquito cycle with House Finches (*Carpodacus mexicanus*), House Sparrows (*Passer domesticus*), Mourning Doves (*Zenaidura macroura*), blackbirds, and some other species as the primary avian hosts and *Cx. tarsalis* as the predominant vector in enzootic cycles in cultivated, irrigated agricultural areas. House Finches, House Sparrows, and Rock Pigeons (*Columba livia*) are the primary avian hosts, and *Cx. pipiens quinquefasciatus* and *Cx. tarsalis* are the principal vector species in transmission cycles in western suburban/urban centers (McLean et al. 1986; Gruwell et al. 2000).

In the south-central and north-central states of the eastern U.S.A. where most of the human epidemics have occurred, human disease is primarily urban-suburban in character because the vectors are the peridomestic and domestic mosquitoes *Cx. p. quinquefasciatus* and *Cx. p. pipiens.* These vectors breed in polluted stagnant water with high organic content such as in sewage or storm water systems or lagoons and even in catch basins within cities. Larvae may also be found in artificial containers such as rainwater barrels, tin cans, and discarded tires. Females with a flight range of up to 0.8 miles feed between dusk and midnight primarily on birds and occasionally on humans. The same urban environments favor the proliferation of host species such as House Sparrows, Rock Pigeons, and other birds that feed and breed among the crowded urban conditions (peridomestic). In addition, some passerine species are closely associated with urban-suburban residential neighborhoods and parks and cemeteries such as American Robin (*Turdus migratorius*), Blue Jay (*Cyanocitta cristata*), Northern Cardinal (*Cardinalis cardinalis*), and Northern Mockingbird (*Mimus polyglottos*), all of which are good reservoir hosts for SLE virus (McLean et al. 1985b; McLean et al. 1993). After SLE virus is introduced into the cities, these peridomestic birds, domestic fowl, and passerine species serve as amplifiers of transmission that can lead to epizootics in the bird populations. Increased transmission and epizootics in birds associated with higher infection rates in vector mosquitoes in the middle of dense human populations create the optimum conditions for the occurrence of human disease and epidemics when some of the infected mosquitoes feed on humans instead of birds. The transmission patterns of SLE virus in Florida are unique because there is an enzootic wild bird-*Cx. nigripalpis* mosquito transmission cycle in rural environments of the state, a mammal-mosquito cycle in a few locations, and in urban areas an epizootic/epidemic cycle involving peridomestic and wild birds species and *Cx. p. quinquefasciatus* mosquitoes (McLean and Bowen 1980; Day and Stark 1999). Some of the primary avian hosts in Florida are the Mourning Dove, Blue Jay, Northern Cardinal, and the House Sparrow.

Virus infections in birds have been associated temporally and spatially with reported human cases in the U.S.A. The overall mean SLE antibody prevalence reported for bird populations analyzed in connection with 10 SLE human epidemics was 18.6%, and certain bird species were positive at higher rates than other species (McLean and Bowen 1980). The relative contribution of various bird species to SLE virus transmission during urban outbreaks is dependent upon their exposure to the virus as determined by antibody prevalence and their density. During three urban SLE epidemics in Texas in the 1960s, Blue Jays had significantly higher antibody prevalences than House Sparrows and yet House Sparrows made a more substantial contribution to the cycling of the virus because of their greater abundance (Lord et al.1974b). Because SLE virus infections in bird populations increase during the summer mosquito transmission season and these amplifications usually precede reported human SLE cases, wild birds have been effectively used for urban surveillance of the disease (Lord et al. 1974a). In the central U.S.A., there is a strong association between human cases and the antibody prevalence in House Sparrows (McLean and Bowen 1980; Monath 1980; McLean et al. 1983; Smith et al. 1983). Following one of the most dramatic years for epidemic SLE in the U.S.A. in 1975, which had 1,815 cases in multiple cities and states (Monath 1980), extensive surveillance networks were established throughout the eastern U.S.A. utilizing the regular sampling and testing of free-ranging wild birds, mostly House Sparrows, and captive sentinel chickens (*Gallus gallus*) to monitor the seasonal appearance and progression of SLE virus activity (Bowen and Francy 1980; McLean and Scott 1979). The city of Memphis, Tennessee, refined urban bird surveillance and directly connected it temporally with mosquito control operations to respond quickly to SLE virus amplification to reduce public health risk (McLean et al. 1983). The states of California and Florida continue to operate an annual SLE surveillance program mostly utilizing sentinel chicken flocks (Reisen et al. 2000; Day 1989).

West Nile Virus

West Nile (WN) virus (*Flavivirus*) was originally isolated in 1937 from a febrile human patient in the West Nile region of Uganda (Smithburn et al. 1940). This *Flavivirus* occurs across a broader distribution range than most of the other arboviruses extending from Africa, the Middle East, Europe, and western Asia and recently in North America. West Nile virus is normally transmitted between birds primarily by bird-feeding (ornithophilic) mosquitoes, although isolations have been reported from mammals, reptiles and amphibians, other mosquitoes, and ticks. This virus has one of the broadest host and vector ranges and historically caused clinical disease in humans and horses as described in reviews by Hayes (1988), Hubalek and Halouzka (1999), and Murgue et al. (2002). McLean et al. (2002) present a historical review of WN virus in livestock and wildlife. Clinical disease in humans from WN virus infection is similar to disease caused by SLE virus although new clinical syndromes (flaccid paralysis) and new methods of transmission (blood transfusion, organ transplant, transplacental, and transmammary) were reported in the U.S.A. in 2002. Clinical disease in equines can be severe, with about a 30% case fatality rate but with a spectrum of clinical signs that have been well described (Murgue et al. 2001; Ostlund et al. 2001).

There are two major genetic lineages of WN virus (Petersen and Roehrig 2001; Scherret et al. 2002). Lineage 1 strains have been isolated throughout its range and contain strains responsible for recent epidemics in humans and epizootics in equines as well as strains also causing mortality in birds in Israel (Isr98) and North America (NY99). Lineage 2 strains are associated with a wide distribution of endemic transmission in Africa and are not known to cause significant human disease or mortality in birds (Malkinson and Banet 2002a; McLean et al. 2002).

Wild birds are the primary hosts for WN virus throughout its geographical distribution as evidenced by the detection of antibody in a broad range of species as well as by a number of virus isolations obtained during field investigations. Therefore, the primary transmission cycle of WN virus involves the regular exchange of virus between mosquitoes, primarily in the genus *Culex*, and wild birds. Infections in many wild bird species produce sufficiently high viremias for several days to subsequently infect susceptible mosquitoes to complete the transmission cycle (Work et al. 1955). Equines and humans are considered incidental or dead-end hosts and do not generally contribute to transmission. Domestic birds are incidental hosts as well because most species, except geese, do not develop sufficient viremias to infect mosquitoes. Domestic geese (*Anser anser anser*) produced viremias sufficient to amplify virus transmission during experimental studies (Swayne et al. 2001) as occurred naturally in Israel in 1999 (OIE 1999). Geese also suffer mortality from both experimental and natural infections. Other mammals, including a few species of wild mammals, have been infected and strains of WN virus isolated, but their role in natural transmission cycles of the virus is unknown. The number and type of avian species involved as hosts and the extent of their involvement depends upon their susceptibility as well as the epidemiological history and current pattern of virus transmission in the geographical region. Specific regional details have been reviewed (Hayes 1988; McLean et al. 2002; Murgue et al. 2002), but we will present some information to contrast avian host involvement in areas with differing epidemiological characteristics from endemic to epidemic rates of transmission and with new introductions. In temperate regions in South Africa, Europe, North America, and the Middle East, data indicate that migratory birds may be important in disseminating WN virus. Interpretation of data is complicated by the existence of cross-reactions between closely related flaviviruses in many of the serological tests that have been used.

West Nile virus has an extensive distribution in Africa, where its presence has been demonstrated by isolation from wild birds, mosquitoes and humans and by serological surveys. A serological survey conducted in an endemic area of the Nile Delta region of Egypt found 40% of the birds and 40% of the mammals positive for neutralizing (Nt) antibody, and WN virus was isolated from two of 44 Rock Pigeons and one of 159 Hooded Crows (*Corvus corone sardonius*) (Taylor et al. 1956). Additional results from field studies in the Sindbis area of the endemic region of Egypt identified Hooded Crows, Cattle Egrets (*Bubulcusibis*), House Sparrows, Laughing (Senegal) Doves (*Streptopelia senegalensis*), and Eurasian Kestrels (*Falco tinnunculus*) as natural hosts for WN virus, with antibody prevalences of 88%, 68%, 57%, 48%, and 100%, respectively (Work et al. 1955). Hooded Crows sampled throughout the Nile Delta confirmed their role as an important host and valuable indicator of virus activity where the antibody prevalence was 3% in nonendemic localities, 33% in intermediate zones, and a 77% average prevalence from eight endemic localities. Experimental infection studies more fully defined the role of Hooded Crows in the epidemiology and ecology of WN virus in Egypt. Crows developed high circulating virus titers following infections with a virus strain (Egypt 101) isolated from a dead pigeon, and these titers remained at high levels for several days until the deaths of the birds (Work et al. 1955). In this experiment, none of the crows survived the infection, and virus was isolated from the brain and spleen of the birds. House Sparrows also developed relatively high titers for several days, whereas herons, doves, and kestrels developed lower viremia titers. Hooded Crows, House Sparrows, and the other three species to a lesser extent were shown to be reservoir competent to infect mosquitoes with the virus strain used.

A survey of wild birds in Israel in 1959–1960 revealed that 14% of 473 birds had WN virus antibody (Akov and Goldwasser 1966), and WN virus was detected in the blood of three European Turtle-Doves (*Streptopelia turtur*) during the summers of 1964–1965, indicating local transmission (Nir et al. 1967). Virus was also isolated from hatching year White Storks (*Ciconia ciconia*) recently arrived from Europe during September to October 1998, suggesting introduction of a WN virus strain from northern temperate foci of summer transmission (Malkinson et al. 2002b). This new WN virus variant appeared in Israel in 1997–1998 and was more virulent for birds and humans, causing a die-off of domestic geese and some mortality in wild birds; a human epidemic occurred in 2000 (Bin et al. 2001).

West Nile virus transmission in northern latitudes in Europe is more typical of seasonal transmission patterns in temperate climates and involves different avian species. In eastern Slovakia during 1971–1973, WN virus was isolated from four wild bird species (Green Sandpiper, *Tringa ochropus;* Black-headed Gull, *Larus ridibundus;* Northern Lapwing, *Vanellus vanellus;* and European Turtle-Dove) and Nt antibody was detected in 11 species of wild birds (Ernek et al.1977). Serological surveys of birds in Czechoslovakia found 9.7% of wild birds with WN virus hemagglutination-inhibition (HI) antibodies in southern Moravia, and 5.5% of 273 House Sparrows from a suburban area had HI antibody during 1995–1997 (Juricova et al. 2000). Experimental infection studies in a variety of birds in Europe such as Northern Pintail *(Anas acuta),* Common Pochard (*Aythya ferina*), and Rooks (*Corvus frugileus*) resulted in prolonged and/or high titer viremias (Hubalek and Halouzka 1996). It was further noted that experimental infection of the Rooks had occasionally resulted in fatal encephalitis and that both viremia and lethality had been recorded following experimental infection of Black-tailed Gulls (*Larus crassirostris*).

In southern temperate areas of South Africa, 2,022 wild birds from 51 species were captured in the plateau area, and 12% of birds in 27 species were positive for WN virus HI antibody, whereas 53% of 322 birds sampled had antibody after a large human outbreak (McIntosh and Jupp 1982). The prevalence of HI and Nt antibody in avian host species during the epidemic were 92% of 24 Olive Thrush (*Turdus olivaceus*), 86% of 72 Laughing Dove (*Streptopelia senegalensis*), 50% of 48 House Sparrow, 40% of 153 Red Bishop (*Euplectes orix*), two of nine Black-fronted Bulbul (*Pycnonotus nigricans*), three of five Red-billed Quelea (*Quelea quelea*), three of nine Masked Weaver (*Ploceus velatus*), and two of two Ring-necked Doves (*Streptopelia capicola*) (McIntosh et al. 1976). Results from experimental infection studies with South African strains of WN virus in 13 common wild avian species from five families demonstrated viremia in all the species, some with high titers sufficient to infect mosquitoes, and none of the birds showed clinical illness (McIntosh et al. 1969a).

In central Africa, more information is available on WN virus infections in mammals than in birds. Virus isolates were obtained from camels and rodents and antibody was detected in a variety of domestic mammals in Nigeria. Few birds were sampled although WN virus was isolated from two Kurrichane Thrushes

(*Turduslibonyanus*). More complete information is available from Madagascar, where WN virus isolates were obtained from Vasa Parrots (*Coracopsis vasa*) and egrets (Ardeidae). Antibody was detected in bats and oxen, and virus and antibody were detected in five species of lemurs (Lemuridae) on the island (McLean et al. 2002). In Asia, 317 birds of 32 species were captured in Changa Manga National Forest of Punjab Province, Pakistan, and 85 (27%) birds from 21 species had Nt antibody to WN virus during 1978 (Hayes et. al. 1982).

Introduction of WN Virus into the Americas

West Nile virus was introduced into the U.S.A. in New York City (NYC) during the early summer of 1999, and this invasion represented a major shift out of its normal geographical distribution in the eastern hemisphere. The virus strain introduced was most closely related to an apparently new WN virus strain (Isr98) from Israel in the Middle East (Lanciotti et al. 1999) that caused some mortality in domestic geese (Swayne et al. 2001) and in migrating White Storks (Malkinson et al. 2002). The introduced strain of WN virus (NY99) appeared to be more virulent, especially to native species of Corvidae, and has become a significant cause of avian mortality in North America (Bernard et al. 2001; McLean 2002). The route or method of entry into the U.S.A. is still unknown, but possible methods include the air transport of infected mosquitoes, infected wild or domestic vertebrates, or infected humans that served as the source to start local transmission in NYC. An infected migratory bird carrying the virus during a transcontinental flight from Europe or the Middle East and introducing it to NYC (Rappole et al. 2000) was an unlikely method because of the low frequency of occurrence of such bird flights, the seasonal timing of the introduction, and the insufficient time for the infected bird to remain viremic and infectious to local mosquitoes upon its arrival in NYC. The weather pattern of a wet spring and hot, dry summer in NYC in 1999 contributed to higher populations of efficient mosquito vector species, *Culex spp.,* likely facilitating the establishment and amplification of WN virus transmission in the NYC area (McLean 2004). Detailed information about the introduction and expansion of the NY99 strain in the U.S.A. is presented in a summary by Roehrig et al. (2002).

The introduced virus initiated an epizootic in the local bird populations, followed by a human epidemic starting in the borough of Queens in NYC (CDC 1999). The epizootic in local bird populations produced a large number of bird deaths, predominantly in American Crows (*Corvus brachyrhynchos*), within the initial introduction site in Queens, New York City, and in an expanding area around New York City. A human epidemic also developed within the introduction site and in the expanded area, with WN virus eventually causing 62 human cases and seven deaths (Table 2.1). The expanded zone was a 161 + km-wide (100+ mile) area (epicenter) in 22 counties in three states surrounding New York City, and one dead crow in Baltimore, Maryland (Figure 2.1) (Eidson et al. 2001a). Only 25 equine cases were reported in the area (Table 2.1) (USDA 2005). Dead crows were reported by the public from August to October in the epicenter, and 700 free-ranging birds of 20 avian species (93% were American Crows) were laboratory confirmed as positive for WN virus (Table 2.1) (Figure 2.1). This information indicated that crows were likely responsible for the geographical expansion of the virus out of the original introduction site in New York City and that several thousand crows may have died from WN virus infection (Eidson et al. 2001b). Relative bird census data from the area showed a decline in the number of crows in the affected zone after the epizootic in 1999 compared to 1998 data (Eidson et al. 2001a). West Nile virus also caused mortality in some captive native and exotic bird species in zoological collections in the area (Steele et al. 2000). An investigation of the outbreak at one of the zoological collections found that 34% of 368 birds in the collection were positive for Nt antibody to WN virus, and 22% of the infected birds developed clinical disease (Ludwig et al. 2002). However, there was a 70% case fatality rate in the clinically ill birds.

Surprisingly, the introduced WN virus survived through the temperate winter of the northeastern U.S.A., where there is no continuous mosquito activity to sustain transmission, and reappeared in American crows in May 2000 within the previous epicenter area around New York City (CDC 2000a). West Nile viral RNA was detected in two pools and virus isolated from a third pool of hibernating *Cx. pipiens* collected in the 1999 epicenter of New York City during January and February 2000 (Nasci et al. 2001b). Infection of over-wintering *Culex* mosquitoes could be an important means of virus survival through the winter and of reinitiation of transmission in the spring. Because of the apparent establishment of WN virus in the U.S.A., an enhanced surveillance network to monitor the geographical dissemination and temporal amplification of the virus was established initially in 2000 in 20 states along the Atlantic and Gulf coasts (CDC 2000b). National guidelines were established for the state and local health agencies, and it was recommended that detection of virus infections in wild birds, sentinel chickens, mosquitoes, domestic animals, and humans be utilized for WN virus surveillance. Because of the high bird mortality occurring from WN virus, particularly in American crows, the testing and reporting of dead birds became an important component of surveillance (see the "Surveillance" section, later in this chapter). The surveillance system was expanded to include all states as the geographical distribution of WN virus expanded and the national guidelines were reviewed and modified each year as needed.

A 10-fold expansion in the distribution of WN virus occurred in the northeastern U.S.A. in 2000 as WN virus rapidly expanded northward from the 1999 epicenter in the New York City area to the Canadian border during the late spring and early summer. West Nile virus–positive birds were then reported westward in New York to Lake Erie during late summer and southward through Virginia to North Carolina in the fall to ultimately include 12 states and the District of Columbia (Figure 2.1). Besides additional human (21) and equine cases (60), a total of 12,961 dead birds were submitted for WN virus testing from 16 states in the state surveillance network, and 4,305 (33%) were virus positive (Table 2.1). American crows comprised 58% (7,580) of the birds submitted and 89% (3,824) of the positive birds (Figure 2.2). Of the 7,580 tested crows, 50% were positive, whereas only 9% (481) of birds from 62 other species tested (5,381) were positive (Marfin et al. 2001). The intensity of transmission among free-ranging crows appeared to be greater within the original epicenter than in other regions; 70% of the dead crows submitted throughout the transmission season from within the epicenter region of Connecticut (Hadler et al. 2001) and 67% of the dead crows tested in the epicenter region of southern New York (Bernard et al. 2001) were WN virus positive compared to the overall 50% infection rate. A few species of wild mammals (Striped Skunk,

Table 2.1. West Nile virus disease in human, equines, and birds in the United States, 1999–2004.

Year	Number States	Human Cases	Human Deaths	Equine Cases	Equine Deaths*	Bird Deaths
1999	4	62	7	25	9	700
2000	12	21	2	60	23	4,305
2001	27	66	8	738	243	7,338
2002	44	4,156	274	15,257	4,577	15,754
2003	47	9,862	264	5,181	1,554	11,597
2004	47	2,470	98	1,341	402	7,331
Total	48	16,702	654	22,602	6,781	47,016

*Estimated overall equine mortality based on a smaller number of cases.

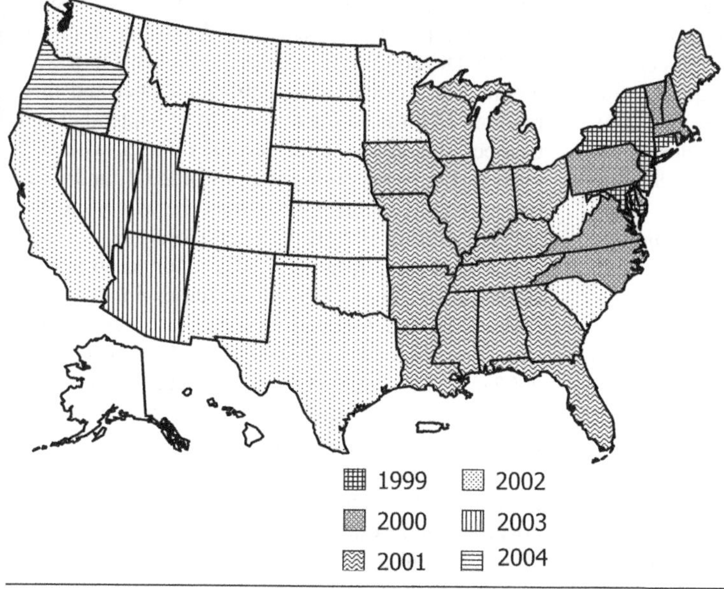

Figure 2.1. The states reported positive for West Nile virus in the continental United States by first year of reporting, 1999–2004.

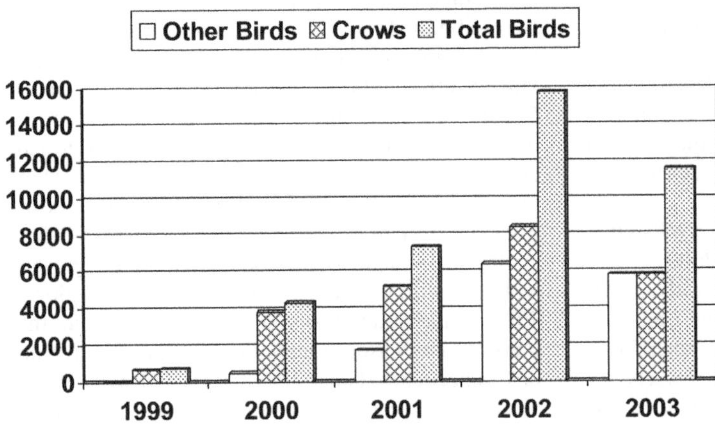

Figure 2.2. The total number of West Nile virus–positive birds, crows, and other species reported in the United States, 1999–2003.

Mephitis mephitis; Eastern Gray Squirrel, *Sciurus carolinensis;* Eastern Chipmunk, *Tamias striatus;* Big Brown Bat, *Eptesicus fuscus;* and Little Brown Bat, *Myotis lucifugus*) were found to be WN virus positive in 2000 (Marfin et al. 2001). Tens of thousands of birds died in 2000, affecting many new species, and the peak in the amplification of transmission (epizootic) in wild bird populations occurred in late summer; 85% of the positive birds were found between July 1 and September 30. *Culex pipiens* was identified as the primary enzootic and epizootic mosquito vector transmitting WN virus among birds during 1999 (Nasci et al. 2001a) and 2000 (Bernard et al. 2001) in the northeastern U.S.A.

West Nile virus again survived through the dormant winter season of 2000–2001 and reappeared in American Crows at sites in five separate states in the northeast in late April and early May 2001, and appeared in a new region in northern Florida in June (CDC 2001a). The new focus of WN virus detected in northern Florida began to quickly expand in all directions, and clinical cases in equines and humans quickly followed in adjacent counties (Blackmore et al. 2003). This virus focus could have been initiated during the fall of 2000 by migratory birds becoming infected in the northeastern states and carrying WN virus south with them during their fall migration to and through Florida. Virus transmission can be maintained through the winter in the warmer Gulf Coast areas of the southeastern states because mosquitoes are active throughout the year. Because mosquito transmission within this WN virus focus was likely occurring weeks before the detection of virus in June 2001, northward-migrating birds could have been infected while traveling through the area in April and May on their way to northern breeding areas and disseminated WN virus to the midwestern states (Godsey et al. 2005). Regardless of how WN virus was disseminated in the U.S.A. in 2001, virus began to be detected in an expanding area from the Northeast, Midwest, and Southeast to eventually encompass 27 states and Ontario, Canada, by the end of the transmission season in November. The original focus in northern Florida gradually expanded throughout that state south to the Florida Keys and into the neighboring states of Georgia and Alabama. The largest outbreak in equines to date occurred in northern Florida with more than 500 equine cases. West Nile virus was detected in the northern states of Ohio, Michigan, Wisconsin, Illinois, and Indiana starting in July and August and continued to expand there throughout the remainder of the transmission season (CDC 2002a). After the initiation of fall bird migration to the south in late August, locations in states along the Mississippi River (which is a major flyway for migratory birds) began detecting WN virus–positive dead birds until all of the states on both sides of the Mississippi River except Minnesota reported positive birds in 2001 (CDC 2002a). The city of Memphis, Tennessee, reported no positive birds until September and then reported 44 birds during the months of September and October. In addition, birds became infected with WN virus in Louisiana during the fall of 2001, and virus transmission continued throughout the winter months and early spring of 2002 (CDC 2002b).

National surveillance for 2001 reported 66 human cases in 10 states, 738 equine cases in 20 states (Table 2.1), and 918 pools of mosquitoes tested positive from 27 mosquito species in 16 states (CDC 2002a; USDA 2005). Of 32,918 dead birds tested, 7,338 (22%) were reported WN virus positive (Table 2.1) from 27 states and the D.C. (Figure 2.1) (CDC 2002a). American Crows comprised 71% (5,161) of the positive birds, and 54% of the crows tested were positive. For the other species, 2,177 birds were tested (29%), but only 9% from these species were positive.

Ontario, Canada, reported WN virus for the first time in wild birds, and 121 (5%) of 2,592 birds tested were positive (Health Canada 2001). Of the species of Corvidae tested in Canada, American Crows were most commonly found WN virus positive (100 of 1,449, 7%), followed by Blue Jays (21 of 1056, 2%).

In 2002, WN virus activity started earlier in the Gulf Coast states, probably because virus activity continued at a low rate throughout the winter season; positive dead birds and equines were detected in Louisiana and Florida during January and February (CDC 2002b). By June, there was a rapid appearance of WN virus activity in new states west of the Mississippi River from Houston, Texas, to North Dakota. A dramatic and enormous geographical expansion of WN virus into western North America occurred in 2002, invading 17 new states (Figure 2.1) and 4 new provinces in Canada (44 states, five provinces in four years). Accompanying this further expansion was a pronounced increase in transmission to humans and equines. The onset of human cases began in Louisiana during the second week of June, and cases increased to an epidemic of 329 cases, peaking the first week of August (CDC 2002b). Nationally, the peak of human cases occurred in late August, with Illinois reporting the most cases (879) and deaths (60). The 2002 human epidemic of 4,156 laboratory-confirmed cases and 284 deaths in the U.S.A. (Table 2.1) (CDC 2002c) was the largest arboviral meningoencephalitis (WNME) epidemic documented in the western hemisphere and the largest ever reported WNME epidemic. The epizootic of 15,257 reported equine cases (Table 2.1) (USDA 2005) with an approximate 30% case fatality rate was also the largest documented equine WN virus outbreak in history. The expansion in distribution and intensity of WN virus was a result of dissemination and amplification of infections in wild birds that was reflected in the continuing high mortality rates. A total of 31,500 dead birds were tested and 15,754 (50%) were found positive (Table 2.1) for WN virus in 94 bird species (Campbell 2003). American Crows, Blue Jays, and other species of Corvidae accounted for 90% of the WN virus–infected birds of the 15,754 laboratory confirmed WN virus–positive birds; 8420 (53%) were crows, about 5,658 were Blue Jays (36%), and 1,667 (11%) were other avian species (Figure 2.2). About 77% of dead crows and 40% of other species tested were WN virus positive, and infected birds were collected from January 10 to November 7 in 43 states and D.C. (Figure 2.1). Only 27% of the 124,854 reported dead birds in 2002 were submitted for testing compared with 50% in 2001. Many political units such as counties throughout the U.S.A. stopped testing dead birds after the first bird was found virus positive; therefore, most birds dying of WN virus, particularly during the peak of transmission during August and September, were never tested or reported. The number of birds dying from WN virus infections in 2002 was significantly greater than the number reported positive.

The geographical expansion of WN virus in NA continued westward in 2003, but to a lesser extent than in 2002. However, virus activity was more intense, especially in a multistate region from west Texas north through the Great Plains States and into Canadian provinces, producing an even larger historic epidemic of this disease (9,862 cases in the U.S.A. [Table 2.1] [Hayes 2004]; and 1,388 in Canada [Health Canada 2005]). Equine cases significantly decreased in the U.S.A. in 2003 to 5,181 (Table 2.1) (USDA 2005), probably as a result of the extensive use of equine vaccines for WN virus and reduced reporting. Colorado reported the most human cases (2,947) in 2003 following a weather pattern of wet spring and hot, dry summer that was similar to the weather pattern that occurred in New York City in 1999 during the successful introduction of WN virus. This weather was optimum for mosquito production, as evidenced by five times more adult mosquitoes being captured in 2003 than the average during the previous five years and for increased WN virus transmission (Pape 2004). A resurgence of WN virus activity also occurred in the eastern states in 2003, where four times more positive dead birds were reported per area than in the central and western states (Hayes 2004). Epizootic transmission of WN virus occurred previously in the eastern states during 1999–2001, which indicates that the virus does not disappear after the initial epizootic in a region. The virus entered and spread through southern Arizona into southern California, most likely by migratory birds from Mexico. Positive birds (96) were reported in California from a five-county area around Los Angeles. The U.S.A. reported 11,597 WN virus–positive birds in 2003 (Table 2.1) including 5,800 American Crows (50% of positive birds) and 3,532 Blue Jays (30%) in 46 states (Figures 2.1 and 2.2) (Hayes 2004). Canada reported a significant increase in WN virus–positive birds (1,632) in 2003 and the addition of two new provinces reporting WN virus activity: New Brunswick in the east and Alberta in the west (Health Canada 2005).

In 2004, Arizona and California were typical of previous states in that epizootic transmission followed the introduction and initial establishment of WN virus during the previous year. Virus activity was intense in Arizona during 2004, and an epidemic of 391 human cases of WN occurred mostly in the Phoenix metropolitan area (Levy 2005). Dead-bird surveillance was not effective in detecting WN virus and evaluating risks in Arizona, partly because there were few highly susceptible bird species such as corvids present in that area. Of the 730 dead birds tested, 98 (13%) were WN virus positive, with sparrows (30) being the most frequently affected. After the 2003 introduction into southern California, positive dead birds were detected first in 2004 in southern California on February 24, seven weeks before any other surveillance event and 11 weeks before the first human case (Kramer 2005). Virus activity began to amplify and expand in this area in April and spread northward to central California in May, to northern California in June, and throughout the state in all counties by September. It seems likely that migratory birds moved WN virus northward in the spring from the Los Angeles area and seeded the virus into new areas, where it became established and amplified enough to be subsequently detected by the surveillance reporting system. Dead-bird surveillance worked well in California in detecting the early appearance and intensity of WN virus transmission. A total of 3,232 positive birds were reported from 58 counties in 2004, compared to 96 birds in five counties in 2003. Positive dead birds were the only surveillance event detected in all 58 counties, was the earliest indication of WN virus activity in 53 (91%) counties, and was the only evidence of WN virus in 22 counties (Kramer 2005). California reported 44% (3,232) of the total birds reported positive for the U.S.A. (7,331) (Table 2.1); 80% of the birds reported for the U.S.A. were corvids and 84% were in California. Even though WN virus activity increased in the far western states, it decreased throughout the rest of the country. The number of counties in the U.S.A. reporting WN virus activity decreased from 1,640 in 2003 to 971 in 2004 (Smith 2005), again despite the increase in California from five to 58 counties reporting positive birds. Generally, WN virus activity in areas east of the Rocky Mountains was reported to be significantly less in 2004 than 2003, probably because of unfavorable weather conditions for virus transmission. Weather data showed that the summer of 2004 was significantly cooler in the U.S.A. (second coldest in the last 20 years), particularly compared to 2003, except in the west region that included Arizona and California and that was similar to the previous five years (NOAA 2005). Mean precipitation for the summer months was next to the highest during the last 20 years, but in the west region of the U.S.A. the 2004 mean precipitation was similar to the mean for the last five years. A combination of a wet and cool summer can greatly reduce mosquito production and activity, lengthen the extrinsic incubation period of the virus in the vector, and affect reproduction and populations of insect eating birds, all of which could reduce WN virus transmission and lower the number of infected birds, equines, and humans in the eastern regions of the U.S.A. In 2004, there was a fourfold reduction in human (2,470) and equine cases (1,341) reported and a 1.6-fold decrease in reported dead birds (7,331) in the U.S.A. An even more significant decline in WN virus activity occurred in Canada in 2004, with only 16 human and 13 equine cases and 445 positive dead birds reported (Health Canada 2005). Virus activity began early in 2005 in a number of states, and at least enzootic transmission will proceed unabated in many regions of NA (CDC 2005).

Following the introduction in New York City in 1999 of this highly virulent NY99 strain of WN virus, it has spread throughout the NA continent in six years about 500 miles north into Canada, 3,000 miles to the west coast, and 3,000 miles south into the Caribbean and Latin America, affecting all 48 continental states of the U.S.A., seven provinces in Canada, Mexico, numerous islands in the Caribbean, and Central America (CA) (Hayes 2004; Mendez-Galvan 2004; Smith 2005). This virus strain has a very broad host range and has affected a total of 47,016 birds (Table 2.1), both free-ranging and captive, of 294 species in 57 families and 24 orders, 22,069 mammals of 25 species from bats to reindeer (including equines), and two species of reptiles in the U.S.A. during the six-year period 1999–2004 (Smith 2005; USGS 2005). American Crows (26,466, 55% of total) were the dominant species found positive for the first three years, and Blue Jays and then magpies became prominent as the virus moved westward from the original introduction site.

During 2001–2004, Canada first detected WN virus in southern Ontario, and the virus then expanded in both directions to seven of ten provinces from Nova Scotia on the Atlantic coast to Alberta in the west (Health Canada 2005). Dead-bird surveillance concentrated on corvids and found that 2,732 of 23,800 birds tested (11.5%) during the four years were WN virus positive, mostly American Crows. The virus was first introduced into the Caribbean in 2001 with a human case on the Cayman Islands (CDC 2001a), and then in Jamaica (Dupuis II et al. 2003) and the Dominican Republic (Komar et al. 2003) in 2002. Antibody prevalences to WN virus in resident birds on Jamaica (17 of 348, 5%) and Dominican Republic (5 of 118, 4%) indicate the establishment of local transmission on these islands after the introduction of the virus by migratory birds from the U.S.A. Introduction of WN virus into Puerto Rico was discovered in 2004 by the detection of antibody-positive equines (CDC 2004). The first indication of WN virus in Mexico was seropositive equines in northern Mexico (Blitvich et al. 2003a; Estrada-Franco et al. 2003) and in other states along the Caribbean coast, including Yucatan, starting in July 2002 (Estrada-Franco et al. 2003). The first dead bird from WN virus was a captive Common Raven (*Corvus corax*) in southern Mexico in the state of Tabasco in 2002 (Estrada-Franco et al. 2003). In 2003, WN virus was active in 24 states with six human cases and 2,630 seropositive equines (Mendez-Galvan 2004). There were 10 WN virus–positive birds confirmed by reverse transcription-polymerase chain reaction (RT-PCR), including three dead birds and 147 seropositive birds from 50 species.

The ecology and epidemiology of the WN virus strain (NY99) introduced into the U.S.A. in 1999 was quite different from what was observed in the Eastern Hemisphere, primarily because of the increased virulence of this virus strain for the naive avian species of North America (McLean et al. 2001). This more virulent strain continues to circulate and expand its distribution in the U.S.A. because the extremely high viremias produced in a number of avian host species, particularly members of the Corvidae family, not only cause significant mortality from infection in these species but also increase the transmission potential to vector mosquito species (Komar et al. 2003). The virus has infected a broad range of vertebrate host species and caused mortality in many of these species, and may be impacting certain avian populations in North America. The virus has consistently occurred in a number of temperate locations for at least four years in the northeastern states. This annual reappearance in the spring in these locations is from local persistence and/or seasonal reintroduction of the virus. The only natural mechanisms documented for the long-term survival of WN virus through periods of no active virus transmission by mosquitoes (for example, during the winter period in temperate climates) are by vertical transmission in mosquitoes. Some evidence in mosquitoes are the isolation of virus from hibernating *Cx. pipiens* mosquitoes in New York City (Nasci et al. 2001a) and the isolation of WN virus from male *Cx. univittatus* complex mosquitoes in Kenya, indicating transovarial transmission within that species (Miller et al. 2000). Other mechanisms are the infection of ticks in which the virus could persist for extended periods (Hoogstraal 1972; Abbassy et al. 1993), and possibly the development of chronically infected birds, as reported for Rock Pigeons following experimental infection (Semenov et al. 1973). Annual introduction of WN virus to previously infected areas or to new locations is likely achieved by infected migratory birds either through direct transport or through sequential steps both northward in the spring and southward in the fall. It is suspected that seasonal movement of WN virus from Africa to Europe occurs annually by migratory birds (Hubalek and Halouzka 1999), and there is evidence of southward movement as well. West Nile virus was isolated from an Nt antibody detected in hatching year White Storks that landed in Israel during the fall migration because of inclement weather (Malkinson et al. 2002). The virus strain isolated from the storks was nearly identical to the dead goose isolate (Isr98) previously mentioned.

Because some migratory bird species are or could be involved as natural hosts for the NY99 strain of WN virus (Komar et al. 2001b; Komar et al. 2003), there are few boundaries that can contain the spread of the virus in the Western Hemisphere. The movement pattern of migratory birds in North America appears to support their apparent role in disseminating WN virus during the last six years across thousands of miles from the New York City introduction site to the western U.S.A. in a north-to-south and south-to-north zigzag fashion. The virus appears to be maintained throughout the year in some semi-tropical locations along the Gulf Coast of the southern states from Florida to California through continuous mosquito activity and transmission (Tesh et al. 2004; Kramer 2005). These foci can serve as a virus source for annual reintroduction to northern states and Canada by spring migrating birds. It is possible that both local persistence and annual reintroduction of WN virus are occurring simultaneously in some locations, and that situation could significantly magnify local transmission. There is previous evidence of the southward transport of arboviruses by migratory birds in the fall (Stamm and Newman 1963; Lord and Calisher 1970) and there is strong evidence that WN virus was disseminated south out of North America by migratory birds. As the virus distribution expands to countries south of the U.S.A. from Mexico to Central America, South America, and the Caribbean, different local patterns of avian infections and mortality will emerge and permanent foci of transmission could be established in tropical environments. These foci could also serve as a source for seasonal movement of WN virus between South America and North America by migratory birds (Rappole et al. 2000).

Recent experimental infection studies of 25 North American native and exotic avian species with the virulent NY99 strain of WN virus found mixed results and revealed some patterns of susceptibility despite the low numbers of birds inoculated (Komar et al. 2003). The duration and titer of viremia varied from extremely high titers and mortality in corvids (crows, jays, and Black-billed Magpies (*Pica pica*); to high viremias and mortality in the Common Grackle (*Quiscalus quiscula*), Ring-billed Gull (*Larus delawarensis*), House Finch, and House Sparrows; and to low viremias and no clinical disease in native and exotic species of Galliformes. passeriform and charadriiform species generally had higher viremias and were more reservoir competent than species in eight other orders of birds. Shedding of WN virus in oral and cloacal secretions was demonstrated, and it led to direct contact transmission between infected and uninfected cagemates. Five of the 15 avian species tested were orally susceptible to WN virus in an aqueous solution, infected mice or House Sparrows, or an infected mosquito. Previous studies demonstrated the extreme susceptibility of American Crows to inoculation with the NY99 strain (nearly 100% mortality of 50 crows in 4–8 days), contact transmission from infected crows to control crows in a free-flying room, and oral transmission from infected mouse carcasses fed to crows (McLean et al. 2001; McLean et al. 2002; R.G. McLean, personal communication). The possible occurrence and significance of direct transmission among crows in nature is unknown.

An outbreak of WN virus in a large captive collection of North American owls in southern Ontario, Canada, further demonstrated differences in species susceptibility. One hundred eight of 235 owls died with an unusual species mortality pattern. There was 100% mortality in northern breeding species (Great Gray Owl, *Strix nebulosa;* Snowy Owl, *Bubo scandiaca;* Northern Hawk Owl, *Surnia ulula;* Boreal owl, *Aegolius funereus;* Northern Saw-whet Owl, *Ae. Acadicus*); intermediate mortality in species with a pan North American breeding range (Great Horned Owl, *Bubo virginianus;* Short-eared Owl, *Asio flammeus;* Long-eared Owl, *A. otus*); and zero mortality in species with a more southerly breeding range (Barn Owl, *Tyto alba;* Burrowing Owl, *Athene cunicularia;* Eastern Screech Owl, *Megascops asio*) (Ganz et al. 2004). In raptors, certain accipiter species such as the Northern Goshawk (*Accipiter gentilis*) seem very susceptible, whereas some species of Falconidae such as the Peregrine Falcon (*Falco peregrinus*) seem less susceptible. All the species of domestic birds tested so far are susceptible to infection with WN virus, but only very young chickens and domestic geese show clinical disease and some mortality. Young chickens (<3 weeks of age) and young geese can amplify transmission by infecting mosquitoes, but older chickens and turkeys produce viremias too low to infect mosquitoes. In the U.S.A., most chickens and commercial turkeys are raised indoors with reduced exposure to vector mosquitoes, and unlike in Israel, the production of domestic geese is small. Domestic birds in the U.S.A. would contribute little to the maintenance and expansion of WN virus compared to wild birds. However, the large domestic goose population in Israel is vulnerable to WN virus infection and could be an important factor in the epidemiology of the disease (Bin et al. 2001).

Murray Valley Encephalitis Virus

Murray Valley encephalitis (MVE) virus (*Flavivirus*) was first identified as the cause of an outbreak of 45 human cases with 19 deaths during the summers of 1950 and 1951 in the Murray Valley of southern Australia even though the virus was originally isolated in 1918 during early work on Australian X disease (Marshall 1988). The next major epidemic occurred in 1974 and involved every mainland state, followed by small epidemics and isolated cases during the ensuing years. Human infections are generally mild with a relatively low morbidity rate of one clinical case for every 800–1,000 infections. Clinical disease in humans begins suddenly with fever, anorexia, and severe headache and proceeds to nausea, vomiting, and diarrhea in about half of the cases. Also about half of the clinical cases develop progressive neurologic signs and lapse into comas and death in 34% of the severe clinical cases. Nervous system disease in horses and fatalities in dogs were noted during periods of MVE virus activity, but clinical cases have not been confirmed. Although viremias are commonly detected in wildlife species, no clinical disease has been reported in wildlife in nature or following laboratory infection.

The virus is closely related to JE virus and distantly related to other members of the JE complex, and unlike many of the flaviviruses in this complex, MVE virus appears to be antigenically stable, with consistent homogeneity among Australian strains. *Culex annulirostris* is the epidemic vector species and may also play an important role in virus maintenance cycles (Marshall 1988). Birds are the primary vertebrate hosts for MVE virus as they are for most of the other flaviviruses in the JE antigenic complex. As with JE virus, water birds are especially important because of their close association with the primary vector species that breeds predominantly in freshwater ponds, swamps, and temporary pools in agricultural areas. During the 1974 epidemic, 55% of Ciconiiformes and 41% of Pelecaniformes were serologically positive for MVE virus, whereas only 4.5% of Anseriformes were positive (Marshall et al.1982a). Rufous (Nankeen) Night Herons (*Nycticorax caledonicus*) had the highest antibody prevalence (88%). There appeared to be a relationship between the breeding activity of Rufous Night Herons and MVE virus activity when combined with abnormally high populations of the mosquito vector, *Cx. annulirostris.* Other species of herons, egrets, cranes, and cormorants as well as other native and feral vertebrates could also be involved in maintenance cycles of MVE virus. Experimental infection studies found the Rufous Night Heron, Little Egret, Intermediate Egret, and White-necked (Pacific) Heron (*Ardea pacifica*) susceptible to MVE virus and capable of infecting the mosquito vector (Boyle et al. 1983a). The Rufous Night Heron and Little Egret developed HI and Nt antibody against MVE virus, reaching a maximum titer between 10–20 days after experimental inoculation, and the specificity of the antibody could be determined from the pattern of cross-reaction among related viruses in the JE antigenic complex (Boyle et al. 1983b). Species of ducks and psittacines, feral pigs, kangaroos, wallabies, and rabbits that were experimentally infected had low titered and erratic viremias despite the finding of antibodies in these species in nature (Marshall 1988).

Kunjin Encephalitis Virus

Kunjin_encephalitis virus (KUN) is a flavivirus in the JE antigenic complex and is closely related to WN virus and more distantly related to MVE virus. This virus coexists with MVE virus in many of the same habitats, vertebrate hosts, and mosquito vectors in Australia (Marshall 1988). Some of the clinical cases during human MVE epidemics were more likely due to KUN virus. In the Murray Valley of southeast Australia in 1984, a severe encephalitis human case was serologically confirmed as KUN virus infection and the virus was isolated from the spinal chord of a moribund horse with encephalomyelitis. Most of the KUN virus isolates have been from mosquitoes from all of the same areas of mainland Australia as MVE virus and from the same mosquito species, especially from the major epidemic vector for both viruses, *Cx. annulirostris.* One difference was the isolation of KUN virus from *Cx. pseudovishnui* in Borneo, where MVE has not been detected. As with MVE and WNV, birds are the primary maintenance and amplifying hosts for KUN virus. The species of water birds serving as KUN virus hosts are similar to MVE virus, such as the Rufous Night Heron, but the bird hosts are spread across more species such as the Yellow Oriole (*Oriolus flavocinctus*). The American Crow was susceptible to experimental infection with KUN virus, and 100% developed viremias with peak titers ranging from 4.2 $\log_{10}$ to 6.1 $\log_{10}$ PFU/mL of serum well below the peak titers of 6.7 $\log_{10}$ to 10.7 $\log_{10}$ PFU/mL of serum in 100% of crows infected with the NY99 strain of WN virus (Brault et al. 2004). Differences in the virulence between these two related flaviviruses was also evident in the contrast in mortality rates of 0% for KUN virus and 100% by day six post-inoculation for WN virus.

Ilheus Virus

Ilheus virus (ILH) is a *Flavivirus* that is currently not identified with any of the serogroups within the genus. The virus is found in forested regions of Central America and South America and generally causes a mild febrile illness in humans with occasional encephalitis (Acha and Szyfres 1987). The virus was originally isolated from mosquitoes (*Aedes* and *Psorophora*) in Ilheus, Brazil, in 1944 and later from other mosquito species in Central America and northern South America. The virus has also been isolated from humans in various countries in South America and from different species of birds in Trinidad and Panama (Karabatsos 1985). Antibody was detected in Agoutis (*Dasyprocta punctata*) in Panama and bats in Trinidad. Recently, ILH virus was isolated from a Double-collared Seedeater (*Sporophila caerulescens*) and Shiny Cowbird (*Molothrus bonariensis*), and antibody was detected in Ruddy Ground-Dove (*Columbina talpacoti*), Diamond Dove (*Geopelia cuneata*), Saffron Finch (*Sicalis flaveola*), and the Shiny Cowbird from the Parque Ecologico do Tiete in Brazil (Pereira-Luiz et al. 2001). Migratory birds such as the Double-collared Seedeaters may be spreading ILH virus to other regions of Brazil.

Rocio Virus

Rocio virus (ROC), an ungrouped *Flavivirus,* was first isolated in southeastern Brazil from a fatal human case with encephalitis during an epidemic of 971 cases during 1975–1976 (Lopes et al. 1978a; Iversson 1989). Individuals involved in outdoor activities of farming and fishing were at greatest risk. The virus produces clinical illness only in humans, and there is no evidence of overt disease in wild animals, but there is some evidence that it killed chickens and pigs during the epidemic of 1975. Neither the enzootic nor the epidemic transmission cycles of this virus have been well defined. However, there is evidence that birds, both wild and domestic, may play a role in the sylvatic and peridomestic cycles, respectively. Studies conducted in the Riberia Valley region of Brazil identified certain common mosquito species. The ROC virus was isolated from a pool of *Ps. ferox* mosquitoes, which were later shown to be a competent vector of ROC virus experimentally, along with *Ae. scapularis* (Mitchell et al. 1981). Rocio virus was isolated from Rufous-collared Sparrows (*Zonotrichia capensis*) and 24% of 153 wild birds captured in a forested area had HI antibodies. Antibodies were also identified from a variety of birds (chickens, ducks, and pigeons), rodents, bats, and marsupials in the epidemic area in 1975 (Lopes et al. 1978b; Iversson 1989). Adult House Sparrows developed viremias with low virus titers, whereas young chickens (<48 hours old) had viremias sufficient to infect vector mosquitoes after experimental infection with the virus (Monath et al. 1978). Wild birds and certain mosquito species appear to be involved in a sylvatic transmission cycle, and chickens could be a domestic reservoir for the virus.

Louping Ill Virus

Louping Ill (LI) virus caused clinical disease in sheep in southern Scotland for centuries, but the virus responsible for the disease and the vector responsible for transmission to sheep, the sheep tick *Ixodes ricinus,* were not discovered until 1931 (Reid 1988). Later, the virus was found to be closely related to other tick-transmitted flaviviruses in the tick-borne encephalitis (TBE) group, although recently LI virus was thought to be an antigenically distinct western subtype of Russian Spring Summer encephalitis complex in the TBE group (Stephenson et al. 1984). The disease is rare in humans and occurs mostly in laboratory and slaughterhouse workers. The virus is endemic in the upland grazing and unimproved pastures that are used for sheep rearing along the western coast of the United Kingdom (U.K.) and in many rural areas of Ireland where the primary tick vector is present. Most species of domestic livestock become infected in the endemic areas, although sheep are at greatest risk and suffer the highest mortality. Infection of wildlife is prevalent in the endemic areas, but most species except the Willow Ptarmigan (Red Grouse) (*Lagopus lagopus scoticus*) have inadequate viremias to infect immature stages of the primary vector tick species (*I. ricinus*) and are thus dead-end hosts for the virus. Small mammals were suspected to play a role in the persistence of LI virus, but field investigations determined that they were relatively unimportant (Gilbert et al. 2000). However, the Mountain or Arctic Hare (*Lepus timidus*) is known to transmit LI virus. The only field evidence of clinical disease in wildlife was the isolation of LI virus from 74% of 31 young Willow Ptarmigan found dead or dying in Scotland (Williams et al. 1963). Experimentally infected Willow Ptarmigan produced sustained viremias for up to five days sufficient to infect immature ticks (Reid 1975), and similar results were found with two related grouse species (Reid et al. 1980); however, these other species suffered 78% and 100% mortality without any evidence of clinical disease. Mortality from experimental infection in Willow Ptarmigan occurred between days 4 and 12 post-inoculation (PI); therefore, many of the grouse could infect ticks prior to their death. Significant natural mortality appears to occur in Willow Ptarmigan populations in some enzootic areas (Reid et al. 1978). To date, only sheep and Willow Ptarmigan have been identified as playing a role in the primary maintenance of the virus in nature. The high susceptibility of the Willow Ptarmigan to LI infection is difficult to explain because both LI virus and grouse have occurred naturally in the U.K. for centuries, but changes in agricultural practices have recently concentrated sheep, grouse, and the tick vector in the traditional highland habitats of the Willow Ptarmigan, suggesting that this host-virus relationship has newly evolved (Reid 1988).

Israel Turkey Meningoencephalitis

Israel Turkey Meningoencephalitis (IT) virus (*Flavivirus*) was isolated from dead, adult domestic turkeys in Israel in 1960 and causes a neuro-paralytic disease in this species. Seasonal outbreaks cause a high morbidity and mortality up to 80% in turkey flocks (Ianconescu 1976). The virus has been isolated from turkeys, *Culex* mosquitoes, and *Culicoides* in Israel and from a turkey in South Africa, although *Culicoides* could not be experimentally infected with IT virus (Braverman and Boorman 1978). The similarity in host range, clinical signs, and pathological changes produced by the virus isolated from turkeys in South Africa in 1978 and the virus isolated previously in Israel, as well as the serological cross-reaction between the two virus isolates, indicate that they are the same virus (Barnard et al. 1980). Antibody against IT virus was found in sera from wild birds in Israel, but the HI antibody detected was only flavivirus specific and could have been antibody against WN virus that was regularly occurring there at the same time (Akov and Goldwasser 1966). The role of wild birds in the transmission cycle of IT virus is not known. Direct transmission among turkeys and commercial Japanese Quail (*Coturnix japonica*) occurs. The virus was attenuated by adapting it to Japanese Quail, and a vaccine was prepared with this attenuated virus that effectively immunized domestic turkeys against the disease (Ianconescu 1976).

Bussuquara Virus

Bussuquara (BSQ) virus is a *Flavivirus* that is probably widespread in the tropical forests of South America. For years it was believed that the principal transmission cycle involved only rodents and mosquitoes, with humans and monkeys being accidental hosts. However, the detection of antibodies against BSQ virus in Amazonian wild birds and the fact that the virus was isolated from two genera of mosquitoes (*Coquillettidia* and *Asethini*) indicated a possible role of wild birds and ornithophilic mosquitoes in the transmission cycle (Karabatsos 1985; Degallier et al. 1992).

Togaviridae

The more than 37 presently recognized viruses and subtypes in the genus *Alphaviruses,* Togaviridae, have been separated into seven complexes (Calisher and Karabatsos 1988).

Alphaviruses are single-stranded, positive-sense RNA viruses containing three structural proteins and a capsid surrounded by a lipoprotein enveloped with surface projections consisting of glycoprotein units. Several studies have indicated that cross immunity may occur between Western Equine Encephalitis (WEE) and other alphaviruses such as Highland J (HJ), EEE, and Venezuelan equine encephalitis (VEE) (Stamm and Kissling 1957; Calisher and Mannes 1975). Alphaviruses in the EEE and WEE virus complexes and some viruses in the Semliki Forest complex have birds as the primary vertebrate hosts, and only these viruses are discussed.

Western Equine Encephalitis

Western equine encephalitis (WEE) virus (*Alphavirus*, Togaviridae) was first isolated from sick horses in 1930 and from a fatal human case eight years later. Periodic epizootics have been reported in Argentina since 1908. Severe outbreaks occurred in several western states of the U.S.A. and Canada from 1930 to 1935; other major epizootics occurred in the north central U.S.A. and the central valley of California between 1937 and 1947, causing thousands of cases of encephalitis in both horses and humans. The WEE epidemics of 1941, 1975, 1977, and 1981 were most severe in the north central U.S.A. and southern Manitoba (Reisen and Monath 1988).

The summer transmission cycle of WEE virus in North America is relatively well understood. It principally involves *Cx. tarsalis* as the primary mosquito vector and passerine birds as the primary vertebrate hosts throughout the western states of the U.S.A. and western provinces of Canada. The WEE virus has been isolated throughout the American continent, and small epizootics or sporadic cases of the disease occur nearly every year. At least 28 mosquito species in six genera have been found to be naturally infected with WEE virus, and 75 species of birds and 12 species of mammals have been found to be naturally positive for WEE virus or antibody. Virus was isolated from 20 species of birds and six species of small, wild mammals (Reisen and Monath 1988). Passerine species of birds, particularly House Finch, House Sparrow, White-crowned Sparrow (*Zonotrichia leucophrys*), Tricolored Blackbird (*Agelaius tricolor*), and a few other species, are the primary avian hosts, and domestic birds (mostly chickens) and perhaps mammals (rodents and Black-tailed Jackrabbits *Lepus californicus*) could be secondary hosts in some locations and certain situations. Extensive studies of mosquito-borne arboviruses were conducted in California for decades, and information on the natural infection of vertebrate hosts with WEE virus for the period of 1943–1987 is contained in a comprehensive summary and review (Reeves 1990). A few abundant summer resident wild bird species were sampled regularly in Kern County, California, and overall WEE virus antibody prevalences were 17%. Domestic birds, particularly chickens and pigeons, were frequently infected and were useful for surveillance.

The annual transmission cycle of WEE virus typically starts with the initiation of transmission in the spring, possibly by early-season mosquitoes such as *Aedes* species or *Culiseta inornata* and Spotted Ground Squirrels (*Spermophilus spilosoma*), Snowshoe Hares (*L. americanus*), and some bird species, particularly in northern latitudes. This early transmission period is followed by gradual amplification in nestling House Sparrows or House Finches in the southwestern and western states by emerging *Cx. tarsalis* mosquitoes during June and July. In the north central states, other avian species may be equally as important as House Sparrows (McLean et al. 1989). Virus transmission continues through the summer among young and adult birds and *Cx. tarsalis* and can subsequently infect a variety of other birds, domestic mammals, and humans if conditions are favorable. Infection of these dead-end hosts, particularly equines, occurs following increased intensity of transmission in the natural bird-mosquito cycle by several weeks. The transmission to mammals increases during late summer because of a seasonal shift in feeding habits of the primary vector from birds to mammals (Reisen and Monath 1988). Virus prevalence in nestling House Sparrows in Hale County, Texas, during 1966–1967 predicted the risk of WEE infection to equines and humans (Holden et al. 1973a) and this predictor could have been used in Richland County, North Dakota, in 1975, but with nestling birds of several other species (McLean et al. 1989).

Mature passeriform and galliform birds as well as nestling sparrows, which occasionally succumb to infection, typically develop high viremias of short duration and rarely develop clinical signs (Hammon and Reeves 1946; Hammon et al. 1951; Holden et al. 1973a, b). Infected birds develop viremias with a sufficiently high titer to infect vector mosquitoes. The WEE virus was serologically implicated as the principal cause of neurological disease in turkeys in Nebraska (Woodring 1957). On one occasion, WEE virus was isolated from experimentally infected birds up to 10 months after inoculation (Reeves et al. 1958). Under certain circumstances and locations, reptiles could serve as a source of WEE virus for local transmission if there are mosquito species present that feed on both reptiles and birds (Sudia et al. 1975). Reptiles could also be an over wintering mechanism for the virus because the Texas Tortoise (*Gopherus berlandieri*) and Garter Snake (*Thamnophis* spp.) developed prolonged viremias sufficient to infect mosquitoes following experimental infection with WEE virus (Bowen 1977).

Highlands J Virus

Highlands J (HJ) virus (*Alphavirus*, Togaviridae) was first isolated in 1960 from two Blue Jays captured in Florida and was originally thought to be an eastern variant of WEE virus (Henderson et al. 1962; Karabatsos et al. 1963). However, it is now considered a distinct virus in the WEE antigenic complex of alphaviruses (Calisher et al. 1980a). Virus and antibodies were also detected in wild birds from south central Florida, Louisiana, Maryland, Massachusetts, Michigan, and New Jersey. Other HJ virus strains were isolated from sentinel mice, bats, and mosquitoes (Karabatsos 1985). The virus appears to coexist with EEE virus in freshwater swamp habitats in the eastern U.S.A. and shares the same enzootic mosquito vector, *Culiseta melanura,* as well as many of the same wild avian host species. During an investigation of an EEE epizootic affecting equines in Michigan in 1980, five HJ virus strains were isolated in addition to six strains of EEE virus from 401 wild birds of 42 species captured (McLean et al. 1985a). However, the HJ antibody prevalence (2.7%) was much lower than the EEE antibody prevalence (30%) in the wild birds sampled, suggesting that the peak in EEE virus activity occurred earlier in the summer than HJ activity. In contrast, three HJ strains were isolated along with five EEE strains from 2,866 wild birds sampled in 1969 during studies at an enzootic focus in a freshwater swamp in eastern Maryland (Dalrymple et al. 1972). The prevalence of HJ antibody was much greater in summer and in permanent resident birds (28–32%) than in transient and winter resident species (2–7%), and the HJ antibody prevalence was similar to the EEE antibody prevalence in these birds. Many surveillance programs for EEE virus in the eastern U.S.A. frequently encounter HJ virus in mosquitoes (Andreadis et al. 1998), and some programs utilize HJ virus activity as a measure of potential EEE virus activity. The virus is considered a veterinary pathogen because it causes disease and some mortality in domestic poultry including turkeys, chickens, and partridges (Ficken et al. 1993; Guy et al. 1994), and it was confirmed as the cause of at least one fatal equine case of encephalitis in Florida (Karabatsos et al. 1988). Previous cases of equine encephalitis in the eastern U.S.A. diagnosed as WEE were more likely caused by HJ virus. It is generally not known to cause clinical disease in humans; however, four patients during an SLE epidemic in Indian River County, Florida, in 1990–1991 were dually infected with SLE and HJ viruses (Meehan et al. 2000). The recent development of a specific, reverse transcriptase-polymerase chain reaction (RT-PCR) test will allow for the rapid and accurate detection of HJ virus in mosquito and vertebrate samples (Whitehouse et al. 2001).

Fort Morgan Virus

Fort Morgan (FM) virus is a member of the WEE antigenic complex (*Alphavirus,* Togaviridae) and is more closely related to HJ virus of the eastern U.S.A. than WEE virus, even though FM virus occurs within the distribution of WEE in the western states (Calisher et al. 1980b). The virus has been isolated only from nestling Cliff Swallows (*Petrochelidon pyrrhonota*) and House Sparrows and from the cimicid Nest or Swallow Bug (*Oeciacus vicarius*) in Colorado (Hayes et al. 1977), South Dakota, Washington, and western Texas. The distribution of FM virus is restricted by its sedentary nature of the vector that serves to locally maintain the virus within swallow nests and infect returning migratory swallows and their young when the nests are reused. This virus has been repeatedly isolated from sick and dead nestling House Sparrows in Colorado that are raised in the bug-infested nests previously built and used by cliff swallows, having a negative effect on the local sparrow populations (Scott et al. 1984). Equines are unaffected by FM virus infections (Calisher and Karabatsos 1988), and no human cases have been reported.

Sindbis Virus

Sindbis (SIN) virus (*Alphavirus,* Togaviridae) was first isolated from *Culex* and *Aedes* mosquitoes and from the blood of a Hooded Crow in the village of Sindbis in northern Egypt in 1952 and has since been reported from Europe, Africa, Asia, and Australia (Niklasson 1989). This broad distribution and the geographical barriers between continents have resulted in two major antigenic subdivisions. The virus causes fever, arthralgia, and rash in humans but no fatal cases have been reported. There is no evidence of clinical disease in domestic or wild animals. Epidemics have been reported in South Africa, and outbreaks of similar diseases caused by Sindbis-like viruses have been reported in Sweden (Ockelbo disease), Finland (Pogosta disease), and the former U.S.S.R. (Karelian fever). No outbreaks have been reported in Australia despite high antibody rates in some areas. Birds are considered to be the principal vertebrate hosts of SIN virus because of numerous virus isolations, high antibody prevalences, and results from experimental studies showing that SIN virus–infected wild birds produce viremias sufficient to infect multiple mosquito species (McIntosh et al. 1969a, b). The virus is maintained primarily in enzootic transmission cycles between birds and mosquitoes. The primary mosquito vectors are ornithophilic species in the *Culex* genus, and some of the bird species from which SIN virus has been isolated are Hooded Crow, Masked-Weaver (*Ploceus velatus*), Eurasian Reed-Warbler (*Acrocephalus scirpaceus*), Black-crowned Night-Heron, European Turtle-Dove, White Wagtail (*Motacilla alba*), and Hill Myna (*Gracula religiosa*). However, SIN virus has also been isolated from some mammals and amphibians and from a variety of *Culex, Mansonia, Aedes, Anopheles,* and *Culiseta* mosquitoes and ticks, suggesting that there are alternative transmission cycles and that other vertebrates could serve as reservoirs for the virus.

Ockelbo virus, a subtype of Sindbis virus, causes Ockelbo disease in humans in Sweden (Espmark and

Kiklasson 1984). Ockelbo virus circulates in a bird-mosquito transmission cycle with several species of *Culex* mosquitoes as the enzootic vectors and a few species of passerine birds as the likely vertebrate hosts (Francy et al. 1989). Sera collected from 324 birds in three orders from the endemic area in Sweden in 1988 found 8% overall Nt antibody prevalence against Ockelbo virus, with the highest prevalence (27%) occurring in five species of Passeriformes (Lundstrom et al.1992). Experimental infection studies determined that young Anseriformes and Galliformes developed viremias of higher titers than adults and these viremias were of sufficient titer to infect enzootic mosquito vectors. Adult Passeriformes, particularly birds in the genera *Turdus* and *Fringilla,* developed viremias of higher titer and of longer duration. These titers were high enough to not only infect enzootic vectors but also to infect bridging vectors to humans (Lundstrom et al. 1993). Information from the field and experimental studies indicate that the passeriform species of Common Chaffinch (*Fringilla coelebs*), Common Song Thrush (*Turdus philomeios*), Redwing (*T. iliacus*), and Fieldfare (*T. pilaris*) play a major role in maintaining and amplifying the virus in Sweden.

Eastern Equine Encephalitis Virus

Eastern equine encephalitis (EEE) virus (*Alphavirus,* Togaviridae) was first isolated during a major epizootic in horses in the coastal areas of the mid-Atlantic states of the eastern U.S.A. in 1933 (Morris 1988). Similar equine epizootics have probably occurred in North America since 1831, and enzootic transmission was likely present for much longer. Additional equine epizootics occurred in the area in 1934 and 1935, and the first human cases were confirmed in New England states in 1938 when EEE virus was isolated from brain tissue. Birds were thought to be involved during the 1935 epizootic, but EEE virus was not isolated from wild birds until a EEE strain was isolated from the Common Grackle (Quiscalus quiscula) in 1950 (Kissling et al. 1951). The distribution of EEE is from eastern Canada, throughout the eastern U.S.A., Caribbean islands, Central America, and to Argentina in South America. No known human outbreaks have occurred outside of North America.

There are two serotypes of EEE virus: the North American serotype, which is found in North America and the northern Caribbean islands; and the South American serotype. Strains from each serotype isolated from migratory birds captured on the Mississippi Delta in the U.S.A. were distinguished by the short-incubation HI test (Calisher et al. 1971). There is obviously some exchange of the serotypes by viremic birds as they migrate between Central America and the Caribbean and North America; however, strains from the South American serotype have not been found established in NA.

Eastern equine encephalitis is less common than the related WEE but is more pathogenic, producing clinical disease and mortality in humans, equines, other domestic animals, exotic game birds and domesticated wild species, and a few native species. Mortality in wild and domestic Ring-necked Pheasants (*Phasianus colchicus*) was first noted in Connecticut in 1938 (Tyzzer et al. 1938), and epornitics occurred in domestic pheasant flocks in New Jersey between 1936 and 1946 as well as in white Pekin ducklings, Rock Partridge (*Alectoris graeca*), and domestic pigeons in a number of states. Epornitics in penned exotic birds, particularly pheasants, are amplified within the flocks after the initial mosquito introduction by bird-to-bird transmission through pecking and cannibalism, with fatality rates of 5 to 75%. Emus (*Dromaius novaehollandiae*) recently introduced into the U.S.A. for commercial farming suffered significant mortality from EEE virus (Tulley et al. 1992). The high virulence of EEE virus in these exotic species contrasts with the generally inapparent clinical infection or benign disease course in native wild species. However, some mortality occurs in native species such as the Whooping Crane (*Grus americana*) (Dein et al. 1986) as well as in a few passerine species (Williams et al. 1971; McLean et al. 1985a). There are apparently two forms of clinical disease in birds. Exotic species such as pheasants and some native species develop a neurotrophic infection with central nervous system (CNS) involvement starting with fever, depression, diarrhea, ataxia, tremors, partial or complete paralysis in one or both legs, prostration, and death. Native bird species and some exotic species such as emus develop viscerotrophic infections that are characterized by lethargy, drooping wings, and ataxia followed by death within 1–3 days with no CNS involvement (Dein et al. 1986; McLean et al. 1995).

Human cases of EEE virus infection are uncommon and sporadic in North America and less frequent in South America. A median of five human cases has been reported per year (ranging from zero to 14) in the U.S.A., and cases have occurred in 20 states although the four states of Florida, Massachusetts, Georgia, and New Jersey have reported the most cases (CDC 1998). One form of human illness is systemic with fever, malaise, arthralgia, and myalgia but no CNS involvement, and complete recovery is common. The encephalitic form is more severe and begins abruptly with high fever, irritability, drowsiness, vomiting, and diarrhea and progresses to convulsions and coma; about one third of the clinical cases with encephalitis are fatal. Equine cases are much more common and are regularly reported in the coastal states of the U.S.A. from Louisiana to Massachusetts each year. Periodic equine outbreaks with infrequent human cases have been reported from Argentina and Brazil, northern South America, Trinidad, and Panama (Monath 1979). Equines develop signs of depression, progressive incoordination, convulsions, and prostration, and more than 75% of the cases with encephalitis die. There are also inland locations where occasional EEE outbreaks occur and where there is sporadic enzootic transmission, such as in upstate New York, Michigan, Ohio, and Wisconsin (Morris et al. 1980; McLean et al. 1985a). The last major outbreak in the U.S.A. occurred in 1996–1997, with 19 human cases reported in eight states and 259 equine cases in 17 states from Texas to Minnesota, New Hampshire, and Florida; 111 equine cases were reported in Florida alone (CDC 1998). A previous EEE outbreak in Florida in 1978 recorded five human and 121 equine cases. A large outbreak occurred earlier in 1978 in the Dominican Republic, with 123 fatal equine cases reported in April (Calisher et al. 1979). The North American serotype of EEE virus was isolated from the brains of two of these horses, suggesting a previous introduction of EEE virus from North America by migratory birds.

In the eastern U.S.A., EEE virus is maintained over a wide geographic area in enzootic foci in freshwater swamp habitats in bird and mosquito enzootic transmission cycles during the summer months in northern latitudes (Dalrymple et al. 1972) and for more extended periods in southern latitudes in the Gulf coastal states (Stamm et al. 1962) and possibly on Caribbean islands. The foci of EEE virus were probably distributed over much larger areas and were bigger in size before the extensive human development and landscape changes that have taken place in the eastern U.S.A., particularly along the coasts. Wild birds (mostly Passeriformes) are the natural hosts and a few mosquito species are the primary enzootic vectors, principally the avian feeding species *Cs. melanura.* The virus is generally confined to these specific wetland areas, and intense amplification of transmission frequently develops during the summer transmission season. The virus escapes from these swamp foci probably during the peak of transmission by either infected mosquitoes or viremic birds to initiate transmission in surrounding areas where other abundant vector species, particularly *Ae. vexans, Ochlerotatus* (formerly *Aedes*) *sollicitans, Cx. nigripalpus,* and *Coquillettidia perturbans,* become infected and transmit EEE virus to humans, horses, and other bird species. Some of these mosquito species feed equally on birds and mammals, making them ideal bridging vectors for the virus from birds to humans and equines and thus potential epizootic vectors in areas around the swamp habitats (McLean et al. 1985a).

It is unknown how EEE virus survives throughout the year in swamp foci where adult mosquitoes are not present during the winter months. In Florida, EEE virus has been isolated every month of the year, suggesting that in at least southern parts of the state virus transmission occurs continuously throughout the year (Bigler et al. 1976). However, some other mechanism(s) of survival through the winter months (over wintering) or reintroduction in the spring is necessary to maintain established foci in the rest of the U.S.A. The virus could survive the winter by vertical transmission in the enzootic vector (*Cs. melanura*) although there is no documented evidence of transovarial transmission in this species, which survives the winter in the larval stage. Other mechanisms could be persistant infections in vertebrate species such as reptiles or amphibians; alternate vectors; or more likely by the annual reintroduction of the virus by birds to these established enzootic swamp habitats. Migratory birds could acquire EEE virus infection during their spring migration from sources in southern Florida, Caribbean islands, or Central America (Calisher et al. 1971; Calisher et al. 1979) and seed the virus into focal sites in a northward-progressing pattern. An alternative mechanism would be recrudescence of latent infections in birds resident in the foci or in returning migratory birds. Some permanent resident birds in a cedar swamp in New Jersey were viremic, and some seroconverted to EEE virus weeks before the first isolation of EEE virus from the enzootic vector (Crans et al. 1994). These viremic birds could have been infected the previous summer, become chronically infected, and relapsed to recirculate virus that was isolated in June. The early-season seroconversions could have occurred in birds with relapsing viremias as well. This source of EEE virus would initiate early-season transmission by infecting emerging enzootic mosquitoes.

Extensive studies conducted in a number of EEE enzootic sites and during epizootics have described the ecological associations of EEE virus transmission in the U.S.A. (Kissling et al. 1954; Stamm 1958; Stamm et al. 1962; Dalrymple et al. 1972; Morris et al. 1973; McLean et al. 1985a; Crans et al. 1994). The EEE virus has been isolated from and antibody detected in the blood of a large number of wild bird species, both resident and migratory. Residence status was a determining factor in the extent of exposure and infection during the transmission season; permanent resident species had much higher antibody prevalences than summer resident species that were higher than winter resident and transient migratory species. Certain species that are associated with the freshwater swamp habitats are consistently involved in transmission and contribute to virus amplification within the EEE foci with antibody prevalences ranging from 17 to 84% in enzootic sites and up to 75 to 100% during epizootics. Some of the species include Blue Jay, Northern Cardinal, Tufted Titmouse (*Parus bicolor*), Carolina Wren (*Thryothorus ludovivianus*), Wood Thrush (*Hyocichla mustelina*), Gray Catbird (*Dumetella carolinensis*), chickadees (*Parus* sp.), vireos (*Vireo* spp.), and to a lesser extent some warblers (*Dendroica* spp. *Seiurus* spp., and so on). Other bird species that frequently become involved after EEE virus activity is seasonally introduced to surrounding upland habitats, particularly in agricultural areas, are American Robin, American Goldfinch (*Spinus tristis*), Song Sparrows (*Melospiza melodia*), House Sparrows, and captive species of exotic game birds and emus (McLean et al. 1985a; Day and Stark 1996).

Venezuelan Equine Encephalitis Virus

Venezuelan equine encephalitis (VEE) virus is an RNA *Alphavirus* of the family Togaviridae with at least 124 known variant strains divided among six antigenic related subtypes (I to VI). Strains in subtype I are most frequently associated with equine epizootics, and human epidemics and large outbreaks have occurred in northern South America (Walton and Grayson 1988). Transmission of VEE viruses occurs almost continuously in parts of tropical and subtropical America, and various distinct VEE variants and subtypes are maintained in natural enzootic foci in a variety of ecologic habitats. Multiple genera of rodents and other orders of mammals (including Vampire Bats, *Desmodus rotundus,* Correa-Giron et al. 1970) as well as more than 114 species of birds have been incriminated as hosts in sylvatic transmission cycles in these foci. Historically, VEE outbreaks in equines and humans have occurred in South America since at least the early 1920s, and the outbreaks were limited especially to Colombia and Venezuela. In general, epizootics in equines begin before human epidemics, and the latest human cases usually end when animal cases cease. During 1969 to 1971, there was a continuous spread of the epidemic strain (VEE-IB) from Columbia and Venezuela to Peru and Ecuador, and then on to Central America, Mexico, and finally southern Texas, covering 4,000 km and causing considerable morbidity and mortality in both humans and equines (Sudia and Newhouse 1975). This was the first recorded invasion of North America by the VEE-IB strain, and during its dramatic spread through a variety of ecological habitats, numerous species of vertebrate hosts and arthropod vectors were involved for the first time in VEE transmission. A massive campaign involving equine quarantine and vaccination and aerial application of insecticides to kill infected mosquitoes confined the northward spread of VEE-IB to southern Texas.

The enzootic transmission of VEE virus occurs mostly among a number of species of small rodents by a variety of mosquito species, but many VEE virus variants have been repeatedly isolated from wild birds in South America and Central America (Bigler and McLean 1973; Sudia and Newhouse 1975). Different wild bird species have been experimentally infected with this virus and show no signs of illness but produce viremias lasting 1–3 days (Bowen and McLean 1977). Wild birds are not only susceptible to small doses of either epizootic or enzootic strains of VEE virus but also are reservoirs for the Tonate variant (III-B) (Chamberlain et al. 1956; Dickerman et al. 1976; Dickerman et al. 1980; Karabatsos 1985). Tonate (TON) virus was originally isolated from a Crested Oropendola (*Psarocolius decumanus*) caught in Tonate, French Guinea, in 1973, and another 14 isolates from blood and/or organs of birds have been reported. Even though previous findings suggest that birds circulate most variants of VEE virus at lower concentrations than do mammals (Bigler and McLean 1973), it has also been observed that during the first 2–4 days post-inoculation, wild birds produce viremias with high enough titers to infect both epizootic and enzootic vector mosquitoes (Bowen and McLean 1977). The detection of HI and Nt antibodies in the serum of eight different bird species from Louisiana (Chamberlain et al. 1956), five bird species (Dickerman et al. 1972) and a Sandwich (Cabot's) Tern (*Sterna sandvicensis*) collected in Corpus Christi, Texas (Sudia et al. 1975), as well as virus isolation from a Long-tailed Hermit (*Phaethornis superciliosus*) from Mexico clearly indicate the involvement of birds in VEE transmission cycles (Kissling et al. 1955). In subsequent studies, Nt antibodies were detected against the Everglades virus (subtype II) in Turkey and Black Vultures (*Cathartes aura* and *Coragyps atratus*), the Great-crested Flycatcher (*Myiarchus crinitus*) and the Common Grackle from the Florida Everglades (Lord et al. 1973), and in 44 wild bird species from southern Texas (Sudia et al. 1975). Even though birds have not yet been considered a major contributor to the local circulation and amplification of this virus, the findings mentioned above suggest that birds could be involved in local and regional movement and in the introduction of VEE virus to new areas.

Ross River Virus

Ross River (RR) virus, a member of the Getah serogroup in the genus *Alphavirus,* Togaviridae, was first isolated in 1965 from three passerine birds (Masked Finch, *Poephila personata;* Brown Flycatcher, *Microeca leucophaea;* and Magpie-Lark, *Grallina*

Cyanoleuca from Queensland, Australia) (Whitehead et al.1968). The ecology and distribution of RR virus has recently been reviewed by Russell (2002). The host range of RR virus is extremely broad but it produces clinical infection only in humans and possibly horses. The clinical disease in humans, "epidemic polyarthritis," is characterized by fever, polyarthralgia, and rash. This mosquito-borne virus is endemic in Australia and parts of New Guinea and in some Pacific islands. Epidemics have been documented in Australia and in the Pacific islands of American Samoa, Fiji, New Caledonia, and Cook Islands (Kay and Aaskov 1989). Ross River virus is the most common mosquito-borne pathogen causing human disease in Australia, with an average of about 5,000 cases reported annually (Russell 2002). More than half of the cases during the period of 1991–1998 were reported from Queensland (Harley et al. 2001). The virus has been isolated from five different genera of mosquitoes, but the most important vector species may be *Cx. annulirostris* because it occurs throughout Australia and the Pacific islands and feeds on a wide variety of animals (Kay and Aaskov 1989). This mosquito breeds mainly in freshwater ponds, swamps, and sewage lagoons although it has rapidly colonized temporary pools in agricultural areas and artificial containers in peridomestic environments. Experimental and field studies have confirmed its vector competence to transmit RR virus.

Despite the initial isolations of RR virus from birds, the principal vertebrates involved in transmission cycles appear to be mammals, particularly large mammals such as kangaroos and wallabies and small mammals such as fruit bats and rodents. Serological surveys of domestic and wild birds in Australia revealed only a low incidence of infection (Doherty et al. 1966; Marshall et al. 1982b). Vertebrate studies conducted during the large epidemic on American Samoa in 1979, where 43.8% of the human population was infected, found that 15–20% of peridomestic dogs and pigs, 5% of chickens, and 3% of rats had RR antibody (Tesh et al. 1981). Experimental infection studies confirmed that marsupials were more competent hosts than placental mammals such as introduced rodents, rabbits, and domestic animals, which in turn were better than birds as amplifying hosts for RR virus (Marshall and Miles 1984; Kay and Aaskov 1989).

Mayaro Virus

Mayaro virus (MAY) in the Semliki Forest complex of alphaviruses was first isolated in 1954 from clinical cases in Trinidad, and a small number of epidemics have been reported from Brazil and Bolivia, with most of the cases associated with forested areas (Pinheiro and LeDuc 1988). Although no fatalities have been reported, the infection is widespread throughout rural areas in northern South America. No clinical disease has been observed in domestic animals or wildlife. The natural vertebrate hosts are thought to be mammals and possibly birds. The only isolate of MAY virus and evidence of infection outside of South America and Trinidad was from a migrating Orchard Oriole (*Icterus spurius*) captured while entering the southern U.S.A. in 1967 during spring migration (Calisher et al. 1974). The virus is likely enzootic in the tropical rain forests where nonhuman primates and other wild animals including birds and a variety of mosquito vectors play an important role in the maintenance and transmission of the virus. However, the role of birds in the ecology of MAY virus in the forested regions of Brazil and other countries in South America is unknown at this time. Uruma virus isolated in Bolivia is considered a strain of Mayaro virus (Herve et al. 1986), and the important role of at least 41 Amazonian bird species in the transmission cycle of this virus has been confirmed (Degallier et al. 1992).

Semliki Forest Virus

Semliki Forest (SF) virus (an *Alphavirus* apparently identical to Kumba virus) was first isolated from mosquitoes in Uganda in 1942 and has been isolated from mosquitoes and antibody detected in humans in the former USSR, India, and southeast Asia. The virus was isolated from Red-headed Quelea (*Quelea erythrops*) in Nigeria and the Central African Republic (CAR), and experimentally inoculated wild birds developed viremia and antibodies (Karabatsos 1985). Antibody was detected in wild birds in Israel (Nir et al. 1969).

Una Virus

Una (UNA) virus is an *Alphavirus* that is maintained in a transmission cycle between at least 10 species of wild birds and a variety of ornithophilic mosquitoes. The role of birds in Brazil was confirmed through the findings of Herve et al. (1986) and Degallier et al. (1992). The original virus isolate was from *Ps. ferox* in Brazil; subsequent isolates were obtained from sentinel mice, horses, and other mosquitoes (*Psorophora spp., Aedes spp., Culex spp., Coquillettidia spp., Wyeomyia spp., and Anopheles spp.*). Antibodies (HI and Nt) were detected in humans (Karabatsos 1985).

Bunyaviridae

Turlock Virus

Turlock (TUR) virus is a single-stranded RNA virus in the genus *Bunyavirus,* Bunyaviridae. It was first isolated from *Cx. tarsalis* mosquitoes collected in Turlock, California, in 1954 and has subsequently been recovered regularly from mosquitoes and birds in North America and South America (Karabatsos 1985). Although TUR virus is a common virus circulating in the Americas, it does not affect humans or domestic animals. Of 328 reported TUR isolates from mosquitoes in the western U.S.A., 305 were obtained from *Cx. Tarsalis,* indicating its importance as the primary vector, and 20 of 21 isolates from vertebrates were from birds (Hayes et al. 1976; Scott et al. 1983a). The avian isolates were predominantly from House Sparrows and a few from House Finches in the western U.S.A. (Holden et al. 1973a), and from two bird species captured near Belem, Brazil (Shope et al. 1966). Viruses in the TUR serogroup have a broad geographical distribution in the western hemisphere from Canada to Ecuador and Brazil and in the eastern hemisphere (Calisher et al. 1984). High HI antibody prevalences against Lednice (LED) virus in this serogroup were found in Mallards, Greylag Goose (*Anser anser*), and Mute Swans (*Cygnus olor*) in southern Moravia in the former USSR (Kolman et al. 1976). Five different passerine species inoculated with TUR virus responded with viremias sufficient to infect mosquitoes and all produced antibody (Scott et al. 1983b). No morbidity or mortality was associated with experimental or natural infections of birds with TUR virus.

Mermet Virus

Mermet (MER) virus is a *Bunyavirus* in the Bunyaviridae family that was originally isolated from a Purple Martin (*Progne subis*) in Massac County, Illinois, in 1964 (Karabatsos 1985). The virus was also isolated from three other wild bird species (Blue Jay, Swainson's Thrush, *Catharus ustulatus;* and Red-winged Blackbird, *Agelaius phoeniceus*) in southern Illinois and from the Northern Cardinal in Texas (Calisher et al. 1969). Antibody (Nt) was detected in a sample of 3,198 birds (mostly House Sparrows) collected in Texas, Mississippi, Tennessee, Ohio, Indiana, and Wisconsin, but no MER antibody was found in birds from Kentucky or Missouri (Calisher et al. 1981). Antibody prevalences varied by location and years and indicated the widespread MER virus activity throughout the central U.S.A. Mermet virus was also isolated from *Cx. pipiens and Cx. restuans* mosquitoes in Memphis, Tennessee, and was isolated in Guatemala. No antibody was detected in paired serum specimens from 966 humans with suspected arboviral infections from the central U.S.A. The primary transmission of MER virus is within a bird-mosquito cycle and no disease has been reported in birds, other animals, or humans.

Itaporanga Virus

Itaporanga (ITP) virus is in the genus *Phlebovirus* (Bunyaviridae) and is closely related to Icoaraci (ICO) virus; the first isolate came from a sentinel mouse (baby Swiss mouse) from Brazil in 1962 (Karabatsos 1985). The virus has been isolated from marsupials, birds, and different nocturnal mosquitoes. Antibodies against this agent have been detected in humans, marsupials, bats, monkeys, and birds (Karabatsos 1985; Herve et al. 1986; Degallier et al. 1992). The virus isolations and the detection of antibodies are interpreted as an indicator that the natural transmission cycle of ITP virus occurs among the vertebrates inhabiting the canopy of the Brazilian forest, such as marsupials, bats, monkeys, and birds. Ground dwelling vertebrates have shown no evidence of infection.

Uukuniemi Virus

Uukuniemi (UUK) virus is a tick-borne arbovirus in the Uukuniemi serogroup, genus *Uukuvirus,* Bunyaviridae that is distributed throughout Europe. The virus was first isolated in Finland from *I. ricinus* ticks in 1959 and characterized as a Bunyamwera serogoup arbovirus in 1969 (Saikku and Brummer-Korvenkontio 1973). An additional 12 strains were isolated in Finland from 12,001 ticks in 1959–1960 as well as six strains from 774 birds in 1963. Further strains of UUK virus were isolated from birds in Finland in 1971 (Saikku 1974). Eight strains were isolated from 579 birds tested, 12.6% of the birds were HI antibody positive to UUK virus, and 10% were infested with immature stages of *I. ricinus* ticks. The peak of virus activity in birds occurred during the period of highest prevalence of tick infestation between June and early July when 37.4% of the birds were parasitized with ticks and 2.7% were viremic. Thrushes and other birds that feed on the ground and share the same habitats with the ticks were more frequently infested with ticks and infected with UUK virus. Since the 1970s, UUK and related viruses in this serogroup have also been isolated from passerine birds and their ectoparasites in other countries: the former USSR, Poland, Hungary, France, Czechoslovakia, Egypt, Pakistan, Australia, and the United States (Calisher and Karabatsos 1988). Wild birds are the principal vertebrate hosts and none of these viruses are known to cause disease in birds, livestock, or humans.

Dugbe Virus

Dugbe (DUG) virus, a tick-borne virus in the genus *Nairovirus,* Bunyaviridae, was originally isolated from *Ambylomma variegatum* ticks removed from cattle in Nigeria in 1964 (Karabatsos 1985) and subsequently isolated from human cases in Central African Republic (CAR) in 1967, 1970, and 1973. It was the most frequently isolated virus among 57 isolates from *A. variegatum* collected from cattle in CAR in 1972–1974. This tick species is the main vector of DUG virus in this African country, with peak abundance during the dry season and the first half of the rainy season. The virus was also isolated from *Boophilus* and *Hylomma* ticks. Dugbe virus infects a high proportion of cattle (70%) in CAR and has been isolated from a bird, rodent, and ticks in Ethiopia during 1974–1976. The role of birds in the transmission and maintenance of DUG virus is unclear at this time.

Tete Serogroup Viruses

Tete serogroup viruses, Tete, Bahig, Matruh, Tsuruse, and Batama, have been isolated from birds, mostly water birds (except one isolate from ticks), in Africa, Europe, and Japan and all are related members of the *Bunyavirus* genus, Bunyaviridae. Two viruses were isolated from ceratopogonid midges in northern Colorado, U.S.A., during field investigations of another arbovirus in the area in 1976–1977 (Calisher et al. 1990). These two viruses were distinct from each other but were identified as members of Tete serogroup. The discovery of these viruses in North America out of their historical range was unexpected, and it was quickly determined that they were infecting local birds, particularly American Coots (*Fulica americana*), Mallards (*Anas platyrhynchos*), House Sparrows, and Rock Pigeons. It is still unknown whether these viruses were recently introduced or were indigenous to Colorado.

Rhabdoviridae

Flanders and Hart Park Viruses

Flanders (FLA) and Hart Park (HP) viruses are closely related viruses in the Hart Park antigenic group of Rhabdoviridae. Both viruses are very common mosquito-borne viruses that likely circulate in bird-mosquito transmission cycles in many parts of North America. These two viruses are frequently isolated from mosquitoes during local and state arbovirus surveillance efforts and are occasionally isolated from wild birds (Karabatsos 1985). There is a close but distinct antigenic relationship between these viruses (Boyd 1972). There is no known disease associated with infections from these viruses, and the only known vertebrate hosts are birds. Flanders virus was originally isolated from *Cs. melanura* mosquitoes collected in Flanders, Suffolk County, New York, 1961, and from the spleen of an ovenbird (*Seiurusaurocapilla*) in New York (Whitney 1964). Flanders virus was isolated from *Cx. pipiens* complex and *Cx. restuans* mosquitoes in the Ohio-Mississippi Basin during 1965–1967 and from the blood of a Northern Cardinal in 1966 and 12 House Sparrows and two Red-winged Blackbirds in 1967 (Kokernot et al. 1969). Nearly all of the birds that were positive for FLA virus were nestlings, and the earliest recovery of virus from nestling House Sparrows was June 9 and the latest was August 16. Flanders virus and not HP virus was routinely isolated from mosquitoes (primarily *Culex*) in Iowa during 1966–1980, and HI antibody to FLA virus was detected in birds (Rowley et al. 1983). The virus was later isolated from mosquitoes from Florida, South Carolina, New York, Canada, Arkansas, and Mexico and from a European Starling in New York and a Magnolia Warbler (*Dendroic amagnolia*) in Michigan (McLean et al. 1985a). Hart Park virus was originally isolated from *Cx. tarsalis* mosquitoes in Kern County, California, in 1955 and was subsequently isolated from mosquitoes and birds from California and other states (Karabatsos 1985). Avian isolates came from House Sparrows, House Finch, Yellow-headed Blackbird (*Xanthocephalus xanthocephalus*), and Tricolored Blackbird (*Aeglaius tricolor*), in California.

Jurona Virus

Jurona (JUR) virus (*Vesiculovirus,* Rhabdoviridae) is an obscure arbovirus first isolated in Brazil from *Haemagogus janthinomys,* the only known mosquito vector (Herve et al. 1986). The natural transmission cycle is believed to involve birds and mosquitoes, in which at least 14 different species of wild birds were found infected as determined by virus and antibody detection (Degallier et al. 1992; Karabatsos 1985). A recent virus isolate obtained from the brain tissue of a dead domestic pigeon in Connecticut, U.S.A., in 2000 was found to be closely related to JUR virus in the *Vesiculovirus* genus (Travassos da Rosa et al. 2002).

Kwatta Virus

Kwatta (KWA) virus is also an obscure member of the genus *Vesiculovirus,* and first isolated in 1964 from mosquitoes (*Culex spp.*) collected in Surinam, South America (Haas et al. 1966). More recent findings suggest that wild birds play an important role in the transmission cycle of this virus (Degallier et al. 1992).

Reoviridae

Umatilla Virus

Umatilla (UMA) virus, an *Orbivirus* in the family Reoviridae, was originally isolated from *Cx. pipiens* collected in Umatilla County, Oregon, in 1969 and later from *Cx. pipiens* and *Cx. tarsalis* from Utah, Texas, and Colorado (Karabatsos 1985). The virus was isolated from a House Sparrow in Texas, and chickens experimentally infected with UMA virus produced viremias, indicating that birds are the likely hosts for the virus. Another virus, Netivot, related to UMA virus was isolated from mosquitoes in Israel (Tesh et al. 1986).

Kemerovo Complex Viruses

Kemerovo (KEM) complex viruses are also in the genus *Orbivirus* and were originally isolated from *I. persulcatus* ticks in the Kemerova region in the west Siberian taiga of the former USSR in 1962 (Karabatsos 1985). Additional isolates have been obtained from ticks, and clinical disease and antibody were confirmed in humans in the USSR and Czechoslovakia (Libikova et al. 1978). Multiple viruses have been isolated and identified from both the eastern and western hemispheres, and four subgroups of viruses were identified in the KEM complex (Yunker 1975). Nine viruses in the KEM antigenic group have been isolated from ticks collected at seabird colonies from eight different geographical locations. Arbroath virus in the KEM group was isolated from female *I. uriae* ticks collected from a dead Atlantic Puffin (*Fratercula arctica*) at Arbroath, Scotland, and from *I. uriae* ticks from the Isle of May, Scotland (Moss and Nuttall 1985; Spence et al. 1985). Kemerovo viruses were also isolated from ticks at a seabird colony in Newfoundland (Oprandy et al. 1988a). Another *Orbivirus* in the KEM group, Mono Lake (ML) virus, was isolated from *A. monolakensis* ticks collected at nests of California Gulls (*Larus californicus*) on islands in an inland lake (Mono Lake), Mono County, California (Schwan et al. 1988). Mono Lake virus was also isolated from the closely related tick, *A. cooleyi,* a parasite of Cliff Swallows in Colorado (Calisher et al. 1988) and a related virus, Sixgun City, from *A. cooleyi* in Colorado and Texas (Yunker et al. 1972). A KEM virus was isolated from a migrating Common Redstart (*Phoenicurus phoenicurus*) in Eurasia (Schmidt and Shope 1971) and Nt antibody was detected in Fieldfares (*Turdus pilaris*) and Dark-throated Thrushes (*T. ruficollis*) as well as rodents (*Clethrionomys* spp.) in the Kemerovo region (Karabatsos 1985). However, little other information is available about virus infections or disease in the avian hosts associated with the tick-borne viruses isolated at seabird colonies.

EPIZOOTIOLOGY

Some virus/vector/vertebrate interactions have unique epidemiological characteristics that can have an impact on human, wild, and domestic animal populations. As in humans, subclinical infections are frequent in wild and domestic animals and occur either as isolated cases that are rarely diagnosed or as epizootics, which can be detected if systematic serological surveys are conducted. The arboviruses of birds are transmitted by different types and species of vectors, have simple to multiple transmission cycles, and may cause clinical disease in a number of incidental hosts (Figure 2.3). Some viruses, such as SLE in North America, have simple transmission cycles involving a few species of avian hosts and a few species of *Culex* mosquitoes as the vectors; humans are the only incidental or dead-end hosts that develop clinical disease. In contrast, a strain of WN virus introduced into North America is much more complicated, with many avian host species involved as well as many mosquito species, and humans, equines, and some wildlife species suffer clinical disease and death. In addition, WN virus may have separate and secondary transmission cycles involving direct transmission between avian species, possible oral transmission from prey to predator, and secondary mosquito transmission cycles involving other vertebrate groups such as mammals and reptiles. However, some arboviruses have different strains of varying virulence for vertebrate hosts, and frequently the strains are of geographic origin. An example is the appearance of a new, more virulent strain of WN virus in Israel in 1998 that for the first time caused noticeable mortality in wild birds and domestic geese (Bin et al. 2001). Other factors that may influence virus virulence to particular hosts are the movement of the virus or the avian host out of their natural ecosystems to new ecosystems. Some examples are the introduction of a virulent strain of WN virus into the U.S.A. from Israel in 1999, causing significant mortality in naïve avian species (Eidson et al. 2001a), and the movement of EEE virus from its specific natural habitat of freshwater swamps in the eastern U.S.A. to surrounding areas, where it causes mortality in some native bird species and exotic game bird species (McLean et al. 1985a). The movement of birds to new ecosystems containing novel viruses can result in increased virulence for these exotic hosts as occurs when exotic birds such as emus are introduced into the U.S.A. and suffer significant mortality from EEE virus (Tulley et al. 1992).

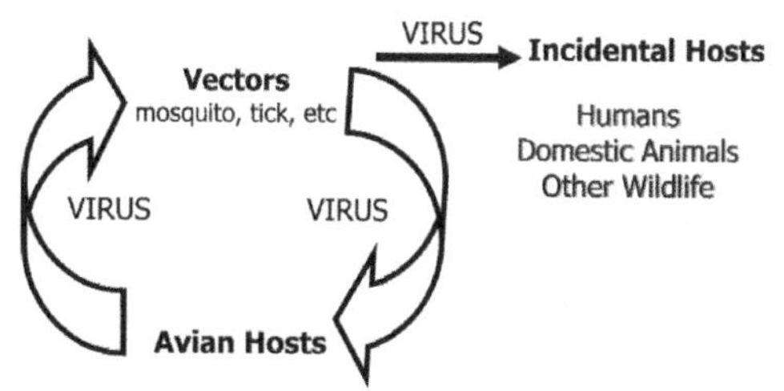

Figure 2.3. General transmission cycle for bird-associated arboviruses.

Arboviruses are transmitted among vertebrates by infected arthropods in two different settings: sylvatic (or rural) and suburban/urban. Arboviruses are maintained by their specific vector(s) in a determined area known as an ecological niche or focus by a transmission chain from infected to susceptible vertebrate hosts (McLean 1991). Transmission can occur as either enzootic in animal populations with almost continuous transmission at a relatively low to moderate frequency, or epizootic when outbreaks occur. The

Table 2.2. Factors that influence the transmission of arboviruses in nature.

Vertebrate Factors	Vector Factors	Environmental Factors
Susceptibility to virus	Susceptibility to virus	Temperature
Competence to infect vector	Competence to transmit	Rainfall
Density and turnover rate	Density and survival rate	Seasonal weather patterns
Attractiveness to vectors	Feeding habits	Wind patterns
Tolerance of vector feeding	Daily activity patterns	Surface water
Daily activity patterns	Flight range	Humidity & soil moisture
Age structure	Age structure	Salinity & water quality
Mobility	Vertical distribution in habitat	Soil type
Seasonal residence status	Geographical distribution	Topography
Ecological association with competent vectors	Ecological association with competent vertebrate hosts	Landscape characteristics
Frequent exposure to vector	Seasonal activity	Vegetation
Vertical distribution in habitat		Habitat type
Geographical distribution		

frequency of transmission of an arbovirus among the susceptible and maintenance hosts is influenced by a number of factors (Table 2.2). An important factor for vectors is population density, which depends on environmental conditions such as temperature, humidity, and surface water that may be constantly, seasonally, or periodically favorable. Other factors that influence transmission are susceptibility to and competence in transmitting viruses, vector activity (diurnal, nocturnal, crepuscular), feeding preferences (habits), flight range, age structure, survival rates, and vector distribution. Important factors for vertebrate hosts are abundance, susceptibility, competence in infecting vectors, attractiveness to vectors, accessibility to and tolerance of vector feeding, activity patterns, age structure, mobility, seasonal presence (residence status) in an area, and geographical distribution. Critical for virus transmission between a specific vector and vertebrate is a close spatial and temporal association (juxtaposition). For example, virus transmission will not occur between a mosquito species and bird species that occur in the exact same location but at different times of the year. Neither will transmission occur between a mosquito species that is active only near the ground and a bird species that is active only in the tree canopy, although both occur at the same time of year and in the same geographical location. A diurnal mosquito species will be inefficient in transmitting viruses between active, diurnal birds, whereas a nocturnal mosquito species can more easily feed on roosting diurnal birds. Some of the characteristics of arboviruses that influence viral transmission, the effects on vertebrate hosts, and laboratory identification are as follows: genomic type, molecular structure, genetic variation or virus strains, phylogenetic relationships, virulence to host cells, and viral proteins that induce host immunity. Some alternate routes of transmission besides by arthropods of some arboviruses are aerosol, contact, tissue, and mechanical transmission.

CLINICAL SIGNS

Clinical signs of arbovirus infections in birds are a result of neurotrophic, viscerotrophic, or sometimes nonrestricted tissue tropisms (preferences) of the infecting virus. Neurotrophic signs occur with central nervous system infection and can consist of depression, partial and then complete paralysis, tremors, and torticollis followed by prostration and death. Pen-raised Ring-necked Pheasants, Rock Partridge, pigeons, white Pekin ducklings, turkeys, and Coturnix Quail (*Coturnix coturnix*) suffered clinical disease with neurotrophic signs and mortality from EEE virus infection U.S.A. (Eleazer et al. 1978). Viscerotrophic infections have occurred with EEE virus in a few bird species such as Whooping Cranes, Glossy Ibis *(Plegadis falcinellus),* and emus. Four of seven Whooping Cranes naturally infected with EEE did not develop any clinical signs before death, whereas the others showed lethargy and ataxia with leg and neck paresis (Dein et al.1986). Some Glossy Ibises and Snowy Egrets *(Egretta thula)* experimentally infected with EEE virus developed clinical signs of lethargy, drooping wings, and ataxia before dying one to three days after signs appeared (McLean et al. 1995).

The introduced virulent strain of WN virus that affected birds at two wildlife facilities in New York City during the epidemic and epizootic in 1999 caused clinical disease, severe pathologic changes, and mortality in a variety of captive and some free-ranging birds (Steele et al. 2000). Clinical signs in captive birds were principally neurotrophic in origin, consisting of ataxia, tremors, abnormal head posture, circling, or convulsions or sometimes just marked depression. Some of the birds became uncoordinated followed by a progressive inability to stand, while others presented with only weakness or sternal recumbency. Natural and experimental WN virus infections in Corvidae presented different patterns of clinical signs and pathogenesis. Natural infections in American Crows, Fish Crows (*Corvus ossifragus*), and captive magpies at the wildlife facilities in New York City showed decreased neurovirulence (Steele et al. 2000); limited viral antigen and mild histological changes were noted in the brain, and the cerebellum was spared. However, severe virus-induced lesions were noted in most major extraneural organs. Experimental infections of American Crows with the 1999 NY strain of WN virus (R.G. McLean personal communication) produced infections similar to the natural infections described above. The infected crows died within four to eight days following inoculation of virus and displayed a variety of clinical signs starting with general weakness and lethargy and then becoming sedentary and perching in a crouched posture followed by a progressive inability to perch, stand, or fly. The infected birds gradually became recumbent and no longer responded normally to danger until death in two to three days after onset of signs. Viral antigen was most intense and pathologic lesions were most severe in kidney, spleen, liver, heart, and brain. Experimental infections of domestic birds did not produce clinical disease in chickens and turkeys but produced clinical signs of depression, weight loss, torticollis, opisthotonus, and death in two-week-old domestic geese (Swayne et al. 2001) similar to what was reported for domestic geese naturally infected in Israel (Malkinson et al. 2002).

Clinical signs of infections from WN virus in equines include rapid onset with ataxia (stumbling or poor coordination), depression or apprehension, weakness of limbs, partial paralysis, muscle twitching, or death (Murgue et al. 2001; Ostlund et al. 2001). Fever is not often observed and fatality rates are about 30–33%. Clinical signs from infections with EEE, VEE, and WEE viruses are similar, but may also include convulsions, prostration, and encephalitis. Fatality rates following clinical disease vary among the viruses with higher rates for EEE (70%) and VEE virus infections. Clinical disease in humans varies among those pathogenic viruses of WN, EEE, WEE, VEE, SLE, JE, MVE, and RR. The majority of infections are subclinical (80% for some viruses) or result in a mild flu-like illness, while others have fever, polyarthralgia, and rash (RR virus). Milder symptoms can include fever, headache, and body aches, nausea, vomiting, and sometimes swollen lymph glands or a skin rash on the chest, stomach, and back. Severe symptoms for WN can include high fever, headache, neck stiffness, stupor, disorientation, coma, tremors, convulsions, muscle weakness, vision loss, numbness, and paralysis. Some clinical cases develop progressive neurologic signs (meningitis or encephalitis) and can lapse into comas and death, with a 10–14% case fatality rate for some flaviviruses and 34–35% for some alphaviruses. Neurological effects may be permanent in survivors (CDC 2005). Many of these viruses cause age-related illness with severe disease and death mostly in the elderly, but some also affect the young age groups (JE) and others at any age (EEE). Clinical disease in humans, domestic animals, and wildlife caused by the various bird-associated arboviruses are listed for various regions of the world (Table 2.3).

PATHOGENESIS AND PATHOLOGY

Specific details of viral pathogenesis and immunology within the hosts are beyond the scope of this chapter and only a simple description of the process is presented here. There are a number of general articles, chapters, and books available on this particular topic (Nathanson 1980; Brinton 2001; Mims et al. 2001; O'Neil et al. 2002). Viral infections in vertebrates progress through defined phases. A typical course of arbovirus infection in birds following the introduction of virus by an arthropod vector is a short period of viremia during the first one to seven days that is mediated by the production and circulation of Nt antibody in the blood (Nathanson 1980). The appearance of clinical signs occurs in some vertebrate species following the viremic phase after virus particles have invaded and multiplied in target tissues. When the virus enters the animal it is carried by the vascular system to tissues or by the lymphatic system to regional lymph nodes where initial replication takes place or replication occurs at the subcutaneous inoculation site. Macrophages are generally the first line of host defense and are more important for certain arboviruses and for certain host species in mediating viral clearance and for the outcome of the infection. Following virus attachment to, entry into, and multiplication within cells, the next generation of virus is released and carried to the vascular system by the lymphatic system. Virus may also replicate in the vascular wall of the small blood vessels initially or secondarily and enter the blood system directly, especially when massive viremias occur. The amount of virus that is replicated depends upon the genetics of the invading virus and the genetics and immunological response of the host. With most of the arboviruses, blood-borne virus

Table 2.3. Arboviruses associated with birds that cause disease in humans, domestic animals, and wildlife.

Region	Arboviruses Affecting Humans	Arboviruses Affecting Domestic Animals	Arboviruses Affecting Wildlife
North America	EEE, SLE, VEE, WEE, WN	EEE, HJ, VEE, WEE, WN	WN, EEE, WEE
Central & South America	EEE, MAY, ROC, SLE, VEE, WEE	EEE, VEE, WEE	
Europe & Western Asia	WN, SIN, TBE, KEM.	WN, LI	LI
Africa & Middle East	WN, SIN	IT, WN	WN
India, Eastern and SE Asia	WN, JE, SIN	JE	
Oceania	KUN, MVE, RR, SIN	MVE, RR	

particles are present almost entirely in the plasma. The host responds to the foreign virus through the production of humoral antibodies by the lymphocytes that neutralize and clear the virus particles from the blood as they are released, usually within about one week after infection. For several days, both virus and antibody may be present in the blood in infectious immune complexes. Generally, infected birds that survive and produce Nt antibodies are protected from future infection with the same or closely related viruses (McLean et al. 1983).

The development of clinical disease is caused by the invasion of virus into the central nervous system and/or other critical organs such as liver, spleen, kidney, and heart with WNV infections (Steele et al. 2000). The probability of tissue invasion and clinical disease increases with the titer of the viremia. Many factors influence the pathogenesis of particular viruses in vertebrate host species (Brinton 2001) including at the molecular level (Brinton 2002). Certain host species are unable to fight off the virus replication and invasion and succumb to the infection, whereas other species are resistant to disease. The differences in responses of individual species or animals are frequently inherited. Unique genes or sets of genes are involved in conferring resistance. A number of host factors such as age, hormone levels, nutritional condition, and immune status can alter the response of the host. Many viruses contain virulence factors that promote viral replication, transmission, and entry and binding to target cells; therefore, the virulence of the infecting virus or strain of virus can vary markedly (Bowen et al. 1980). The strain (NY1999) of WN virus introduced into the U.S.A. in 1999 is particularly virulent to naïve bird species in the western hemisphere compared to WN virus strains circulating in Africa and Europe to native birds in the eastern hemisphere (McLean et al. 2002). A recent experimental infection study of historic (KEN 3829) and recent (NY99) strains of WN virus and a related strain (KUN) from Australia demonstrated significant differences in susceptibility and mortality of American crows (Brault et al. 2004). The dose of virus and route of infection are critical in determining the outcome of the infection.

Since WNV was introduced to NA in 1999, there have been numerous publications describing pathological changes and tissue distribution of WNV antigen in a variety of avian species following natural or experimental infection (Senne et al. 2000; Steele et al. 2000; Swayne et al. 2000, 2001; Fitzgerald et al. 2003; Josan et al. 2003; Bertelsen et al. 2004; Gancz et al. 2004; Weingartl et al. 2004; Wunschmann et al. 2004a, 2004b, 2005; Gibbs et al. 2005; Gancz et al. 2006).

Based on these reports, it is clear that there are no lesions pathognomonic for WNV infection and the virus can affect virtually any body organ system. Lesions have been described in the central nervous system (CNS), liver, spleen, kidney, heart, lung, pancreas, proventriculus, intestine, and in some species also in the eye, peripheral nervous system, adrenal gland, gonads, bone marrow, and integument. The pattern of location, intensity, and chronicity of lesions appears to reflect the clinical course of the disease. Thus highly susceptible species such as crows (Wunschmann et al. 2004b) or northern North American owl species (Gancz et al. 2004, 2006) that die rapidly following a short incubation period may have few or no observable lesions at necropsy except perhaps scattered tissue hemorrhage, hepato- or splenomegaly, or acute hepatic necrosis. These species tend to have large amounts of WNV antigen in the blood and widely distributed in major organs, and the histological changes are peracute to acute with minimal inflammatory response. Acute single-cell to coalescing necrosis in organs such as spleen and liver or heart are commonly observed but usually with minimal inflammation. In the CNS there may be few or many scattered glial nodules or in some cases only a few vascular changes but prominent WNV antigen within neurons. It is likely that these birds die before they mount an extensive inflammatory response.

Birds that survive longer have more pronounced lesions. These typically include lymphoplasmacytic and histiocytic encephalitis, necrotizing and lymphoplasmacytic myocarditis, and often inflammation in major parenchymal organs and even thyroid glands, gonads, and peripheral nerves. Encephalitis, myocarditis, and pancreatitis are the most frequent lesions reported, and in some species such as the Red-tailed hawk (*Buteo jamaicensis*) and the Cooper's Hawk (*Accipiter cooperii*) there may also be endophthalmitis (Wunschmann et al. 2004a).

Birds that survive days to months develop chronic lesions of encephalitis and pancreatitis and often the main organ affected is the myocardium. In these cases a diagnosis of WNV may be difficult because viral antigen maybe sparse and difficult to find using IHC.

In viremic birds, WNV antigen is likely to be present in many organs and tissues, but in birds with chronic disease it may be difficult to detect. In such birds, careful examination of the kidney, CNS, heart, pancreas, and submucosal ganglia of the digestive tract is required for antigen detection. Patterns of WNV antigen distribution in tissues may differ between species but also may be variable within birds of the same species. In corvids, experimentally infected with WNV, it was shown that the antigen distribution pattern changes as a function of time post infection. For example, viral antigen was detected in kidney macrophages at three days post infection (dpi), and in tubular epithelium at 4 dpi. Interspecies differences were also noted, with involvement of glomeruli in Blue Jays (*Cyanocitta cristata*) but not in American Crows (*Corvus brachyrhynchos*) (Weingartl et al. 2004). The reasons for these differences in lesion pattern distribution, host responses, and disease susceptibility between species and even between individuals is not known.

DIAGNOSIS

Vertebrates produce complex antibody responses following arbovirus infections and thus the laboratory tests used to detect antibody may be difficult to interpret. The IgM antibody appears to be more specific than IgG antibody, but both may cross react with closely related viruses, adding to the diagnostic problems in identifying the infecting virus. Serology is seldom used for specific diagnosis in wild, free-ranging birds because rarely are acute and convalescent serum specimens collected and available to detect a diagnostic rise in antibody titer. However, a single serum specimen with high antibody titer (McLean et al. 1983) or the presence of IgM antibody in an acute serum of domestic chickens (Calisher et al. 1986) can be diagnostic in some circumstances. Serology can be used to diagnose arbovirus infections in captive birds (sentinels or birds in zoological collections) because multiple blood samples can be obtained to detect conversions from negative to positive or to detect a diagnostic rise in antibody titer associated with a known infection. However, the development and use of WN virus monoclonal antibodies in an epitope blocking, enzyme-linked immunosorbent assay (ELISA) has allowed the detection of WN virus-specific antibody in single serum specimens from captive (Hall et al. 1995) and wild birds (Blitvich et al. 2003b; Jozan et al. 2003).

Laboratory confirmation of infection is by identification of a virus or specific antibody against a virus. Whole blood, serum, or tissue samples are taken for virus isolation and/or direct testing of tissues for viral antigen and for antibody testing (serology). Specimens taken for testing should be processed immediately or frozen at a suitable temperature until they can be tested. The general laboratory procedures used for testing vertebrate hosts for arboviruses are reviewed by Beaty et al. (1989), Roehrig (1999), and Kramer and Bernard (2001).

Virus isolation is attempted in a variety of cell culture types or by intracerebral inoculation of suckling white mice. The arboviruses produce cytopathic effects in cells or form plaques in cell culture and generally kill baby mice. Virus isolates can be confirmed by direct fluorescent antibody (FA) or by indirect fluorescent antibody (IFA) testing of infected cell cultures with monoclonal antibody (Ostlund et al. 2001), virus neutralization tests with known antisera (Calisher et al. 1989), and reverse transcription-polymerase chain reaction (RT-PCR) (Lanciotti et al. 2000).

Serological assays include screening tests that can rapidly test large numbers of blood samples but generally cannot distinguish between closely related viruses (for example, WN and SLE viruses in the JE virus complex). A confirmatory test is generally required to identify the specific viral antibody. The three types of screening tests commonly used are the HI test, the indirect immunofluorescent antibody (IFA) assay, and the enzyme immunoassay (EIA) or ELISA. The HI was the primary test used for screening vertebrate sera for a number of years and still remains a viable technique because of its low cost and ease of use (Clarke and Casals 1958). The IFA was also a standard test to detect arbovirus antibody, particularly in humans, and was recently modified to detect IgM antibody against WN virus (Kulas et al. 2001). The

ELISA format has replaced the HI test in many laboratories because of its larger capacity and rapidity of testing. A number of different ELISA (or EIA) formats have been developed for testing bird sera. To determine recent infections in sentinel chickens, IgM antibodies can be detected by immunoglobulin M capture enzyme-linked immunosorbent assay (MAC-ELISA) (Calisher et al. 1986; Sahu et al. 1994; Johnson et al. 2003). However, IgM antibody in birds is present generally for a much shorter duration (3–4 weeks or less) and the duration can vary by the infecting virus and possibly by the bird species (Boyle et al. 1983b; Johnson et al. 2003). An indirect EIA for detecting IgG antibodies to SLE and WEE viruses in sentinel chickens was developed as part of the California statewide arbovirus surveillance program (Reisen et al. 1993) and was modified in 1992 for the use of filter paper strips to collect blood samples (Reisen et al. 1994). An ELISA (Olsen et al. 1991) and a rapid dot immunoassay (Oprandy et al. 1988b) to detect EEE and SLE antibody in sentinel chickens were also developed. Wild bird sera in California were tested for arbovirus antibody by a direct EIA using a multispecies, anti-avian conjugate (Chiles and Reisen 1998). A recently developed indirect IgG ELISA is being used to test wild and captive bird sera for WN virus antibody in New York and other locations (Ebel et al. 2002). An epitope-blocking ELISA has been used as a WN virus-specific antibody test for wild bird studies (Ringia et al. 2004). If other flaviviruses may be present, an epitope-blocking ELISA using a flavivirus-specific monoclonal antibody (6B6C-1) can be used to screen sera for flavivirus antibody (for example, both WN and SLE viruses) followed by the epitope-blocking ELISA with the WN virus-specific monoclonal antibody (3.1112G) to test only the flavivirus antibody positives (Root et al. 2005). The plaque-reduction neutralization test (PRNT) is the standard test for confirmation of virus-specific antibodies (Calisher et al. 1989) and is used for regular testing of avian sera in some laboratories (Komar et al. 2001a), but some cross-reactivity still occurs with closely related viruses. Typically, Nt antibody titers to WN virus are fourfold higher than to the other flaviviruses, but for some blood samples, differences cannot be demonstrated and they are designated as flavivirus-antibody positive only. The PRNT is also used to confirm positive sera detected in the IgG ELISA and in the epitope-blocking ELISA for detection of flavivirus antibody and sometimes in combination. A serial virus neutralization test using a LD_{50} in intra-cranially inoculated baby mice has been used to identify virus-specific antibody (Beaty et al. 1989).

The laboratory tests on dead or sacrificed animals are virus isolation from tissues similar to tests on serum described above and the detection of antigen in tissues. The methodology used for testing birds for WN virus infections is described as an example because avian mortality from arboviruses is most pronounced with this virus and the antigen detection tests developed for WN virus in North America are the most recent. For directly testing tissues, the FA test with flavivirus monoclonal antibody for screening tissues or with WN virus-specific monoclonal antibody for virus identification can be used on frozen sections or fixed tissues. Immunohistochemistry (IHC) of formalin-fixed tissues was used to identify WN virus in tissues of positive birds and to describe tissue tropism (Steele et al. 2000). The IHC was further used by a number of state laboratories to test birds for surveillance, realizing that this test using polyclonal antibody was only a preliminary screening test to distinguish flaviviruses and that a confirmation test was needed. However, the IHC could be used in laboratories not certified as Biosafety level 3, which was required for working with live WN virus. An in situ hybridization probe (pWNV-E) was used to identify WN virus from other related viruses (Steele et al. 2000). A standard reverse transcription-polymerase chain reaction (RT-PCR) and a real-time RT-PCR (TaqMan) are used to test RNA extracted from animal tissues for detection of WN viral antigen (Lanciotti et al. 2000) during routine WN virus surveillance. In New York State in 2000, tissues from dead birds were initially tested by TaqMan RT-PCR with a primer-probe set (Bernard et al. 2001). To confirm the results, a second TaqMan primer-probe set was used along with the standard RT-PCR. Virus isolation in cell culture and virus identification by the FA test with WN virus-specific monoclonal antibody was also used for confirmation. WN virus infection was confirmed as positive by at least two of the different test results. High throughput RNA detection systems were added to increase the volume of WN virus testing (Shi et al. 2001). In testing suspect dead birds, brain, heart, kidney, or spleen were the tissues consistently found positive by multiple procedures (IHC, VI, RT-PCR) (Steele et al. 2000; Kramer and Bernard 2001).

Testing oral (nasopharyngeal) swabs from carcasses of dead crows and Blue Jays for WN virus infection has been suggested to replace necropsy and tissue removal for virus testing because virus can be detected in oral and cloacal swabs taken from these species (Komar et al. 2002). A rapid field diagnostic test using dipstick technology (VecTest™) was recently developed and approved for testing mosquitoes for arboviruses and identifying WN, SLE, and other viruses separately or in combination (Ryan et al. 2003). The VecTest™ has also been used as a rapid, field test for detecting virus in oral and cloacal swabs from selected avian species, mostly in species of corvids (Komar et al. 2002; Lindsay et al. 2003). This test has the specificity of the RT-PCR but is a little less sensitive. Test sensitivity is likely related to the titre of virus in secretions. It was highly sensitive for detecting WNV antigen in oral and cloacal secretions from northern North American owl species dead of WNV but had low sensitivity for southern North American owl species and raptors, likely due to different species' susceptibility patterns to WNV and viral shedding (Gancz et al. 2004). Both of these tests can detect dead or inactive viruses (Nasci et al. 2001b), which is advantageous in extending the detection period but disadvantageeous in knowing whether an active infection occurred or in isolating a virus for confirmation and further studies. The type and combination of laboratory tests used by different laboratories are dependent upon the objectives of the testing, the types of specimens received, the sensitivity and specificity needed, and the rapidity of results required. Laboratory resources, training, and availability of reagents may limit the types of laboratory tests used.

IMMUNITY

Although many arboviruses are quite distinct and the pathogenesis varies with the virus and host species, the immune responses of birds to arboviruses are similar. A general description will be given and more detailed information can be obtained from a number of sources (Beaty et al. 1989; Thomas 1993; Brinton 2001; Szomolanyi-Tsuda et al. 2002). Nonspecific immune mechanisms (interferon, macrophages, and natural killer cells) respond rapidly to a viral infection, often controlling it, but also activate the specific immune response. The virus-specific humoral and cellular immune responses are usually effective in combating viral infections by restricting the spread of the virus. Humoral antibody is produced in response to a viral infection. The first class of immunoglobulin produced immediately after infection is IgM antibody, which contains both Nt and HI antibodies (Beaty et al. 1989). The IgG class of antibody is produced several days after IgM and also contains both HI and Nt antibodies. Generally IgM antibody is short lived in avian species for most arboviruses, although the duration of IgM antibody appears to be longer in WN virus–infected birds (Johnson et al. 2003). However, IgG antibody persists much longer, usually for the life of the bird. The detection of circulating IgG antibody may decline over time, but because of immune memory of antibody, birds respond to a second viral exposure with a rapid and extensive anamnestic antibody response to the same virus (McLean et al. 1983) and to a lesser extent to exposures to closely related viruses. The anamnestic response prevents clinical signs in vertebrate hosts and limits the titer of secondary viremias because secondary humoral antibody increases rapidly (Tesh et al. 2002). Vaccines produce humoral antibodies and immune memory and are effective in the same way by protecting animals from natural exposure to viruses.

SURVEILLANCE

Most arboviruses for which birds are the primary vertebrate hosts and mosquitoes are the principal vectors are transmitted seasonally. Bird populations experience seasonal variation in and amplification of virus infections because of seasonal changes in abundance of both mosquitoes and birds in specific locations or habitats. The mosquito species that sustain and amplify transmission among birds may also be the source of virus for mammalian hosts subsequently, and in some locations; other mosquito species serve as bridging vectors to move the virus from a primary bird-mosquito transmission cycle to secondary hosts. The local amplification in transmission among birds usually precedes transmission to secondary hosts that develop clinical disease, such as humans and equines. Public health and animal health programs utilize this fact to establish active surveillance of free-ranging birds or captive sentinel birds to provide early warning of impending risk to human and/or domestic animal populations (Bowen and Francy 1980; McLean et al. 1983; McLean 1991; Moore et al. 1993).

The type, extent, and frequency of surveillance depend upon the objectives and resources available. The characteristics of avian hosts that make them useful sentinels to detect, monitor, and track arbovirus transmission in surveillance programs are listed in Table 2.2, but also include ease of capture and handling and the fact that they should reflect the virus activity in the surveillance area (McLean 1991). Avian species useful for local surveillance programs will vary depending upon the geographical location, local habitats, avian characteristics influencing interactions with local vector species, local abundance and distribution, local vector competence for the virus, and possibly the virulence of local virus strains (Bowen et al. 1980). An avian species may be suitable in one location and setting but not in another. For example, House Sparrows were the best sentinel species in several Texas cities (Holden et al. 1973a; Lord et al. 1974b) and Memphis, Tennessee (McLean et al. 1983), but not in Chicago, Illinois (McLean and Bowen 1980). A local survey can determine the avian species most frequently exposed to the arbovirus of concern and which species are the most suitable to serve as sentinels. For example, serologic testing of sentinel bird species for WN virus antibody in association with a small human epidemic in 2000 on Staten Island, New York, identified captive pigeons and several wild passerine bird species as possible candidates for use in active WN virus surveillance programs (Komar 2001).

Periodic sampling of free-ranging or captive sentinel birds can be used effectively, separately or in combination with other surveillance methods depending on the specific arbovirus, situation, objectives, resources, and the training and experience of the technical staff conducting the program. Studies have shown that the seasonal rise in antibody prevalence in both free-ranging birds and captive sentinels occurs in association with but usually prior to human cases of arboviruses and thus can serve as an early warning of impending human risk (Bowen and Francy 1980; McLean et al. 1983; Smith et al. 1983). In the U.S.A., sentinel chickens have been used extensively and successfully for years in California, Florida, and other states; free-ranging house sparrows together with captive chickens are used in Memphis, Tennessee (McLean et al. 1983); and free-ranging birds in Los Angeles (Gruwell et al. 2000). Some surveillance programs utilize the collection and testing of vector mosquito species alone or in combination with avian surveillance to monitor virus activity and predict human health risk. Recently, surveillance for SLE and WEE viruses in California utilized three methods simultaneously during 1996–1998 (virus isolations from vector mosquito species, seroconversions in sentinel chickens, and seroprevalence in wild birds) to regularly monitor virus activity in three regions of the state (Reisen et al. 2000). This study found that sentinel chickens were the most sensitive indicator of arbovirus activity in California. Marking with leg bands and serial sampling of free-ranging birds can be an effective method for locally monitoring arboviruses and for understanding the epidemiology, as demonstrated during a SLE virus surveillance program in Los Angeles (Gruwell et al. 2000). Experimental studies found that older chickens appear to be suitable as captive sentinels for WN virus surveillance because they become readily infected but produce viremias too low to infect mosquitoes.

Surveillance programs designed and implemented to monitor WN virus introduced into the U.S.A. in 1999 followed traditional methods except for the collection and testing of dead, free-ranging birds, particularly crows and jays (CDC 2001b). This virulent strain of WN virus caused significant mortality in some North American birds (Eidson et al. 2001a). The mortality was used to develop a dead bird surveillance program to detect the presence and distribution of the virus as it expanded from the original introduction site in New York City to 48 states by the fall of 2004. The use of dead birds for public health surveillance of mosquito-borne avian viruses was a new and unique method for WN virus because other avian viruses of public health importance in North America, such as SLE, EEE, and WEE viruses, do not produce significant bird mortality in native species and thus other less effective surveillance methods are utilized for these viruses (Moore et al. 1993). Through public education and communication efforts, sick and dead birds were observed and reported by the public to local public health and wildlife personnel, who collected the birds for virus testing. Tissues from these birds were tested for WN virus by state public health and federal laboratories. Positive dead birds, particularly crows, became an early warning system for increased risk of WN virus transmission (Eidson, et al. 2001b) and predicted human cases in 2002 (Guptill et al. 2003). The testing results on dead birds were summarized for each county in every cooperating state and when combined with the results from sentinel bird, mosquito, equine, and human surveillance became the nationwide surveillance program starting in 2000 (CDC 2000b). The county surveillance data were accumulated by each state and reported weekly to a national database, ArboNET, developed and implemented by the Centers for Disease Control and Prevention (Marfin et al. 2001). This database was part of the cooperative WN surveillance system designed to provide an early warning system to detect the appearance and seasonal reappearance of the virus in a location, to provide weekly information on the geographical and temporal spread of the virus, to identify areas of increased human risk, and to develop strategies to prevent or minimize infections in humans or domestic animals. The U.S. Geological Survey regularly prepared national maps to display the weekly updated surveillance data, and the maps can be found at the following Web site: http://cindi.usgs.gov/hazard/event/west_nile/west_nile. html. The national surveillance system has continued and expanded with minor modifications during the last six years and now includes all states.

Canada prepared for the potential invasion of West Nile virus and developed a WNV surveillance plan similar to the approach in the U.S.A., and implemented an animal, human, and mosquito surveillance program. Dead-bird surveillance concentrated on corvid testing. The virus was first detected in Ontario, Canada, in 2001 and during the next four years, WNV activity expanded in both directions to seven of 10 provinces from Nova Scotia on the Atlantic coast to Alberta in the west (Health Canada 2005. West Nile Virus Surveilance Information Web site: www.phacaspc.gc.ca/wnv-vwn/index.html).

The particular method or combination of methods selected for arbovirus surveillance need to be tested, modified to meet local needs and resources, and verified for sensitivity and specificity before being fully implemented. Newly developed rapid and specific tests allow for quick assessment of arbovirus activity to provide timely information on public health risk and for the immediate determination of the need to initiate appropriate prevention and control measures.

WILDLIFE POPULATION IMPACTS

Avian mortality from infection with arboviruses occurs with only a few of the viruses and generally causes limited mortality with little impact on natural populations of birds. As explained in the etiology description of viruses above, some viruses such as EEE and WEE cause mortality in very specific exotic avian species, particularly in captive game birds or domestic flocks, or in some highly susceptible species such as the Whooping Crane with EEE virus. Some viruses such as EEE cause sporadic mortality in low numbers for some native species, and LI virus causes more intense mortality in certain locations in several grouse species. However, the NY99 strain of WN virus in North America is the exception because it has affected nearly 300 avian species, causing severe mortality in many corvid species. High mortality rates from WN virus have been reported in some corvid and raptor species throughout the U.S.A. and Canada as well as specific die-offs in Greater Sage Grouse (Centrocercus urophasianus) and American White Pelicans (Pelecanus erythrorhynchus), but the impacts on wild bird populations are poorly documented.

An impact of WN virus on local populations of birds was observed in some localities such as the NYC area, but no significant declines have been detected yet by the regional population trend data. Local American crow populations suffered estimated mortality rates from the virus at 43% of 216 birds observed in three different states in 2002. The highest mortality was documented in central Illinois, where 68% of 28 radio-tagged crows died from confirmed WN virus infection during the summer transmission season (Yaremych et al. 2003). Crow mortality from WN virus infection in a local New York crow population was 37% of 68 birds (McGowan et al. 2003). Estimated mortality in an Oklahoma study population was observed at about 40% of 120 crows in 2002 (Caffrey et al. 2003) and 65% of 78 crows in this population in 2003 (Caffrey et al. 2005).

There were 11 die-offs of American White Pelicans from WN virus of 10 to 2,864 birds each for a total of 9,322 birds documented at wildlife refuges in seven states in the north central U.S.A. during 2002–2003 (Rocke et al. 2005). A large die-off with approximately 95% mortality was observed among the 10,000+ nestlings at a breeding colony in North Dakota in 2003. Only the carcasses submitted and tested toward the end of the mortality event were confirmed as WN virus positive. The apparent high susceptibility of juvenile American White Pelicans to WN virus and the cause of this susceptibility remain to be determined; however, the potential impact of WN virus on future pelican populations must be considered. Some mortality of Greater Sage-Grouse, a declining and threatened species in western North America, was caused by WN virus in free-ranging populations in Montana, Wyoming, and Alberta, Canada, in 2003 (Naugle et al. 2004). Of 22 radio-marked females from four study sites that could be tested, 18 (82%) died from WN virus infection. In addition, serum collected from 112 Greater Sage-Grouse from those areas after the outbreaks were all antibody negative, suggesting a low survival rate following WN virus infection. Experimental studies confirmed the high susceptibility and mortality in Greater Sage-Grouse from WN virus infection; 100% mortality occurred in second-year birds with a 3.7 day mean survival time (Clark et al. unpubl. data).

Information on the impact of WN virus on bird populations is meager because the spatial distribution and intensity of outbreaks of WN virus in birds have not been fully quantified and the cause of many outbreaks have been suspected but not confirmed to be WN virus. The population data from the national monitoring bird surveys and surveillance data on bird mortality from WN virus are too imprecise to detect direct impacts but may be useful for long-term trends in declines associated with WN virus. Analyses of data from two separate winter bird monitoring surveys, Christmas bird counts and project feeder watch, have been conducted to examine potential impacts of WN virus on populations of birds (Caffrey and Peterson 2003a; Bonter and Hochachka 2003). The only notable or suggested declines documented were local and patchy declines for American crows and several other species. Local populations of American crows in the New York City area continued to decline by as much as 90% following the 1999–2000 WN virus outbreaks (Chu et al. 2003). Detailed and precise field studies are needed to measure actual effects of WN virus on local and regional populations to determine real mortality rates and effects on populations.

PREVENTION AND CONTROL

Because there is no treatment for virus infections in individual birds, prevention and control is the only solution to protect birds. Effective prevention and control of arbovirus epizootics and epidemics can best be accomplished with an integrated approach to target the most vulnerable components of the transmission cycles (Moore et al. 1993; CDC 2000b). Most control efforts have concentrated on reducing vector populations because vectors represent local virus transmission, are easier to locate and target, are susceptible to a variety of chemicals or agents, occur in greater abundance around human population centers where the risk of epidemic disease is highest, and have little appeal to or sympathy from the public. Frequently, long-term and short-term vector control programs have been used with varying success. Long-term mosquito control programs are designed to limit the breeding of mosquitoes through source reduction and treatment of breeding sites to kill the larval stage. Habitat management of wetland areas, draining and removal of breeding sites and containers (used tires, buckets, cans, and so on) in urban/suburban areas and residential yards, and application of biological and chemical products, all targeted at the larval stages of mosquitoes, have been successful in reducing local production of adult mosquitoes that feed on vertebrate hosts. These mosquito-control efforts can reduce and minimize virus transmission in an area if done early in the transmission season and if conducted thoroughly and appropriately, but will not eliminate transmission, particularly among wild birds. However, the reduced amount of transmission can modify the risk to associated human and domestic animal populations. The most effective long-term management of mosquito populations is through an integrated pest management program that includes source reduction of breeding sites, providing a community water system (to avoid local storage of water in containers), maintaining sewage waste systems, managing irrigation systems in good working condition, implementing public education for personal protection from biting mosquitoes, and conducting insecticide treatments for larval and adult mosquito control when necessary. Occasionally, short-term control of adult mosquitoes using ground or aerial application of ultra-low volume insecticides may be needed to stop a developing epidemic or reduce the risk of an impending epidemic by killing as many as possible of the virus-infected adult mosquitoes that could transmit virus to humans.

Personal protection measures are the most effective in preventing direct contact with vectors such as culicoid midges, phlebotomine flies, ticks, and also mosquitoes (CDC 2000b; see Web site at www.cdc.gov/ncidod/dvbid/westnile/index.htm). Some of the useful methods to prevent or reduce virus transmission by vectors are the following: installing screens on doors and windows and/or bed netting to prevent contact with flying insects; wearing clothes with long pants and long sleeves to reduce vector contact (including impregnating clothes with repellants); using repellants on exposed body parts when active in areas with elevated vector populations; checking for and removing ticks immediately upon returning from tick-infested sites; and reducing outdoor activities during the early evening hours when vector mosquito species are most active. Educating the public about source reduction around their residences and how to reduce their risks of exposure to vectors through the use of personal protection activities and measures will improve the success of the program.

Population control or management of the avian host populations that support arbovirus transmission would appear to be an effective method of controlling disease transmission and preventing epidemics. In reality, bird control would be an ineffective method in preventing human disease except for the long-term management of peridomestic species in urban environments, and would be impractical and unpopular in most circumstances. The long-term population management of urban bird species (peridomestic species) such as House Sparrows, pigeons, and possibly Canada Geese (*Branta canadensis*) in the U.S.A. could be accomplished through habitat modification to reduce nesting sites, elimination of food sources, and egg destruction or treatment (to make eggs nonviable) for nesting geese. To be effective, these control efforts must be community wide, intense, and sustainable. Few cities have even attempted any comprehensive and integrated control programs. Most other avian host species for the arboviruses, except colonial roosting species such as crows, gulls, blackbirds, and starlings, would be difficult and impractical to control. The colonial species congregate in large roosting flocks, particularly during the winter months, and have been controlled locally with chemical compounds (Boyd and Hall 1987; Seamans and Belant 1999). However, because local populations of these species are able to rebound quickly by influx of birds from surrounding areas and through reproduction, control is only temporary. Control of avian hosts in environments other than in urban settings or in bird congregation sites would be difficult, ineffective, and generally unacceptable to the public. The long-term environmental management of the habitats supporting peridomestic bird species could lower the intensity of urban transmission of arboviruses and thus diminish but not eliminate the risk of human disease. Emergency, short-term control of birds to reduce or stop a human epidemic would also not be effective because it would occur after the peak in the epizootic in the bird populations was detected and most likely after the peak in the human epidemic. Multiple human cases are usually not recognized early in the course of epidemics, and bird control could actually increase the risk of human disease. Infected adult mosquitoes would feed more frequently on humans if fewer birds were available as blood sources. Mosquito control is a more effective and practical method and thus the best alternative.

The use of vaccines to prevent infections and prevent, minimize, or control epizootics has a long history of use with some of the bird-associated arboviruses that affect domestic animals (Monath 1988). Equine vaccines against VEE, EEE, and WEE viruses (including a trivalent vaccine for all three) are available, and all of these vaccines, except VEE vaccine produced in Central and South America, are killed-virus vaccines that require annual boosters to remain effective. A killed, whole WN virus vaccine and a recombinant canarypox WN virus vaccine have been licensed and are available in the U.S.A. (USDA 2005) and new WN virus vaccines for equines are under development. An experimental DNA WN virus vaccine showed some success in protecting birds against WN virus challenge (Turell et al. 2003). The killed, WN virus vaccine has also been used (legally off label) in the U.S.A. in an effort to protect valuable birds in zoological collections from infection and mortality. An attenuated, commercial vaccine derived from Israel Turkey Meningoencephalitis virus was used to immunize domestic geese to protect them from WN virus, but protection was limited to 39–72% under field conditions. Subsequently, an attenuated WN virus variant has been used successfully to protect geese against a wild-type field isolate of WN virus in Israel (Lustig et al. 2000). Heterologous flavivirus vaccines were protective against fatal WN virus infections in an animal model (Tesh et al. 2002). Human vaccines to protect high-risk groups such as the elderly against WN virus infection are under development (Monath 2001). Vaccines are also available to protect the human population against JE virus in Japan, China, and other southeast Asian countries as well as for visitors to those countries (Monath 2002).

MANAGEMENT IMPLICATIONS

The impact of arbovirus infections on bird species and populations is generally minimal and causes little long-term effect, thus requiring no management needs, with a few exceptions. The primary and major exception is WN virus, but EEE and WEE viruses cause mortality in captive-reared exotic bird species such as emus, Ring-necked Pheasants, and other game bird species. Management of these problems can generally be achieved by integrated pest management of mosquito populations in the immediate vicinity of the rearing facilities, but more specifically through the use of virus vaccines and improved husbandry practices. The management of the impact of WN virus on captive domestic and wild birds can also be achieved by local mosquito control and mosquito-proof caging for valuable birds, and eventually with the use of effective vaccines. The effects of WN virus on populations of free-ranging

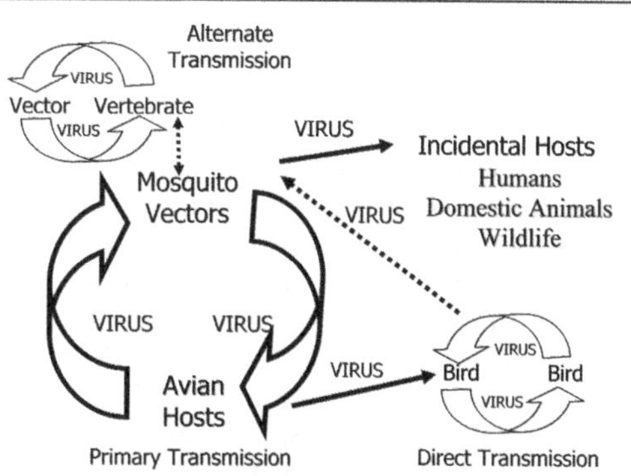

Figure 2.4. Routes of transmission for West Nile virus in North America.

birds are extensive, and management will be very difficult. The various routes of transmission for WN virus present additional complexities and challenges (Figure 2.4). Certainly area mosquito control programs can reduce the intensity of virus transmission among birds in certain locations and reduce mortality somewhat in those susceptible species, but these control programs will be limited and implemented only in urban/suburban environments. Specific management schemes for species at high risk, such as the Greater Sage Grouse, can be designed to protect local populations through habitat modifications of high risk sites, mosquito larval control at small isolated water sources within grouse habitats, and capture and hand vaccination if necessary. Vaccines for use in wild bird species are being tested, and new vaccines and delivery methods can be developed if resources become available.

UNPUBLISHED DATA

Larry Clarke, National Wildlife Reserach Center, WS/APHIS/USDA, Fort Collins, CO, U.S.A.

LITERATURE CITED

Abbassy, M.M., M. Osman, and A.S. Marzouk. 1993. West Nile virus (Flaviviridae: *Flavivirus*) in experimentally infected Argas ticks *(Acari: Argasidae). The American Journal of Tropical Medicine and Hygiene* 48:726–737.

Acha, P.N., and B. Szyfres. 1987. *Zoonoses and communicable diseases common to man and animals.* Pan American Health Organization, Washington D.C., U.S.A., p. 963.

Akov, Y., and R. Goldwasser. 1966. Prevalence of antibodies to arboviruses in various animals in Israel. *Bulletin of the World Health Organization* 34:901–909.

Andreadis, T.G., J.F. Anderson, and S.J. Tirrell-Peck. 1998. Multiple isolations of eastern equine encephalitis and highlands J viruses from mosquitoes (Diptera:

Culicidae) during a 1996 epizootic in southeastern Connecticut. *Journal of Medical Entomology* 35: 296–302.

Barnard, B.J.H., S.B. Buys, J.H. Du-Preez, S.P. Geyling, and H.J. Venter. 1980. Turkey meningoencephalitis in South Africa. *Onderstepoort Journal of Veterinary Research* 47:89–94.

Beaty B.J., C.H. Calisher, and R.E. Shope. 1989. Arbovirus. In *Diagnostic procedures for viral, reckettsial and chlamydial infections,* 6th Ed., N.H. Schmidt, and R.W. Emmons (eds.). American Public Health Association, Washington D.C., U.S.A., p. 797–856.

Bernard, K.A., J.G. Maffei, S.A. Jones, E.G. Kauffman, G.D. Ebel, A.P. Dupuis II, K.A. Ngo, D.C. Nicholas, D.M Young, P-Y Shi, V.L. Kulasekera, M. Eidson, D.J. White, W.B. Stone, NY State West Nile Virus Surveillance Team, and L.D. Kramer. 2001. West Nile Virus Infection in Birds and Mosquitoes, New York State, 2000. *Emerging Infectious Diseases* 7:679–685.

Bertelsen, M.F., R.A. Olberg, G.J. Crawshaw, A. Dibernardo, L.R. Lindsay, M. Drebot, and I.K. Barker. 2004. West Nile virus infection in the eastern loggerhead shrike (*Lanius ludovicianus migrans*): pathology, epidemiology, and immunization. *Journal of Wildlife Diseases* 40:538–542.

Bigler, W.J., and R.G. McLean. 1973. Wildlife as sentinels for Venezuelan equine encephalomyelitis. *Journal of the American Veterinary Medical Association* 163:657–661.

Bigler, W.J., E. Lassing, E. Buff, C. Prather, E.C. Beck, and G.L. Hoff. 1976. Endemic eastern equine encephalomyelitis in Florida: A twenty-year analysis, 1955–1974. *The American Journal of Tropical Medicine and Hygiene* 25:884–890.

Bin, H., Z. Grossman, S. Pokamunski, M. Malkinson, L. Weiss, P. Duvdevani, C. Banet, Y. Weisman, E. Annis, D. Gandaku, V. Yahalom, M. Hindyieh, L. Shulman, and E. Mendelson. 2001. West Nile fever in Israel 1999–2000: from geese to humans. In *West Nile Virus: Detection, Surveillance, and Control. Annals of New York Academy Sciences* 951:127–142.

Blackmore, C.G.M., L.M. Stark, W.C. Jeter, R.L. Oliveri, R.G. Brooks, L.A. Conti, and S.T. Wiersma. 2003. Surveillance results from the first West Nile virus transmission season in Florida, 2001. *The American Journal of Tropical Medicine and Hygiene* 69:141–150.

Blitvich, B.J., I. Fernandez-Salas, J.F.Contreras-Cordero, N.L. Marlenee, J.I. Gonzalez-Rojas, N. Komar, D.J. Gubler, C.H. Calisher, and B.J. Beaty. 2003a. Serologic evidence of West Nile virus infection in horses, Coahuila State, Mexico. *Emerging Infectious Diseases* 9:853–856.

Blitvich, B.J., N.L. Marlenee, R.A. Hall, C.H. Calisher, R.A. Bowen, J.T. Roehrig, N. Komar, S.A. Langevin, and B.J. Beaty. 2003b. Epitope-blocking enzyme-linked immunosorbent assays for the detection of serum antibodies to West Nile virus in multiple avian species. *Journal of Clinical Microbiology* 41:1041–1047.

Bonter, D.N., and W.M. Hochachka. 2003. Declines of chickadees and corvids: possible impacts of West Nile virus. *American Birds* p. 22–25.

Bowen, G.S. 1977. Prolonged western equine encephalitis viremia in the Texas tortoise (*Gopherus berlandieri*). *The American Journal of Tropical Medicine and Hygiene* 26:171–175.

Bowen, G.S., and R.G. McLean. 1977. Experimental infection of birds with epidemic Venezuelan encephalitis virus. *The American Journal of Tropical Medicine and Hygiene* 26:808–814.

Bowen, G.S., and D.B. Francy. 1980. Surveillance. In *St. Louis Encephalitis,* T.P. Monath (ed.). American Public Health Association, Washington D.C., p. 473–499.

Bowen, G.S., T.P. Monath, G. E. Kemp, J.H. Kerschner, and L.J. Kirk. 1980. Geographic variation among St. Louis encephalitis virus strains in the viremic responses of avian hosts. *The American Journal of Tropical Medicine and Hygiene* 29:1411–1419.

Boyd, F.L., and D.I. Hall. 1987. Use of DRC-1339 to control crows in three roosts in Kentucky and Arkansas. *Proceedings of Eastern Wildlife Damage Control Conference* 3:3–7.

Boyd, K.R. 1972. Serological comparisons among Hart Park virus and strains of Flanders virus. *Infection and Immunity* 5:933–937.

Boyle, D.B., R.W. Dickerman, and I.D. Marshall. 1983a. Primary viremia responses of herons to experimental infection with Murray Valley encephalitis, Kunjin and Japanese encephalitis viruses. *Australian Journal of Experimental Biology and Medical Science* 61: 655–664.

Boyle, D.B., R.W. Dickerman, and I.D. Marshall. 1983b. Primary antibody responses of herons to experimental infection with Murray Valley encephalitis and Kunjin viruses. *Australian Journal of Experimental Biology and Medical Science* 61:665–674.

Brault, A.C., S.A. Langevin, R.A. Bowen, N.A. Panella, B.J. Biggerstaff, B.R. Miller, and N. Komar. 2004. Differential virulence of West Nile strains for American crows. *Emerging Infectious Diseases* 10:2161–2168.

Braverman, Y., and J. Boorman. 1978. Unsuccessful attempts to infect Culicoides with Israel turkey virus. *Acta Virologica* 22:429.

Brinton, M.A. 2001. Host factors involved in virus replication. West Nile Virus: Detection, Surveillance, and Control. *Annals of New York Academy Sciences* 951: 207–219.

Brinton, M.A. 2002. The molecular biology of West Nile virus: A new invader of the Western Hemisphere. *Annual Review of Microbiology* 56:371–402.

Buescher, E.L., W.F. Scherer, H.E. McClure, J.T. Rosenberg, M. Yoshii, and Y. Okada. 1959. Ecologic studies of Japanese encephalitis virus in Japan. IV. Avian infection. *The American Journal of Tropical Medicine and Hygiene* 8:678–688.

Burke, D.S., and C.J. Leake. 1988. Japanese encephalitis. In *The arboviruses: Epidemiology and Ecology.* Vol. III, T.P. Monath (ed.). CRC Press, Inc. Boca Raton, FL, U.S.A., pp. 63–92.

Caffrey, C., and C.C. Peterson. 2003a. West Nile virus may not be a conservation issue in northeastern United States. *American Birds,* pp. 14–21.

Caffrey, C., T.J. Weston, and S. C. R. Smith. 2003b. High mortality among marked crows subsequent to the arrival of West Nile virus. *Wildlife Society Bulletin* 31:870–872.

Caffrey, C., S.C.R. Smith, and T.J. Weston. 2005. West Nile virus devastates an American crow population. *The Condor* 107:128–132.

Calisher, C.H., R.H. Kokernot, J.G. DeMoore, K.R. Boyd, J. Hayes, and W.A. Chappell. 1969. Arbovirus studies in the Ohio-Mississippi Basin, 1964–1967. VI. Mermet: A Simbu-group Arbovirus. *The American Journal of Tropical Medicine and Hygiene* 18:779–788.

Calisher, C.H., K.S.C. Maness, R.D. Lord, and P.H. Coleman. 1971. Identification of two South American strains of eastern equine encephalomyelitis virus from migrant birds captured on the Mississippi Delta. *American Journal of Epidemiology* 94: 172–178.

Calisher, C.H., E. Gutierrez, K.S.C. Maness, and R.D. Lord. 1974. Isolation of Mayaro virus from a migrating bird captured in Louisiana in 1967. *Bulletin of the Pan American Health Organization* 7:243–248.

Calisher, C.H., and K.S. Maness. 1975. Laboratory studies of Venezuelan equine encephalitis in equines, Texas, 1971. *Journal of Clinical Microbiology* 2:198–205.

Calisher, C.H., E. Levy-Koening, C.J. Mitchell, F.A. Cabrera, L. Cuevas, and J.E. Pearson. 1979. Eastern equine encephalitis in the Dominican Republic. 1978. *Bulletin of the Pan American Health Organization* 13:380–390.

Calisher, C.H., R.E. Shope, W. Brandt, J. Casals, N. Karabatsos, F.A. Murphy, R.G. Tesh, and M.E. Wiebe. 1980a. Proposed antigenic classification of registered arboviruses. I. Togaviridae, Alphavirus. *Intervirology* 14:229–232.

Calisher, C.H., T.P. Monath, D.J. Muth, J.S. Lazuick, D.W. Trent, D.B. Francy, G.E. Kemp, and F.W. Chandler. 1980b. Characterization of Fort Morgan virus, an Alphavirus of the western equine encephalitis virus complex in an unusual ecosystem. *The American Journal of Tropical Medicine and Hygiene* 29: 1428–1440.

Calisher, C.H., S.J. Ahmann, P.R. Grimstad, J.G. Hamm, and M.A. Parsons. 1981. Distribution and prevalence of Mermet virus infections in the central United States. *The American Journal of Tropical Medicine and Hygiene* 30:473–476.

Calisher, C.H., J.S. Lazuick, K.L. Wolff, and D.J. Muth. 1984. Antigenic relationships among Turlock serogroup Bunyaviruses as determined by neutralization tests. *Acta Virologica* 28:148–151.

Calisher, C.H., H.N. Fremount, W.L. Veseley, A.O. el-Kafrawi, and M.I. Mahmud. 1986. Relevance of detection of immunoglobulin M antibody response in birds used for arbovirus surveillance. *Journal of Clinical Microbiology* 24:770–774.

Calisher, C.H., T.G. Schwan, J.S. Lazuick, R.B. Eads, and D. B. Francy. 1988. Isolation of Mono Lake virus (Family Reoviridae, Genus *Orbivirus,* Kemerovo serogroup) from *Argas cooleyi* (Acari: Argasidae) collected in Colorado. *Journal of Medical Entomology* 25:388–390.

Calisher, C.H., and N. Karabatsos. 1988. Arbovirus serogroups: definition and geographic distribution. In *The arboviruses: epidemiology and ecology,* Vol. I, T.P. Monath (ed.). CRC Press, Inc. Boca Rotan, FL, U.S.A., pp. 19–57.

Calisher, C.H., N. Karabatsos, J.M. Dalrymple, R.E. Shope, J.S. Porterfield, E.G. Westaway, and W. E. Brandt. 1989. Antigenic relationships between flaviviruses as determined by cross-neutralization tests with polyclonal antisera. *Journal of General Virology* 70:37–43.

Calisher, C.H., R.G. McLean, H.G. Zeller, D.B. Francy, N. Karabatsos, and R.A. Bowen. 1990. Isolation of the Tete serogroup Bunyaviruses from Ceratopogonidae collected in Colorado. *The American Journal of Tropical Medicine and Hygiene* 43:319–318.

Campbell, R. 2003. Summary of West Nile virus activity, U.S.A., 2002. Fourth National Conference on West Nile virus in the United States. Centers for Disease Control and Prevention. [Online.] Retrieved from the World Wide Web: www.cdc.gov/ncidod/dvbid/westnile/conf/index.htm.

CDC, Centers for Disease Control and Prevention. 1998. Arboviral infections of the central nervous system—United States, 1996–1997. *Morbidity and Mortality Weekly Report* 47:517–522.

CDC, Centers for Disease Control and Prevention. 1999. Outbreak of West Nile-like viral encephalitis—New York, 1999. *Morbidity and Mortality Weekly Report* 48:845–849.

CDC, Centers for Disease Control and Prevention. 2000a. West Nile virus activity—New York and New Jersey, 2000. *Morbidity and Mortality Weekly Report* 49:640–642.

CDC, Centers for Disease Control and Prevention. 2000b. Guidelines for surveillance, prevention, and control of West Nile virus infection—United States. *Morbidity and Mortality Weekly Report* 49:25–28.

CDC, Centers for Disease Control and Prevention. 2001a. West Nile virus activity—Eastern United States, 2001. *Morbidity and Mortality Weekly Report* 50:617–619.

CDC, Centers for Disease Control and Prevention. 2001b. Epidemic/epizootic West Nile virus in the United States: Revised guidelines for surveillance, prevention and control. [Online.] Retrieved from the World Wide Web: www.cdc.gov/ncidod/dvbid/westnile/resources/wnv.

CDC, Centers for Disease Control and Prevention. 2002a. West Nile virus activity—United States, 2001. *Morbidity and Mortality Weekly Report* 51:497–501.

CDC, Centers for Disease Control and Prevention. 2002b. West Nile virus activity—United States, August 8–14, 2002, and Louisiana, January 1–August 7, 2002. *Morbidity and Mortality Weekly Report* 51:681–683.

CDC, Centers for Disease Control and Prevention. 2002c. Provisional surveillance summary of the West Nile virus epidemic—United States, January–November 2002. *Morbidity and Mortality Weekly Report* 51:1129–1133.

CDC, Centers for Disease Control and Prevention. 2004. West Nile virus activity—United States, November 9–16, 2004. *Morbidity and Mortality Weekly Report* 53: 1071–1072.

CDC, Centers for Disease Control and Prevention. 2005. Domestic Arboviruses and West Nile Virus. [Online.] Retrieved from the World Wide Web: www.cdc.gov/ncidod/dvbid/index.htm.

Chamberlain, R. W., R.E. Kissling, D.D. Stamm, D.B. Nelson, and R.K. Sikes. 1956. Venezuelan Equine encephalomyelitis in wild birds. *American Journal of Hygiene* 63:261–273.

Chamberlain, R.W. 1980. History of St. Louis Encephalitis. In *St. Louis Encephalitis,* T.P.Monath (ed.). American Public Health Association, Washington D.C., U.S.A., pp. 3–61.

Chiles, R.E., and W.K. Reisen. 1998. A new enzyme immunoassay to detect antibodies to arboviruses in the blood of wild birds. *Journal of Vector Ecology* 23:123–135.

Chu, M., W. Stone, K.J. McGowan, A.A. Dhondt, W.M. Hochachka, and J.E. Therrien. 2003. West Nile file. *Birdscope* (Winter): 10–11.

Clarke, D.H., and J. Casals. 1958. Techniques for hemagglutination and hemagglutination-inhibition with arthropod-borne viruses. *The American Journal of Tropical Medicine and Hygiene* 7:561–573.

Correa-Giron, P., C.H. Calisher, and G. M. Baer. 1970. Epidemic strain of Venezuelan equine encephalomyelitis from a vampire bat captured in Oaxaca, Mexico, 1970. *Science* 175:546–547.

Crans, W.J., D.F. Caccamise, and J.R. McNelly. 1994. Eastern equine encephalomyelitis virus in relation to the avian community of coastal cedar swamp. *Journal of Medical Entomology* 31:711–728.

Dalrymple, J.M., O.P. Young, B. F. Eldridge, and P.K. Russell. 1972. Ecology of arboviruses in a Maryland freshwater swamp. III. Vertebrate hosts. *American Journal of Epidemiology* 96:129–140.

Day, J.F. 1989. The use of sentinel chickens for arbovirus surveillance in Florida. *Journal of Florida Anti-Mosquito Association* 60:56–61.

Day, J.F., and L.M. Stark. 1996. Eastern equine encephalitis transmission to emus in Volusia County, Florida: 1992 through 1994. *Journal of American Mosquito Control Association* 12:429–436.

Day, J.F., and L.M. Stark. 1999. Avian serology in a St. Louis encephalitis epicenter before, during and after a wide-spread epidemic in south Florida, U.S.A. *Journal Medical Entomology* 36:614–624.

Degallier, N., A.P.A. Travassos da Rosa, J.M.C. da Silva, S.G. Rodrigues, P.F.C. Vasconcelos, J.F.S. Travassos da Rosa, G. Pereira da Silva, R. Pereira da Silva. 1992. As aves como hospedeiras de arbovirus na Amazonia Brasileira. *Boletin Museu Paraense Emilio Goeldi, Servicos Zoologicos* 8:69–111.

Dein, F.J., J.W. Carpenter, G.G. Clark, R.J. Montali, C.L. Crabbs, T.F. Tsai, and D.E. Docherty. 1986. Mortality of captive whooping cranes caused by eastern equine encephalitis virus. *Journal of the American Veterinary Medical Association* 189:1006–1010.

Dickerman, R.W., W.F. Scherer, A.S. Moorhouse, E. Toaz, M.E. Essex and R.E. Steel.1972. Ecologic studies of Venezuelan encephalitis virus in southern Mexico. VI. Infection of wild birds. *The American Journal of Tropical Medicine and Hygiene* 21:66–78.

Dickerman, R.W., C.M. Bonacorsa and W.F. 1976. Viremia in young herons and ibis infected with Venezuelan encephalitis virus. *American Journal of Epidemiology* 104:678–683.

Dickerman, R.W., M.S. Martin, and E.A. Dipaola. 1980. Studies on Venezuelan encephalitis in migrating birds in relation to possible transport of virus from South to Central America. *The American Journal of Tropical Medicine and Hygiene* 29:269–276.

Doherty, R.L., B.M. Gorman, R.H. Whitehead, and J. Carley. 1966. Studies of arthropod-borne virus infections in Queensland. V. Survey of antibodies to Group A arboviruses in man and other animals. *Australian Journal of Experimental Biology and Medical Science* 44:365–378.

Dupuis II, A.P., P.P. Marra, and L.D. Kramer. 2003. Serologic evidence of West Nile virus transmission, Jamaica, West Indies. *Emerging Infectious Diseases* 9:860–863.

Ebel, G.D., A.P. Dupuis II, D. Nicholas, D. Young, J. Maffei, and L.D. Kramer. 2002. Detection by enzyme-linked immunosorbent assay of antibodies to West Nile virus in birds. *Emerging Infectious Diseases* 8:979–982.

Endy, T.P., and A. Nisalak. 2002. Japanese encephalitis virus: Ecology and epidemiology. In *Japanese encephalitis and West Nile viruses,* J.S. Mackenzie, A.D.T. Barrett, and V. Deubel (eds.). Springer-Verlag, Berlin, Germany, pp. 11–48.

Eidson, M., N. Komar, F. Sorhage, R. Nelson, T. Talbot, F. Mostashari, R. McLean, and the West Nile Virus Avian Mortality Surveillance Group. 2001a. Crow deaths as a sentinel surveillance system for West Nile virus in the Northeastern United States, 1999. *Emerging Infectious Diseases* 7:615–620.

Eidson, M., L. Kramer, W. Stone, Y. Hagiwara, K. Schmit, and The New York State West Nile Virus Avian Surveillance Team. 2001b. Dead bird surveillance as an early warning system for West Nile virus. *Emerging Infectious Diseases* 7:631–635.

Eleazer, T.H., H.G. Blalock, J.H. Warner Jr., and J.E. Pearson. 1978. Eastern equine encephalomyelitis outbreak in coturnix quail. *Avian Diseases* 22:522–525.

Ernek, E., O. Kozuch, J. Nosek, J. Teplan, and C. Folk. 1977. Arboviruses in birds captured in Slovakia. *Journal of Hygiene, Epidemiology, Microbiology, and Immunology* 21:353–359.

Espmark, A., and B. Kiklasson. 1984. Ockelbo disease in Sweden: epidemiological, clinical, and virological data from the 1982 outbreak. *The American Journal of Tropical Medicine and Hygiene* 33:1203–1211.

Estrada-Franco, J.G., R. Navarro-Lopez, D.W.C. Beasley, L. Coffey, A.S. Carrara, A. Travassos da Rosa, T. Clements, E. Wang, G.V. Ludwig, A.C. Cortes, P.P. Ramirez, R.B. Tesh, A.D.T. Barrett, and S. C. Weaver. 2003. West Nile virus in Mexico: Evidence of widespread circulation since July 2002. *Emerging Infectious Diseases* 9:1604–1607.

Ficken, M.D., D.P. Wages, J.S. Guy, J.A. Quinn, and W.H. Emory. 1993. High mortality of domestic turkeys associated with Highlands J virus and eastern equine encephalitis virus infections. *Avian Diseases* 37:585–590.

Fitzgerald, S.D., J.S. Patterson, M. Kiupel, H.A. Simmons, S.D. Grimes, C.F. Sarver, R.M. Fulton, B.A. Steficek, T.M. Cooley, J.P. Massey, and J.G. Sikarskie. 2003. Clinical and pathologic features of West Nile virus infection in native North American owls (Family *strigidae*). *Avian Diseases,* 47:602–610.

Francy, D.B., T.G. Jaenson, J.O. Lundstrom, E.B. Schildt, A. Espmark, B. Henriksson, and B. Niklasson. 1989. Ecologic studies of mosquitoes and birds as hosts of Ockelbo virus in Sweden and isolation of Inkoo and Batai viruses from mosquitoes. *The American Journal of Tropical Medicine and Hygiene* 41:355–363.

Gancz, A.Y., I.K. Barker, R. Lindsay, A. Dibernardo, K. McKeever, and B. Hunter. 2004. West Nile virus outbreak in North American Owls, Ontario. 2002. *Emerging Infectious Diseases* 10:2135–2142.

Gancz, A.Y., D.G. Campbell, I.K. Barker, R. Lindsay, and B. Hunter. 2004. Detecting West Nile virus in owls and raptors by antigen-capture assay. *Emerging Infectious Diseases* 10:2204–2206.

Gancz, A., I.K. Barker, D. Smith, R. Lindsay, and B. Hunter. 2006. Pathology and tissue distribution of West Nile virus in North American owls (family: Strigidae). *Avian Pathology* (in press, February issue) 35.

Gibbs, S.E., A.E. Ellis, D.G. Mead, A.B. Allison, J.K. Moulton, E. W. Howerth, and D.E. Stallknecht. West Nile virus detection in organs of naturally infected blue jays (*Cyanocitta cristala*). *Journal Wildlife Diseases* 41:354–362.

Gilbert, L., L.D. Jones, P.J. Hudson, E.A. Gould, and H.W. Reid. 2000. Role of small mammals in the persistence of Louping-ill virus: field survey and tick co-feeding studies. *Medical Veterinary Entomology* 14:277–282.

Godsey, M.S., M.S. Blackmore, N.A. Panella, K. Burkhalter, K. Gottfried, L.A. Halsey, R. Rutledge, S.A. Langevin, R. Gates, K.M. Lamonte, A. Lambert, R.S. Lanciotti, C.G.M. Blackmore, T. Loyless, L. Stark, R. Oliveri, L. Conti, and N. Komar. 2005. West Nile virus Epizootiology in the Southeastern United States, 2001. *Vector-Borne and Zoonotic Diseases* 5:82–89.

Gruwell, J. A., C. L. Fogarty, S. G. Bennett, G. L. Challet, K. S. Vanderpool, M. Jozan, and J. P. Webb, Jr. 2000. Role of peridomestic birds in the transmission of St. Louis encephalitis virus in southern California. *Journal of Wildlife Diseases* 36:13–34.

Guptill, S.C., K.G. Julian, G.L. Campbell, S.D. Price, and A.A. Marfin. 2003. Early-season avian deaths from West Nile virus as warnings of human infection. *Emerging Infectious Diseases* 9: 483–484.

Guy, J.S., H.J. Barnes, and L.G. Smith. 1994. Experimental infection of young broiler chickens with eastern equine encephalitis virus and Highlands J virus. *Avian Diseases* 38:572–582.

Haas, R.A., A.H. Jonkers, and D.W. Heinemann. 1966. Kwatta virus, a new agent isolated from *Culex* mosquitoes in Surinam. *The American Journal of Tropical Medicine and Hygiene* 15:954–957.

Hadler, J., R. Nelson, T. McCarthy, T. Andreadis, M.J. Lis, R. French, W. Beckwith, D. Mayo, G. Archambault, and M. Cartter. 2001. West Nile Virus surveillance in Connecticut in 2000: An intense epizootic without high risk for severe human disease. *Emerging Infectious Diseases* 7:636–642.

Hall, R.A., A.K. Broom, A.C. Hartnett, M.J. Howard, and J.S. MacKenzie. 1995. Immunodominant epitopes on the NS1 protein of Murray Valley encephalitis and Kunjin viruses serve as targets for a blocking ELISA to detect virus-specific antibodies in sentinel animal serum. *Journal of Virological Methods* 51:201–210.

Hammon, W. McD., and B. F. Howitt. 1942. Epidemiological aspects of encephalitis in the Yakima Valley, Washington: mixed St. Louis and Western equine types. *American Journal of Hygiene* 35:163–185.

Hammon, W. McD., and W.C. Reeves. 1946. Western equine encephalitis virus in the blood of experimentally inoculated chickens. *Journal of Experimental Medicine* 83:163.

Hammon, W. McD., W.C. Reeves, and G.E. Sather. 1951. Western Equine and St. Louis encephalitis viruses in the blood of experimentally infected wild birds and epidemiological implications of findings. *Journal of Immunology* 67:357–367.

Hanna, J.N., S.A. Ritchie, D.A. Phillips, J. Shield, M.C. Bailey, J.S. Mackenzie, M. Poidinger, B.J. McCall, and P.J. Mills. 1996. An outbreak of Japanese encephalitis in the Torres Strait, Australia, 1995. *Medical Journal of Australia* 165:256–260.

Hanna, J.N., S.A. Ritchie, D.A. Phillips, J. M. Lee, S.L. Hills, A.F. Vandenhurk, A.T. Pyke, C.A. Johansen, and J.S. Mackenzie. 1999. *Medical Journal of Australia* 170:533–536.

Harley, D., A. Sleigh, D. Bossingham, S. Ritchie, and G. Williams. 2001. Ross River virus disease from a north Queensland public health perspective. *Arbovirus Research of Australia* 8:180–185.

Hayes, C.G., S. Baqar, T. Ahmed, M.A. Chowdhry, and W.K. Reisen. 1982. West Nile virus in Pakistan. 1. Sero-epidemiological studies in Punjab Province. *Transactions of the Royal Society of Tropical Medicine and Hygiene* 76:431–436.

Hayes, C.G. 1988. West Nile Fever. In *The Arboviruses: Epidemiology and Ecology,* Vol. V, T.P. Monath (ed.). CRC Press, Inc. Boca Raton, FL, U.S.A., pp. 59–88.

Hayes, N. 2004. Summary of West Nile virus activity, United States 2003. Fifth National Conference on West Nile virus in the United States. Centers for Disease Control and Prevention. [Online.] Retrieved from the World Wide Web: www.cdc.gov/ncidod/dvbid/westnile/conf/index.htm.

Hayes, R.O., D.B. Francy, J.S. Lazuick, G.C. Smith, and R.H. Jones. 1976. Arbovirus surveillance in 6 states during 1972, U.S.A. *The American Journal of Tropical Medicine and Hygiene* 25:463–476.

Hayes, R.O., D.B. Francy, J.S. Lazuick, G.C. Smith, and E.P.J. Gibbs. 1977. Role of the cliff swallow bug (*Oeciacus vicarius*) in the natural cycle of a western equine encephalitis-related alphavirus. *Journal of Medical Entomology* 14:257–262.

Health Canada. 2001. West Nile virus surveillance information. Population and Public Health Branch. [Online.] Retrieved from the World Wide Web: www.hc-sc.gc.ca/pphb-dgspsp/wnv-vwn/index.html.

Health Canada. 2005. West Nile Virus Surveillance Information. [Online.] Retrieved from the World Wide Web: http://www.phac-aspc.gc.ca/wnv-vwn/index.html.

Henderson, J.R., N. Karabatsos, A.T.C. Bourke, R.C. Walis, and R.M. Taylor. 1962. A survey for arthropod-borne viruses in south-central Florida. *The American Journal of Tropical Medicine and Hygiene* 11:800–810.

Herve, J.P., N. Degallier, A.P.A. Travassos da Rosa, F.P. Pinheiros, and G.C. Sa Filho. 1986. Arboviroses: aspectos ecologicos, 409–437. In *Instituto Evandro Chagas, 50 anos de contribuicao as ciencias biologicas e a medecina tropical,* Vol. 1. Ed.Fundacao Servicios de Saude publica, Belem, 529 pp.

Holden, P., R.O. Hayes, C.J. Mitchell, D.B. Francy, J.S. Lazuick, and T.B. Hughes. 1973a. House sparrows, *Passer domesticus* (L.), as hosts of arboviruses in Hale County, Texas. I. Field studies 1965–1969. *The American Journal of Tropical Medicine and Hygiene* 22:244–253.

Holden, P., D.B. Francy, C.J. Mitchell, R.O. Hayes, J.S. Lazuick, and T.B. Hughes. 1973b. House sparrows, *Passer domesticus* (L.), as hosts of arboviruses in Hale County, Texas. II. Laboratory studies with western equine encephalitis virus. *The American Journal of Tropical Medicine and Hygiene* 22:254–262.

Hoogstraal, H. 1972. Birds as tick hosts and as reservoirs and dissemination of tick-borne infectious agents. *Wiad Parazitologia* 18:4–6.

Hubalek, Z., and J. Halouzka. 1996. Arthropod–borne viruses of vertebrates in Europe. *Acta Scientiarum Naturalium Academiae Brno* 30:95.

Hubalek, Z., and J. Halouzka 1999. West Nile Fever—A reemerging mosquito-borne viral disease in Europe. *Emerging Infectious Diseases* 5:643–650.

Iaconescu, M. 1976. Turkey meningoencephalitis: A general review. *Avian Diseases* 20:135–138.

Iversson, L.B. 1989. Rocio Encephalitis. In *The Arboviruses: Epidemiology and Ecology.* Vol. IV, T.P. Monath (ed.). CRC Press, Inc. Boca Raton, FL, U.S.A., pp. 77–92.

Johnson, A.J., S. Langevin, K.L. Wolff, and N. Komar. 2003. Detection of anti-West Nile virus immunoglobulin M in chicken serum by an enzyme-linked immunosorbent assay. *Journal of Clinical Microbiology* 41:2002–2007.

Jozan, M., R. Evans, R. McLean, R. Hall, B. Tangredi, L. Reed, and J. Scott. 2003. Detection of West Nile virus infection in birds in the United States by blocking ELISA and immunohistochemistry. *Vector-borne Zoonotic Diseases* 3:99–110.

Juricova, Z., I. Literak, and J. Pinowski. 2000. Antibodies to arboviruses in house sparrows (*Passer domesticus)* in the Czech Republic. *Acta Veterinaria* 69:213–215.

Karabatsos, N., A.T.C. Bourke, and J.R. Henderson. 1963. Antigenic variation among strains of western equine encephalomyelitis virus. *The American Journal of Tropical Medicine and Hygiene* 12:408–412.

Karabatsos, N., (ed). 1985. *International Catalogue of Arboviruses Including Certain Other Viruses of*

Vertebrates, 4th Ed., American Society of Tropical Medicine and Hygiene, San Antonio, TX, U.S.A., 1147 pp.

Karabatsos, N., A.L. Lewis, C.H. Calisher, A.R. Hunt, and J.T. Roehrig. 1988. Identification of Highland J virus from a Florida horse. *The American Journal of Tropical Medicine and Hygiene* 39:603–606.

Kay, B.H., and J.G. Aaskov. 1989. Ross River virus (epidemic polyarthritis). In *The Arboviruses: Epidemiology and Ecology.* Vol. IV. T.P. Monath (ed.). CRC Press, Inc. Boca Raton, FL, U.S.A., pp. 167–176.

Kissling, R.E., H. Rubin, R.W. Chamberlain, and M.E. Eidson. 1951. Recovery of virus of eastern equine encephalomyelitis from blood of a Purple Grackle. *Proceedings of Society for Experimental Biology and Medicine* 77:398–399.

Kissling, R.E., R. W. Chamberlain, R.K. Sikes, and M.E. Eidson. 1954. Studies on the North American arthropod-borne encephalitides. III. Eastern equine encephalitis in wild birds. *American Journal of Hygiene* 60:251–265.

Kissling, R.E., R.W. Chamberlain, D.B. Nelson, and D.D. Stamm. 1955. Studies on the North American arthropod-borne encephalitides. VIII. Equine Encephalitis studies in Louisiana. *American Journal of Hygiene* 88:233–254.

Kokernot, R.H., J. Hayes, R.L. Will, B. Radivojevic, K.R. Boyd, and D.H.M. Chan. 1969. Arbovirus studies in the Ohio-Mississippi Basin, 1964–1967: III. Flanders virus. *The American Journal of Tropical Medicine and Hygiene* 18:762–767.

Kolman, J.M., C. Folk, K. Hudec, and G.N. Reddy. 1976. Serologic examination of birds from the area in southern Moravia for the presence of antibodies against arboviruses of the groups Alphavirus, Flavivirus, Uukuniemi virus, Turlock virus, and Bunyamwera virus supergroup. Part 2: Wild living birds. *Folia Parasitologica Ceske Budejovice* 23:251–255.

Komar, N. 2001. West Nile virus surveillance using sentinel birds. In *West Nile Virus: Detection, Surveillance, and Control.* Annals of New York Academy Sciences 951:58–73.

Komar, N., N.A. Panella, J.E. Burns, S.W. Dusza, T.M. Mascarenhas, and T.O. Talbot. 2001a. Serologic evidence for West Nile virus infection in birds in the New York City vicinity during an outbreak in 1999. *Emerging Infectious Diseases* 7:621–625.

Komar, N., J. Burns, C. Dean, N.A. Panella, S. Dusza, and B. Cherry. 2001b. Serologic evidence for West Nile virus infection in birds in Staten Island, New York, after an outbreak in 2000. *Vector Borne Zoonotic Diseases* 1:191–196.

Komar, N., R. Lanciotti, R. Bowen, S. Langevin, and M. Bunning. 2002. Detection of West Nile virus in oral and cloacal swabs collected from bird carcasses. *Emerging Infectious Diseases* 8:741–742.

Komar, N., S. Langevin, S. Hinten, N. Nemeth, E. Edwards, D. Hettler, B. Davis, R. Bowen, and M. Bunning. 2003. Experimental infection of North American birds with the New York 1999 strain of West Nile virus. *Emerging Infectious Diseases* 9:311–322.

Komar, O., M.B. Robbines, K. Klenk, B.J. Blitvich, N.L. Marlenee, K.L. Burkhalter, D.J. Gubler, G. Gonzalvez, C.J. Pena, A.T. Peterson, and N. Komar. 2003. West Nile virus transmission in resident birds, Dominican Republic. *Emerging Infectious Diseases* 9:1299–1302.

Kramer, L.D., and K.A. Bernard. 2001. West Nile virus infection in birds and mammals. In *West Nile Virus: Detection, Surveillance, and Control. Annals of New York Academy Sciences* 951:84–93.

Kramer, V. 2005. West Nile virus activity in California in 2004. Sixth National Conference on West Nile virus in the United States. Centers for Disease Control and Prevention. [Online.] Retrieved from the World Wide Web: www.cdc.gov /ncidod/dvbid/westnile/conf/index.htm.

Kulas, K.E., V.L. Demarest, C.S. Franchell, and S.J. Wong. 2001. Use of an arboviral immunofluorescent assay in screening for West Nile virus. In *West Nile Virus: Detection, Surveillance, and Control.* Annals of New York Academy Sciences 951:357–360.

Lanciotti, R.S., J.T. Roehrig, V. Deubel, J. Smith, M. Parker, K. Steele, K.E. Volpe, M.B. Crabtree, J. Scherret, R. Hall, J. Mackenzie, C.B. Cropp, B. Panigraphy, M. Malkinson, N. Komar, H.M Savage, W. Stone, T. McNamara, and D.J. Gubler. 1999. Origin of the West Nile virus responsible for an outbreak of encephalitis in the northeastern United States. *Science* 286: 2333–2337.

Lanciotti, R.S., A.J. Kerst, R.S. Nasci, M.S. Godsey, C.J. Mitchell, H. M. Savage, N. Komar, N.A. Panella, B.C. Allen, K.E. Volpe, B.S. Davis, and J.T. Roehrig. 2000. Rapid detection of West Nile virus from human clinical specimens, field-collected mosquitoes, and avian samples by a TaqMan reverse transcriptase-PCR assay. *Journal of Clinical Microbiology* 38:4066–4071.

Levy, C. 2005. West Nile virus in Arizona. Sixth National Conference on West Nile virus in the United States. Centers for Disease Control and Prevention. [Online.] Retrieved from the World Wide Web: www.cdc.gov/ncidod/dvbid/westnile/conf/index.htm.

Libikova, H., F. Heinz, D. Ujhazyova, and D. Stunzner. 1978. Orbiviruses of the Kemerovo complex and neurological diseases. *Medical Microbiology and Immunology* 116:255–263.

Lindsay, R., I. Barker, G. Nayar, M. Drebot, S. Calvin, C. Scammell, C. Sachvie, T. Scammell-La Fleur, A. Dibernardo, M. Andonova, and H. Artsob. 2003. Rapid antigen-capture assay to detect West Nile virus in dead corvids. *Emerging Infectious Diseases* 9:1406–1410.

Lopes, O.de S., T.L.M. Coimbra, L. de A. Sacchetta, and C.H. Calisher. 1978a. Emergence of a new arbovirus disease in Brazil. I. Isolation and characterization of the etiologic agent, Rocio virus. *American Journal of Epidemiology* 107:444–449.

Lopes, O.de S., L.DE A. Sacchetta, T. L. M. Coimbra, G.H. Pinto and C.M. Glasser. 1978b. Emergence of a new arbovirus disease in Brazil. II. Epidemiologic studies on 1975 epidemic. *American Journal of Epidemiology* 108:394–401.

Lord, R.D., and C.H. Calisher. 1970. Further evidence of southward transport of arboviruses by migratory birds. *American Journal of Epidemiology* 92:73–78.

Lord, R.D., C.H. Calisher, and T.H. Work. 1973. Ecological investigations of vertebrate hosts of Venezuelan equine encephalomyelitis virus in south Florida. *The American Journal of Tropical Medicine and Hygiene* 22:116–123.

Lord, R.D., C.H. Calisher, W.A. Chappell, W.R. Metzger, and G.W. Fischer. 1974a. Urban St. Louis encephalitis surveillance through wild birds. *American Journal of Epidemiology* 99:360–363.

Lord, R.D., C.H. Calisher, and W.P. Doughty. 1974b. Assessment of bird involvement in three urban St. Louis encephalitis epidemics. *American Journal of Epidemiology* 99:364–367.

Ludwig, G.V., P.P. Calle, J.A. Mangiafico, B.L. Raphael, D.K. Danner, J.A. Hile, T.L. Clippinger, J.F. Smith, R.A. Cook, and T. McNamara. 2002. An outbreak of West Nile virus in a New York City captive wildlife population. *The American Journal of Tropical Medicine and Hygiene* 67:67–75.

Lundstrom, J.O., M.J. Turell, and B. Niklasson. 1992. Antibodies to Ockelbo virus in three orders of birds (Anseriformes, Galliformes and Passeriformes) in Sweden. *Journal of Wildlife Disease* 28:44–147.

Lundstrom, J.O., M.J. Turell, and B. Niklasson. 1993. Viremia in three orders of birds (Anseriformes, Galliformes and Passeriformes) inoculated with Ockelbo virus. *Journal of Wildlife Disease* 29:189–195.

Lustig, S., U. Olshevsky, D. Ben-Nathan, B.E. Lachmi, D. Kobiler, E. Israeli, and U. Olshevsky. 2000. A live attenuated West Nile virus strain as a potential veterinary vaccine. *Viral Immunology* 13:401–410.

Mackenzie, J.S., A.D.T. Barrett, and V. Deubel. 2002. The Japanese encephalitis serological group of flaviviruses: a brief introduction to the group. In *Japanese Encephalitis and West Nile Viruses,* J.S. Mackenzie, A.D.T. Barrett, and V. Deubel (eds.). Springer-Verlag, Berlin, Germany, pp. 1–10.

Malkinson, M., and C. Banet. 2002. The role of birds in the ecology of West Nile virus in Europe and Africa. In *Japanese Encephalitis and West Nile Viruses,* J.S. Mackenzie, A.D.T. Barrett, and V. Deubel, (eds.). Springer-Verlag, Berlin, Germany, pp. 309–322.

Malkinson, M., C. Banet, Y.Weisman, S. Pokamunski, R. King, M-T Drouet, and V. Deubel. 2002. Introduction of West Nile virus in the Middle East by migrating white storks. *Emerging Infectious Diseases* 8:392–397.

Marfin, A.A., L.R. Petersen, M. Eidson, J. Miller, J. Hadler, C. Farello, B. Werner, G.L. Campbell, M. Layton, P. Smith, E. Bresnitz, M. Cartter, J. Scaletta, G. Obiri, M. Bunning, R.C. Craver, J.T. Roehrig, K.G. Julian, S.R. Hinten, D.J. Gubler, and the ArboNET Cooperative Surveillance Group. 2001. Widespread West Nile Virus Activity, Eastern United States, 2000. *Emerging Infectious Diseases* 7:730–735.

Marshall, I.D., G.M. Woodroofe, and S. Hirsch. 1982a. Viruses recovered from mosquitoes and wildlife serum collected in the Murray Valley of South-eastern Australia, February 1974. *Australian Journal of Experimental Biology and Medical Science* 60:457–470.

Marshall, I.D., B.K. Brown, K. Keith, G.P. Gard, and E. Thibos. 1982b. Variation in arbovirus infection rates in species of birds sampled in a serological survey during an encephalitis epidemic in the Murray Valley of South-eastern Australia, February 1974. *Australian Journal of Experimental Biology and Medical Science* 60:471–478.

Marshall, I.D., and J.R. Miles. 1984. Ross River virus and epidemic polyarthritis. *Current Topics of Vector Research* 2:31–56.

Marshall, I.D. 1988. Murray Valley and Kunjin encephalitis. In *The Arboviruses: Epidemiology and Ecology,* Vol. III. T.P. Monath (ed.). CRC Press, Inc. Boca Raton, FL, U.S.A., pp. 151–189.

McGowan, K.J., A.B. Clark, and D.A. Robinson. Quoted in Caffrey, C., T.J. Weston, and S.C.R. Smith. 2003. High mortality among marked crows subsequent to the arrival of West Nile virus. *Wildlife Society Bulletin* 31:870–872.

McIntosh, B.M., D.B. Dickinson, and G.M. McGillivray. 1969a. Ecological studies on Sindbis and West Nile viruses in South Africa. V. The response of birds to inoculation of virus. *South African Journal of Medical Science* 34:77–82

McIntosh, B.M., W. Madsen, and D.B. Dickinson. 1969b. Ecological studies on Sindbis and West Nile viruses in South Africa. VI. The antibody response of wild birds. *South African Journal of Medical Science* 34:83–91

McIntosh, B.M., P.G. Jupp, I. Dos Santos, and G.M. Meenehan. 1976. Epidemics of West Nile and Sindbis viruses in South Africa with *Culex (Culex) univittatus Theobald* as vector. *South African Journal of Medical Science* 72:295–300.

McIntosh, B.M., and P.G. Jupp. 1982. Ecological studies on West Nile virus in southern Africa, 1965–1980. In *Proceedings 3rd Symposium Arbovirus Research in Australia,* pp. 15–17.

McLean, R.G., and T.W. Scott. 1979. Avian hosts of St. Louis encephalitis virus. Proceedings Eighth Bird

Control Seminar. Bowling Green State University, Bowling Green, OH, U.S.A., pp. 143–155.

McLean, R.G., and G.S. Bowen. 1980. Vertebrate hosts. In *St. Louis Encephalitis,* T.P. Monath (ed.). American Public Health Association, Washington D.C.,U.S.A., pp. 381–450.

McLean, R.G., J. Mullenix, J. Kerschner, and J. Hamm. 1983. The house sparrow (*Passer domesticus*) as a sentinel for St. Louis encephalitis virus. *The American Journal of Tropical Medicine and Hygiene* 32:1120–1129.

McLean, R.G., G. Frier, G.L. Parham, D.B. Francy, T.P. Monath, E.G. Campos, A. Therrien, J. Kerschner, and C.H. Calisher. 1985a. Investigations of the vertebrate hosts of eastern equine encephalitis during an epizootic in Michigan, 1980. *The American Journal of Tropical Medicine and Hygiene* 34:1190–1202.

McLean, R.G., D.B. Francy, and E.G.Campos. 1985b. Experimental studies of St. Louis encephalitis in vertebrates. *Journal of Wildlife Diseases* 21:85–93.

McLean, R.G., J.P. Webb, E.G. Campos, J. Gruwell, D.B. Francy, D. Womeldorf, C.M. Myers, T.H. Work, and M. Jozan. 1986. Antibody prevalence of St. Louis encephalitis virus in avian hosts in Los Angeles, California. *Journal of the American Mosquito Control Association* 4:524–528.

McLean, R.G., R.B. Shriner, L.J. Kirk, and D.J. Muth. 1989. Western equine encephalitis in avian populations in North Dakota, 1975. *Journal of Wildlife Diseases* 25:481–489.

McLean, R.G. 1991. Arboviruses of wild birds and mammals. *Bulletin of the Society for Vector Ecology* 16:3–16.

McLean, R.G., Kirk, L.J., Shriner, R.B., and Townsend, M. 1993. Avian hosts of St. Louis encephalitis virus in Pine Bluff, Arkansas, 1991. *The American Journal of Tropical Medicine and Hygiene* 49:46–52.

McLean, R.G., W.J. Crans, D.F. Caccamise, J. McNelly, L.J. Kirk, and C.H. Calisher. 1995. Experimental infection of wading birds with eastern equine encephalitis virus. *Journal of Wildlife Diseases* 31:502–508.

McLean, R.G., S.R. Ubico, D.E. Docherty, W.R. Hansen, L. Sileo, and T.S. McNamara. 2001. West Nile virus transmission and ecology in birds. In *West Nile Virus: Detection, Surveillance, and Control. Annals of New York Academy Sciences* 951:54–57.

McLean, R.G. 2002. West Nile virus. A threat to North American avian species. *Transactions 67th North American Wildlife Natural Resource Conference* pp. 62–74.

McLean, R.G., S.R. Ubico, D. Bourne, and N. Komar. 2002. West Nile virus in livestock and wildlife. In *Japanese Encephalitis and West Nile Viruses,* J.S. Mackenzie, A.D.T. Barrett, and V. Deubel (eds.). Springer-Verlag, Berlin, Germany, pp. 271–308.

McLean, R.G. 2004. West Nile Virus: Impact on Crow Populations in the United States, R.M. Timm and W.P. Gorenzel, (eds.). *Proceedings 21st* Vertebrate Pest Conference, Univ. Calif., Davis, CA. pp. 180–184.

Meehan, P.J., D.L. Wells, W. Paul, E. Buff, A. Lewis, D. Muth, R. Hopkins, N. Karabatsos, and T.F. Tsai. 2000. Epidemiological features of and public health response to a St. Louis encephalitis epidemic in Florida, 1990-1. *Epidemiology and Infection* 125:81–188.

Mendez-Galvan, J.F. 2004. West Nile virus in Latin America. Fifth National Conference on West Nile virus in the United States. Centers for Disease Control and Prevention. [Online.] Retrieved from the World Wide Web: www.cdc.gov/ncidod/dvbid/westnile/conf/index.htm.

Miller, B.R., R.S. Nasci, MS. Godsey, H.M. Savage, J.J. Lutwama, R.S. Lanciotti, and C.J. Peters. 2000. First field evidence for natural vertical transmission of West Nile virus in *Culex univittatus* complex mosquitoes from Rift Valley Province, Kenya. *The American Journal of Tropical Medicine and Hygiene* 62:240–246.

Mims, C.A., A. Nash, and J. Stephen. 2001. *Mims' Pathogenesis of Infectious Disease,* 5th ed. Academic Press, Inc., San Diego, CA, U.S.A., 474 pp.

Mitchell, C.J., D.B. Francy, and T.P. Monath. 1980. Arthropod vectors. In *St. Louis Encephalitis,* T.P. Monath (ed.). American Public Health Association, Washington D.C., U.S.A., pp. 313–379.

Mitchell, C.J., T.P. Monath, and C.B. Cropp. 1981. Experimental transmission of Rocio virus by mosquitoes. *The American Journal of Tropical Medicine and Hygiene* 30:465–472.

Monath, T.P., G.E. Kemp, C.B. Cropp, and G.S. Bowen. 1978. Experimental infection of house sparrows (*Passer domesticus*) with Rocio virus. *The American Journal of Tropical Medicine and Hygiene* 27:1251–1254.

Monath, T.P. 1979. Arthropod-borne encephalitides in the Americas. *Bulletin of the World Health Organization* 57:513–534.

Monath, T.P. 1980. Epidemiology. In *St. Louis Encephalitis,* T.P. Monath (ed.). American Public Health Association, Washington D.C., U.S.A., pp. 239–312.

Monath, T.P., (ed.). 1988. *The Arboviruses: Epidemiology and Ecology.* Vols. 1–5. CRC Press Inc., Boca Raton, FL, U.S.A., 1319 pp.

Monath, T.P. 2001. Prospects for the development of a vaccine against the West Nile virus. In *West Nile Virus: Detection, Surveillance, and Control. Annals of New York Academy Sciences* 951:1–12.

Monath, T.P. 2002. Japanese encephalitis vaccines: Current vaccines and future prospects. In *Japanese Encephalitis and West Nile Viruses,* J.S. Mackenzie, A .D. T. Barrett, and V. Deubel (eds.). Springer-Verlag, Berlin, Germany, pp. 105–138.

Moore, C.G., R.G. McLean, C.J. Mitchell, R.S. Nasci, T.F. Tsai, C.H. Calisher, A.A. Marfin, P.S. Moore, and

D.J. Gubler. 1993. *Guidelines for Arbovirus Surveillance Programs in the United States.* Centers for Disease Control and Prevention, Fort Collins, CO, U.S.A., 83 pp.

Morris, C.D., E. Whitney, T.F. Bast, and R Deibel. 1973. An outbreak of eastern equine encephalomyelitis in upstate New York during 1971. *The American Journal of Tropical Medicine and Hygiene* 22:561–566.

Morris, C.D., M.E. Corey, D.E. Emord, and J.J. Howard. 1980. Epizootiology of eastern equine encephalomyelitis virus in upstate New York, U.S.A. I. Introduction, demography, and natural environment of an endemic focus. *Journal of Medical Entomology* 17:442–452.

Morris, C.D. 1988. Eastern equine encephalomyelitis. In *The arboviruses: epidemiology and ecology,* Vol. III, T.P. Monath (ed.). CRC Press, Boca Raton, FL, U.S.A., pp. 1–20.

Moss, S.R., and P.A. Nuttall. 1986. Isolation of orbiviruses and uukuviruses from puffin ticks. *Acta Virologica* 29:158–161.

Murgue, B., S. Murri, S. Zientara, B. Durand, J-P Durand, and H. Zeller. 2001. West Nile outbreak in horses in southern France, 2000: The return after 35 years. *Emerging Infectious Diseases* 7: 692–694.

Murgue, B., H. Zeller, and V. Deubel. 2002. The ecology and epidemiology of West Nile virus in Africa, Europe and Asia. In *Japanese Encephalitis and West Nile Viruses,* J.S. Mackenzie, A.D.T. Barrett, and V. Deubel (eds.). Springer-Verlag, Berlin, Germany, pp.195–221.

Nasci, R.S., D.J. White, H. Stirling, J. Oliver, T.J. Daniels, R.C. Falco, S. Campell, W.J. Crans, H.M. Savage, R.S. Lanciotti, C.G. Moore, M. S. Godsey, K.L. Gottfried, and C.J. Mitchell. 2001a. West Nile virus isolates from mosquitoes in New York and New Jersey, 1999. *Emerging Infectious Diseases* 7:626–630.

Nasci, R.S., H.M. Savage, D.J. White, J.R. Miller, B.C. Cropp, M.S. Godsey, A.J. Kerst, P. Bennett, K. Gottfried, and R.S. Lanciotti. 2001b. West Nile Virus in over wintering *Culex* mosquitoes, New York City, 2000. *Emerging Infectious Diseases* 7:742–744.

Nathanson, N. 1980. Pathogenesis. In *St. Louis Encephalitis,* T.P. Monath (ed.). American Public Health Association, Washington D.C., U.S.A., pp. 201–236.

Naugle, D.E., C.L. Aldridge, B.L. Walker, T.E. Cornish, B.J. Moynahan, M.J. Holloran, K. Brown, G.D. Johnson, E.T. Schmidtmann, R.T. Mayer, C.Y. Kato, M.R. Matchett, T.J. Christiansen, W.E. Cook, T. Creekmore, R.D. Falise, E.T. Rinkes, and M. S. Boyce. 2004. West Nile virus: pending crisis for greater sage-grouse. *Ecology Letters* 7:704–713.

Niklasson, Bo. 1989. Sindbis and Sindbis-like viruses. In *The Arboviruses: Epidemiology and Ecology,* Vol. IV, T.P. Monath (ed.). CRC Press, Boca Raton, FL, U.S.A., pp. 167–176.

Nir, Y., G. Goldwasser, G. Lasowski, and A. Avivi. 1967. Isolation of arboviruses from wild birds in Israel. *American Journal of Epidemiology* 86:372–378.

Nir, Y., Y. Lasowski, A. Avivi, and R. Goldwasser. 1969. Survey for antibodies to arboviruses in the serum of various animals in Israel during 1965-1966. *The American Journal of Tropical Medicine and Hygiene* 18:416–422.

NOAA, National Oceanic Atmospheric Administration. 2005. National Climatic Data Center, Asheville, NC, U.S.A. [Online.] Retrieved from the World Wide Web: www.lwf.ncdc.noaa.gov/oa/climate/research/cag3/cag3.html.

OIE, Office International des Epizooties (1999) West Nile fever in Israel in geese. *Disease Information* 12:166.

O'Leary, D.R., A.A. Marfin, S. P. Montgomery, A.M. Kipp, J.A. Lehman, B.J. Biggerstaff, V.L. Elko, P.D. Collins, J.E. Jones, and G.L. Campbell. 2004. The epidemic of West Nile virus in the United States. 2002. *Vector-borne and Zoonotic Diseases* 4:61–70.

Olsen, J.G., T.W. Scott, L.H. Lorenz, and J.L. Hubbard. 1991. Enzyme immunoassay for detection of antibodies against eastern equine encephalomyelitis virus in sentinel chickens. *Journal of Clinical Microbiology* 29:1457–1461.

O'Neil, S.P., W-J. Shieh, and S.R. Zaki. 2002. Pathology and pathogenesis of virus infections. In *Immunology of Infectious Diseases,* S.H.E. Kaufmann, A. Sher, and R. Ahmed (eds.). American Society for Microbiology Press, Washington, D.C., U.S.A., pp. 307–328.

Oprandy, J.J., T.G. Schwan, and L. Main. 1988a. Tick-borne Kemerovo group arboviruses in a Newfoundland seabird colony. *Canadian Journal of Microbiology* 34:782–786.

Oprandy, J.J., J.G. Olson, and T.W. Scott. 1988b. A rapid dot immunoassay for the detection of serum antibodies to eastern equine encephalomyelitis and St. Louis encephalitis viruses in sentinel chickens. *The American Journal of Tropical Medicine and Hygiene* 38:181–186.

Ostlund, E.N., R.L. Crom, D.D. Pedersen, D.J. Johnson, W.O. Williams, and B.J. Schmitt. 2001. Equine West Nile encephalitis, United States. *Emerging Infectious Diseases* 7:665–669.

Pape, J. 2004. West Nile virus in Colorado, 2003. Fifth National Conference on West Nile virus in the United States. Centers for Disease Control and Prevention. [Online.] Retrieved from the World Wide Web: www.cdc.gov/ncidod/dvbid/westnile/conf/index.htm.

Petersen, L.R., and J.T. Roehrig. 2001. West Nile virus: A reemerging global pathogen. *Emerging Infectious Diseases* 7:611–614.

Pereira-Luiz, E., A. Suzuki, T.L. Moraes-Coimbra, R. Pereira de Souza, and E.L. Bocato-Chamelet. 2001.

Ilheus arbovirus in wild birds (*Sporophila caerulescens* and *Molothrus bonariensis*). *Revista de Saude Publica* 35:119–123.

Pinheiro, F.P., and J.W. LeDuc. 1988. Mayaro virus disease. In *The Arboviruses: Epidemiology and Ecology,* Vol. III, T.P. Monath (ed.). CRC Press, Boca Raton, FL, U.S.A., pp. 137–150.

Rappole, J.H., S.R. Derrickson, and Z. Hubaleck. 2000. Migratory birds and spread of West Nile virus in the western hemisphere. *Emerging Infectious Diseases* 6:319–328.

Reeves, W.C., G.A. Hutson, R.E. Bellamy, and R.P. Scrivani. 1958. Chronic latent infections of birds with western equine encephalomyelitis virus. *Proceedings of the Society of Experimental Biology and Medicine* 97:733–736.

Reeves, W.C. 1990. *Epidemiology and control of mosquito-borne arboviruses in California, 1943–1987.* California Mosquito Vector Control Association, Sacramento, CA, U.S.A.

Reid, H.W. 1975. Experimental infection of red grouse with louping-ill virus (*Flavivirus* group). I. The viraemia and antibody response. *Journal of Comparative Pathology* 85:223–229.

Reid, H.W., J.S. Duncan, J.D. Phillips, R. Moss, and A. Watson. 1978. Studies of louping-ill virus (*Flavivirus* group) in wild red grouse (*Lagopus lagopus scoticus*). *Journal of Hygiene* 81:321–329.

Reid, H.W., R. Moss, I. Pow, and D. Buxton. 1980. The response of three grouse species (*Tetrao urogallus, Lagopus mutus, Lagopus lagopus*) to louping-ill virus. *Journal of Comparative Pathology* 90:257–263.

Reid, H.W. 1988. Louping-Ill. In *The arboviruses: epidemiology and ecology,* Vol. III, T.P. Monath (ed.). CRC Press, Boca Raton, FL, U.S.A., pp. 117–135.

Reisen, W.K., and T.P. Monath. 1988. Western equine encephalomyelitis. In *The Arboviruses: Epidemiology and Ecology,* Vol. V, T.P. Monath (ed.). CRC Press, Boca Raton, FL, U.S.A., pp. 89–138.

Reisen, W.K., J. Lin, S.B. Presser, B. Enge, and J. Hardy. 1993. Evaluation of new methods for sampling sentinel chickens for antibodies to WEE and SLE viruses. *Proceedings of California Mosquito and Vector Control Association* 61:33–36.

Reisen, W.K., S.B. Presser, J. Lin, B. Enge, J.L. Hardy, and R.W. Emmons. 1994. Viremia and serological responses in adult chickens infected with western equine encephalomyelitis and St. Louis encephalitis viruses. *Journal of the American Mosquito Control Association* 10:549–555.

Reisen, W.K., J.O. Lundstrom, T.W. Scott, B.F. Eldridge, R.E. Chiles, R. Cusack, V.M. Martinez, H.D. Lothrop, D. Gutierrez, S.E. Wright, K. Boyce, and B.R. Hill. 2000. Patterns of avian seroprevalence to western equine encephalomyelitis and Saint Louis encephalitis viruses in California, U.S.A. *Journal of Medical Entomology* 37:507–527.

Ringia, A.M., B.J. Blitvich, H-Y Koo, M. Van de Wyngaerde, J.D. Brawn, and R.J. Novak. 2004. Antibody prevalence of West Nile virus in birds, Illinois, 2002. *Emerging Infectious Diseases* 10:1120–1124.

Rocke, T., K. Converse, C. Meteyer, and R. McLean. 2005. The impact of disease in American White Pelicans in North America. *Waterbirds* 28 (Special Publication 1):87–94.

Roehrig, J.T. 1999. Arboviruses. In *Clinical Virology Manual.* S. Specter, R.L. Hodinka and S.A. Young (eds.). 3rd ed. American Society for Microbiology, Washington D.C., pp. 356–373.

Roehrig, J.T., M. Layton, P. Smith, G.L. Campbell, R. Nasci, and R.S. Lanciotti. 2002. The emergence of West Nile virus in North America: Ecology, epidemiology, and surveillance. In *Japanese Encephalitis and West Nile Viruses,* J.S. Mackenzie, A.D.T. Barrett, and V. Deubel (eds.). Springer-Verlag, Berlin, Germany, pp. 223–240.

Root, J.J., J.S. Hall, R.G. McLean, N.L.Marlenee, B.J. Beaty, J. Gansowski, and L. Clark. 2004. Serologic evidence of exposure of wild mammals to flaviviruses in the central and eastern United States. *The American Journal of Tropical Medicine and Hygiene* 72:622–630.

Rowley, W.A., G. J. Hunt, and D.C. Dorsey. 1983. Flanders virus activity in Iowa, U.S.A. *Journal of Medical Entomology* 20:409–413.

Russell, R.C. 2002. Ross River virus: Ecology and distribution. *Annual Review of Entomology* 47:1–31.

Ryan, J., K. Dave, E. Emmerich, B. Fernandez, M. Turell, J. Johnson, K. Gottfried, K. Burkhalter, A. Kerst, A. Hunt, R. Wirtz, and R. Nasci. 2003. Wicking assays for the rapid detection of West Nile and St. Louis encephalitis viral antigens in mosquitoes (Diptera: Culicidae). *Journal of Medical Entomology* 40:95–99.

Sahu, S.P., A.D. Alstad, D.D. Pedersen and J.E. Pearson. 1994. Diagnosis of eastern equine encephalomyelitis virus infection in horses by immunoglobulin M and G capture enzyme-linked immunosorbent assay. *Journal of Veterinary Diagnostic Investigation* 6:34–38.

Saikku, P., and M. Brummer-Korvenkontio. 1973. Arboviruses in Finland. II. Isolation and characterization of Uukuniemi virus, a virus associated with ticks and birds. *The American Journal of Tropical Medicine and Hygiene* 22:390–399.

Saikku, P. 1974. Passerine birds in the ecology of Uukuniemi virus. *Medical Biology* 52:98–103.

Scherret, J.H., J.S. Mackenzie, R.A. Hall, V. Deubel, and E.A. Gould. 2002. Phylogeny and molecular epidemiology of West Nile and Kunjin viruses. In *Japanese Encephalitis and West Nile Viruses,* J.S. Mackenzie, A.D.T. Barrett, and V. Deubel (eds.). Springer-Verlag, Berlin, Germany, pp. 373–390.

Schwan, T.G., J.J. Oprandy, and A.J. Main. 1988. Mono Lake virus infecting *Argas* ticks (Acari: Argasidae) associated with California gulls breeding on islands in Mono Lake, California. *Journal of Medical Entomology* 25:381–387.

Scott, T.W., R.G. McLean, D.B. Francy, and C.S. Card. 1983a. A simulation model for the vector-host transmission system of a mosquito-borne avian virus, Turlock (Bunyaviridae). *Journal of Medical Entomology* 20:625–640.

Scott, T.W., R.G. McLean, D. B. Francy, C.J. Mitchell, and C.S. Card. 1983b. Experimental infections of birds with Turlock virus. *Journal of Wildlife Diseases* 19:82–85.

Scott, T.W., G.S. Bowen, T.P. Monath. 1984. A field study of the effects of Fort Morgan virus, an arbovirus transmitted by swallow bugs, on the reproductive success of cliff swallow and symbiotic house sparrows in Morgan County, Colorado, 1976. *The American Journal of Tropical Medicine and Hygiene* 33:981–991.

Schmidt, J.R., and R.E. Shope. 1971. Kemerovo virus from a migrating common redstart of Eurasia. *Acta Virologica* 15:112.

Seamans, T., and J.L. Belant. 1999. Comparison of DRC-1339 and alpha-chloralose to reduce herring gull populations. *Wildlife Society Bulletin* 27:729–733.

Semenov, B.F., S.P. Chunikhin, V.I. Karmysheva, and N.I. Iakovleva. 1973. Study of chronic forms of arbovirus infections in birds. 1. Experiments with West Nile, Sindbis, Bhadja, and Sicilian mosquito fever viruses. *Vestnick Akademii Meditsinskikh* Nauk SSSR 28:79–83.

Senne, D.A., J.C. Pedersen, D.L. Hutto, W.D. Taylor, B.J. Schmitt, and B. Panigrahy, 2000. Pathogenicity of West Nile virus in chickens. *Avian Diseases* 44:642–649.

Shi, P-Y., E.B. Kauffman, P. Ren, A. Felton, J.H. Tai, and A.P. Dupuis II, et al. 2001. High throughput detection of West Nile virus RNA. *Journal of Clinical Microbiology* 39:1264–1271.

Shope, R.E., A.H.P. de Andrade, G. Bensabath, O.R. Causey, and P.S. Humphrey. 1966. The epidemiology of EEE, WEE, SLE, and Turlock viruses, with special reference to birds, in a tropical rain forest near Belem, Brazil. *American Journal of Epidemiology* 84:467–477.

Smith, G.C., D.B. Francy, E.G. Campos, P. Katona, and C.H. Calisher. 1983. Correlation between human cases and antibody prevalence in house sparrows during a focal outbreak of St. Louis encephalitis in Mississippi, 1979. *Mosquito News* 43:322–325.

Smith, T. 2005. National West Nile virus surveillance summary, United States, 2004. Sixth National Conference on West Nile virus in the United States. Centers for Disease Control and Prevention. [Online.] Retrieved from the World Wide Web: www.cdc.gov/ncidod/dvbid/westnile/conf/index.htm.

Smithburn, K.C, T.P. Hughes, A.W. Burke, and J.H. Paul. 1940. A Neurotrophic virus isolated from the blood of a native of Uganda. *The American Journal of Tropical Medicine* 20:471–492.

Soman, R.S., F.M. Rodrigues, S.N. Guttikar, and P.Y.Guru. 1977. Experimental viraemia and transmission of Japanese encephalitis virus by mosquitoes in ardeid birds. *Indian Journal of Medical Research* 66:709–718.

Spence, L.P. 1980. St. Louis encephalitis in tropical America. In *St. Louis Encephalitis,* T.P. Monath (ed.). American Public Health Association, Washington D.C., U.S.A., pp. 451–471.

Spence, R.P., K.A. Harrap, and P.A. Nuttall. 1985. The isolation of Kemerovo group orbiviruses and Uukuniemi group viruses transmitted by ticks from the Isle of May, Scotland. *Acta Virologica* 29:129–136.

Stamm, D.D., and Kissling KE. 1957. The influence of reciprocal immunity on eastern and western equine encephalomyelitis infection in horses and English sparrows. *Journal of Immunology* 79:342.

Stamm, D.D. 1958. Studies on the ecology of equine encephalomyelitis. *American Journal of Public Health* 48:328–335.

Stamm, D.D., R.W. Chamberlain, and W.D. Sudia. 1962. Arbovirus studies in south Alabama, 1957–1958. *American Journal of Hygiene* 76:61–81.

Stamm, D.D., and R.J. Newman. 1963. Evidence of southward transport of arboviruses from the U.S. by migratory birds. *Annals of Microbiology* 11:123–133.

Steele, K.E., M.J. Linn, R.J. Schoepp, N. Komar, T.W. Geisbert, R.M. Manduca, P.P. Calle, B.L. Raphael, T.L. Clippinger, T. Larsen, J. Smith, R.S. Lanciotti, N. A. Panella, and T.S. McNamara. 2000. Pathology of fatal West Nile virus infections in native and exotic birds during the 1999 outbreak in New York City, New York. *Veterinary Pathology* 37:208–224.

Stephenson, J.R., J.M. Lee, and P.D. Wilton-Smith. 1984. Antigenic variation among members of the tick-borne encephalitis complex. *Journal of General Virology* 65:81–89.

Sudia, W.D., and V.F. Newhouse. 1975. Epidemic Venezuelan equine encephalitis in North America: A summary of virus-vector-host relationships. *American Journal of Epidemiology* 101:1–13.

Sudia, W.D., R.G. McLean, V.F. Newhouse, J.G. Johnston, Jr., D.L. Miller, H. Trevino, G.S. Bowen, and G. Sather. 1975. Epidemic Venezuelan equine encephalitis in North America in 1971: vertebrate field studies. *American Journal of Epidemiology* 101:36–50.

Swayne, D.E., J.R. Beck, C.S. Smith, W-J. Shieh, and S.R. Zaki. 2001. Fatal encephalitis and myocarditis in young domestic geese (Anser anser domesticus) caused by West Nile virus. *Emerging Infectious Diseases* 7:751–753.

Szomolanyi-Tsuda, E, M.A. Brehm, and R.M. Welsh. 2002. Acquired immunity against viral infections. In *Immunology of Infectious Diseases,* S.H.E. Kaufmann, A. Sher, and R. Ahmed (eds.). American Society for Microbiology Press, Washington, D.C., U.S.A., pp. 247–265.

Taylor, R.M., T.H. Work, H.S. Hurlbut, and F. Rizk. 1956. A study of the ecology of West Nile Virus in Egypt. *The American Journal of Tropical Medicine and Hygiene* 5:579–620.

Tenbroeck, C. 1938. Birds as possible carriers of the virus of equine encephalomyelitis. *Archives of Pathology* 25:759.

Tesh, R.B., R.G. McLean, D.A. Shroyer, L. Rosen, and C. H. Calisher. 1981. Ross River virus (Togaviridae: Alphavirus) infection (epidemic polyarthritis) in American Samoa. *Transactions Royal Society of Tropical Medicine and Hygiene* 75:426–431.

Tesh, R.B., J. Peleg, I. Samina, J. Margalit, D.K. Bodkin, R.E. Shope, and D. Knudson. 1986. Biological and antigenic characterization of Netivot virus, an unusual new Orbivirus recovered from mosquitoes in Israel. *The American Journal of Tropical Medicine and Hygiene* 35:418–428.

Tesh, R.B., A.P.A. Travassos da Rosa, H. Guzman, T.P. Araujo, and S.Y. Xiao. 2002. Immunization with heterologous flaviviruses protective against fatal West Nile encephalitis. *Emerging Infectious Diseases* 8:245–251.

Tesh, R.B., R. Parsons, M. Siirin, Y. Randle, C. Sargent, H. Guzman, T. Wuithiranyagool, S. Higgs, D.L. Vanlandingham, A.A. Bala, K. Haas, and B. Zerinque. 2004. Year-round West Nile virus activity, Gulf Coast region, Texas and Louisiana. *Emerging Infectious Diseases* 10:1649–1652.

Thomas, D.B. 1993. In *Viruses and the Cellular Immune Response.* Marcel Dekker, New York, NY, U.S.A., 524 pp.

Travassos da Rosa, A.P.A., T.N. Mather, T. Takeda, C.A. Whitehouse, R.E. Shope, V.L. Popov, H. Guzman, L. Coffey, T.P. Araujo, and R.B. Tesh. 2002. Two new Rhabdoviruses (Rhabdoviridae) isolated from birds during surveillance for arboviral encephalitis, Northeastern United States. *Emerging Infectious Diseases* 8:614–618.

Tsai, T.F., and C.J. Mitchell. 1988. St. Louis encephalitis. In *The Arboviruses: Epidemiology and Ecology,* Vol. IV, T.P. Monath (ed.). CRC Press, Boca Raton, FL, U.S.A., pp. 113–143.

Tulley, T.N. Jr., S.M. Shane, R.P. Poston, J.J. England, C.C. Vice, D.Y. Cho, and B. Panigrahy. 1992. Eastern equine encephalitis in a flock of emus (*Dromaius novaehollandiae*). *Avian Diseases* 36:808–812.

Turell, M.J., M. Bunning, G.V. Ludwig, B. Ortman, J. Chang, T. Speaker, A. Spielman, R. McLean, N. Komar, R. Gates, T. McNamara, T. Creekmore, L. Farley, and C.J. Mitchell. 2003. DNA vaccine for West Nile virus infection in fish crows (*Corvus ossifragus*). *Emerging Infectious Diseases* 9:1077–1081.

Tyzzer, E.E., A.W. Sellards, and B.L. Rennett. 1938. The occurrence in nature of equine encephalomyelitis in the ring-necked pheasant. *Science* 88:505–506.

USDA, United States Department of Agriculture. 2005. West Nile virus in equines in the United States, 1999–2004. Veterinary Services, APHIS, USDA. [Online.] Retrieved from the World Wide Web: www.aphis.usda.gov/lpa/issues/wnv/wnv.html.

USGS, National Wildlife Health Center. 2005. West Nile virus. [Online.] Retrieved from the World Wide Web: www.nwhc.usgs.gov/research/west_nile/west_nile.html.

Ubico, S.R., and R.G. McLean. 1995. Serologic prevalence of viruses from neotropical bats from Guatemala. *Journal of Wildlife Diseases* 31:1–9.

Walton, T.E., and M.A. Grayson, 1988. Venezuelan equine encephalomyelitis. In *The Arboviruses: Epidemiology and Ecology.* Vol. IV, T.P. Monath (ed.). CRC press, Inc. Boca Raton, FL, U.S.A., pp. 203–231.

Weingartl, H.M., J.L. Neufeld, J. Copps, and P. Marszal. 2004. Experimental West Nile virus infection in blue jays (*Cyanocitta cristata*) and crows (*Corvus brachyrhynchos*). *Veterinary Pathology* 41:362–370.

Whitehead , R.H., R.L. Doherty, R. Domrow, H.A. Stanfast, and E.J. Wetters. 1968. Studies of the epidemiology of arthropod-borne virus infections at Mitchell River mission, Cape York Peninsula, North Queensland. III. Virus studies of wild birds, 1964–67. *Transactions Royal Society of Tropical Medicine and Hygiene* 62:439–445.

Whitehouse, C.A., A. Guibeau, D. McGuire, T. Takeda, and T.N. Mather. 2001. A reverse transcriptase-polymerase chain reaction assay for detecting Highlands J virus. *Avian Diseases* 45:605–611.

Williams, H., H. Thorburn, and G.S. Ziffo. 1963. Isolation of louping-ill from the red grouse. *Nature* 200:193.

Williams, J.E., O.P. Young, D.M. Watts, and T.J. Reed. 1971. Wild birds as eastern (EEE) and western (WEE) equine encephalitis sentinels. *Journal of Wildlife Diseases* 7:188–194.

Whitney, E. 1964. Flanders strain, an Arbovirus newly isolated from mosquitoes and birds of New York State. *The American Journal of Tropical Medicine and Hygiene* 13:123–131.

Woodring, F.R. 1957. Naturally occurring infection with western equine encephalomyelitis in turkeys. *Journal of American Veterinary Medical Association* 130:511.

Work, T.H., H.S. Hurlbut, and R.M. Taylor. 1955. Indigenous wild birds of the Nile Delta as potential West Nile circulating reservoirs. *The American Journal of Tropical Medicine and Hygiene* 4:872–878.

Wunschmann, A., J. Shivers, J. Bender, L. Carroll, S. Fuller, M. Saggese, A. van Wettere, and P. Redig. 2004a. Pathologic findings in red-tailed hawks (*Buteo jamaicensis*) and Cooper's hawks (*Accipiter cooper*) naturally infected with West Nile virus. *Avian Diseases* 48:570–580.

Wunschmann, A., J. Shivers, L. Carroll, and J. Bender. 2004b. Pathological and immunohistochemical findings in American crows (*Corvus brachyrhynchos*) naturally infected with West Nile virus. *Journal of Veterinary Diagnostic Investion* 16:329–333.

Wunschmann, A., J. Shivers, J. Bender, L. Carroll, S. Fuller, M. Saggese, A. vaan Wettere, P. Redig. 2005. Pathologic and immunohistochemical findings in goshawks (*Accipiter gentilis*) and great horned owls (*Bubo virginianus*) naturally infected with West Nile virus. *Avian Diseases* 49:252–259.

Yaremych, S.A., R.E. Warner, P.C. Mankin, J.D. Brawn, A. Raim, and R. Novak. 2003. West Nile virus causes high mortality in a free-ranging population of American crows (*Corvus brachyrhynchos*). *Emerging Infectious Diseases* 10:709–711.

Yunker, C.E., C.M. Clifford, L.A. Thomas, J. Cory, and J.E. George.1972. Isolation of viruses from swallow ticks, *Argas cooleyi,* in the southwestern United States. *Acta Virologica* 16:415–421.

Yunker, C.E. 1975. Tick-borne viruses associated with seabirds in North America and related islands. *Medical Biology* 53:302–311.

3
Avian Herpesviruses

Erhard F. Kaleta and Douglas E. Docherty

INTRODUCTION

Avian Herpesviruses (HV) cause a variety of disease conditions in birds, and those individuals that recover tend to establish latent infections for prolonged times. In many cases concomitant infections by other agents, debilitating environmental factors, and social or reproductive stress contribute to the development of variable forms of overt diseases and to occasional epizootics that may result in significant mortalities (Vindevogel and Duchatel 1997). With rare exceptions, HV-induced diseases never threaten the existence of well-established populations (Davison 2002). In contrast, losses mainly affect the offspring of some individual pairs or eliminate variable numbers of birds at any age from a population (Gerlach 1994).

Vertical transmission of HV from parents to offspring through the egg has not been reported and arthropod vectors are not required for bird-to-bird transmission. Because HV are quite sensitive to inactivation outside their natural hosts, mechanical vectors play only a minor role in virus dissemination (Ritchie 1995; Phalen 1997).

Avian HV have a worldwide distribution and have been isolated from diseased as well as healthy appearing but latently infected wild, captive, and domestic birds. Because well-planned surveillance studies for the discovery of HV have neither been designed nor implemented, data on regional distribution, host ranges, and rates of morbidity and mortality are presently not available. Screening for HV should be part of health monitoring programs for wild birds (Kaleta 1998, 1999). It is intended in this chapter to provide a broad but condensed overview of the consolidated knowledge on the ever-increasing variety of free-living birds naturally infected by HV. Emphasis is placed more on the host aspect in terms of signs, lesions, and diagnosis and less on the divergent molecular and other *in vitro* properties of the HV. HV have been recorded in more than 100 species of free-living birds (Heinrichs 1992). Although the known host range is biased by variable intensities of virological examinations, it appears that most isolates are derived from old and new world parrots, various species of pigeons, owls, and falcons. It is impossible within the scope of this chapter to name all affected bird species and their manifold disease expressions. Duck plague (duck virus enteritis), an important HV disease of waterfowl, is not discussed in this chapter but is covered in detail in Chapter 4, "Duck Plague."

SYNONYMS

So far, only a few diseases caused by HV have been given specific names. Some diseases have been named in honor of scientists who provided the first description of a defined disease entity (for example, Marek's disease of chickens, Pacheco's parrot disease, Smadel's disease of pigeons). Names also have been derived from prominent pathological lesions (for example, hepatosplenitis in various owls, laryngotracheitis in fowl and pheasants), and identified histological lesions (for example, inclusion body disease of falcons, eagles, and cranes). Quite a number of diseases and their respective viruses remain so far as nameless orphans.

HISTORY

In history, the intellectual approach to birds—as to any living matter—differs markedly. All existing life was interpreted as a donation of God. Any disease and death represented a punishment of God or a machination of the Devil. For these reasons no factual need was seen to differentiate between various etiologies of diseases and causes of death. Aristotle (389–322 B.C.), one of the first natural scientists, in Ancient Greece tried to find answers to questions such as where birds evolved, how they live, and their migration destinations. Also, the Roman writers on natural history,

Cajus Plinius Secundus the Older (A.D. 23–79) and Lucius Iunius Moderatus Columella (A.D. 4–73), describe a large number of free-living and domestic birds, along with their husbandry conditions, breeding, and brooding, and also common diseases in domestic and wild birds. These texts are approximately 2,000 years old, and the information on signs and lesions is limited and difficult to associate with presently well-defined etiologically oriented descriptions. They indicate that wild and domestic bird mortality was noted at these times and was recognized as disease.

A hallmark in aviculture, avian medicine, and falconry is the detailed and colorfully illustrated book *De arte venandi cum avibus* (*On the Art to Hunt With Falcons*) by Emperor Fredericius II (1212–1250), which was written in Latin and has been translated in many languages. The book was produced around the year 1245 in Italy. The illustrated book provides splendid information on all issues of falconry and summarizes the current knowledge on trapping, maintenance, feeding, signs for health and bodily condition, and training methods of various species of captive falcons. Detailed descriptions or illustrations of ailments or diseases are obviously lacking.

The Swiss natural scientist Konrad Gesner collected all available information of his time on wild and domestic animals and published the wealth of data in three large volumes in Latin in 1555. One volume is devoted to birds; in it he described many bird species and mentioned which birds are useful not only as sources of food but also as medical remedies for humans.

With the development of histological techniques and the concept of cellular pathology by Rudolf Virchov (1821–1902) in the second half of the nineteenth century, well-defined descriptions of microscopic lesions were possible for the first time in medical history. It took until the beginning of the twentieth century for the first concise account of signs and histopathology of a disease with HV etiology.

Josef Marek, a veterinarian working in Budapest, Hungary, described in 1907 an infectious disease with inflammatory lesions in peripheral nerves and differentiated his findings from vitamin B deficiencies. The newly described disease was associated with lameness and tumor formation in several breeds of domestic chickens. May and Tittsler (1925) described a severe respiratory disease in chickens that is now known as infectious laryngotracheitis (ILT) of fowl, pea fowl, Guinea fowl, and pheasants (Kaleta and Redmann 1997).

Genesio Pacheco and Otto Bier (1930), both researchers at the Instituto Biologico in Sao Paulo, Brazil, published a report on a highly lethal epizootic disease among different species of parrots. The etiologic agent was filterable, which differentiated the disease from psittacosis. It took until 1975 to firmly establish the herpes viral etiology (Simpson et al. 1975).

A severe HV-induced disease in racing pigeons used for military purposes was described by Joseph E. Smadel et al. (1945), working in a U.S. Army medical establishment of the Rockefeller Institute for Medical Research in New York.

Hugo Burtscher, working as a veterinary pathologist in the University of Vienna, Austria, provided histological evidence in 1965 that a common lethal disease in various species of free-living owls was caused by an HV. For this disease of owls, he coined the term "hepatosplenitis infectiosa strigum" and stressed that the newly discovered viral disease needed to be differentiated from avian tuberculosis. Later, he and his associates described the isolation of an HV in cell cultures and made a number of successful transmission experiments in owls (Burtscher 1965, 1968; Burtscher and Schumacher 1966; Burtscher and Sibalin 1975). All HV obtained from birds of the order Strigiformes produce distinct cytopathic changes in cell cultures (Schettler 1969; Kaleta 1998). Differences in type and duration of development of these changes exist and can be verified by differences in plaque types (Kaleta et al. 1980b; Sallmann 1991; Schroeder 1992).

More recently, additional infections and diseases with HV etiology were described and confirmed by virus isolation and typing. These are in the Prairie Falcon (*Falco mexicanus*), Red-headed Falcon (*F. chiquera*), and Peregrine Falcon (*F. peregrinus*) by Mare and Graham (1973), in a Little Pied Cormorant (*Halietor melanoleucos*) by French et al. (1973), in Sudan Crowned Cranes (*Balearica pavonina*) and Demoiselle Cranes (*Anthropoides virgo*) by Burtscher and Gruenberg (1979) in Europe, and by Docherty and Henning (1980) and Docherty and Romaine (1983) in North America affecting Sandhill Cranes (*Grus canadensis*), Japanese Cranes (*Grus japonensis*), Paradise Cranes (*Anthropoides paradisea*), and Hooded Cranes (*Grus monacha*). Further HV were detected by Forster et al. (1989) in Demoiselle Cranes in Europe, a Black Stork (*Ciconia nigra*) (Kaleta et al. 1980d), a group of Northern Bobwhite (*Colinus virginianus*) (Kaleta et al. 1980a), a Bald Eagle nestling (*Haliaeetus leucocephalus*) by Docherty et al. (1983), American White Storks (*Ciconia ciconia*) by Kaleta and Kummerfeld (1983), a Black-footed Penguin (*Spheniscus demersus*) by Kincaid and Cranfield (1988), a toucan of unknown species by Charlton et al. (1990), a Satyr Tragopan (*Tragopan satyra*) by Günther et al. (1997), and in various passerine birds summarized by Kaleta (1998), as listed in Table 3.1.

Table 3.1. Herpesviruses-induced diseases in birds, natural hosts, and geographic distribution.

Name of Disease	Natural Hosts	Present Geographic Distribution	References (First Report and Present Situation)
Marek's disease	Red Jungle Fowl (*Gallus gallus* [*G. g.*] *bankiva*), Ceylon Jungle Fowl (*G. g. lafayettii*)	SE Asia	Weiss and Biggs 1972 Cho and Kenzy 1975 Marek 1907
	All breeds of domestic hybrid chickens (*G. g.* forma dom.)	Worldwide	Calnek and Witter 1997 Dutton et al. 1973
	Japanese quail (*Coturnix coturnix japonica*), Domestic turkey (*Meleagris gallopavo*)		Pennycott and Venogupal 2002
Infectious laryngotracheitis	Domestic, fancier & backyard chickens (*G. gallus* forma dom.)	Worldwide N America Japan	May and Tittsler 1925 Bagust and Guy 1997 Crawshow and Boycott 1982
	Indian Peafowl (*Pavo cristatus*) Helmeted Guineafowl (*Numida meleagris*), several pheasants	Europe N America	Watanabe and Ohmi 1983 Kaleta and Redmann 1997
Pacheco's parrot disease	Almost all psittacine birds of the order Psittaciformes	S America N America World-wide	Pacheco and Bier 1930 Simpson et al. 1975 Krautwald et al. 1988 Horner et al. 1992 Gough and Alexander 1993 Gerlach 1994 Magnino et al. 1996
Smadel's disease of pigeons	Feral, urban, and domestic Rock Pigeons (*Columba livia*)	N America S America Europe Europe, Asia Australia Africa	Smadel et al. 1945 Toro et al. 1999 Marthedal and Jylling 1966 Vindevogel et al. 1975, 1984 Boyle and Bennington 1973 Pollard and Marais 1983

(Continued)

Table 3.1. *(Coninued)*

Name of Disease	Natural Hosts	Present Geographic Distribution	References (First Report and Present Situation)
Hepatosplenitis infectiosa strigum, syn. Inclusion body hepatitis	Great Horned Owl (*Bubo* [*B.*] *virginianus*), Eurasian Eagle-Owl (*B. bubo*), Forest Eagle-Owl (B. nipalensis), Barred Eagle-Owl (*B. sumatranus*), Eastern Screech-Owl (*Otus asio*), Brown Fish-Owl (*Ketupa* [*K.*] *zeylonensis*), Buffy Fish-Owl (*K. ketupa*), Snowy Owl (*Bubo scandiaca*), Fishing Owl (*Scotopelia* sp.) Brown Wood-Owl (*Strix* [*S.*] *leptogrammica*), Tawny Owl (*S. aluco*), Spectacled Owl (*Pulsatrix* [*S.*] *perspicilla*), Eurasian Pygmy-Owl (*Glaucidium passerinum*), Little Owl (*Athene noctua*), Boreal Owl (*Aegolius funereus*), Northern Long-eared Owl (*Asio otus*)	N America Europe	Mare and Graham 1973 Burtscher 1965, 1968 Schettler 1969 Herceg and Huber 1972 Green and Shillinger 1935, 1936 Sileo et al. 1975 Drüner 1978 Burtscher and Schumacher 1966 Heidenreich and Kaleta 1978 Bürki et al. 1973
None	Barn Owl (*Tyto alba*)	Europe	Glünder et al. 1991 Gómez-Villamandos et al. 1995
Falcon & Eagle HV	Falcons of Subfamily Falconinae, Eagles of Family Accipitridae and Bald Eagle (*Haliaeetus leucocephalus*)	N America N America Europe	Ward et al. 1971 Mare and Graham 1973 Docherty et al. 1983 Mozos et al. 1994 Ramis et al. 1994 Sander 1995
Lake Victoria Cormorant HV	Lake Victoria Cormorant (*Phalacrocorax melanoleucos*)	Australia	French et al. 1973
Inclusion body disease of cranes	Black Crowned-Crane (*Balearica pavonica*) Demoiselle Crane (*Anthropoides virgo*) Blue Crane (Grus [G.] paradisea), Sandhill Crane (*G. canadensis*) Red-crowned Crane (*G. japonensis*) Hooded Crane (*G. monacha*)	Austria Austria N America France & Germany Japan	Burtscher and Grünberg 1975 Burtscher and Grünberg 1979 Docherty and Henning 1980 Förster et al. 1989 Suzuki et al. 1997
None	Northern Bobwhite (quail) (*Colinus virginianus*)	Germany	Kaleta et al. 1980a
None	Black Stork (*Ciconia* [*C.*] *nigra*), White Stork (*C.ciconia*)	Germany	Kaleta et al. 1980d

	Abdim's stork (*C. abdimii*)	Germany Spain	Kaleta and Kummerfeld 1983 Gómez-Villamandos et al. 1998
None	Black-footed Penguin (*Spheniscus demersus*)	N America	Kincaid and Cranfield 1988
None	Toucan (unknown species)	N America	Charlton et al. 1990
None	Satyr Tragopan (*Tragopan satyra*)	Germany	Günther et al. 1997
None	Order Passeriformes: Northern Cardinal (*Cardinalis cardinalis*) Gouldian Finch (*Chloebia gouldinae*) Superb Starling (*Lamprotornis superbus*) White-rumped Munia (*Lonchura striata*) Great Tit (*Parus major*) Island Canary (*Serinus canaria* forma domestica) Bronze Mannikin (*Lonchura cucullatus*) Zebra Finch (*Taeniopygea guttata*) Red-cheeked Cordonbleu (*Uraeginthus bengalus*)	Europe, America, Africa, SE Asia	Schönbauer and Köhler 1982 Mueller 1990 Blumenstein 1993 Desmid et al. 1991 Gravendyck 1996 Kaleta 1998 Wellehan et al. 2003

DISTRIBUTION

Because most of the HV have a relatively narrow host range under natural conditions, the geographic distribution of HV follow the natural habitats of affected bird species. In migrating birds, the geographical distribution can reach enormous proportions, extending from northern Alaska to South America or northern regions of Europe and Asia to Africa or southern parts of Asia.

Natural bird migration and modern international transport of exotic birds contribute to worldwide dissemination of HV and make meaningful statements on the occurrence of HV in regional habitats increasingly difficult.

Cracraft (2000) attempted to use fossil records of currently extinct avian species to gain information on the origin and dispersion of modern birds. The author came to the conclusion that the temporal history of neornithes are derived from birds that had lived on the Gondvana prior to the Cretaceous-Tertiary extinction event, which is supposedly due to the Chicxulub meteorite impact on Yucatan peninsula, Mexico. A co-evolution rather than a switch from "old to new" host species appears to be more likely for birds and their herpes viruses (Davison 2002).

HOST RANGE

At least one natural host is known for each of the HV isolated from wild birds. Determination of host range is difficult in wild species because of legal and ethical restrictions in keeping wildlife for experimental purposes, as well as practical considerations including unknown origin and health status of the birds. Conducting large-scale transmission experiments for the assessment of the complete host range, reproduction of clinical signs, and pathogenesis are unlikely given these considerations. The postulates laid down by Henle and Koch to establish a firm cause-effect-relationship between a characterized HV and a defined form of disease in a given bird species are rarely fulfilled.

A successful "take" of a natural or experimental infection depends on the presence of an antigen(s) on the surface (envelope) of a virus and the presence of a matching receptor(s) on the cellular surface of the respiratory or intestinal tracts of a potential host. Both preconditions might be fulfilled in many species of birds, but due to geographic separation of birds, were not historically significant.

As indicated, the complete natural host range of most HV is not known. It appears that the range of natural hosts is very narrow for some HV, but others affect many different bird species belonging to the same or to unrelated families or even orders. It is very likely that captive birds originating from different continents will be exposed to HV that were formerly endemic to only one geographic region.

The Suid Herpesviruses 1 (SHV 1) cause a generally mild disease in swine and some other mammals. If SHV 1 is experimentally transmitted to chickens or pigeons, severe disease including mortality occurs. This is the only known mammalian HV that also infects birds (Vindevogel and Duchatel 1997).

ETIOLOGY

Herpesviruses (HV) of birds contain an inner core of linear double stranded DNA, an icosahedral (a polyhedron having 20 faces) capsid, a tegument, and on the outside a lipid containing envelope with surface projections (Mettenleiter 2003). Electron microscopic size estimates of the complete virion range from 102 to 200 nm (Figure 3.1). The relatively large genome (124 to 235 kbp depending on the virus species) encodes for many different internal as well as glycosylated and nonglycosylated surface proteins (Mettenleiter 2003, 2004). These outer membrane proteins account for *in vivo* differences in host susceptibility and *in vitro* for various degrees of cross neutralization.

All avian HV isolated from domestic birds are presently grouped into the subfamily Alphaherpesvirinae. However, many listed isolates from wild birds have not been studied in great detail. Therefore, 10 of the listed avian HV were not assigned to any of the three subfamilies or to the already established herpesvirus genera or species (Roizman 1996; Minson et al. 2000). These viruses remain unassigned to any of the subfamilies but are tabulated as members of the family Herpesviridae (Minson et al. 2000).

Several genes code for the primary and three-dimensional structure of the outer membrane proteins and the surface projections of virions (Roizman 1996; Mettenleiter 2003). The differences in antigenicity result in production of monospecific serum antibodies. These can be used in cross neutralization tests for the differentiation of isolates and for the formulation of serotypes (Kaleta et al. 1980b).

The results of serotyping seem to correspond well with the cleavage pattern of purified DNA after digestion with restriction endonucleases (Günther et al. 1997; Schroeder-Gravendyck 1999), thus making the analysis of restriction fragment length polymorphism a valuable tool for basic virus characterization and epidemiological research (Tomaszewski et al. 2001, 2003).

EPIZOOTIOLOGY

Sources and Reservoirs

Modes and duration of excretion, stability of the shed HV in the environment, and routes of entry vary

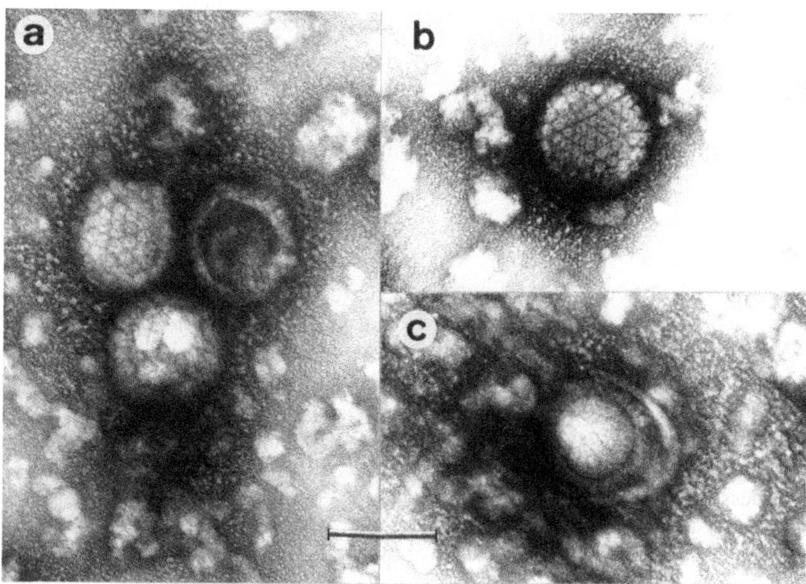

Figure 3.1. Electron micrographs of HV particles contrasted with uranylacetate. Concentrated supernatant fluids of CEF cultures that were inoculated with an HV obtained from a Snowy Owl (*Bubo scandiaca*). (a) and (b) non-enveloped nucleocapsids displaying triangular arrangement of hollow capsomers; (c) HV particle with partially visible envelope. Bar represents 100 nm.

greatly between isolates and hosts. In general, the path of virus excretion is associated with the predominant type of clinical signs and lesions. Thus, sources of infection might be virus containing cells that originate from the feather follicle epithelium (Marek's disease), mucosal cells and saliva of the pharynx, conjunctival cells and lacrimal fluids, and droppings that originate from the gut and kidneys. During the viremic phase, virus is also present in blood-filled feather quills (Gravendyck et al. 1998).

Transmission

Inhalation of virus-containing dust derived from feathers, nasal excretions, saliva, nasal discharge, urine, and feces is the predominant way of transmission from bird to bird. Adults that feed their offspring with crop-milk (feral and domestic pigeons, some psittacine birds) experience an activation of their latent infection in the oropharyngeal region during egg incubation and transmit the HV via crop-milk to their newly hatched offspring. Vectors are not required for transmission, and vertical transmission has never been unequivocally proven.

Life History

Most natural infections are acquired during early life. Latency may thereafter exist for prolonged times from brooding to adulthood, which may result in morbidity and mortality at any time of life. A prerequisite for disease development is, in adult birds, an activation of latency by endogenous or exogenous factors. The trigeminal ganglia are the site of latency of infectious laryngotracheitis virus (Bagust et al. 1986; Hughes et al. 1991; Williams et al. 1992) and duck viral enteritis (Shawky and Schat 2002). Peripheral blood lymphocytes of storks are, in addition to the trigeminal ganglia, the site of prolonged virus persistence (Kaleta and Kummerfeld 1986).

Environmental Limitations

Natural dispersal and also migration of birds limit the horizontal spread within a susceptible population. Gathering on feeding grounds or use of common sources of drinking water and any other aggregation of wild birds results in accumulation of excreted HV and enhances the likelihood for horizontal, predominantly aerogenic infections. Ultraviolet radiation by sunlight along with elevated temperatures and low humidity results in reduction or inactivation of infectivity of HV in the natural habitats of birds. Common surface disinfectants containing organic acids, aldehydes, glyoxal, and tensides inactivate the infectivity of avian HV at concentrations of 0.5% within 30 minutes at room temperature (Wagner 1993).

Prevalence and Intensity

There is little if any reliable data published from field studies on the prevalence and intensity of HV-associated infections. In general, wild birds kept in captivity, including rehabilitation or breeding centers for future release, are more likely to have outbreaks than are free-living populations.

CLINICAL SIGNS

Several major obstacles make it difficult to record signs of disease in free-living wild birds: (a) observed affected birds tend to "hide" their signs of disease; (b) sick birds may hide themselves to escape predation and consequently escape observation; (c) birds that are active only during evening twilight, such as owls, sit immobile during daytime and cannot be properly observed during darkness; (d) detailed and prolonged monitoring of individuals within larger groups of birds is difficult to perform unless several observers or video recording or other technical aids are available; (e) single birds are difficult to follow unless they are individually marked; (f) small, gregarious birds living normally in brushlands or in high trees can disappear from the examined groups without being noticed; (g) predators may easily catch sick birds before final stages of disease are developed and noticed; (h) different organ systems might be involved during the progression of a disease, hampering recognition of the same bird by displayed signs.

The chronology of the development of signs is known only for a few thoroughly studied HV in some bird species. These signs may comprise a broad spectrum of signs ranging from nonspecific to almost pathognomonic (Table 3.2). In individual birds, signs may change from respiratory or enteric to neurological. Although the knowledge of clinical signs is scarce and often anecdotal or circumstantial, there are a few diseases caused by HV that can be recognized based on clinical signs.

Marek's disease (MD) has been recorded in both domestic fancy (hobby) and commercial hybrid chickens and in free-living jungle fowl (Weiss and Biggs 1972; Cho and Kenzy 1975) and in various breeds of Japanese Quail (*Coturnix coturnix japonica*) following contact exposure to MDV shedding chickens (Dutton et al. 1973). In chickens, several forms of disease develop after an incubation period of approximately four to 10 weeks. These include mostly unilateral lameness of wings or legs, aberrant vocalization, and dehydration and emaciation, which finally end in cachexia and death. In some of the older chickens, depigmentation of the iris associated with irregularly shaped pupils finally leads to panophthalmia and subsequent complete blindness. Also, multiple, palpable nodular tumors in the skin or internal organs may develop, which are associated with general deterioration of activity and health. Some birds remain subclinically infected and play a major role as latent carriers and in virus shedding and transmission to gallinaceus birds (Calnek and Witter 1997).

Colwell et al. (1973) isolated from kidneys of apparently healthy wild turkeys living in four geographic regions of Florida HV that were antigenetically indistinguishable from HV isolates obtained from domestic turkeys. None of the isolates caused disease in domestic turkeys (Witter and Schat 2003). However, the turkey is susceptible to virulent MD virus derived from chickens (Voelkel, 2003) and display anorexia, paleness and reduced growth rates (Coudert et al. 1995; Davidson et al. 1996; Pennycott and Venugopal 2002).

Infectious laryngotracheitis (ILT) is predominantly seen in adult domestic hybrid chickens and in fancier chickens, Indian Peafowl, Guineafowl, and various species of pheasants (Bagust and Guy 1997; Kaleta and Redmann 1997). The highest losses occur in pheasants of the genera *Chrysolophus, Crossoptilon, Lophophorus, Syrmaticus,* and *Argusianus.* Mild respiratory or no signs develop in pheasants of the genera *Gennaeus, Hierophasis,* and *Phasianus.* It is noteworthy that such signs of disease and mortality are seen not only after exposure to virulent field strains of ILT virus but also after vaccination with or deliberate exposure to licensed attenuated live vaccines (Kaleta and Redmann 1997). The term "attenuated" of the vaccinal ILT virus applies only to the domestic chickens and not to any other avian species (Crawshaw and Boycott 1982; Kaleta and Redmann 1997).

The acute form of ILT is characterized by severe tracheal rales and bloody discharge from the beak and nostrils. Mortality is due to suffocation and/or bacterial and fungal complications (Kaleta and Redmann 1997). The chronic form of ILT is associated with general weakness, inflammation of the sinus infraorbitales, serous nasal discharge, and slightly increased mortality (Bagust and Guy 1997).

Pacheco's parrot disease (PPD) was first described near Sao Paulo, Brazil, in free-ranging Amazon parrots (Pacheco and Bier 1930). As a consequence of international trade in trapped psittacine birds, the disease is now diagnosed worldwide in bird collections, zoos, and breeding and trading centers (Kaleta et al. 1980c; Gerlach 1994; Ritchie 1995; Magnino et al. 1996; Phalen 1997; Steinke and Mundt 1997). The sources of infection are in most cases newly introduced, latently infected carriers and prolonged shedders, which appear to be relatively resistant to disease. These are, in particular, South American conures (Phalen 1997) such as the Patagonian Conure (*Cyanoliseus patagonus*), Nanday

Table 3.2. Predominant clinical signs for recognized herpesviruses diseases of birds and routes of HV excretion. (For the predominant host species for each disease, see Table 3.1.)

Disease or Infection	Predominant Clinical Signs	Routes of Virus Excretion	Comments
Marek's disease and Turkey HV infection	Neurologic, respiratory signs, tumors in skin	Feather follicle epithelium	Enhanced HV excretion during moulting
Infectious Laryngo-tracheitis in Guineafowl Indian Peafowl and some pheasants	Increased mortality, respiratory signs, conjunctivitis, suffocation possible	Bloody discharge from nostrils and beak	Pronounced respiratory rales, signs of suffocation
Pacheco's parrot disease (PPD)	Lethargy, increased mortality, papilloma in pharynx, cloaca, yellow-greenish feces	Feces, discharge from pharynx, growing feather quills	Wide-spread, enzootic disease in captive psittacine birds
Smadel's disease of columbiform birds	Increased squab mortality, in adults: sialiths in palate mucosa	Crop-milk, pharynx excretions with *Trichomonas* sp. Likely	Enhanced HV shedding during brooding of squabs, coinfection
Hepatosplenitis of owls	Enhanced mortality, pharyngitis	Pharynx excretions, feces	Only in owls with orange or yellow iris
Barn owl HV infection	Enhanced mortality	Unknown	
Inclusion body hepatitis of falcons and eagles	Sudden mortality, Lethargy, enteritis	Unknown	Some birds received HV positive pigeons as prey
Lake Victoria cormorant HV	Unknown	Unknown	
Inclusion body disease in cranes	Enhanced mortality, enteritis, lethargy	Feces	
Northern Bobwhite HV infection	Enhanced mortality, lethargy	Feces	
Black and White Stork HV infection, also in Abdim's Stork	Subclinical infections frequent, sudden mortality without previous signs, vomiting, hypothermia, diphtheric white plaques on choanae, occasionally hemorrhagic enteritis	Feces likely	Long-term viremia in captive and free-living storks
Toucan HV infection	Sudden death, decreased appetite	Unknown	Contact to macaws, which died on PPD
Tragopan HV infection	Sudden death	Unknown	
Passeriform HV infections	Subclinical infections frequent, sudden mortality, conjunctivitis, CNS involvement, severe respiratory distress, enteritis	Pharynx, feces	Latency is frequent, differentiation from canary poxvirus necessary

Conures (*Nandayus nenday*), and possibly also Blue-crowned (*Aratinga acuticaudata*) and Maroon-bellied Conures (*Pyrrhura frontalis*).

Horizontal infection of healthy psittacine birds is likely because birds that recently returned from trade fairs or exhibitions may develop the disease and become the source of virus for lateral spread to susceptible psittacine birds. The incubation period in natural outbreaks appears to be highly variable, but reliable estimates indicate periods between four to 10 days. The disease affects birds of any age and sex. Mortality may reach 30 to 50% of all psittacines (Kaleta 1990; Gómez-Villamandos et al. 1991; Gerlach 1994; Ritchie 1995; Phalen 1997; Kaleta 1999). However, differences in morbidity and mortality rates among species have been noted. Macaws, amazons, cockatoos, and African Gray Parrots (*Psittacus erithacus*) are highly susceptible. The disease begins usually with nonspecific signs such as lethargy, ruffled feathers, and reduced food intake. More prominent signs are yellowish or light-green watery feces. Mortality begins after a short period of illness of less than one to three days. As a late sequelae, reconvalescent birds may develop papilloma-like tumors in the cloaca and in the pharyngeal region (Phalen 1997; Johne et al. 2002; Styles et al. 2004, 2005).

Differences in morbidity and mortality rates in psittacine birds between natural outbreaks do not necessarily reflect differences in virulence of the involved virus or species-associated susceptibility. Dose, route of infection, and host-associated factors (general health and immune status, age, concomitant subclinical infections, sexual and environmental stress) have a bearing on the severity of signs and lesions and on the rates of mortality.

Experimental transmission studies with well-defined herpesviruses preparations are rare (Ritchie 1995). In addition, birds used in these studies might be of variable origin and of uncertain health and immune status. Thus, only circumstantial evidence suggests differences in virulence of the HV isolates studied so far, and the same is likely true for apparent differences in susceptibility of psittacine birds to infection.

Smadel's disease (pigeon herpesviruses infection) is presently seen world wide in any breed of young squabs or immunocompromised adult pigeons (Vindevogel and Duchatel 1997; Raue et al. 2005). Subclinical infections are present in almost every racing and fancier pigeon loft, whereas pigeon HV is less frequently found in free-living and urban pigeons (Toro et al. 1999). Infected squabs appear weak, do not grow, display extended abdomens, and die as emaciated nestlings. The immunosuppressive circovirus (Todd 2000) may aggravate signs, losses, and lesions (Abadie et al. 2001; Raue et al. 2005) Forms of the disease in adult pigeons are less frequently seen. Such pigeons have a history of poor performance during flight or beauty competitions, suffer from parasite infections, and have occasional respiratory or enteric problems (Steinmetz 1995). Small, solid, greyish foci, termed sialiths by Zwart et al. (1983), develop close to the palate's choanal cleft.

The eagle and falcon HV were detected for the first time in North America (Ward et al. 1971, Mare and Graham 1973, 1975; Kocan et al. 1977; Potgieter et al. 1979; Docherty et al. 1983) and subsequently in several European countries (Blandford and Keymer 1987; Sallmann 1991; Villforth 1995, Sander 1995). Signs are mostly nonspecific and may consist of lethargy, regurgitation, loss of body weight, and diarrhea. The duration of the disease varies between several hours and a few days. Falcon HV has also been isolated from clinically normal-appearing falcons (Sander 1995). Circumstantial evidence suggests that both HV associated subclinical infection and overt disease in eagles and in falcons occur infrequently (Heinrichs 1992, Villforth 1995; Sander 1995; Hatt et al. 1996; Heidenreich 1996; Morishita et al. 1997).

Owl Herpesviruses infection results in a highly lethal disease of owls first described by Green and Shillinger (1936) in the U.S.A. and later in Europe as "Hepatosplenitis infectiosa strigum, HSiS" by Burtscher (1965) and Schettler (1969). The isolate from Schettler was characterized by Lee et al. (1972) in more detail and found to be different from five other avian herpesviruses (Marek's disease virus, turkey herpesviruses, laryngotracheitis virus, Lake Victoria cormorant virus, and duck enteritis virus). Clinical signs of the hepatosplenitis of owls are rather nonspecific. Northern Eagle Owls (Bubo bubo) display diphtheric lesions along the choanal cleft. These alterations are frequently super infected by *Trichomonas* spp. or bacteria (Figure 3.2).

Clinical illness in owls ranges between a few hours and a few days. Sudden losses in owls of the Genera *Bubo, Otus, Ketupa, Strix, Pulsatrix, Glaucidium, Athene, Aegolius,* and *Asio* are frequent, making the HSiS the most often diagnosed viral disease of owls. It has been frequently noted that only owls with a yellow to orange iris are susceptible to owl HV, whereas owls of the genus *Tyto* that have a brown iris appear to be resistant (Burtscher and Sibalin 1975; Heidenreich and Kaleta 1978). As a rare sequelae of a previous HV infection, a unilateral keratitis and conjunctivitis may develop; an example is depicted in Figure 3.3, which shows a Little Owl (*Athene noctua*) with a keratitis and conjunctivitis of one eye.

An HV possibly antigenetically unrelated to the "classical" HSiS viruses of Strigidae has been isolated from a Barn Owl (*Tyto alba*) in Germany (Glünder et al. 1991). Clinical signs consisted of lethargy, emaciation, and reluctance to move. A disease that was

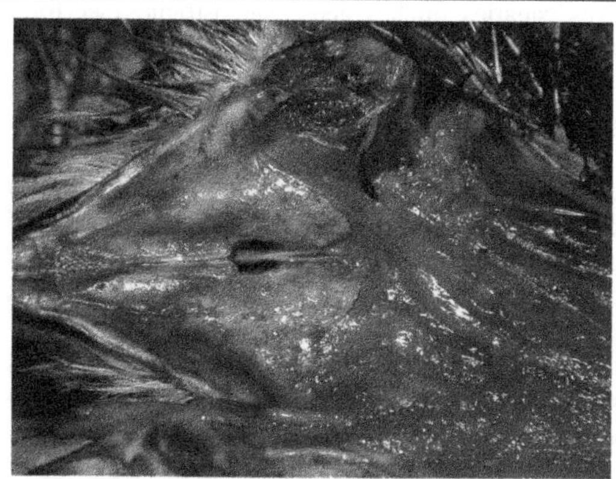

Figure 3.2. Wild-caught adult Northern Eagle Owl (*Bubo bubo*). Severe lesions of the palate mucosa on both sides of the choanal cleft. Swabs taken from the lesion yielded both a herpesviruses and *Trichomonas* spp., following cultivation in CEF cultures.

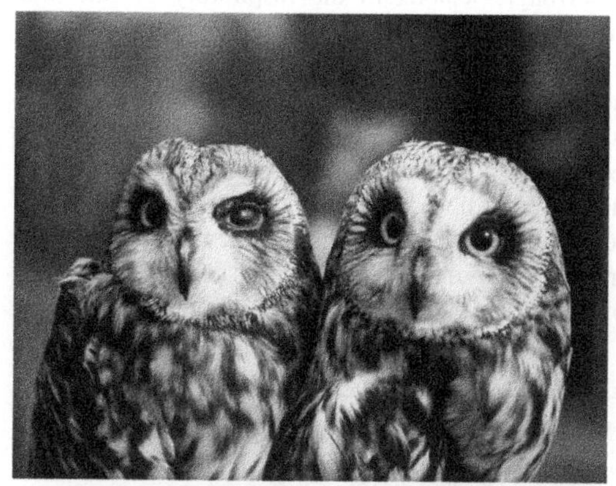

Figure 3.3. Pair of captive Little Owls (*Athene noctua*). The bird on the left displays a keratitis on its left eye. HV was isolated in CEF cultures from the swab that was taken from the cornea and conjunctiva of the affected eye.

similar in signs, gross pathology, histology, and electron microscopy was described by Gómez-Villamandos et al. (1995) in Barn Owls (*Tyto alba*) in southern Spain. The cormorant HV was isolated only once from a nestling Little Pied Cormorant in New South Wales, Australia, by French et al. (1973). No information was provided in that report on signs of disease. Subsequent studies in other regions have so far yielded no further isolations from birds of the genus *Phalacrocorax* (Kaleta 1998). Gómez-Villamoandos et al. (1998) mention a cormorant (*Phalacrocorax* sp. of unidentified species) in conjunction with a large HV-induced die-off in American White Storks (*Ciconia ciconia*) but provide no details on signs and lesions.

The crane HV were first isolated in Austria (Burtscher and Grünberg 1975) from livers and spleens of dead Sudan Crowned and Demoisselle Cranes (*Balearica pavonina* and *Anthropoides virgo*). These birds were anorexic, had diarrhea, and separated from each other and sat on their hock joints with closed eyes.

In March of 1978 a captive crane mortality event due to a HV occurred in Wisconsin, U.S.A. The mortality occurred in a crowded nonbreeder population and involved Sandhill (*Gurus (G.) Canadensis),* Japanese (*G. japonensis),* Hooded (*G. monacha*) and Stanley (*Anthropoides paradisea*) Cranes (Docherty and Henning, 1980). This nonbreeder population also included Saurus (*G. antigone*), Common (*G. grus*), Brolga (*G. rubicunda*), White-naped (*G. vipio*), and Desmoiselle (*Anthropoides virgo*) Cranes. Cold, wet, and crowded conditions may have precipitated the event. A subsequent serologic follow-up to the outbreak (Docherty and Romaine 1983) revealed that exposure to the HV may have occurred in 1975 (approximately 2 1/2 years before the event), that preexisting antibody may have allowed individual cranes to survive, and that crane host reaction may vary by species. American Coots (*Fulica americana*) and young Pekin ducklings were experimentally susceptible to infection with this isolate, whereas white leghorn chicks and Muscovy Ducks were resistant (Docherty and Henning 1980).

In France and Germany, Förster et al. (1989) isolated HVs from Demoiselle Cranes, and in Japan, Suzuki et al. (1997) cultured a HV from a Japanese Crane (*Grus japonensis*). Affected species belonged to the genera *Grus* in the U.S.A. and Japan, and *Anthropoides* and *Balearica* in Europe. The sudden appearance of the crane herpesviruses at almost the same time in various areas of the world raises many questions regarding the identity and modes of spread of these isolates. The development of a monoclonal antibody to crane HV that can be used in immunohistochemical studies and in a competitive ELISA may have value in further characterizing the crane HV and lead to a better understanding of its natural history (Letchworth et al. 1997).

HV was isolated from Northern Bobwhite from a single epizootic in Europe with high mortality that was preceded by nonspecific signs of disease (Kaleta et al. 1980a). The quail isolate and the crane HVs obtained from France and Austria cross neutralize *in vitro* (Förster et al. 1989) and yield strikingly similar but not identical bands in agarose gels after digestion of purified DNAs with the restriction enzymes BamH I, EcoR I, Sal I, Hind III, and Kpn I (Günther et al. 1997).

Reports on clinical signs in Black Storks (*Ciconia nigra*) and American White Storks from Germany (Kaleta and Kummerfeld 1983; 1986 and Kaleta et al. 1983) are restricted to lethargy and anorexia a few days prior to death. However, most of the HV isolates were obtained from peripheral blood leukocytes of storks that were clinically normal but remained viremic for years (Kaleta and Kummerfeld 1986).

Clinical signs in three- to four-month-old American White Storks and in White-bellied Storks (*Ciconia abdimii*) of various ages ranged from sudden death to general depression, lack of appetite, drooping wings, and in some cases hemorrhagic diarrhea (Gómez-Villamandos et al. 1998). An HV from a tragopan (unknown species, subfamily Gallinae of the order Phasianiformes) has been characterized by Günther et al. (1997), but data on signs were not mentioned.

Charlton et al. (1990) discovered an HV in a toucan (Order Piciformes but unidentified species) that was ill and had decreased appetite. The bird had contact with psittacine birds suffering from PPD. Additional details were not available.

Numerous HV have been isolated from various bird families of the order Passeriformes, which comprises more than 4,000 bird species. The HV-positive birds were either found dead or in the final stages of disease. Clinical signs in these birds typically consisted of respiratory distress and soft droppings. Several isolations were also made from clinically healthy birds. The families involved were Estrildae, Paridae, Ploceidae, Serinidae, and Lampronidae (Blumenstein 1993; Gravendyck 1996; Kaleta 1998).

PATHOGENESIS

In contrast to detailed *in vitro* and *in vivo* pathogenicity studies in domestic birds, virtually nothing is known about the genesis of lesions in free-living birds. Extrapolations and vague assumptions of analogies are necessary to interpret disease development and the final outcome of natural infections in free-ranging birds (Ramis et al. 1996).

Because many healthy birds remain viremic or persistently infected for prolonged periods of time, it can be concluded that some often undetermined stress factors, internal or environmental, must alter the host-virus balance to allow the development of clinical signs followed by the development of lesions and mortality (Ritchie 1995; Ramis et al. 1996; Phalen 1997). This concept of stress-induced disease in latently infected wild birds appears to be reasonable, but experimental proof does not yet exist. Several reports describe concurrent infections with immunosuppressive circoviruses in psittacines, pigeons, Laughing (Senegal) Doves, canaries, finches, geese, and ostriches (see Todd 2000). The detrimental immunosuppressive effect of natural circovirus infections has been demonstrated in pigeons (Raue et al. 2005).

Most dead birds likely die during the viremic phase of the disease, and HV can be isolated from most tissues including bone marrow. Gravendyck et al. (1998) examined 52 different tissues obtained from 18 dead psittacine birds from a spontaneous die-off of Pacheco's parrot disease and found them HV positive with the exceptions of feather vanes and pancreas. Similar studies and analogous results were obtained in other bird species (Kaleta 1998).

PATHOLOGY

Gross Pathology

Because the duration of overt disease is in most cases short, the birds are generally in good bodily condition, and muscle development and fat tissue deposits are normal. The most prominent pathological lesions can be grouped into three categories. These include: (a) hemorrhagic lesions in the respiratory or intestinal tracts. For example, gallinaceous birds with ILT develop a necrotizing and often hemorrhagic tracheitis and waterfowl dead of duck plague (duck virus enteritis) often have ring-like hemorrhagic and subsequently necrotic lesions of annular bands in the small intestine and pin-point hemorrhages, ulceration, and erosion of the mucosa of the esophagus; (b) necrotic lesions in the large parenchymal organs such as liver (Figure 3.4), spleen, kidney, and bone marrow and pharynx. The

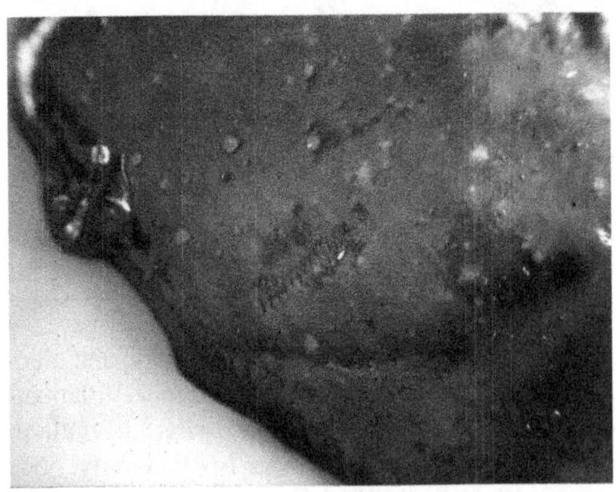

Figure 3.4. Liver from a wild-caught Northern Eagle Owl (*Bubo bubo*) (different bird from that shown in Figure 3.2), demonstrating multiple pinpoint white foci of necrosis on the outer surface caused by owl herpesviruses.

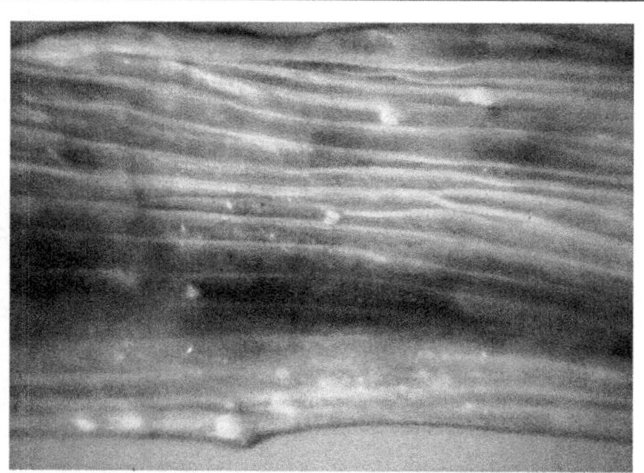

Figure 3.5. Northern Eagle Owl (same bird as in Figure 3.2) with multiple focal areas of necrosis along the longitudinal folds of the esophagus caused by owl herpesviruses.

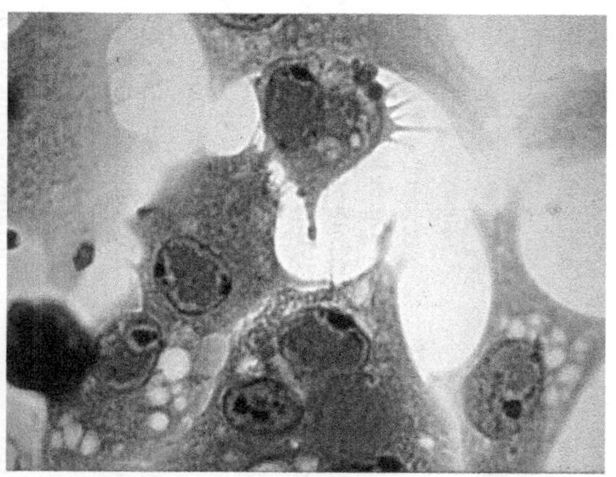

Figure 3.6. Chicken embryo fibroblast coverslip culture that was inoculated with an HV obtained from a Northern Eagle Owl and stained with H & E. Note intranuclear inclusions that are surrounded by a clear halo.

examination of bone marrow is often overlooked at necropsy. In addition, small necrotic foci are apparent along the longitudinal folds of the esophagus in some species such as the Northern Eagle Owl, shown in Figure 3.5; (c) neoplastic lesions in parenchymal organs and nerves of chickens affected with Marek's disease. Table 3.3 summarizes the most prevalent lesions in a variety of avian species.

Microscopic Pathology

All avian herpesviruses induce focal necrosis in parenchymal organs and intranuclear inclusion bodies of Cowdry type A in infected tissues and cell cultures (Figure 3.6). These lesions may occur in any large parenchymal organs (liver, spleen, kidney) and in epithelial cells of the respiratory and digestive tracts (Table 3.3). Necrotic lesions in visceral organs are usually focal and acute, with little or no inflammatory response. Epithelial cells within or adjacent to necrotic foci may contain intranuclear inclusion bodies.

Hemorrhagic lesions in the upper respiratory tract consist initially of loss of ciliated epithelium and focally detached respiratory epithelium, and progress to submucosal hemorrhage and occasionally to secondary infections with bacteria, fungi, and yeasts. Epithelial cells may contain intranuclear inclusion bodies.

Electron Microscopy

Viral particles with morphologic characteristics of herpesviruses can be detected in ultrathin sections of tissues containing focal necrosis and in infected cells with inclusion bodies adjacent to the areas of necrosis. Occasionally, single virus particles are scattered throughout the cytoplasm of these cells (Ramis et al. 1992, 1994, 1996; Gómez-Villamandos et al. 1995).

DIAGNOSIS

Diagnostic laboratories use one or more of the following criteria to establish a diagnosis of herpesviruses: (a) replication in chicken embryos with subsequent development of lesions such as stunted embryos, necrotic alterations in liver and spleen, and pock formation on the chorio-allantoic membrane; (b) replication in cell cultures of avian origin with the formation of cytopathic effects such as the development of round refractile cells or small syncytia; (c) sensitivity of the isolate to treatment with lipid solvents such as chloroform or ether; (d) inhibition but not complete prevention of virus replication by halogenated desoxyribonucleosides such as iodo- or bromodeoxyuridine; (e) lack of agglutination of infectious allantoic fluids or cell culture supernatants with chicken red blood cells; (f) negative contrast electron microscopy (Kaleta 1998).

Diagnosis on the basis of clinical signs (Table 3.2) is at best suggestive but not pathognomonic for any HV-induced disease. Exceptions are palpable tumors of the skin and large tumors in the viscera in cases of MD in chickens, bloody oronasal discharge in pheasants, guinea fowl, or pea fowl that are affected with ILT, and the tiny sialiths in the palate mucosa of pigeons with Smadel's disease.

Gross pathology may support suspicions made on clinical grounds as in cases of MD and ILT (Eskens et al. 1994), but in these cases as well as birds presented with necrotic lesions, further diagnostic work is needed for confirmation (Table 3.3).

Histological detection of intranuclear inclusions is suggestive of a herpesviruses etiology but needs

Table 3.3. Diseases caused by avian Herpesviruses: macroscopic and microscopic lesions and differential diagnosis.

Disease or Infection	Gross Pathology	Histopathology	Differential Diagnosis
Marek's disease	Emacination, enlarged peripheral nerves, tumors in many organs	Lymphocyte infiltration of nerve tissue, lymphoid-cell tumors	Tumors due to avian retroviruses, tumors of unknown etiology
Infectious laryngotracheits	Anemia, blood clots in trachea, lung	Detached respiratory epithelium, hemorrhages, intranuclear inclusions in epithelial cells	Newcastle disease, highly pathogenic avian influenza, infectious bronchitis, respiratory toxins
Pacheco's parrot disease (PPD)	Enlarged liver, spleen, kidney, hemorrhagic enteritis, pale bone marrow, papillomas in pharynx and cloaca	Focal necrosis in liver, spleen, kidney, bone marrow, intranuclear inclusions	Any cause of increased mortality, enteric or systemic infections, chlamydiosis, aspergillosis
Smadel's disease of columbiform birds	Squabs: anorexia, enlarged liver, spleen, kidney. Adults: pharyngitis	Squabs and adults: necrosis and lymphocytic infiltrates in liver, spleen, kidney, intranuclear inclusions	Trichomononiasis, spironucleosis, bacterial infections: salmonellosis, pasteurellosis
Hepatosplenitis of owls	Anemia, enlarged liver, spleen, kidney, pale bone marrow, external and intestinal and renal parasites	Necrosis in liver, spleen, kidney, bone marrow, intranuclear inclusions, developmental stages of renal coccidia	Trauma due to crashes, shot projectiles, intestinal coccidiosis, tuberculosis, pasteurellosis
Barn owl HV infection	Anemia, enlarged liver, spleen, kidney, pale bone marrow	Necrosis in liver, spleen, kidney, bone marrow, intranuclear inclusions	Trauma due to crashes, bacterial infections, aspergillosis
Inclusion body hepatitis of falcons and eagles	Anemia, emacination, enlarged liver, spleen, kidney	Necrosis in liver, spleen, kidneys, intranuclear inclusions	Trauma due to crashes, shot, fungal and bacterial infections
Lake Victoria cormorant HV infection	Unknown	Unknown	Unknown
Inclusion body disease of cranes	Enlarged liver, spleen, kidney, enteritis	Necrosis in liver, spleen, kidneys, intranuclear inclusions	Fungal infections, poisons, bacterial infections
Northern Bobwhite HV infection	Enlarged liver and spleen with whitish foci, ulcerative enteritis	Multiple necrosis, perivascular lymphocytic infiltrates	Aviadenovirus of serotype 1, (Quail bronchitis) clostridial infection, intestinal parasites
Black and white stork HV infections	Enlarged liver, spleen, pharyngitis, pale bone marrow	Necrosis in liver and spleen, intranuclear inclusions	Trauma, shot, bacterial and fungal infections
Toucan HV infection	Liver and spleen enlarged, liver yellow and friable, enteritis	Hepatocellular necrosis, marginated chromatin, intranuclear inclusions	Pacheco's parrot disease, chlamydiosis
Tragopan HV infection	Unknown	Unknown	Unknown
Passeriform HV infections	Poor bodily condition, pharyngitis, hyperemic lung, enteritis	Hemorrhages in trachea, lung, intranuclear inclusions	Canary poxvirus infection, yersiniosis, listeriosis, salmonellosis, coccidiosis

discrimination from other viral infections (adenoviruses, parvoviruses, and circoviruses) that also produce intranuclear inclusion bodies (Ramis et al. 1992).

The method of choice, the "gold standard," for an accurate diagnosis is virus isolation and subsequent characterization. The criteria for the selection of the appropriate tissue for virus isolation depends on the virus and bird species involved and on whether live or dead birds are to be tested (Kaleta 1998). In sick, healthy, and even dead birds in the viremic stage, blood containing feather quills can be pulled and the content used as an inoculum (Gravendyck et al. 1998). From dead birds, approximately 10% (w/v) homogenates from tissues containing focal lesions in parenchymal organs can be used.

Various cell cultures of avian origin, namely chicken embryo fibroblast (CEF) monolayers or cultures prepared from chicken embryo livers or kidneys are suitable and are the most promising route for virus isolation attempts. The cytopathic effect will develop within one week and consist of roundish refractile single cells or small syncytia in focal arrangement. Altered cells will subsequently detach and lyse.

Egg inoculation in 10-day-old embryonated chicken eggs via the chorioallantoic membrane (CAM) is performed in some laboratories. Within one week post infection, lesions will develop on the CAM and also in the embryo. The inoculated CAM will contain white foci of variable size (Figure 3.7). Confirmation of the viral etiology is achieved by histological detection of intranuclear inclusions and/or in ultrathin sections by electron microscopy. The examination of the embryo will reveal focal necrosis mainly in the liver and spleen but also in the mucosa of the palate bone.

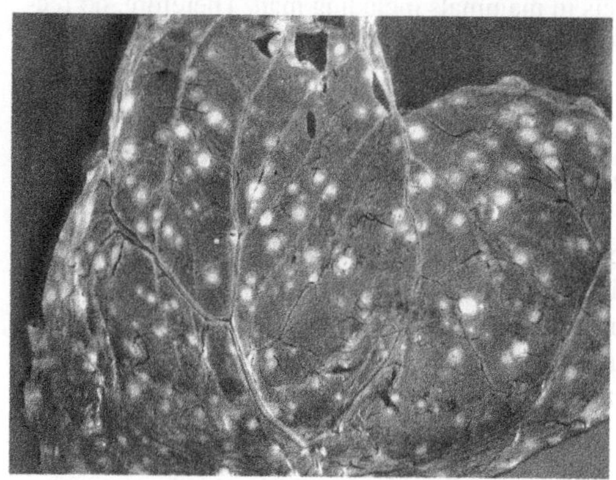

Figure 3.7. Chorioallantoic membrane of a chicken embryo inoculated with an HV from the Northern Eagle Owl shown in Figure 3.2. Multiple pox-like lesions of different sizes are visible throughout the ectodermal layer of the membrane.

Following inoculation of embryos with material from pigeons, falcons, or owls, a diphtheric pharyngitis is also visible (Sallmann 1991). The inoculation of embryos with separated blood leukocytes obtained from live birds results also in pock-like lesions.

Verification of the HV is achieved by determining viral properties that are easily performed *in vitro*, or by PCR using degenerate consensus primers (VanDevanter et al. 1996). Initial investigations include tests for chloroform sensitivity and inhibition of CPE formation by cultivating infected cultures in the presence of halogenated desoxyribonucleosides such as bromin- or iodine-desoxyribonucleoside. HV do not agglutinate chicken erythrocytes. Partially purified and concentrated supernatant fluids from heavily infected cell cultures yield upon negative staining and electron microscopic examination single or groups of particles with HV morphology (Figure 3.1). These include an envelope of variable diameter and a capsid and capsomers consistent with all members of the family herpesviridae. Negative staining of cell-culture-grown HV is possible, but due to the generally low number of viral particles, false negative results are likely.

In recent years, several PCRs were developed for rapid and specific detection of avian HV. VanDevanter et al. (1996) and Ehlers et al. (1999) described a consensus primer PCR targeted to the herpesviral DNA polymerase that uses degenerative primers in a nested format. Tomaszewski et al. (2001) used partially sequenced psittacine HVs and constructed several primer sets. These authors concluded that psittacine HVs consist of generically heterogeneous subpopulations that form at least four genotypes (Tomaszewski et al. 2003, 2004).

The detection of serum antibodies in neutralization tests with the homologous virus is possible for all HV. The presence of antibodies confirms previous exposure or vaccination. Negative results of antibody testing should be carefully interpreted (Kaleta and Druener 1976). No detectable antibody titer means (a) erroneous testing with a heterologous, antigenetically unrelated HV, (b) no exposure to HV, and (c) no antibody synthesis occurred following exposure or vaccination. It should also be noted that no straightforward correlation exists between antibody titers and the degree of protection.

Differential Diagnoses

Any case needs a complete and thoroughly performed necropsy examination, checks for external and internal (including blood) parasites, and subsequent laboratory examinations. The latter should include plating of tissues for bacteria, yeasts, and fungi, a complete set of tissues for histology, and several organs (skin and blood containing feather quills, brain, respiratory organs, liver, spleen, kidney, cecal tonsils, cloacal content) for virus isolation attempts.

Major causes of diseases that appear to be similar to that caused by HV are listed in Table 3.3. It is obvious that the differential diagnoses vary from bird to bird species. Common to almost all free-living birds are the agents causing psittacosis or ornithosis (chlamydiosis; Kaleta and Taday 2003). Work with dead birds needs special precautions for this reason because chlamydiosis is a zoonotic disease.

Almost all birds are susceptible to avian paramyxovirus 1 (PMV1), the cause of Newcastle disease in domestic and free-living birds (Kaleta and Baldauf 1988; Lierz et al. 2002). Avian influenza A viruses are frequently isolated from diseased or latently infected wild birds (Hergarten 1994). Hemorrhages in intestines including proventriculus, respiratory tract, and internal organs can be caused by velogenic Newcastle disease virus (Alexander 1997) and highly pathogenic avian influenza A viruses (Easterday et al. 1997). On occasion, avian adenovirus of group II (Massi et al. 1993) and a number of toxic substances, trauma, or mycotoxins (Olson et al. 1995; Mikaelian et al. 1997; Hoffman et al. 1998; Hoerr 1997; Julian and Brown 1997) can induce hemorrhages and macroscopic lesions similar to HV infections.

HV-induced necrotic foci in parenchymatous organs are macroscopically similar to granulomatous and necrotizing lesions caused by bacterial diseases such as salmonellosis, listeriosis, campylobacteriosis, pasteurellosis, and tuberculosis (Scope 1999). The North American strain of West Nile virus can produce a hepatosplenitis in some species of owls that is indistinguishable macroscopically from owl herpesviruses (Gancz et al. 2004).

In passeriform birds, the lung manifestation of poxvirus infection (Bolte et al. 1999) may produce similar clinical signs, high rates of mortality, and macroscopic lesions as would infection with the Serinid HV-1. In one outbreak, Serinid HV-1 was isolated from young canaries, which were vaccinated against pox yet developed signs like the pulmonary form of canary pox. The supposedly poorly vaccinated birds were in fact suffering from an HV infection (Kaleta, unpubl. data).

IMMUNITY

Most birds that recover from an HV-induced disease and also latently infected birds have detectable humoral antibodies. However, these serum antibodies do not in all cases protect against recurrent disease, and some recovered birds have only low levels or no detectable serum antibodies (Ritchie 1995; Phalen 1997). Thus, antibody assays have little merit in detecting previous exposure or evaluating immunity. However, neutralization tests are useful for antigenic differentiation of various HV isolates (Kaleta et al. 1980b).

So far, attenuated live virus vaccines have been developed only for the successful control of Marek's disease, infectious laryngotracheitis in chickens, and duck viral enteritis in anatiform birds. No attenuated live virus containing vaccine is available for the control of any of the HV in free-living or caged birds. The detection of a plaque variant of low pathogenicity within a wild-type of a pigeon HV isolate (Sallmann 1991) may make it a promising vaccine virus candidate.

Noninfected psittacine birds can be protected against infection by formol-inactivated adjuvanted vaccines (Kaleta and Brinkmann 1993; Ritchie 1995). Because differences in antigenicity of psittacine HV are well established (Krautwald et al. 1988; Horner et al. 1992; Gravendyck et al. 1996; Phalen 1997; Günther et al. 1997; Tomaszewski et al. 2001), the autogenous vaccines provide best protection against the homologous virus. However, it needs to be admitted that detailed chronologic follow-up studies to determine the duration and degree of immunity in terms of resistance to challenge in various psittacine birds have not been performed.

PUBLIC HEALTH CONCERNS

None of the known avian HVs are transmissible to mammals. No report in the scientific literature contains data linking avian HV to any adverse health effects in mammals including man. Therefore, no recognizable public health concerns exist.

DOMESTIC ANIMAL HEALTH CONCERNS

It is possible that Marek's disease HVs could be transmitted from Red and Ceylon Jungle Fowl (*Gallus gallus* and *Gallus lafayettei*) to domestic chickens and vice versa. However, no report on such an event is available (Calnek and Witter 1997). Virulent field virus and also attenuated live infectious laryngotracheitis virus can spread from free-living pheasants, Common Peafowl (*Pavo cristatus*), and Helmeted Guineafowl (*Numida meleagris*) to domestic chickens, and possibly also to domestic and free-living Northern Bobwhite because all these birds are susceptible to infection and develop severe forms of disease (Kaleta and Redmann 1997).

Docherty and Henning (1980) have shown that the U.S.A. crane HV isolate is transmissible to and causes mortality in white Pekin ducklings and adult American Coots. In contrast, white leghorn chicks and Muscovy Ducks were resistant to experimental infection. This important example demonstrates that at least the crane HV that originated from wild birds can cause disease in domestic birds.

Due to the generally anticipated narrow host range of most of the other HV, horizontal spread from free-living to domestic birds seems unlikely.

WILDLIFE POPULATION IMPACTS

Evidence suggests that the HV causing Pacheco's parrot disease was originally restricted to psittacine birds in South America (Pacheco and Bier 1930; Simpson et al. 1975). Due to increasing intercontinental transport of birds, the psittacine HV has been spread globally, and these viruses have been detected in many species of psittacine birds that have their original habitat in continents other than South America (Gerlach 1994; Ritchie 1995; Phalen 1997).

Wildlife monitoring in Australia has not provided evidence that wild and captive cockatoos and other psittacine birds have been exposed to psittacine HV (Raidal et al. 1998). Appropriate evidence from other continents is either lacking or inconclusive. However, the possibility of HV to spread from exotic captive psittacines to indigenous birds does exist.

In Europe, several attempts were made to repopulate at least some areas with captive-bred Northern Eagle Owls (*Bubo bubo*). These trials met for many years with failure until all candidates for release were tested for the presence of owl HV and only the serologically negative birds used for release (Barkhoff 1987). Since that decision, the free-living population of *Bubo bubo* is well established and expanding.

Pigeons persistently infected with HV (Vindevogel and Pastoret 1993; Johannknecht et al. 2000) were repeatedly incriminated as a source of disease in eagles, falcons, and owls (Ritchie 1995; Phalen 1997). Epidemiological data and circumstantial evidence (close time-effect relationship) indicate that birds of prey may contract the HV by ingestion of HV-infected pigeons. However, more recent evidence from molecular studies provided data that indicate that not all pigeon HV are identical with HV obtained from eagles, falcons, and owls (Aini et al. 1993; Günther et al. 1997). Further molecular studies on HV isolates from pigeons used as prey and affected/diseased birds of prey are needed to clarify this important issue. If no other sources of food are available for birds of prey, pigeon carcasses should be fed with the head removed. Because healthy appearing pigeons harbor latent HV in trigeminal ganglia and pharynx, feeding of pigeons without the head would clearly reduce the risk of HV transmission.

It appears from the available information that none of the HV discussed in this chapter threatens well-established populations of free-ranging birds. On the other hand, the possibility should be considered that a viral infection and simultaneous occurrence of detrimental environmental factors will have an impact on the number of birds and on the degree of their dispersion. Separation of viral versus environmental effects on the bird's health status might be difficult to determine.

TREATMENT AND CONTROL

No licensed drugs are available for the treatment of HV-induced diseases in domestic and free-living birds. However, the compounds acyclovir and gancyclovir, which are recommended for the treatment of cutaneous herpetic lesions in people (Hirsch et al. 1997), may be tried. Northon et al. (1991) were able to reduce overall morbidity and mortality with acyclovir in Quaker Parakeets. Data on the use of this drug to treat or to prevent overt disease following exposure have been in some cases encouraging and in other cases disappointing. The recommended oral dose is 80 mg/kg body weight three times a day followed by 25 mg/kg intramuscularly for one day, and thereafter for about one week 1 mg/kg orally in drinking water or mixed in food.

Studies on the effect of acyclovir on the inhibition of HV multiplication in cell cultures demonstrate great differences in sensitivity between several HV isolates (Thiry et al. 1983). Experimental data confirms the existence of these differences in the sensitivity of various isolates to the action of acyclovir *in vitro* (Kaleta unpubl. data).

A number of different chemical compounds such as caffeolylics and flavanoids yielded significant reductions in virus replication *in vitro* (Köenig and Dustmann 1985). Also, studies *in vitro* with various preparations that were purified from propolis that were collected from honey bees in North America, Asia, and Europe yielded significant rates in reduction of viral replication (Kaleta 1991). Further studies are needed to evaluate the effectiveness of these and other candidates for the treatment of diseased birds.

Autogenous vaccines were prepared and successfully used to control disease and mortality in outbreaks of Pacheco's parrot disease in captive psittacine birds (Kaleta and Bueno Brinkmann 1993) and in captive falcons (Wernery et al. 1999). These vaccines resulted in seroconversion and subsequent reduction of losses in vaccinated birds. However, well-designed vaccination and challenge experiments to test for safety/innocuity and potency—as in domestic birds—meet with several technical problems. Among others, birds for this type of experimentation need to be free of PPD and other ailments, need to be from the same avian species as the future target birds, and are expensive (Ritchie 1995, Wernery et al. 1999). However, one inactivated and adjuvanted PPD vaccine was licensed in the U.S.A. This vaccine contains a PPD virus that was originally isolated by Simpson et al. (1975) and is antigenetically related to isolates obtained from PPD outbreaks in Great Britain (Gough and Alexander 1993) and Germany (Schroeder-Gravendyck 1999). In view of the well established antigenic heterogeneity of psittacine HVs, a potent vaccine should be prepared from seed viruses representing all known PPD serotypes (Gravendyck et al. 1996; Tomaszewski et al. 2001, 2003, 2004; Johne et al. 2002). The best choice is at present to prepare autogenous vaccines from completely inactivated virus that was obtained from the same outbreak and an adjuvant that is well tolerated by the various vaccinees.

Attenuated live virus vaccines against HV-induced diseases of domestic birds such as Marek's disease, duck virus enteritis, and laryngotracheitis do not protect against challenge by any of the HV in free-living birds.

MANAGEMENT IMPLICATIONS

Ornithologists and avian pathologists of any specialization are aware of the fact that rather limited information is presently available on infectious diseases and their impact on bird life. Therefore, a comprehensive management plan directed to the following issues are of paramount importance:

a. Any diseased and dead bird should be thoroughly examined and the causes of death determined.
b. Only birds that have been proven to be free of infectious agents, HV in particular, should be prepared for release.
c. Publication of solid data and international exchange of information on experiences should be encouraged.
d. Following HV-associated mortality events in captive birds, the possibility of latent carriers among the survivors should be acknowledged. This possibility can be addressed through depopulation or quarantine.
e. Ring-banded birds that were vaccinated with an attenuated live virus should be released into the wild with great care. The attenuated virus may be shed into the environment and infect species for which it was not intended, with unknown possibly harmful consequences.
f. If a mortality event occurs in an area where large numbers of birds had aggregated, the area should be decontaminated if at all possible.

ACKNOWLEGEMENTS

The mentioned scientific names and those in English-American language are mostly identical with the names that the various authors provided in their publications. Some additional scientific names and occasionally in cases of discrepancies the names given here were obtained from J. F. Clements, *Birds of the World. A Checklist,* 5th Ed., Facts On File, Inc., New York City, New York, 1981, plus supplement provided by http://www.ibispub.com/updates.html, in June 2005.

The books published by C. G. Sibley and B. L. Monroe (1991, *Distribution and Taxonomy of Birds of the World,* Yale University Press) and H. E. Wolters (1975–1982, *Die Vogelarten der Erde,* Paul Parey, Hamburg and Berlin, 1982) were also consulted to solve some language queries.

The generous support of the libraries of the Justus-Liebig-Universität Giessen and the Stiftung tierärztliche Hochschule Hannover during retrieval of rather remote publications is gratefully acknowledged.

Last but not least, the staff members of the Clinique for Birds, Reptiles, Amphibians and Fish at the University of Giessen, Germany, in particular the valuable assistance of the veterinarians Brigitte M. Bönner and Sabine Jäger, is highly appreciated.

LITERATURE CITED

Abadie, J. F. Nguyen, C. Groizeleau, N. Amenna, B. Fernandez, C. Guereaud, L. Guigand, P. Robart, B. Lefebvre, and M. Wyers. 2001. Pigeon circovirus infection: pathological observations and suggested pathogenesis. *Avian Pathology* 30:149–158.

Aini, I., L.M. Shih, A.E. Castro, and Y.C. Zee. 1993. Comparison of herpesvirus isolates from falcons, pigeons and psittacines by restriction endonuclease analysis. *Journal of Wildlife Diseases* 29:196–202.

Alexander, D.J. 1997. Newcastle disease and other avian paramyxoviridae infections. In *Diseases of Poultry,* 10th Ed. B.W. Calnek, H.J. Barnes, C.W. Beard, L.R. McDougald, and Y.M. Saif (eds.). Iowa State University Press, Ames, Iowa, U.S.A., pp. 541–569.

Aristotle, 350 B.C.E. The history of animals. Translated by D'Arcy W. Thompson. http://classics.mit.edu/Aristotle/history_anim.html.

Bagust, T.J., B.W. Calnek, and K.J. Fahey. 1986. Gallid-1 herpesvirus infection in chicken. 3. Reinvestigation of the pathogenesis of infectious laryngotracheitis in acute and early post-acute respiratory disease. *Avian Diseases* 30:179–190.

Bagust, T.J., and J.S. Guy. 1997. Laryngotracheitis. In *Diseases of Poultry,* 10th Ed. B.W. Calnek, H.J. Barnes, C.W. Beard, L.R. McDougald, and Y.M. Saif (eds.). Iowa State University Press, Ames, Iowa, U.S.A., pp. 527–539.

Barkhoff, M. 1987. Die Krankheiten des Uhus (Bubo bubo) und ihre Bedeutung für die Wiedereinbürgerung in die Bundesrepublik Deutschland. Veterinary Medical Dissertation, Giessen, Germany, 203 pp.

Blandford, T.B., and I.F. Keymer. 1987. Inclusion body hepatitis in captive birds of prey (Falco spp.) in Great Britain. *Berichte der Internationalen Tagung über Zootiere* 29:97–100.

Blumenstein, V. 1993. Isolierung und biologische Eigenschaften von sechs neuen Herpesviren aus verschiedenen Sperlingsvögeln (Passeriformes). Veterinary Medical Dissertation, Giessen, Germany, 135 pp.

Bolte, A.L., J. Meurer, and E.F. Kaleta. 1999. Avian host spectrum of avipoxviruses. *Avian Pathology* 28: 415–432.

Burtscher, H. 1965. Die virusbedingte Hepatosplenitis infectiosa strigum. I. Mitteilung: Morphologische Untersuchungen. *Pathologia Veterinaria* 2:227–255.

Burtscher, H. 1968. Die virusbedingte Hepatosplenitis infectiosa strigum. II. Mitteilung: Kultur- und Infektionsversuche. *Zentralblatt für Veterinärmedizin B* 15:540–554.

Burtscher, H., and A. Schumacher. 1966. Morphologische Untersuchungen zur Virusätiologie der Hepatosplenitis strigum. *Pathologia Veterinaria* 3:506–528.

Burtscher, H. and W. Grünberg. 1975. Epizootische Virushepatitis bei Kranichen (Balearica pavonina L. und Anthropoides virgo L., 1758). Diseases of zoo animals. In *Proceedings of the XVIIth International Symposium,* June 1975, Tunis, Tunisia, pp. 277–279.

Burtscher, H., and M. Sibalin. 1975. Host spectrum and virus distribution in infected owls of herpesvirus strigis. *Journal of Wildlife Diseases* 11:164–169.

Burtscher, H., and W. Grünberg 1979. Herpesvirus-Hepatitis bei Kranichen (Aves: Gruidae). I. Pathologische Befunde. *Zentralblatt für Veterinärmedizin B* 26:561-569.

Calnek, B.W. and R.L. Witter. 1997. Marek's disease. In *Diseases of Poultry,* 10th Ed. B. W. Calnek, H.J. Barnes, C.W. Beard, L.R. McDougald, and Y.M. Saif (eds.). Iowa State University Press, Ames, Iowa, U.S.A., pp. 369–413.

Charlton, B.R., B.C. Barr, A.E. Castro, P.L. Davis, and B.J. Reynolds. 1990. Herpes viral hepatitis in a toucan. *Avian Diseases* 34:787–790.

Cho, B.R. and S.G. Kenzy. 1975. Virologic and serologic studies of zoo birds for Marek's disease virus infection. *Infection and Immunity* 11:809–814.

Colwell, W.M., C.F. Simpson, L.E. Williams Jr., and D.J. Forrester. 1973. Isolation of a herpesvirus from wild turkeys in Florida. *Avian Diseases* 17:1–11.

Columella, L.I.M. Undated. *De re rustica, liber octavus. Reprint 1983.* Artemis Verlag, München und Zürich, Vol. II, pp. 228–329.

Coudert, F., A. Vauillaume, M. Wyers and F.X. Le Gros. 1995. Une nouvelle pathologie chez la dinde—la maladie de Marek. In *Proceedings Journées de la Recherche Avicole,* March 28–30, Anger, France, pp. 164–166.

Cracraft, J. 2000. Avian evolution, Gondwana biogeography and the Cretaceous-tertiary mass extinction event. In *Proceedings of the Royal Society, London B* 268:459–469.

Crawshaw, G.J., and B.R. Boycott. 1982. Infectious laryngotracheitis in peafowl and pheasants. *Avian Diseases* 26:397–401.

Davidson, I., Y. Weisman, S. Perl, and M. Malkinson. 1996. Differential diagnosis of avian tumors by PCR and a case of MDV-1 in turkeys. In *Current research on Marek's disease,* Silva, R.F., H.H. Cheng, P.M. Coussens, L.F. Lee, and L.F. Velicer (eds.). *Proceedings of the 5th International Symposium on Marek's Disease*. September 7–11 1996, East Lansing, Michigan, U.S.A., pp. 311–316.

Davison, A.J. 2002. Evolution of herpesviruses. *Veterinary Microbiology* 86:69–88.

Docherty, D.E., and D.J. Henning. 1980. The isolation of a herpesvirus from captive cranes with inclusion body disease. *Avian Diseases* 24:278–283.

Docherty, D.E., R.I. Romaine, and R.L. Knight. 1983. Isolation of a herpesvirus from a bald eagle nestling. *Avian Diseases* 27:1162–1165.

Docherty, D.E., and R.L. Romaine. 1983. Inclusion body disease of cranes: A serological follow-up to the 1978 die-off. Avian Diseases 27:830–835.

Dutton, R.L., S.G. Kenzy, and W.A. Becker. 1973. Marek's disease in the Japanese quail (Coturnix coturnix japonica). *Avian Diseases* 17:139–143.

Easterday, B.C., V.S. Hinshaw, and D.A. Halvorson. 1997. Influenza. In *Diseases of Poultry,* 10th Ed., B.W. Calnek, H.J. Barnes, C.W. Beard, L.R. McDougald, and Y.M. Saif (eds.). Iowa State University Press, Ames, Iowa, U.S.A., pp. 583–605.

Ehlers, B., K. Borchers, C. Grund, K. Frölich, H. Ludwig, and H.-J. Buhk. 1999. Detection of new polymerase genes of known and potentially novel herpesviruses by PCR with degenerative and deoxyinosine-substituted primers. *Virus Genes* 18:211–220.

Eskens, U., E.F. Kaleta, and G. Unger. 1994. Eine Herpesvirus-bedingte Enzootie—Pachecosche Papageienkrankheit—in einem *Psittazidenbestand. Tieraerztliche Praxis* 22:542–553.

Förster, S., C. Chastel, and E.F. Kaleta. 1989. Crane hepatitis viruses. *Journal of Veterinary Medicine B* 36:433–441.

Fredericius Secundus, De arte venandi cum avibus, cited in Stresemann, E. 1996. *Die Entwicklung der Ornithologie von Aristoteles bis zur Gegenwart.* Aula-Verlag, Wiesbaden, Germany, pp. 1–24.

French, E.L., H.G. Purchase, and K. Nazerian. 1973. A new herpesvirus isolated from a nestling cormorant (Phalacrocorax melanoleucos). *Avian Pathology* 2:3–15.

Gancz, A.Y., I.K. Barker, D. Smith, R. Lindsay, and B. Hunter. 2006. Pathology and tissue distribution of West Nile virus in North American owls (family: Strigidae). *Avian Pathology* (in press, February issue) 35.

Gerlach, H. 1994. Herpesviridae. In *Avian Medicine: Principles and Application.* B.W. Ritchie, G.J. Harrison, and L.R. Harrison (eds.). Wingers Publishing, Inc. Lake Worth, Florida, U.S.A., pp. 874–885.

Gesner, K. 1555. Reprints from 1669 and 1981. In *Vollkommenes Vogelbuch.* Schlütersche Verlagsanstalt, Hannover, Germany, 450 pp.

Glünder, G., O. Siegmann, and W. Kohler. 1991. Krankheiten und Todesursachen bei einheimischen Wildvögeln. *Journal of Veterinary Medicine B* 38:241–262.

Gómez-Villamandos, J.C., E. Mozos, M.A. Sierra, A. Fernández, and F. Díaz. 1991. Mortality in psittacine birds resembling Pacheco's disease in Spain. *Avian Pathology* 20:541–547.

Gómez-Villamandos, J.C., A. Méndez, J. Martín de las Mulas, J. Hervás, and M. A. Sierra. 1995. Histological and ultrastructural study of an unusual herpesvirus infection in owls (*Tyto alba*). *The Veterinary Record* 136:614–615.

Gómez-Villamandos, J.C., J. Hervás, F.J. Salguero, M.A. Quevedo, J.M. Aguilar, and E. Mozos. 1998. Haemorrhagic enteritis associated with herpesvirus in storks. *Avian Pathology* 27:229–236.

Gough, R.E. and D.J. Alexander. 1993. Pacheco's disease in psittacine birds in Great Britain 1987–1991. *The Veterinary Record* 132:113–115.

Gravendyck, M., S. Tritt, H. Spenkoch-Piper, and E.F. Kaleta. 1996. Antigenic diversity of psittacine herpesviruses: cluster analysis of antigenic differences obtained from cross-neutralization tests. *Avian Pathology* 25:345–357.

Gravendyck, M. 1996. Isolierung und biologische Eigenschaften eines neuen Herpesvirus aus einem Dreifarbenglanzstar (Lamprotornis superbus Rüppel, 1845) sowie Versuche zur Differenzierung von Herpesviren aus Passeriformes durch Restriktionsendonukleasen. Veterinary Medical Dissertation, Giessen, Germany, 114 pp.

Gravendyck, M., E. Balks, A.S. Schröder-Gravendyck, U. Eskens, H. Frank, R.E.M. Marschang, and E. F. Kaleta. 1998. Quantification of the herpesvirus content in various tissues and organs, and associated post mortem lesions of psittacine birds which died during an epornithic of Pacheco's parrot disease (PPD). *Avian Pathology* 27:4788–489.

Green, R.G., and J.E. Shillinger. 1935. A virus disease of owls. *Journal of Immunology* 29:68–69.

Green, R.G., and J.E. Shillinger. 1936. A virus disease of owls. *American Journal of Pathology* 12:405–410.

Günther, B.M.F., B.G. Klupp, M. Gravendyck, J.E. Lohr, T.C. Mettenleiter and E.F. Kaleta. 1997. Comparison of the genomes of 15 avian herpesvirus isolates by restriction endonuclease analysis. *Avian Pathology* 26:305–316.

Hatt, J.-M, R. Baumgartner, and E. Isenbügel. 1996. Diagnostik und medizinische Betreuung von Greifvögeln in einer Zusammenstellung der Fälle von 1985–1994. *Schweizer Archiv für Tierheilkunde* 138: 434–440.

Heidenreich, M. 1996. In *Greifvögel. Krankheiten, Haltung, Zucht.* Blackwell Wissenschafts-Verlag, Berlin, Wien, Oxford, 294 pp.

Heidenreich, M. and E.F. Kaleta. 1978. Hepatosplenitis infectiosa strigum: Beitrag zum Wirtsspektrum und zur Übertragbarkeit des Eulen-Herpesvirus. *Fortschritte der Veterinärmedizin* 28:198–203.

Heinrichs, M.A. 1992. Herpesvirus-induzierte Infektionen und Krankheiten bei nicht domestizierten Vogelarten—eine vergleichende Literaturstudie. Veterinary Medical Dissertation. Giessen, Germany 385 p.

Hergarten, G. 1994. Influenza A: aviäres Wirtsspektrum, Symptomatik und Organ-läsionen sowie ein Vergleich biologischer Eigenschaften neuerer H1N1-Isolate aus Puten und Schweinen. Veterinary Medical Dissertation, Giessen, Germany. 286 pp.

Hirsch, M.S., J.C. Kaplan, and R.T.D'Aquila. 1997. Antiviral agents. In *Viral pathogenesis.* Nathanson, N. (Ed.-in-Chief). Lippincott–Raven, Philadelphia, New York, U.S.A., pp. 401–411.

Hoerr, F.J. 1997. Poisons and toxins. Mycotoxikoses. In *Diseases of poultry,* 10th ed. B.W. Clanek, H.J. Barnes, C.W. Beard, L.R. McDougald, and Y.M. Saif (eds.). Iowa State University Press, Ames, Iowa, U.S.A., pp. 951–979.

Hoffman, D.J., M.J. Melancon, P.N. Klein, J.D. Eisemann, and J.W. Spann. 1998. Comparative developmental toxicity of planar polychlorinated biphenyl congeners in chickens, American kestrels, and common terns. *Environmental Toxicology and Chemistry* 17:747–757.

Horner, R.F., M.E. Parker, E.F. Kaleta, and l. Prozzesky. 1992. Isolation and identification of psittacid herpesvirus 1 from imported psittacines in South Africa. *Journal of the South African Veterinary Association* 63:59–62.

Hughes, C.S., R.M. Williams, F.T.W. Jordan, J.M.Bradbury, M. Bennett, and R.C. Jones. 1991. Latency and reactivation of infectious laryngotracheitis virus. *Archives of Virology* 121:213–218.

Johne, R., A. Konrath, M.-E. Krautwald-Junghanns, E.F. Kaleta, H. Gerlach, and H. Müller. 2002. Herpesviral, but no papovalviral sequences, are detected in cloacal papillomas of parrots. *Archives of Virology* 147:1869–1880.

Julian, R.J. and T.P. Brown. 1997. Other toxins and poisons. In *Diseases of Poultry,* 10th Ed. B. W. Calnek, H.J. Barnes, C.W. Beard, L.R. McDougald, and Y.M. Saif (eds.). Iowa State University Press, Ames, Iowa, U.S.A., pp. 979–1005.

Johannknecht, S., U. Wernery, and C.H. Grund. 2000. Relation of falconid and columbid herpesvirus isolates. In *Proceedings of the XIIth Conference on Bird Diseases,* Munich, Germany pp. 145–152.

Kaleta, E.F. 1990. Herpesviruses of birds. A review. *Avian Pathology* 19:193–211.

Kaleta, E.F. 1991. Einfluβ von Propolis der Honigbiene (Apis mellifera L., 1758) auf die Vermehrung einer Klein- und einer Groβplaque-Variante des Tauben-Herpesvirus in vitro. *Tierärztliche Umschau* 46: 553–556.

Kaleta, E.F. 1998. Herpesviruses of free-living and pet birds. In *A Laboratory Manual for the Isolation and Identification of Avian Pathogens,* 4th Ed. D.E. Swayne, J.R. Glisson, M.W. Jackwood, J.E. Pearson, and W.M. Reed (eds.). American Association of Avian Veterinarians, Kennett Square, Pennsylvania, U.S.A., pp. 129–136.

Kaleta, E.F. 1999. Virale Erkrankungen. In *Kompendium der Ziervogelkrankheiten.* E.F. Kaleta and M.-E. Krautwald-Junghanns (eds.). Schlütersche GmbH & Co. KG Verlag und Druckerei, Hannover, Germany, pp. 269–311.

Kaleta, E.F. and K. Druener. 1976. Hepatosplenitis infectiosa strigum und andere Krankheiten der Greifvögel und Eulen. *Fortschritte der Veterinärmedizin* 25:173–180.

Kaleta, E.F., H.-J. Marschall, G. Glünder, and B. Stiburek. 1980a. Isolation and serological differentiation of a herpesvirus from bobwhite quail (Colinus virgianus L. 1758). *Archives of Virology* 66:359–364.

Kaleta, E.F., U. Heffels, U. Neumann, and T. Mikami. 1980b. Serological differentiation of 14 avian herpesviruses by plaque reduction tests in cell cultures. In *Proceedings of the 2nd International Symposium of Veterinary Laboratory Diagnosticians,* Vol. 1. Lucerne, Switzerland. June 24–26,pp.38–41.

Kaleta, E.F., H.-J. Marschall, U. Heffels, and T. Mikami. 1980c. Nachweis eines Herpesvirus bei Amazonen (Amazona aestiva und A. ochrocephala). *Zentralblatt für Veterinärmedizin B* 27:405–411.

Kaleta, E.F., T. Mikami, H.-J. Marschall, U. Heffels, M. Heidenreich, and B. Stiburek. 1980d. A new herpesvirus isolated from black storks (Ciconia nigra). *Avian Pathology* 9:301–310.

Kaleta, E.F. and N. Kummerfeld. 1983. Herpesvirus and Newcastle disease virus in white storks (Ciconia ciconia). *Avian Pathology* 12:347–352.

Kaleta, E.F., and N. Kummerfeld. 1986. Persistent viraemia of a cell-associated herpesvirus in white storks (Ciconia ciconia). *Avian Pathology* 15:447–453.

Kaleta, E.F., and C. Baldauf 1988. Newcastle disease in free-living and pet birds. In: *Newcastle Disease,* D.J. Alexander (ed.). Kluwer Academic Publishers, Boston, Dordrecht, London, pp. 197–246.

Kaleta, E.F., and M. Bueno Brinkmann. 1993. An outbreak of Pacheco's parrot disease in a psittacine bird collection and an attempt to control it by vaccination. *Avian Pathology* 22:785–789.

Kaleta, E.F., and T. Redmann 1997. Die infektiöse Laryngotracheitis bei Huhn, Pfau und Fasan sowie Möglichkeiten und Grenzen ihrer Bekämpfung durch attenuierte Lebendimpfstoffe. *Tierärztliche Praxis* 25:605–610.

Kaleta, E.F., and E.M.A. Taday. 2003. Avian host range of Chlamydophila spp. based on isolation, antigen detection and serology. *Avian Pathology* 32:435–462.

Kincaid, A. L., and M. Cranfield. 1988. Herpesvirus-like infection in black-footed penguins (*Spheniscus demersus*). *Journal of Wildlife Diseases* 24:173–175.

Kocan, A.A., L.N.D. Potgieter, and K.M. Kocan. 1977. Inclusion body disease of falcons (herpesvirus infection) in an American kestrel. *Journal of Wildlife Diseases* 13:199–201.

Koenig, B., and J.H. Dustmann. 1985. The caffeolylics as a new family of natural antiviral compounds. *Naturwissenschaften* 72:659–661.

Krautwald-Junghanns, M.-E., S. Foerster, W. Herbst, B. Schildger, and E.F. Kaleta. 1988. Nachweis eines neuen Herpesvirus bei einem ungewöhnlichen Fall von Pachecoscher Krankheit bei Amazonen und Graupapageien. *Journal of Veterinary Medicine B* 35:415–420.

Lee, L.F., R.L. Armstrong, and K. Nazerian. 1972. Comparative studies of six avian herpesviruses. *Avian Diseases* 16:799–805.

Letchworth, G.J., J.R. Fishel, and W. Hansen. 1997. A monoclonal antibody to inclusion body disease of cranes virus enabling specific immunohistochemistry and competitive ELISA. *Avian Diseases* 41:808–816.

Lierz, M., T. Gübel, and E.F. Kaleta. 2002. Vorkommen von Chlamydophila psittaci, Falkenherpesvirus und Paramyxovirus 1 bei geschwücht oder verletzt aufgefundenen Greifvögeln und Eulen. *Tieraerztliche Praxis* 30 (K):139–144.

Magnino, S., G. Conzo, A. Fioretti, L. F. Menna, T. Rampin, G. Sironi, M. Fabbi, and E.F. Kaleta. 1996. An outbreak of Pacheco's parrot disease in psittacine birds recently imported to Campania, Italy: Isolation of psittacid herpesvirus 2. *Journal of Veterinary Medicine B* 43:631–637.

Mare, C.J., and D.L. Graham. 1973. Falcon herpesvirus, the etiologic agent of inclusion body disease of falcons. *Infection and Immunity* 8:118–126.

Mare, C.J., and D.L. Graham. 1975. Pathogenicity and host range of the falcon herpesvirus. In *Proceedings of the 3rd International Wildlife Disease Conference,* Munich, Germany pp. 471–482.

Marek, J. 1907. Multiple Nervenentzündung (Polyneuritis) bei Hühnern. *Deutsche Tierärztliche Wochenschrift* 15:417–421.

Massi, P.D. Gelmetti, G. Sironi, A. Lavazza,, M. Dottori, and S. Pascucci. 1993. Haemorrhagic disease of guinea fowls. Its presence in Italy. *Zootecnica International* 4:75–76.

May, H.G., and R.P. Tittsler. 1925. Tracheo-laryngitis in poultry. *Journal of the American Veterinary Medical Association* 67:229–231.

Mettenleiter, T.C. 2003. Herpesviren—vom Genom zur Erkrankung. *Leopoldina* (R. 3) 49:501–512.

Mettenleiter, T.C. 2004. Budding events in herpesvirus morphogenesis. *Virus Research* 106:167–180.

Mikaelian, I., F. Gauthier, R. Higgins, R. Claveau, and D. Martineau. 1997. Primary causes of death in wild birds in Quebec. *Médicine Vétérinaire du Quebec* 27:94–102.

Minson, A.C., A. Davidson, R. Eberle, R.C. Desrosiers, B. Fleckenstein, D.J. McGeoch, P.E. Pellet, B. Roizman, and D.M.J. Studdert. 2000. Family Herpesviridae. In *7th Report of the International Committee on Taxonomy of Viruses*. Springer Verlag, Wien und New York, pp. 203–225.

Morishita, T.Y., P.A. Pyone, and D.L. Brooks. 1997. A survey of diseases of raptorial birds. *Journal of Avian Medicine and Surgery* 11:77–92.

Northon, T.M., J. Gaskin, G.V. Kollias, B. Homer, C.H. Clark, and R. Wilson. 1991. Efficacy of acyclovir against herpesvirus infection in Quaker parakeets. *American Journal of Veterinary Research* 52:2007–2009.

Olson, G.H., J.W. Carpenter, G.F. Gee, N.J. Thomas, and F.J. Dein. 1995. Mycotoxin-induced disease in captive whooping cranes (*Grus americana*) and sandhill cranes (*Grus canadensis*). *Journal of Zoo and Wildlife Medicine* 26:569–576.

Pacheco, G. and O. Bier. 1930. Epizootie chez perroques du Bresil. Relations avec la psittacose. *C. R. Seances Societie Biologie* 105:109–111.

Pennycott, T.W. and K. Venogupal, 2002. Outbreak of Marek's disease in a flock of turkeys in Scotland. *The Veterinary Record* 150:277–279.

Phalen, D.N. 1997. Viruses. In *Avian medicine and surgery,* Altman, R. B., S. L. Clubb, G. M. Dorrestein, and K. Quesenberry (eds.). W. B. Saunders Company, Philadelphia, U.S.A., pp. 281–322.

Plinius, C.S. (*23 and † 79), *Naturalis historiae, liber X.* Artemis Verlag, München und Zürich, pp. 16–238.

Potgieter, L.N.D., A.A. Kocan, and K.M. Kocan. 1979. Isolation of a herpesvirus from American Kestrel with inclusion body disease. *Journal of Wildlife Diseases* 15:143–149.

Raidal, S.R., G.M. Cross, E. Tomaszewski, D.l. Graham, and D.N. Phalen. 1998. A serologic survey for avian polyomavirus and Pacheco's disease virus in Australian Cockatoos. *Avian Pathology* 27:263–268.

Ramis, A., D. Fondevila, J. Tarres, and L. Ferrer. 1992. Immuncytochemical diagnosis of Pacheco's disease. *Avian Pathology* 21:523–527.

Ramis, A., N. Majo, M. Pumarola, D. Fondevila, and L. Ferrer. 1994. Herpesvirus hepatitis in two Eagles in Spain. *Avian Diseases* 38:197–200.

Ramis, A., J. Tarrés, D. Fondevilla, and L. Ferrer. 1996. Immunocytochemical study of the pathogenesis of Pacheco's parrot disease in budgerigars. *Veterinary Microbiology* 52:49–61.

Raue, R., V. Schmidt, M. Freick, B. Reinhardt, R. Johne, L. Kamphausen, E.F. Kaleta, H. Müller, and M.-E. Krautwald-Junghanns. 2005. A disease complex associated with pigeon circovirus infection, young pigeon disease syndrome. *Avian Pathology,* accepted.

Ritchie, B.W. 1995. *Avian Viruses, Function and Control.* Wingers Publishing, Inc., Lake Worth, Florida, U.S.A., 515 pp.

Roizman, B. 1996. Herpesviridae. In *Fields Virology,* B.N. Fields, D.N. Knipe, P.M. Howley et al. (eds.). Lippincott-Ravens Publishers, Philadelphia, U.S.A., pp. 2221–2230.

Sallmann, M. 1991. Untersuchungen an zwei Plaquevarianten aus einem Herpes-virusisolat einer Brieftaube (*Columba livia,* var. *domestica,* Gmelin, 1789). Veterinary Medical Dissertation. Giessen, Germany, 83 pp.

Sander, O. 1995. Untersuchungen über die Herpesvirus-Infektionen der Greifvögel (Falconiformes und Accipitriformes) sowie vergleichende Unterwuchungen an 5 Isolaten aus verschiedenen Greifvögeln. Veterinary Medical Dissertation. Giessen, Germany, 92 pp.

Schettler, C.H. 1969. Eine infektiöse Leberentzündung (Hepatitis) der Eulen. *Tierärztliche Umschau* 24:163–167.

Schönbauer, M. und H. Köhler. 1982. Über eine Virusinfektion bei Prachtfinken (Estrildidae). *Kleintierpraxis* 27:149–152.

Schroeder, D. 1992. Untersuchungen über die Hepatosplenitis infectiosa strigum sowie vergleichende Studien an Herpesvirusisolaten aus Uhu (*Bubo bubo*) und Schnee-Eule (*Nyctea scandiaca*). Veterinary Medical Dissertation. Giessen, Germany, 90 pp.

Schroeder-Gravendyck, A.S. 1999. Isolierung und Charakterisierung von 10 neuen Herpesviren aus Psittaziden sowie Versuche zur Differenzierung von insgesamt 31 Psittaciden-Herpesviren mittels Restriktionsendonukleasen. Veterinary Medical Dissertation. Giessen, Germany, 147 pp.

Scope, A. 1999. Bakterielle Erkrankungen. In *Kompendium der Ziervogelkrank-heiten.* Kaleta, E.F. and M.-E. Krautwald-Junghanns (eds.). Schlütersche

GmbH & Co KG Verlag und Druckerei, Hannover, Germany, pp. 229–250.

Shawky, S. and K.A. Schat. 2002. Latency sites and reactivation of duck enteritis virus. *Avian Diseases* 46:308–313.

Simpson, C.F., J.E. Hanley, and J.M. Gaskin. 1975. Psittacine herpesvirus infection resembling Pacheco's parrot disease. Journal of Infectious Diseases 131:390–396.

Smadel, J.E., E.B. Jackson, and J.W. Harman. 1945. A new virus disease of pigeons. I. Recovery of the virus. *Journal of Experimental Medicine* 81:385–398.

Steinke, A. and S. Mundt. 1997. Ausbruch der Pachecoschen Papageienkrankheit in einer privaten Papageienhaltung. *Der Praktische Tierarzt* 78:548–557.

Steinmetz, D. 1995. Serologische Untersuchungen zur Verbreitung von Antikörpern gegen ein Tauben-Herpesvirus unter Berücksichtigung der Flugleistung von Brieftauben in Südhessen. Veterinary Medical Dissertation, Giessen.

Styles, D.K., E.K. Tomaszewski, L.A. Jaeger, and D.N. Phalen. 2004. Psittacid herpesviruses associated with mucosal papillomas in neotropical parrots. *Virology* 325:24–35.

Styles, D.K., E.K. Tomaszewski, and D.N. Phalen. 2005. A novel psittacid herpesvirus found in African grey parrots (Psittacus erithacus erithacus). *Avian Pathology* 34:150–154.

Suzuki, H., T. Taniguchi, T. Ogawa, S. Shichiri, and F. Hashizaki. 1997. Pathology of cranes with suspected herpesvirus infection. *Journal of the Japan Veterinary Medical Association* 50:327–332.

Thiry, E., H. Vindevogel, P. Leroy, P.-P. Pastoret, A. Schwers, B. Brochier, Y. Anciaux, and P. Hoyois. 1983. *In vivo* and *in vitro* effect of acyclovir on pseudorabies virus, infectious bovine rhinotracheitis virus and pigeon Herpesvirus. *Annales Recherches Vétérinaire* 14:239–245.

Todd, D. 2000. Circovirus: immunosuppressive threats to avian species: a review. *Avian Pathology* 29:373–394.

Tomaszewski, E., G. van Wilson, W.L. Wigle, D.N. Phalen. 2001. Detection and heterogeneity of herpesviruses causing Pacheco's parrot disease. *Journal of Clinical Microbiology* 39:533–538.

Tomaszewski, E.K., E.F. Kaleta, and D.N. Phalen. 2003. Molecular phylogeny of the psittacid herpesviruses causing Pacheco's disease: correlation of genotype with phenotypic expression. *Journal of Virology* 77:11260–11267.

Tomaszewski, E.K., M. Gravendyck, E.F. Kaleta, and D.N. Phalen. 2004. Genetic characterization of a herpesvirus isolate from a Superb Starling (Lamprotornis superbus) as a psittacid herpesvirus genotype 1. *Avian Diseases* 48:212–214.

Toro, H., C. Saucedo, C. Borie, R.E. Gough, and H. Alcaíno. 1999. Health status of free-living pigeons in the city of Santiago. *Avian Pathology* 28:619–623.

VanDevanter, D.R., P. Warrener, L. Bennett, E.R. Schultz, S. Coulter, R.L. Garber, and T.M. Rose. 1996. Detection and analysis of diverse herpesviral species by consensus primer PCR. *Journal of Clinical Microbiology* 34:1666–1671.

Villforth, Y.M. 1995. Krankheiten und Todesursachen von Greifvögeln und Eulen. Veterinary Medical Dissertation, Giessen, Germany, 208 pp.

Vindevogel, H., P.P. Pastoret, and E. Thiry. 1984. Latency of pigeon herpesvirus 1. Latent herpesvirus infections in Veterinary Medicine. In *Current Topics in Veterinary Medicine and Animal Sciences.* Martinus Nijhof Publisher. Amsterdam, 300 pp.

Vindevogel, H. and P.P. Pastoret. 1993. Herpesvirus infections of pigeons and wild birds. In *Virus Infections of Birds,* J. B. McFerran and M. S. McNulty (eds.). Elsevier Science Publishers B. V. Amsterdam, London, New York, Tokyo, pp. 91–106.

Vindevogel, H. and J.P. Duchatel. 1997. Miscellaneous herpesvirus infections. In *Diseases of Poultry,* 10th Ed. B.W. Calnek, J.H. Barnes, C.W. Beard, L.R. McDougald, and Y.M. Saif (eds.). Iowa State University Press, Ames, Iowa, U.S.A., pp. 757–761.

Voelckel, K. E. 2003. Beitrag zur Klärung der Marek-Herpesvirus-Ätiologie einer mit Allgemeinsymptomen und Tumoren einhergehenden Krankheit der Mastputen mittels klinischer, pathologischer, histologischer, virologischer, serologischer und molekularbiologischer (PCR) Methoden. Veterinary Medical Dissertation, Giessen, Germany.

Von Bülow, V. 1971. Diagnosis and certain biological properties of the virus of Marek's disease. *The American Journal of Veterinary Research* 32:1275–1288.

Wagner, U. 1993. Vergleichende Untersuchungen zur Empfindlichkeit verschiedener aviärer Herpesvirusisolate gegenüber chemischen Desinfektions-mitteln. Veterinary Medical Dissertation. Giessen, Germany, 140 pp.

Ward, F.P., D.G. Fairchild, and J. V. Vuicich. 1971. Inclusion body hepatitis in prairie falcon. *Journal of Wildlife Diseases* 7:120–124.

Weiss, R.A. and P.M. Biggs. 1972. Leukosis and Marek's disease virus of feral red jungle fowl and domestic fowl in Malaya. *Journal of the National Cancer Institute* 39:1713–1725.

Wernery, U., R. Wernery, and J. Kinne. 1999. Production of a falcon herpesvirus vaccine. Berliner und Münchener Tieraerztliche Wochenschrift 112:339–344.

Williams, R.A., M. Bennett, J.M. Bradbury, R.M. Gaskel, R.C. Jones, and F. T. W. Jordan. 1992.

Demonstration of sites of latency of infectious laryngotracheitis virus using polymerase chain reaction. *Journal of General Virology* 73:2415–2420.

Witter, R.L., and K.A. Schat. 2003. Marek's disease. In *Diseases of Poultry,* 11th Ed., Y.M. Saif, H.J. Barnes, J.R. Glisson, A.M. Fadly, L.R. McDougald, D.E. Swayne (eds.). Iowa State University Press, Ames, Iowa, U.S.A., pp. 407–465.

Zwart, P., J. v.d. Sluis, and J.W.E. Stam. 1983. Sialolithen (weisse Punkte) im Munddach bei Tauben. Berichte der III. *Tagung über Vogelkrankheiten,* March 2/3, Munich, Germany, pp. 39–45.

4
Duck Plague (Duck Virus Enteritis)

Wallace R. Hansen and Richard E. Gough

INTRODUCTION

Duck plague is an acute, contagious disease of waterfowl caused by a herpesvirus classified as Anatid herpesvirus 1 of the subfamily alphaherpesvirinae (Roizman et al. 1992). Duck plague is primarily a disease of domestic ducks and has become of concern for wild waterfowl in the United States only since the late 1960s (Sandhu and Leibovitz 1997; Friend 1999b; Converse and Kidd 2001). Infections not only cause mortality but also result in significant economic loss due to the reproductive impacts of declining egg production, fertility, and hatchability. Catastrophic outbreaks have caused major economic impacts in Asia (Jansen and Kunst 1964a) and the subcontinent of India (Duraiswami et al. 1979) in countries that depend on duck breeding for meat and egg production for economic survival. This disease has also affected the commercial duck farms of Europe and the U.S.A.

Other than scattered, infrequent mortality, the impact of this disease on migratory waterfowl populations is virtually unknown. Most duck plague outbreaks within North America and Great Britain are associated with backyard flocks, zoological and ornamental waterfowl collections, and wild, nonmigratory resident waterfowl (Gough 1984; Converse and Kidd 2001). Waterfowl surviving virus infection can become lifelong asymptomatic virus carriers and shedders (Burgess et al. 1979) providing virus reservoirs for future disease outbreaks.

SYNONYMS

Duck plague, duck virus enteritis (U.S.A.), eendenpest (Dutch), peste du canard (French), entenpest (German), kacsapestis (Hungarian), peste delle anatre (Italian), mor kachen (Czechoslovakia), and anatid herpesvirus.

HISTORY AND DISTRIBUTION

Duck plague was described for the first time in domestic waterfowl in the Netherlands in 1923 and reported as a strain of fowl plague virus (avian influenza) adapted specifically for ducks (Baudet 1923). De Zeeuw (1930) reported on additional duck-specific mortality on adjacent farms and even though experimentally inoculated chickens, rabbits, and pigeons were resistant to infection with the virus, the disease was still thought to be fowl plague. Bos (1942) referred to the disease as duck plague and considered it caused by a new virus that was pathogenic for ducks but failed to cause disease in chickens, pigeons, rabbits, guinea pigs, rats, or mice. In 1949 the viral agent was isolated and shown to be different from other known bird viruses, and the name duck plague was proposed for the new disease agent at the XIVth International Veterinary Congress in London (Jansen 1968). Duck plague was suspected in France in 1949 (Lucam 1949) and China in 1958 (Jansen and Kunst 1964a). Jansen (1968) speculated that the significant duck mortality in India in 1944 and 1945 could have been duck plague. India reported duck plague in 1963 (Mukerji et al. 1963) and Belgium in 1964 (Devos et al. 1964). Other European countries have since reported duck plague, including England (1972), Germany (1973), Hungary (1973), Italy (1973), Denmark (1983), Austria (1985), and Spain (1998) (Figure 4.1). Asian countries that have reported duck plague include Vietnam (1969), Thailand (1976), Taiwan (1978), Bangladesh (1978), Indonesia, and Malaysia. The first duck plague outbreak was reported in the U.S.A. in 1967 (Leibovitz and Hwang 1968) and in Canada in 1974 (Hanson and Willis 1976). Duck plague was recently suspected in Brazilian zoo collections in 2005 (Saidenberg, pers. comm.), but has not been reported in Australia, despite ongoing surveillance, nor in Africa.

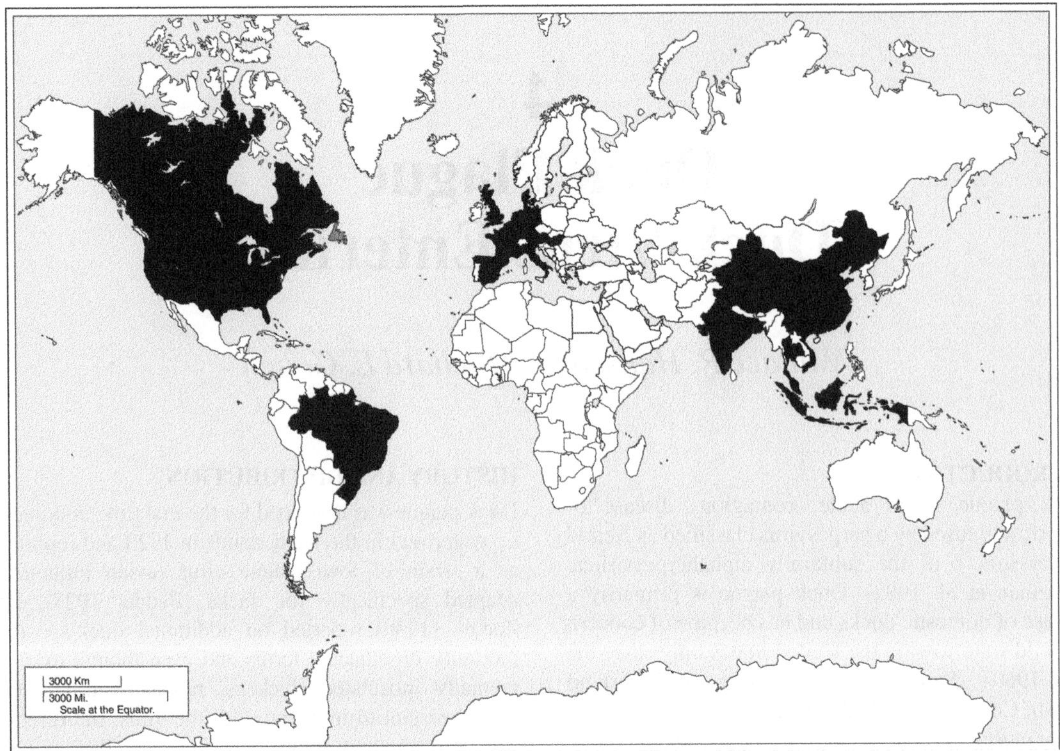

Figure 4.1. Global distribution of reported duck plague mortality events by country.

The origin of duck plague is unknown, but because the first outbreaks in the Netherlands in 1923 and 1930 were misdiagnosed, it is likely that this new disease was not recognized as a cause of duck mortality in other countries. The virus may have already been geographically scattered in Europe and Asia at the time of discovery.

How the disease became distributed in Europe and Asia is not clear because disease reports were sporadic and no link was made to a common source. The long intervals between early duck plague outbreaks in the Netherlands suggested that the disease was recently introduced and slowly became established over the first 30 years as the time periods between outbreaks decreased (Jansen 1961). Duck mortality was reported to be associated with the presence of open water (Jansen 1961) and not in large commercial duck farms where ducks were raised on dry soil and allowed to drink from troughs (Jansen 1961). It was suggested that co-mingling of free-range ducks with other ducks on pasture in adjacent farms likely facilitated disease spread, and that wild waterfowl should be considered as possible disease carriers in the Netherlands (DeZeeuw 1930). Movement of waterfowl breeding stock between countries probably also contributed to the disease distribution as reported in Hungary (Ferenc et al. 1982). There were no historical reports of mortality in wild migratory waterfowl due to duck plague in Europe or Asia, a situation that continues today.

Duck plague was first identified in North America in 1967, affecting the commercial duck producers of Long Island, New York (Leibovitz and Hwang 1968). A recent comprehensive review of duck plague in the U.S.A. has been published by Sandhu and Leibovitz (1997). The New York State and United States Department of Agriculture (USDA), Agricultural Research Service regulatory officials designated the Long Island duck disease duck virus enteritis, which was more descriptive of the condition than the term duck plague (Title-9, Code of Federal Regulations). The disease spread across commercial duck farms on Long Island and to captive flocks of waterfowl in Maryland and Pennsylvania in 1969 (Walker et al. 1970). Dead wild waterfowl, associated with mortality in commercial flocks, were also found infected with duck plague in 1967 (Walker et al. 1970). Following quarantine, depopulation, decontamination, and vaccination of waterfowl on affected farms, the disease was declared eradicated from commercial ducks in Suffolk County, Long Island in April 1970 by the USDA

(USDA news release 1079–70). In April and May 1970 duck plague reappeared in captive Muscovy Ducks (*Cairina moschata*) in Pennsylvania and a wild American Black Duck (*Anas rubripes*) on Long Island (Goldstein et al. 1971). In 1972 duck plague appeared for the first time on the West coast in a mixed population of resident and wild waterfowl at the Palace of Fine Arts in San Francisco, California (Snyder et al. 1973). In 1973 duck plague appeared in the Midwest in wild migratory waterfowl at Lake Andes, South Dakota (Friend and Pearson 1973), captive waterfowl at a zoo in St. Paul, Minnesota (NWHC unpub. data), and in captive waterfowl in Coloma, Wisconsin (Jacobson et al. 1976).

The Lake Andes duck plague outbreak that killed 42,000 Mallards was the largest of only two major mortality events from duck plague reported for wild waterfowl in North America (Friend and Pearson 1973). The other occurred in the Finger Lakes region of New York during 1994 and killed 1,150 waterfowl, primarily American Black Ducks (Converse and Kidd 2001). Since 1967, duck plague outbreaks have continued to occur mostly in captive or wild, nonmigratory waterfowl in the Northeast, Chesapeake Bay, South Central, and South Western California in the U.S.A., with slow expansion to other states in recent years (Friend 1999b; Converse and Kidd 2001). Duck plague is considered endemic in domestic waterfowl in many Asian countries including China, Vietnam, Thailand, Bangladesh, and India. The distribution of duck plague is shown in Figure 4.1.

HOST RANGE

Duck plague is a disease of birds of the Order Anseriformes, Family Anatidae (ducks, geese, and swans). A wide range of waterfowl species are susceptible to duck plague virus infection (Table 4.1) (Van Dorssen and Kunst 1955; Dardiri and Butterfield 1969; Montali et al. 1976; Gough 1984; Gough and Alexander 1990; Spieker et al. 1996; Converse and Kidd 2001). Experimental studies have shown that waterfowl species vary in susceptibility to duck plague virus. Van Dorssen and Kunst (1955) found Northern Pintails (*Anas acuta*) and European Green-winged Teal (*Anas crecca crecca*) resistant to disease after virus infection, but they did produce antibodies. In contrast, Converse and Kidd (2001) reported Green-winged Teal mortality due to duck plague. Spieker et al. (1996) reported a similar resistance of Northern Pintails when inoculated with high doses, >3.5 $\log_{10}$ plaque-forming units (PFU), of a virulent virus isolate. The investigators also reported a range of susceptibilities to duck plague for the other species of wild waterfowl tested, with Blue-winged Teal (*Anas discors*) demonstrating extreme sensitivity resulting in 50% mortality when infected with 0.01 $\log_{10}$ PFU of virus. Based on experimental inoculation studies, waterfowl range from most to least susceptible to virus infection as measured by mortality in the following order: Blue-winged Teal > Redhead (*Aythya americana*) = Wood Duck (*Aix sponsa*) > Gadwall (*Anas strepera*) = Muscovy Duck > American Black Duck > Canada Goose (*Branta canadensis*) = Mallard (*Anas platyrhynchos*) > Northern Pintail. A list of waterfowl species and an indication of their relative susceptibility to duck plague virus based on 25 years of mortality records from the Wildfowl and Wetland Trust (WWT), Slimbridge, England is presented in Table 4.1.

Nonwaterfowl species have been found to be resistant to duck plague virus. Herring Gulls (*Larus argentatus*) and Black-headed Gulls (*Larus ridibundus*) did not die from experimental virus infection and failed to produce antibodies to the virus (Van Dorssen and Kunst 1955). Attempts to infect adult chickens and pigeons (Bos 1942) or Brown-headed Cowbirds (*Molothrus ater*) (Dardiri and Butterfield 1969) were also unsuccessful. Attempts to infect mammals including rabbits, guinea pigs, rats, or mice have been unsuccessful (Bos 1942).

A recent report by Salguero et al. (2002) reported that two species of coots, the Eurasian Coot (*Fulica atra*) and Red-knobbed Coot (*Fulica cristata*) may be susceptible to duck plague infection based on gross lesions and histopathology of two dead birds found with Mallards that were also suspected of being infected with duck plague virus. No laboratory tests were done to verify the presence of duck plague virus. In duck plague die-offs in waterfowl at the WWT in England, lesions of duck plague have never been identified in Eurasian Coots (Brown, pers. comm.). Additional experimental work is required to determine the susceptibility of coots to duck plague virus infection.

Duck plague virus replicates only in cell cultures from avian species in the orders Anseriformes and Galliformes (Kocan 1976; Attanasio et al. 1980) and it does not replicate in mammalian cell cultures derived from humans, monkeys, or fish (Attanasio et al. 1980).

ETIOLOGY

The name Anatid herpesvirus 1 was suggested by Roizman et al. (1973). The duck plague virus is a herpesvirus assigned to the Alpha herpesvirus sub-family (Roizman et al. 1992). It has a nucleocapsid diameter of 75 μ and an envelope diameter of 181 μ (Breese and Dardiri 1968). The viral genome is dsDNA with a molecular weight of 119×10^6 Daltons and a GC content of 64.3% (Gardner et al. 1993). The virus does not agglutinate red blood cells from chicken, duck, horse, or sheep (Jansen and Kunst 1949).

The gel banding patterns of DNA fragments generated by restriction enzyme (RE) cleavage of genomes from duck plague virus strains offer a possible method

Table 4.1. Wild waterfowl species of the family Anatidae naturally and experimentally susceptible to duck plague virus infection.

Common Name (species)	Mortality	Method of Bird Infection: Natural		Experimental		References
		Died	PCR[a]	Died	Carrier	
Magpie Goose (*Anseranas semipalmata*)	L[b]	+[b]	+[w]			
Black-bellied Whistling Duck (*Dendrocygna autumnalis*)		+				Converse et al. (2001)
Plumed Whistling-duck (*Dendrocygna eytoni*)		+[b]				
Fulvous Whistling-duck (*Dendrocygna bicolor*)		+[b]				
West Indian Whistling-duck (*Dendrocygna arborea*)		+[b]				Gough (1984)
Black Swan (*Cygnus atratus*)		+				Snyder et al. (1973)
						Gough (1984)
Tundra Swan (*Cygnus columbianus bewickii*)	M	+[b]	+[w]			
Whooper Swan (*Cygnus cygnus*)			+[w]			
Mute Swan (*Cygnus olor*)	M	+[b]		+		Leibovitz (1971)
						Van Dorssen & Kunst (1955)
Corscoroba Swan (*Coscoroba coscoroba*)	M	+[b]				Gough (1984)
Bean goose (*Anser fabalis*)				+		Van Dorssen & Kunst (1955)
Pink-footed Goose (*Anser brachyrhynchus*)		+[b]				
Greater White-fronted Goose (*Anser albifrons*)					+	Leibovitz (1971)
Greylag (*Anser anser anser*)		+[b]				
Greater Snow Goose (*Chen caerulescens atlanticus*)		+[b]				
Ross's Goose (*Chen rossii*)		+[b]				Gough (1984)
Emperor Goose (*Chen canagica*)		+[b]				
Hawaiian Goose (*Branta sandvicensis*)	L	+[b]				
Canada Goose (*Branta canadensis*)	L	+[b]	+[m]	+	+	Leibovitz (1971)
						Burgess et al. (1979)
						Spieker et al. (1996)
Aleutian Canada Goose (*Branta canadensis leucopareia*)			+[w]			
Dusky Canada Goose (*Branta canadensis occidentalis*)		+[b]				
Richardson's Canada Goose (*Branta canadensis hutchinsii*)		+[b]				
Barnacle Goose (*Branta leucopsis*)		+[b]				
Brant (*Branta bernicla orentalis*)		+[b]				
Cape Barren Goose (*Cereopsis novaehollandiae*)	H	+[b]	+[w]			
Blue-winged Goose (*Cyanochen cyanopterus*)	H	+[b]				Gough (1984)
Andean Goose (*Chloephaga melanoptera*)	H	+[b]				
Upland Goose (*Chloephaga picta leucoptera*)	H	+[b]				
Kelp Goose (*Chloephaga hybrida*)	H	+[b]				
Ashy-headed Goose (*Chloephaga poliocephala*)	H	+[b]	+[w]			

Ruddy-headed Goose (*Chloephaga rubidiceps*)	H	+[b]				
Orinoco Goose (*Neochen jubata*)	H	+[b]				
Egyptian Goose (*Alpochen aegyptiacus*)	H	+[b]				Snyder et al. (1973)
						Gough (1984)
Ruddy Shelduck (*Tadorna ferruginea*)	H	+[b]	+[w]			
South African Shelduck (*Tadorna cana*)	H	+[b]				
Australian Shelduck (*Tadorna tadornoides*)	H	+[b]				
Paradise Shelduck (*Tadorna variegata*)	H	+[b]	+[w]			
Common Shelduck (*Tadorna tadorna*)	H	+[b]		+		Van Dorssen & Kunst (1955)
						Gough (1984)
Radjah Shelduck (*Tadorna radjah*)	H	+[b]	+[w]			
Flightless Stemerduck (*Tachyeres pteneres*)	H	+[b]				
Falkland Steamerduck (*Tachyeres brachypterus*)	H	+[b]				
Spur-winged Goose (*Plectropterus gambensis*)	H	+[b]				Gough (1984)
Muscovy Duck (*Cairina moschata*)	H	+[b]				
White-winged Duck (*Cairina scutulata*)	H	+[b]	+[w]			
Hartlaub's Duck (*Pteronetta hartlaubii*)	H	+[b]				Van Dorssen & Kunst (1955)
Wood Duck (*Aix sponsa*)	M	+[b]		+		Snyder et al. (1973)
						Spieker et al. (1996)
						Snyder et al. (1973)
Mandarin Duck (*Aix galericulata*)	M	+[b]	+[w]			
Maned Duck (*Chenonetta jubata*)	L	+[b]	+[w]			
Brazilian Teal (*Amazonetta brasiliensis brasiliensis*)	M	+[b]	+[w]			
Brazilian Teal (*Amazonetta brasiliensis ipecutiri*)	M	+[b]				
African Black Duck (*Anas sparsa sparsa*)	H	+[b]	+[w]			
Eurasian Wigeon (*Anas penelope*)	L	+[b]		+		Van Dorssen & Kunst (1955)
American Widgeon (*Anas americana*)	L	+[b]				Snyder et al. (1973)
Chiloe Wigeon (*Anas sibilatrix*)	L	+[b]				
Falcated Duck (*Anas falcata*)	M	+[b]	+[w]			
Gadwall (*Anas strepara strepara*)	L	+[b]	+[w]	+		Van Dorssen & Kunst (1955)
						Spieker et al. (1996)
						Converse et al. (2001)
Baikal Teal (*Anas Formosa*)	M	+[b]				
Green-winged Teal (*Anas crecca carolinensis*)		+	+[w]			Converse et al. (2001)
Green-winged Teal (*Anas crecca crecca*)					–	Van Dorssen & Kunst (1955)
Speckled Teal (*Anas flavirostris oxyptera*)			+[w]			
Cape Teal (*Anas capensis*)	M	+[b]				

(*Continued*)

Table 4.1. (Continued)

Common Name (species)	Mortality	Method of Bird Infection: Natural Died	Natural PCR[a]	Experimental Died	Experimental Carrier	References
Gray Teal (*Anas gibberifrons gracilis*)		+				Montali et al. (1976)
Chestnut Teal (*Anas castanea*)	M	+[b]	+[w]			
Brown Teal (*Anas chlorotis*)	M	+[b]				
Mallard (*Anas platyrhynchos platyrhynchos*)	H	+[b]	+[w, m]	+	+	Leibovitz (1971) Burgess et al. (1979) Spieker et al. (1996)
Mallard (*Anas platyrhynchos diazi*)		+[b]				
Laysan Duck (*Anas laysanensis*)	H	+[b]	+[w]			
Hawaiian Duck (*Anas wyvilliana*)	H	+[b]	+[w]			
Mottled Duck (*Anas fulvigula*)	H	+[b]				Converse et al. (2001)
American Black Duck (*Anas rubripes*)	H	+[b]	+[w]	+	+	Leibovitz (1971) Montali et al. (1976) Burgess et al. (1979)
Yellow-billed Duck (*Anas undulata undulata*)	H	+[b]	+[w]			
Meller's Duck (*Anas melleri*)	H	+[b]	+[w]			Gough (1984)
Spot-billed Duck (*Anas poecilorhyncha zonorhyncha*)	H	+[b]				
Spot-billed Duck (*Anas poecilorhyncha poecilorhyncha*)			+[w]			
Pacific black Duck (*Anas superciliosa rogersi*)	H	+[b]	+[w]			
Philippine Duck (*Anas luzonica*)	H	+[b]	+[w]			Gough (1984)
Spectacled Duck (*Anas specularis*)		+[b]				
Crested Duck (*Anas s. specularioides*)	M	+[b]				
Northern Pintail (*Anas acuta*)			+[w]	–	+	Van Dorssen & Kunst (1955) Burgess et al. (1979) Spieker et al. (1996)
Yellow-billed Pintail (*Anas georgica georgica*)	H	+[b]	+[w]			
White-cheeked Pintail (*Anas bahamensis*)	M	+[b]				
Red-billed Duck (*Anas erythrorhyncha*)	M	+[b]				
Puna Teal (*Anas puna*)			+[w]			
Silver Teal (*Anas versicolor fretensis*)	M	+[b]				
Hottentot Teal (*Anas hottentota*)			+[w]			
Garganey (*Anas querquedula*)			+[w]	+		Leibovitz (1971)
Blue-winged Teal (*Anas discors*)		+[b]	+[w]	+		Wobeser (1987) Spieker et al. (1996)

					Converse et al. (2001)
Cinnamon Teal (*Anas cyanoptera septentrionalium*)		+	+[w]		Converse et al. (2001)
Red Shovler (*Anas platalea*)	L	+[b]	+[w]		
Cape Shoveler (*Anas smithii*)	L	+[b]	+[w]		
Australian Shoveler (*Anas rhynchotis rhynchotis*)		+[b]			
Australian Shoveler (*Anas rhynchotis variegata*)		+[b]	+[w]		
Northern Shoveler (*Anas clypeata*)		+		+	Van Dorssen & Kunst (1955)
					Gough (1984)
Pink-eared Duck (*Malacorhynchus membranaceus*)		+[b]			
Marbled Teal (*Marmaronetta angustirostris*)		+[b]	+[w]		
Southern Pochard (*Netta erythrophthalma erythrophthalma*)		+[b]	+[w]		
Common Pochard (*Aythya ferina*)		+[b]		+	Van Dorssen & Kunst (1955)
Canvasback (*Aythya valisineria*)		+			Snyder et al. (1973)
Redhead (*Aythya americana*)		+		+	Converse et al. (2001)
					Spieker et al. (1996)
Tufted Duck (*Aythya fuligula*)		+[b]		+	Van Dorssen & Kunst (1955)
New Zealand Scaup (*Aythya novaeseelandiae*)		+[b]			
Greater Scaup (*Aythya marila*)		+			Leibovitz (1971)
Lesser Scaup (*Aythya affinis*)		+			Snyder et al. (1973)
Common Eider (*Somateria mollissima*)	H	+[b]		+	Van Dorssen & Kunst (1955)
King Eider (*Somateria spectabilis*)		+			Converse et al. (2001)
Common Goldeneye (*Bucephala clangula*)		+			Pearson and Cassidy (1997)
					Montali et al. (1976)
Barrow's Goldeneye (*Bucephala islandica*)		+			ProMed Mail (2005)
Bufflehead (*Bucephala albeola*)		+			Leibovitz (1971)
					Montali et al. (1976)
Hooded Merganser (*Lophodytes cucullatus*)		+[b]			Converse et al. (2001)
Red-breasted Merganser (*Mergus serrator*)		+[b]	+[w]*Q*		
Common Merganser (*Mergus merganser merganser*)	L	+[b]	+[w]		Montali et al. (1976)
Ruddy Duck (*Oxyura jamaicensis*)		+			Converse et al. (2001)

Key: + = positive test for duck plague virus or animal died from virus infection; – = animal survived duck plague virus infection.

[a] Cloacal samples positive for duck plague virus by nested polymerase chain reaction (PCR) collected from clinically healthy captive and local wild birds at The Wildfowl and Wetlands Trust (WWT) (w), Slimbridge, England and Maryland (m), U.S.A. W. Hansen.

[b] Information on waterfowl mortality from duck plague at the WWT since 1978 provided by M. J. Brown, Animal Health Officer, Slimbridge, England. Symbols show species sensitivity to duck plague virus infection based on annual mortality records over 25 years as high (H), Medium (M), or low (L) at the WWT.

for sub-typing and tracking virus movement. The duck plague vaccine and field viruses have shown variable and distinct gel banding patterns from each other and other herpesviruses (Gunther et al. 1997; Gough and Hansen 2000). Some RE pattern differences that have been reported are probably due to the host and/or passage history of the Holland vaccine strain used (Gunther et al. 1997). Genomes from field virus isolates from the U.S.A. and U.K. produced different numbers and molecular sizes of some RE bands. In fact the genome pattern of the U.K. field isolate has more similarity to the Dutch vaccine strain than to the Lake Andes, South Dakota isolate (Gough and Hansen 2000). Vijaysri et al. (1997) reported differences in genome band numbers for local duck plague isolates in India when compared to other published reports. A few single nucleotide substitutions were found in duck plague virus genomes of field isolates from different geographical locations that either create or eliminate RE cleavage sites, changing the gel banding pattern. Amplification of a specific viral DNA region containing a genetic variation with polymerase chain reaction (PCR) and cleaving the cDNA product with RE provides a rapid epidemiological tool for tracking different subtypes of the duck plague virus (Hansen, unpubl. data).

Virus Stability

The infectivity of duck plague virus is more stable at lower environmental temperatures and more alkaline pH levels. The virus remains infectious longer when incubated at 4°C than 22°C when virus stabilizers (calf serum, bovine albumin, gelation, or glycerin) are added to the suspension medium (Hansen, unpubl. Data). At −15°C, virus viability declined rapidly, but glycerin and bovine serum provided the best virus stabilization. The Lake Andes strain of duck plague virus showed minimal decline in titer when inoculated into filtered water from outbreak sites in South Dakota and held at 4°C for 60 days in the laboratory (Wolf and Burke 1982). Virus titre of duck plague virus inoculated into unfiltered water declined steadily to low levels by 30 days and were barely detectable at 60 days. Investigators suggested that unknown particulate matter, including bacteria, in natural water may increase virus inactivation or nonspecifically bind the virus preventing detection. Attempts to recover virus from environmental samples collected at the sites of disease outbreaks have not been reported.

Virus held at 50°C for 90 minutes had a significant loss in titer to barely detectable levels, and at 56°C virus was completely inactivated in 10 minutes (Hess and Dardiri 1968). Investigators found that virus infectivity was stable at pH 7, 8, 9, less stable at pH 6, 5, 10, with immediate inactivation at pH 3 and 11. Desiccation of a virus suspension at 22°C resulted in complete inactivation by nine days.

Antigenic Type and Virulence

Only one antigenic type or serotype of duck plague virus has been identified based on cross protection studies with field isolates in waterfowl (Jansen and Kunst 1967a), or by *in vitro* virus neutralization comparisons with other herpesviruses using reference homologous and heterologous sera in cell culture (Dardiri 1975; Kaleta 1998). Although most scientific publications support the idea of a single virus serotype, a recent report from Vietnam indicates that there may be two serotypes or major subtypes of duck plague virus in that country (Bensink et al. 2004). Careful examination of field isolates from other geographic regions may uncover similar or additional antigenic variations.

Isolates of duck plague virus can vary in their ability to cause mortality in the same or different waterfowl species. Virus recovered in the Netherlands from duck plague outbreaks in 1959 killed <80% of experimentally infected ducks compared to 100% mortality for the original O strain of virus (Jansen 1961), indicating that the virus became less virulent over time. Field strains of virus in the U.S.A. have shown variation in their virulence for specific waterfowl species (Spieker et al. 1996). Similarly, Vietnamese field isolates that were co-circulating ranged from avirulent to causing 100% mortality when Pekin ducklings were inoculated (Tu et al. 2004). The minimum infective dose required to cause mortality in waterfowl previously naive to duck plague virus varies with the route of infection, the virulence of the virus isolate, the age of the waterfowl species infected (Spieker et al. 1996), and the number of serial passages in a laboratory host species (Jansen 1968).

EPIZOOTIOLOGY

Carrier State

The first experimental evidence for a persistent duck plague virus carrier state was suggested in 1969 when duck plague virus was isolated from the cloaca of Lesser Scaup (*Aythaya affinis*), Pekin ducks and Mallards (*Anas platyrhynchos*) 17 days post infection (Dardiri and Butterfield 1969) and from cloacal and esophageal samples from Pekin ducks 45 days post infection (Dardiri 1970). Subsequently, duck plague virus was shown to establish a long-term carrier state in waterfowl following both experimental and natural exposure (Burgess et al. 1979). Naturally exposed American Black Ducks and Canada Geese (*Branta canadensis*) were transferred to a containment facility where they shed virus for several years. Experimentally infected Mallards, Gadwalls (*Anas strepera*), and

Northern Pintails shed duck plague virus for more than a year. Experimentally infected carrier waterfowl were able to transmit virus vertically via the egg in Muscovy, Pekin, and Mallard ducks (Burgess and Yuill 1981). Investigations found that depending on the virus isolate and the duck species used, vertical transmission of virus had variable effects on fertility and hatchability of eggs. All the ducklings hatched from eggs laid by carrier waterfowl were found to be shedding small amounts of virus in their feces, suggesting that vertical transmission may be a mechanism for virus maintenance in wild waterfowl.

Transmission

The primary method for natural duck plague virus transmission is direct contact between virus-shedding and susceptible waterfowl or contact with a virus-contaminated environment, especially water (Sandhu and Leibovitz 1997). Successful experimental infections have occurred following nasal, oral, or cloacal inoculation as well as intravenous, subcutaneous, or intramuscular injection of virus. Cloacal inoculation has proven to be the best method for establishing the carrier state (Burgess and Yuill 1982). Vertical transmission of duck plague virus by asymptomatic carrier waterfowl has been shown experimentally (Burgess and Yuill 1982). The hatchlings were asymptomatic virus carriers that were also capable of shedding virus.

Studies by Burgess and Yuill (1981) have demonstrated the presence of virus in both the eggs and progeny of persistently infected ducks. Vertical transmission of duck plague virus likely occurs under natural conditions (Richter and Horzinek 1993), particularly as the seasonality of duck plague outbreaks coincide with the breeding season of waterfowl.

Mechanical transmission of virus by hematophagus arthropods feeding on duck plague viremic ducks may be possible (Jansen 1961; Dardiri 1970); however, there is no field or laboratory evidence to support this theory.

Seasonality

The highest number of disease events occur in the U.S.A. primarily from late winter to late spring, with 86% reported from March to June (Friend 1999b; Converse and Kidd 2001). Similar seasonal appearances of duck plague outbreaks were reported in the Netherlands (Jansen 1968) and the U.K. (Gough 1984; Gough and Alexander 1990). In Brazil, duck plague has been seen in November through February, which are Brazil's spring and summer (Saidenberg, pers. comm.). In the U.S.A., seasonal weather changes in the spring of the year facilitate virus transmission by crowding waterfowl in limited open water along migration routes (Friend and Pearson 1973). Stress due to spring migration, onset of breeding season, or social interactions with local waterfowl probably contributes to virus shedding by carriers. Testing cloacal samples for duck plague virus using nested PCR indicated that there was a gradual decline in the number of captive or wild nonmigratory waterfowl shedding virus from a high in May to a low in September in Maryland during surveillance in 1998 (Hansen, unpubl. data). This finding is consistent with that of investigators who found that undefined seasonal factors influenced the quantity of duck plague virus shed by experimentally infected carrier waterfowl over the same months (Burgess and Yuill 1983). The virus therefore seems to have a seasonal latent period in carrier waterfowl under natural conditions that is reactivated annually when stimulated by environmental or physiological changes. However, when both naturally and experimentally infected carrier waterfowl were removed from seasonal cues in a light-controlled laboratory, waterfowl shed virus periodically throughout the year for several years (Burgess et al. 1979).

Virus Reservoir

When duck plague was first seen in the U.S.A. in 1967, serological surveys indicated that the virus was new to the area because virus exposure was concentrated around sites where disease outbreaks had occurred, and it was not found in local free-flying waterfowl nor in other geographical areas of the U.S.A. (Dardiri and Hess 1967). However, because antibodies were found in domestic waterfowl at the same time on the farm where the first disease signs and lesions were discovered, it is believed that the virus had arrived before the first cases appeared (Newcomb 1968). Many theories were proposed on how and when the virus entered the U.S.A. (Leibovitz and Hwang 1968; Newcomb 1968), but the matter remains unresolved.

The presence of duck plague specific antibodies in wild waterfowl in Britain preceded disease outbreaks in domestic birds (Asplin 1970), indicating that virus was likely present before the first cases were reported in 1972 (Hall and Simmons 1972). Dardiri and Butterfield (1969) concluded that the duck plague virus maintained by small numbers of asymptomatic healthy carrier birds was transmitted to other susceptible waterfowl populations in the area, initiating new disease outbreaks.

The wild Mallard has been identified as one of the primary waterfowl species associated with the annual initiation of duck plague die-offs, especially in Britain (Van Dorssen and Kunst 1955; Gough et al. 1987). In both the U.S.A. and U.K. domestic ducks including the Muscovy have been most frequently affected during duck plague mortality events (Gough 1984; Converse and Kidd 2001). Expanding populations of resistant nonmigratory Mallards and Canada Geese in urban areas of the U.S.A. may be providing ideal reservoir populations for this disease. Duck plague virus has been detected in healthy, wild, nonmigratory Mallards and Canada Geese in regions of the U.S.A. that have recurrent die-offs (Hansen, unpubl. data). Local nonmigratory waterfowl and especially waterfowl raised for release in regulated shooting areas provide the best candidates for maintaining duck plague virus in nature. The survival rate of released waterfowl is less than that of wild waterfowl (Stanton et al. 1992), so repetitive releases of imported or locally produced young birds are done to replenish the declining released population. Such releases provide repeated opportunities for introduction of virus from infected premises. Local sanctuaries in city parks, suburban areas, or wildlife refuges that support local production and expansion of nonmigratory waterfowl also promote birds with longer life spans, thereby favoring virus maintenance.

In recent years duck plague disease events in the U.S.A. have been reported in new geographic locations as well as reappearing at sites of previous outbreaks (Friend 1999b). Isolated cases of mortality in wild waterfowl have been reported (Wobeser and Docherty 1987), but studies to date have failed to prove the virus is established in native migratory populations of waterfowl (Brand and Docherty 1984). Despite this, some researchers believe that the virus has become established (Pearson and Cassidy 1997) and that the inability to detect duck plague in migratory waterfowl may reflect the technology used rather than the presence or absence of the virus. Previous surveys used less sensitive traditional detection methods (Hansen et al. 1999). Field studies using nested PCR technology demonstrated that duck plague field virus was present in nonmigratory waterfowl populations of Maryland even though no cases of disease were reported in the area during the survey (Hansen, unpubl. data).

The mortality rate of waterfowl at risk during duck plague outbreaks appears to decrease over time when they occur repeatedly in the same region. Initial outbreaks in domestic ducks in the U.S.A., Europe (Netherlands and Hungary), India, and Thailand resulted in high mortality whereas subsequent outbreaks showed lower mortality rates (Jansen 1961; Mukerji et al. 1963; Suwathanaviroj et al. 1977; Ferenc et al. 1982). The initial outbreak on a commercial duck farm in the U.S.A. resulted in higher mortality (50%) than later outbreaks (<5%) before vaccination was initiated (Leibovitz and Hwang 1968). Prior to the 1950s mortality rates of 90–100% were reported in the Netherlands (Jansen 1961), but rates were lower in subsequent outbreaks. Jansen (1961) demonstrated differences in virulence between the original and new virus isolates as the cause for reduced mortality in subsequent disease outbreaks in the Netherlands.

In the two largest wild waterfowl outbreaks, mortality was higher at Lake Andes, South Dakota, in 1973, with 42% mortality of Mallards at risk than in the Finger Lakes region of New York in 1994, with 2% waterfowl mortality. High mortality rates may have been due to crowding of waterfowl into areas with limited open water during winter. However, the high mortality may also reflect the introduction of duck plague virus into a new geographic region with historically naive waterfowl populations. The declines in mortality in recent years may reflect establishment of a changing virus-host relationship by sequential passages through natural hosts over time, favoring adaptation to a carrier state.

CLINICAL SIGNS

Clinical signs can vary with virulence of the virus strain, species, sex, age, and immune status of the affected host. Signs include depressed activity, ruffled unpreened feathers, labored breathing, ataxia (lack of coordination), photophobia, extreme thirst, anorexia (lack of appetite), ocular and nasal (sometimes bloody) discharge, watery diarrhea with bloody vent, prolapsed penis in males, and drop in egg production (Friend 1999b). In field situations, wild migratory waterfowl may display some or none of these signs, although observing subtle signs such as ocular and nasal discharges in birds on lakes can be difficult.

PATHOGENESIS

The natural portal of entry of duck plague virus is through the oral cavity or cloaca as large concentrations of virus are excreted into pond and lake water. The incubation period varies depending on host factors and the pathogenicity of the virus and will range from three to seven days in domestic birds and up to 14 days in wild waterfowl (Sandhu and Leibovitz 1997). In the highly susceptible species, such as some species of teal and Muscovy Ducks, the incubation period ranges from five to 10 days. In other waterfowl, such as Mute Swans (*Cygnus olor*) and Mallard, the incubation period may be significantly longer. The primary site of virus replication is in the mucosa of the digestive tract, in particular the esophagus and cloaca (Islam and Khan 1995). Thereafter, a viremic phase occurs associated with increased vascular permeability, resulting in numerous petechial hemorrhages in various organs, particularly the liver, spleen, thymus, and bursa of Fabricius. Viral antigen and nucleocapsids can be detected in the nuclei and cytoplasm of epithelial cells, macrophages, and lymphocytes (Richter and Horzinek 1993).

Detailed chronological pathogenesis studies using PCR to track the progression of virulent duck plague virus in experimentally and naturally infected ducks showed that the route of infection influenced the sequence of tissues infected and the incubation time

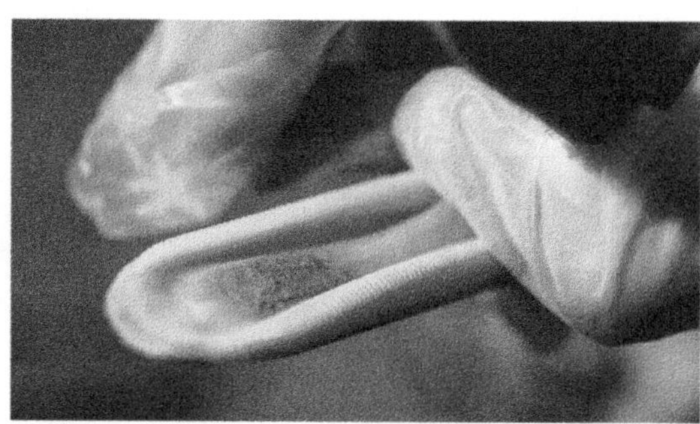

Figure 4.2. Lesion occasionally found under the tongue of some infected waterfowl. Photo by James Runningen.

required for virus appearance (AnChun et al. 2004; XiaoYan et al. 2004). The brain, liver, spleen, bursa of Fabricius, and thymus were PCR positive for viral DNA at two hours post infection in naturally infected ducks (AnChun et al. 2004). The chronology of infected tissues in naturally infected ducks was the liver, lungs, blood, excrement, spleen, brain, leg muscles, thoracic muscles, and kidneys (XiaoYan et al. 2004). All tissues sampled were positive at 12 hours post infection. Similar virus distribution was reported for vaccinated ducks (AnChun et al. 2004; AnChun et al. 2005; XiaoYan et al. 2004).

Waterfowl that survive primary infection may become persistently infected and excrete virus for long periods. American Black Ducks and Canada Geese surviving a natural infection of duck plague were monitored for virus persistence, and virus was isolated from cloacal swabs of some of the birds for more than four years (Burgess et al. 1979). Herpesviruses can remain latent in nerves and nerve ganglia, and during periods of stress virus may migrate down nerve roots and induce herpetic lesions of epithelium. Some persistently infected birds had erosions near the orifices of the sublingual salivary glands, which are in close proximity to the trigeminal nerve. Duck plague virus can be latent in the trigeminal nerve of carrier ducks and be reactivated by co-cultivation with susceptible cells (Shawky and Schat 2002). The nerves in other tissues such as the cloaca may serve as virus transporters when latent infections are reactivated in periodic virus shedders.

PATHOLOGY

Most waterfowl dying of duck plague die while in good body condition with ample deposits of fat and well-developed pectoral muscles. In general, there are variable amounts of hemorrhage in the heart and liver, and focal necrosis in the liver. The most distinctive differences occur along the digestive tract, reflecting species differences in the distribution of lymphoid tissue (Leibovitz 1969). The gross pathology of this disease has been studied extensively in domestic waterfowl and Mallard Ducks (Leibovitz 1969; Leibovitz 1971; Sandhu and Leibovitz 1997).

Mallards show the full spectrum of duck plague lesions. Oral erosions under the tongue (Figure 4.2) may be found near the opening of the sublingual salivary gland in a few waterfowl species including Mallards, American Black Ducks, and Northern Pintails following natural or experimental infections (Burgess et al. 1979).

In Mallards, esophageal lesions vary from focal hemorrhage and necrosis to a crusty, yellow pseudomembrane overlying necrotic epithelium (Figure 4.3A). Hemorrhages and necrosis may be present at the esophageal-proventricular junction, the mucosal surface of the lower intestine (Figure 4.3B), and in the transverse annular bands (Figure 4.3C and D) that reflect the distribution of gut-associated lymphoid tissues in the species. In adult females there may be extensive hemorrhage in ovarian tissues and free blood in the body cavity. Hemorrhages and necrosis are usually present in the cloaca, on the liver and heart (Figure 4.3F and G).

The gross pathology in other wild waterfowl species can be highly variable (Leibovitz 1969; Montali et al. 1976; Spieker 1978; Wobeser 1987). The most common lesions include necrotic lesions in the esophagus, necrosis of the lymphatic tissue (annular bands and discs), focal necrosis in the liver, and petechial hemorrhages on the epicardium and the surface of the liver, spleen, and pancreas, but their appearance varies by species (Brown pers. comm.). Hemorrhage of the annular bands was reported in naturally infected Wood Ducks (Montali et al. 1976) but these lesions were not reproduced in experimentally infected birds (Spieker 1978; Wobeser 1987). In contrast in the Canada Goose, hemorrhagic and necrotic lymphoid discs (Figure 4.3E) are scattered in groups along the small intestinal tract appearing as 0.5 to 1.5 cm button-like structures with raised, rounded borders and depressed necrotic centers (Leibovitz 1969; Locke, pers. comm.). In the American Black Duck, hemorrhages along the intestinal tract are usually punctiform and distributed along the length of the intestine. Diphtheritic esophagitis is the most common lesion found in swans (Keymer and Gough 1986). The extent of duck plague gross lesions that develop under field conditions appears to be influenced by the ambient temperature. The classical gross pathology seen at Lake Andes, South Dakota, in January and in the Finger Lakes region of New York in February are not typically seen in warmer climates in

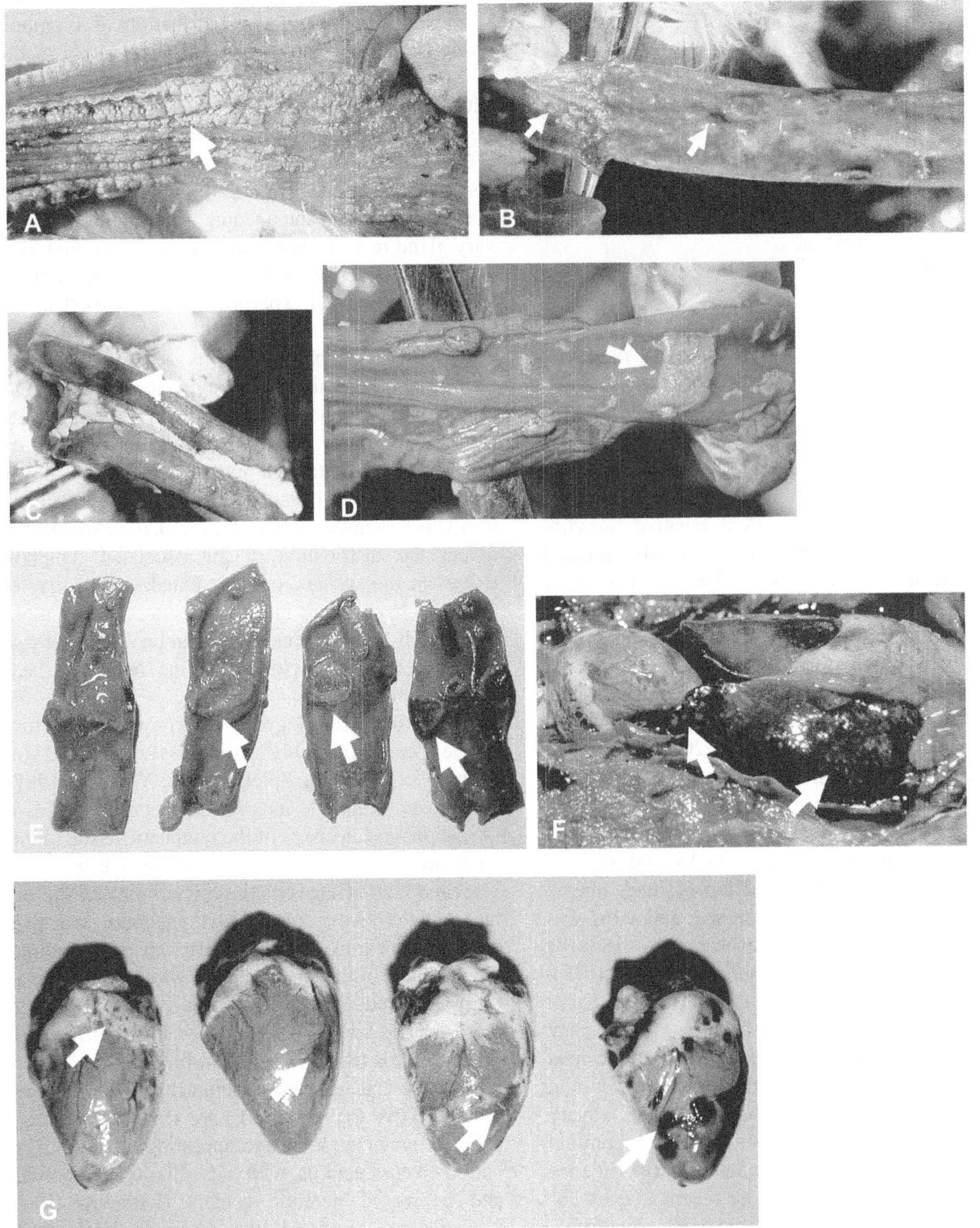

Figure 4.3. Appearance of major lesions of duck plague: (A) cheesy, raised plaques along the longitudinal folds of the esophagus, proventriculus; (B) inside the mucosal surface of the lower intestine; (C) external appearance of hemorrhagic bands in Mallard intestine; (D) the same lymphoid bands when the intestine is open; and (E) similar lymphoid button-like discs inside Canada Goose intestine; (F) necrotic spots on the liver; and (G) varying degrees of hemorrhage on the heart surface. Photo A by Steve Schmitt; D by James Runningen; the rest by Milton Friend.

comparable species (ProMed 2005; Saidenberg, pers. comm.).

In Muscovy Ducks, often the only lesions present are focal hemorrhages and necrosis in the cloaca (NWHC, unpubl. data). Blue-winged Teal and Wood Ducks may succumb without developing any visible lesions (Spieker 1978; Wobeser 1987). These latter observations reinforce the need for a thorough investigation of the entire waterfowl digestive tract when duck plague is suspected, with supporting attempts at virus isolation and or PCR identification of the virus from tissues.

Histological changes in affected tissues have been examined extensively in domestic and a few species of wild waterfowl (Leibovitz 1971; Sandhu and Leibovitz 1997; Yuan et al. 2005). Inclusion bodies are often present in the nucleus and cytoplasm of infected epithelial cells that have sloughed from or are adjacent to areas of ulceration and erosion (esophagus, intestine, bile duct epithelium) as well as in other affected organs (spleen, thymus, bursa of Fabricius, liver) with accumulations of enveloped virus particles in the nucleus, cytoplasm, and intracellular spaces.

DIAGNOSIS

Virus Isolation and Identification

Although a presumptive diagnosis of duck plague can be made on the basis of clinical, gross, and histopathological findings, confirmation can be made only by virus isolation or detection of viral antigen. Primary cell cultures derived from duck or goose embryos have been used and evaluated for sensitivity and suitability for isolation of duck plague virus, and Muscovy Duck embryo liver cells appear to be the most suitable (Woolcock 1998). Appropriate techniques for cell culture preparation and replication of duck plague virus have been reviewed (Schat and Purchase 1998; Woolcock 1998). Blind passages of inoculated cell cultures are often required to isolate duck plague virus from field samples.

Embryonated duck eggs have also been used to isolate duck plague virus. Inoculation onto the chorioallantoic membrane of 10- to 14-day-old embryonated Pekin or Muscovy Duck eggs produces embryo mortality and CAM lesions. Serial blind passages may be required before embryo mortality occurs. This method is relatively insensitive, time consuming, and expensive. Some Asian countries still use this method for duck plague diagnosis because of duck egg availability, and it is recommended as a diagnostic option by the World Organization for Animal Health (OIE) (Woolcock 2004).

Some laboratories have used duckling inoculation and protection tests to confirm the presence of duck plague virus in submitted samples. This method is undoubtedly sensitive, particularly if Muscovy ducklings are used, but may be considered expensive, time consuming, or unethical by laboratories as a means of diagnosing duck plague. Viral antigen detection by enzyme linked immunosorbent assay (ELISA), dot immunobinding assay, and immunofluoresence and immunoperoxidase techniques have also been described; these techniques are not routinely available in many parts of the world (Woolcock 1998) but are gaining acceptance in Asian countries (Morrissy et al. 2004; Kumar et al. 2004b; Kumar et al. 2005).

Duck plague specific antibody can be detected by serum neutralization tests in cell cultures or duck eggs. More rapid ELISA tests such as the indirect antibody test and the competitive ELISA are being used to find evidence for virus infection in domestic flocks in Asia (Morrissy et al. 2004; Kumar et al. 2004a).

More recently, PCR techniques have been described for the detection and identification of duck plague isolates (Plummer et al. 1998; Hansen et al. 1999; Pritchard et al. 1999; Hansen et al. 2000). For duck plague diagnosis, DNA extracts from cloacal swabs or tissue suspensions from dead waterfowl are tested with primers that locate a conserved region of the duck plague viral genome (Hansen et al. 2000). The PCR test is highly sensitive, specific, rapid, and easy to perform. Both a standard and nested duck plague PCR, which is 10-fold more sensitive, have been used to detect carriers of duck plague virus that are shedding virus in populations of both captive and wild, nonmigratory waterfowl (Hansen et al. 2000). Detecting waterfowl that have a latent infection would require testing of nerve cells containing the sequestered viral DNA. Duck plague PCR technology is gaining acceptance as a diagnostic as well as a research tool in other countries including China and Vietnam (AnChun et al. 2004; Phuc et al. 2004) and is a recommended method for the identification of duck plague by the OIE (Woolcock 2004).

Differential Diagnoses

Although the seasonal occurrence of duck plague outbreaks and the gross pathology are virtually pathognomonic of the disease, differentiation from the following diseases is required. Duck virus hepatitis causes hemorrhagic liver lesions in young ducklings (Woolcock and Fabricant 1997) similar to those caused by duck plague in young birds. Goose and Muscovy Duck parvovirus infections are also associated with hemorrhagic lesions in very young birds (Gough 1997). Avian cholera (*Pasteurella multocida*) and high pathogenicity strains of avian influenza can also produce hemorrhages and necrosis in susceptible waterfowl (Friend 1999a; Woolcock 1998).

Early duck plague lesions can sometimes be confused with those caused by the nematode *Capillaria contorta*. In fact, the two disease agents can occur together and viral isolation is essential to identify duck plague (Locke, personal communication.).

Serologically and genetically different herpesviruses that present a similar pathological picture to duck plague have been described in other countries (Kaschula 1950; Reece et al. 1987; Ketterer et al. 1990; Gough and Hansen 2000). Accurate identification and characterization of herpesviruses associated with waterfowl mortality should be carried out because complacency could allow a new or more virulent herpesvirus to become established in waterfowl populations.

IMMUNITY

Some waterfowl species have natural resistance to infection (Spieker et al. 1996), whereas others can become infected and die rapidly before the immune system can respond. Immunity to duck plague infection in waterfowl has been reviewed by Dardiri (1975). Virus virulence, exposure dose, the species of waterfowl, and individual host variation all play a role in the waterfowl antibody response. The ability of the bird to develop a strong neutralizing antibody response is important in protection. Several species of domestic ducks from sites where natural duck plague mortality had occurred had high titers of neutralizing antibodies, indicating that they had survived virus exposure (Dardiri and Butterfield 1969). Pekin and Mallard ducks that survived experimental infection with virulent field virus also produced high neutralizing antibody titers 38 to 58 days post infection (Dardiri and Butterfield 1969; Dardiri and Gailunas 1969).

Vaccination can produce lifelong immunity for domestic ducks, but it seems to provide only variable protection for wild waterfowl species (Jansen and Wemmenhove 1966; Butterfield and Dardiri 1969b). Ducklings and breeder ducks do not produce high neutralizing antibody titres immediately following initial vaccination (Toth 1971a); however, the vaccinated birds are resistant to virus challenge before antibody can be detected, suggesting that interferon or some other protective antiviral product may be produced immediately following vaccination (Jansen 1964; Toth 1970). A low-level anamnestic antibody response can be detected following a second vaccination, but challenge of the vaccinated birds with a field strain of virus results in a much higher anamnestic response (Butterfield and Dardiri 1969b; Toth 1971a). Neutralizing antibody levels usually peak at about six weeks and decline to low or nondetectable levels 10 to 12 weeks post vaccination.

Lin et al. (1984) used passive immunization of birds with anti-duck plague antibody to show that antibody plays an important role in waterfowl resistance to duck plague infection. The importance of antibody in protection from virus infection is supported by the work of Goldberg et al. (1990). However, the level of serum neutralizing antibody does not accurately reflect waterfowl resistance to virus challenge (Jansen and Wemmenhove 1966; Butterfield and Dardiri 1969b; Dardiri 1975). Some waterfowl with low antibody levels may resist virus challenge, whereas others with higher antibody levels may succumb. Pekin ducks resisted virus challenge one year after vaccination despite low levels of serum antibodies (Jansen and Wemmenhove 1966). Breeder ducks with 3.5 $\log_{10}$ of neutralizing antibody can pass maternal antibody to ducklings; however, the maternal protection diminishes rapidly by 13 days post hatch (Toth 1971a). The presence of high serum antibody levels also does not prevent virus shedding from the esophagus or cloaca of infected waterfowl (Dardiri 1970).

PUBLIC HEALTH CONCERNS

Duck plague virus has not been reported to infect mammals (Bos 1942) and there is no evidence to suggest that duck plague virus poses a risk to humans.

DOMESTIC ANIMAL HEALTH CONCERNS

Outbreaks of duck plague in domestic ducks and geese have occurred following contact with wild waterfowl and aquatic environments shared with wild waterfowl (Gough et al. 1987; Sandhu and Leibovitz 1997). In commercial duck flocks and game farms, strict biosecurity is essential to prevent contact with wild waterfowl, particularly with Mallards, which are the species most likely to be shedding virus. In Asia, where duck plague is considered endemic and free-range duck farming practices are used, vaccination of domestic ducks is routinely used to protect flocks (Hossain et al. 2004; Trung et al. 2004). Contact with infected wild waterfowl is much more difficult to control in ornamental waterfowl collections and wildlife rescue centers. Outbreaks in wildlife hospitals and rescue centers in Great Britain have frequently been attributed to the introduction of birds either incubating duck plague or excreting the virus (Gough and Alexander 1990).

WILDLIFE POPULATION IMPACTS

Little is known about the impacts of duck plague on migratory waterfowl populations. Mortality has been the most visible and measurable indicator reported. Only three known duck plague outbreaks in the U.S.A. have involved migratory waterfowl. The largest outbreak, at Lake Andes, a South Dakota wildlife refuge, in 1973 caused the highest mortality with an estimated 42% of 100,000 Mallards and 3% of the 9,000 Canada Geese at risk of dying (Friend and Pearson 1973). The other two outbreaks were both in the state of New York in 1967 and 1994, the latter at Keuka Lake involving 1,150 waterfowl, primarily American Black Ducks (Converse and Kidd 2001). In 1967 a die-off of approximately 100 waterfowl, mostly Mallards and American Black Ducks, occurred at Flanders Bay, Long Island, New York. There have not been any reports of impacts of duck plague in wild birds in other parts of the world. This may be a result of a lack of awareness or limited surveillance.

The real impact of this disease on migratory waterfowl may be subclinical infections that could affect annual duckling production for some species. Adverse effects on certain reproductive parameters including egg fertility and hatchability were more severe in Muscovy Ducks than Mallards that were experimentally infected with certain strains of duck plague virus (Burgess and Yuill 1981). Extrapolation of these limited experimental studies to wild waterfowl in general is difficult due to the wide range of susceptibilities exhibited by different waterfowl species and known differences in the biological characteristics of field strains of duck plague virus. Further, the prevalence of virus carrier birds in wild waterfowl populations is unknown (Brand and Docherty 1984).

More field research is required to fully understand the epizootiology and the virus-host interactions of duck plague in wild, migratory waterfowl that are being increasingly managed. Understanding these interactions will provide conservation agencies and wildlife managers with better scientific-based information to assist in managing the waterfowl resource in the future.

TREATMENT AND CONTROL

Treatment and control strategies for duck plague in North America are controversial, and opinions differ regarding the status of duck plague. Available scientific information needs to be supplemented with additional field studies using improved, sensitive molecular techniques.

The only prevention for duck plague is vaccination. A modified-live virus vaccine was first developed in the Netherlands by attenuation through serial passage of the virus in embryonated chicken eggs or primary cultures derived from chicken and duck embryos (Jansen 1964). Vaccination has been used successfully in the commercial duck industry in the Netherlands and the U.S.A. (Jansen 1968; Toth 1970; Toth 1971a). Several countries, including China, Vietnam, India, Thailand, Pakistan, and Bangladesh, have successfully utilized the Holland duck plague vaccine or developed their own modified-live virus vaccines from local isolates to combat duck plague in their economically important duck industries (Bordolai et al. 1994; Cheng et al. 1996; Kulkarni et al. 1998). Laboratory studies in domestic ducks have indicated that following vaccination, resistance to challenge occurs very rapidly (Jansen 1964; Richter and Horzinek 1993).

Vaccination has also been used in prevention or to interrupt a disease outbreak in captive ornamental flocks. In the U.K., annual spring vaccination with a modified-live duck plague vaccine in collections of ornamental waterfowl has been effective for a number of years in reducing losses from the disease at the WWT (Gough and Brown, unpubl. data). Vaccine has also been used in the U.S.A. to limit duck plague outbreaks and prevent future occurrences in a zoological collection (Montali et al. 1976; ProMed 2005).

In general, modified-live vaccines produce better protection from challenge when compared to inactivated vaccines (Jansen et al. 1963; Butterfield and Dardiri 1969a). However, delivery of an inactivated virus in an adjuvant has produced challenge protection equivalent to a modified-live vaccine (Shawky and Sandhu 1997). Use of the modified-live vaccine licensed by USDA in the U.S.A. is regulated by individual state authorities, usually the state veterinarian. The vaccine was originally intended for use in commercial breeder ducks, and it is not approved for use in migratory waterfowl that fall under the responsibility of the Fish and Wildlife Service through the Migratory Bird Treaty Act (16 USAC. 703–712) and the Fish and Wildlife Act of 1956.

Whether the vaccine interference phenomenon described by Jansen (1964) occurs in all waterfowl species has not been determined, but the efficacy of the vaccine varies for some wild waterfowl species. An unpublished study done by the New York Department of Public Health, Center for Laboratories and Research demonstrated this variation when wild waterfowl were vaccinated according to the manufacturer's recommendations for domestic waterfowl (NWHC, unpubl. data). Vaccinated Wood Duck, Blue-winged Teal, Gadwall, Mallard, Northern Pintail, and Canvasback (*Aythya valisineria*) had a range of mortality from 100% to 11% respectively when challenged with the Lake Andes strain of duck plague virus, and Northern Pintails that are normally resistant to Lake Andes virus infection (Spieker et al. 1996) became susceptible to virus challenge, with a 38% mortality rate.

There has always been a concern that the modified-live vaccine may revert to virulence. The work of Jansen and Kunst (1967b) indicated that back passage of the vaccine strain in duck eggs did not revive virulence for susceptible waterfowl; however, in a separate study duck egg passage was used to revive vaccine potency (Bhattacharya et al. 1977).

Whether the modified live vaccine can produce carrier waterfowl that can transmit virus to contacts remains controversial. Contact controls placed with vaccinated ducks did not produce antibody and remained susceptible to challenge with virulent virus, suggesting that the vaccine virus was not spread by the vaccinates (Jansen and Kunst 1964b; Toth 1971a). In a similar study, unvaccinated controls were comingled with virus-challenged vaccinated waterfowl. The control birds did not develop detectable neutralizing antibody nor were they able resist challenge with virulent duck plague virus, suggesting that the vaccinates did not transmit the challenge virus to the controls (Toth 1971b). In contrast, field studies in the U.K. have found that vaccinated captive waterfowl can become carriers of either the vaccine or field strains of virus and that wild waterfowl that frequented the site were shedding the vaccine virus (Hansen, unpubl. data). In the U.S.A., wild, nonmigratory waterfowl and captive-raised and released Mallards were found to be shedding either vaccine or field duck plague viruses, but the source of the vaccine virus was unknown (Hansen, unpubl. data). There is also evidence from field surveys of wild nonmigratory waterfowl that horizontal transmission of the vaccine virus occurs from vaccinates to wild waterfowl (Hansen, unpubl. data), raising questions on possible virus reversion to virulence and concern that vaccine virus will permit more susceptible wild waterfowl species to become concurrent field virus carriers.

Persistently infected carrier waterfowl can become superinfected with a second duck plague virus strain, resulting either in mortality or protection depending on the combination of initial and challenge viruses used and the route of exposure (Burgess and Yuill 1982). These results suggest that carrier waterfowl naturally infected by a less virulent virus strain may be protected from mortality when reexposed. It is unknown whether the use of modified-live vaccines could serve a similar role by expanding the number of field virus carrier waterfowl in nature.

Prevention of duck plague outbreaks would be difficult in wild, especially migratory waterfowl. Jansen and Kunst (1964c) used a modified-live vaccine in drinking water that was efficacious in domestic waterfowl, providing a delivery method that could be applied to wild birds. The use of inactivated vaccines for vaccination of wild waterfowl populations would not be currently feasible (Shawkey and Sandhu 1997).

Strict biosecurity is essential in preventing the introduction of duck plague into collections of susceptible, ornamental waterfowl. Outbreaks of duck plague in wild waterfowl hospitals and rescue centers can be significantly reduced with good management and the provision of a stress-free environment. Outbreaks of duck plague in waterfowl sanctuaries and zoological collections have been attributed to overcrowding, poor hygiene, contaminated water, and the introduction of birds incubating or shedding duck plague virus. Where outbreaks occur in valuable ornamental collections of waterfowl, mortality can be reduced by removing birds from any potentially contaminated water and housing them in isolated accommodations. They should be tested and proven not to be virus carriers before being mixed with new birds (Gough 1984; Hansen et al. 2000).

Disease control efforts in captive and wild waterfowl have utilized depopulation of all exposed or potentially exposed birds from a die-off site, with few follow-up studies to verify the effectiveness of the methods (Brand and Docherty 1988). Due to the difficulty in detecting duck plague carrier waterfowl post epizootic, depopulation is the best control method. As the epizootiology of this disease is studied further, better management strategies will be developed. Advances in technology will provide more rapid diagnostic methods for detection of virus carrier waterfowl, possibly allowing selective removal and testing of valuable or endangered birds from virus-exposed ornamental populations.

MANAGEMENT IMPLICATIONS

Decreasing the occurrence of duck plague in commercial, domestic, and captive waterfowl can be achieved by practicing sound management strategies for prevention and control. Ducks should be housed to discourage comingling with wild waterfowl. Managers should be alert to changes in the general health of the managed waterfowl population, and any dead birds should be submitted to an accredited diagnostic laboratory for rapid diagnosis. Vaccination of commercial or ornamental birds may be considered. Biosecurity practices should be developed to protect captive waterfowl from exposure to duck plague virus and prevent virus from spreading if disease does occur. Captive releases of waterfowl that would have contact with wild birds should be discouraged. Winter dispersal of large concentrations of wild waterfowl should be promoted, large concentrations of waterfowl in heavily used bodies of water should be avoided, and collecting dead waterfowl for proper diagnosis and disposal should be encouraged.

UNPUBLISHED DATA/PERSONAL COMMUNICATIONS

Martin J. Brown, The Wildfowl and Wetlands Trust, Slimbridge, Gloucestershire, GL2 7BT, United Kingdom.

Richard Gough, Veterinary Laboratories Agency, Waybridge, Surrey KT15 3NB, United Kingdom.

Wallace R. Hansen, National Wildlife Health Center, USA Geological Survey, 6006 Schroeder Rd., Madison, United States.

Louis Locke, National Wildlife Health Center, USA. Geological Survey, 6006 Schreoder Rd., Madison, Wisconsin, United States.

National Wildlife Health Center, U. S. Geological Survey, 6006 Schroeder Rd., Madison, Wisconsin, United States.

Andre Saidenberg, Ornithopathology Research Group, Sao Paulo State University, Campinas, Brazil.

LITERATURE CITED

AnChun, C., W. MingShu, L. Fei, S. Yong, Y. GuiPing, H. XiaoYing, X. Chao, L. YongHong, W. Ming, Z. WeiGuang, and J. RenYong. 2005. Distribution and excretion of duck plague virus attenuated Cha strain in vaccinated ducklings. *Chinese Journal of Veterinary Science* 25:231–233.

AnChun, C., W. MingShu, L. Fei, S. Yong, Y. GuiPing, H. XiaoYing, X. Chao, L. YongHong, Z. WeiGuang, W. Ming, J. RengYong, and C. XiaoYue. 2004. The preliminary application of PCR in research of clinical diagnosis and mechanisms of immunity and pathology of duck plague virus (DPV). *Chinese Journal of Virology* 20:364–370.

Asplin, F.D. 1970. Examination of sera from wildlife for antibodies against the viruses of duck plague, duck hepatitis and duck influenza. *Veterinary Record* 87:182–183.

Attanasio, R., R. Olson, and J.C. Johnson. 1980. Improvement in plaquing methods for the enumeration of anatid herpesvirus (duck plague virus). *Intervirology* 14:245–252.

Baudet, A.E.R.F. 1923. Een sterfte onder eenden in Nederland, veroorzaakt door een filtreerbaar virus (vogelpest) = Mortality in ducks in the Netherlands caused by a filtrable virus (fowl plague). *Tijdschrift voor Diergeneeskunde* 50:455–459.

Bensink, Z., J. Meers, N.T.K. Dinh, N.V. Dung, N.T.L. Huong, K.V. Phuc, D. Hung, and P. Spradbrow. 2004. Antigenic relatedness of duck plague viruses isolated in Vietnam. In *Proceedings of the 2003 Control of Newcastle Disease and Duck Plague in Village Poultry Workshop,* No. 117, J. Meers, P.B. Spradbrow, and T. D. Tu (eds.). Australian Center for International Agricultural Research, Canberra, Australia, pp. 71–76.

Bhattacharya, A.K., K.K. Maulik, S.P. Chandra Chowdhury, and P.C.B. Dasgupta. 1977. Revival of duck plague vaccine virus (chick embryo adapted modified strain) by back passing in embryonated duck eggs. *Indian Journal of Animal Health* 16:123–127.

Bordolai, G.K., B.R. Boro, A. Mukit, K. Sharma, and G.N. Dutta. 1994. Adaptation and attenuation of duck plague virus for vaccine production. *Indian Veterinary Journal* 71:639–644.

Bos, A. 1942. Weer nieuwe gevallen van eendenpest = Again new cases of duck plague. *Tijdschrift voor Diergeneeskunde* 69:372–381.

Brand, C.J., and D.E. Docherty. 1984. A survey of North American migratory waterfowl for duck plague (duck virus enteritis) virus. *Journal of Wildlife Diseases* 20:261–266.

Brand, C.J., and D.E. Docherty. 1988. Post-epizootic surveys of waterfowl for duck plague (duck virus enteritis). *Avian Diseases* 32:722–730.

Breese Jr., S. S., and A. H. Dardiri. 1968. Electron microscope characterization of duck plague virus. *Virology* 34:160–169.

Burgess, E.C., J. Ossa, and T.M. Yuill. 1979. Duck plague:a carrier state in waterfowl. *Avian Diseases* 23:940–949.

Burgess, E.C., and T.M. Yuill. 1981. Vertical transmission of duck plague virus (DPV) by apparently healthy DPV carrier waterfowl. *Avian Diseases* 25:795–800.

Burgess, E.C., and T.M. Yuill. 1982. Superinfection in ducks persistently infected with duck plague virus. *Avian Diseases* 26:40–46.

Burgess, E.C., and T.M. Yuill. 1983. The influence of seven environmental and physiological factors on duck plague virus shedding by carrier mallards. *Journal of Wildlife Diseases* 19:77–81.

Butterfield, W.K., and A.H. Dardiri. 1969a. Serologic and immunologic response of ducks to inactivated and attenuated duck plague virus. *Avian Diseases* 13:876–887.

Butterfield, W.K., and A.H. Dardiri. 1969b. Serologic and immunologic response of wild waterfowl vaccinated with attenuated duck plague virus. *Bulletin of the Wildlife Disease Association* 5:99–102.

Cheng, A.C., M.S. Wang, H.M. Cui, D.H. Liao, and X.Y. Chen. 1996. Study on a bivalent attenuated vaccine against duck plague and duck virus hepatitis. *Acta Veterinaria et Zootechnica Sinica* 27:466–474.

Converse, K.A., and G.A. Kidd. 2001. Duck plague epizootics in the United States, 1967–1995. *Journal of Wildlife Diseases* 37:347–357.

Dardiri, A.H. 1970. Transmission and certain disease features of duck plague. In *Proceedings 14th World's Poultry Congress.* Madrid, Spain, pp. 209–219.

Dardiri, A.H. 1975. Duck viral enteritis (duck plague) characteristics and immune response of the host. *American Journal of Veterinary Research* 36:535–538.

Dardiri, A.H., and W.K. Butterfield. 1969. The susceptibility and response of wild waterfowl to duck plague virus. *Acta Zoologica et Pathologica Antverpiensia* 48:373–383.

Dardiri, A.H., and P. Gailunas. 1969. Response of pekin and mallard ducks and Canada geese to experimental infection with duck plague virus. *Bulletin of the Wildlife Disease Association* 5:235–247.

Dardiri, A.H., and W.R. Hess. 1967. The incidence of neutralizing antibodies to duck plague virus in serums from domestic ducks and wild waterfowl in the United States of America. *In Proceedings 71st Annual Meeting of the U S Livestock Sanitation Association.* Phoenix, Arizona, pp. 225–237.

Devos, A., N. Viaene, and M. Staelens. 1964. Eendenpest in Belgie. *Vlaams Diergeneeskundig Tijdschrift* 33:260–266.

De Zeeuw, F.A. 1930. Nieuwe gevallen van eendenpest en de specificiteit van het virus. *Tijdschrift voor Diergeneeskunde.* 57:1095–1098.

Duraiswami, J., M.P. Rajendran, M. John, and M. Ganesamurthy. 1979. Duck plague in Tamil Nadu. *Indian Veterinary Journal* 56:1–5.

Ferenc, V., P. Vilmos, L. Sandor, and K. Pal. 1982. A kacsapestis (duck plague) elofordulasa kacsaallomanyokban. *Magyar Allatorvosok Lapja* 37:171–182.

Friend, M. 1999a. Avian Cholera. *In Field Manual of Wildlife Diseases: General Field Procedures and Diseases of Birds,* M. Friend and C.J. Franson (eds.). U.S. Geological Survey, National Wildlife Health Center, Madison, Wisconsin, pp. 75–92.

Friend, M. 1999b. Duck plague. In *Field Manual of Wildlife Diseases: General Field Procedures and Diseases of Birds,* M. Friend and C.J. Franson (eds.). U.S. Geological Survey, National Wildlife Health Center, Madison, Wisconsin, pp. 141–151.

Friend, M., and G.L. Pearson. 1973. Duck plague (duck virus enteritis) in wild waterfowl. In *Proceedings 53rd Annual Conference of the Western Association of State Game and Fish Commissioners.* Salt Lake City, Utah, pp. 315–325.

Gardner, R., J. Wilkerson, and J. C. Johnson. 1993. Molecular characterization of the DNA of Anatid herpesvirus 1. *Intervirology* 36:99–112.

Goldberg, D.R., T.M. Yuill, and E.C. Burgess. 1990. Mortality from duck plague virus in immunosuppressed adult mallard ducks. *Journal of Wildlife Diseases* 26:299–306.

Goldstein, H.E., R. Allen, R.A. Bankowski, F. G. Buzzell, L.C. Grumbles, J.E. Hanley, R. Houge, A. E. Janawicz, T.L. Landers, S.A. Moore, H.E. Nadler, B.S. Pomeroy, W. Scholfield, J.B. Thomas, J. W. Walker, J.B. Roberts, and C.W. Wilder. 1971. Transmissible diseases of poultry committee:Updating of the duck virus enteritis (DVE) situation in the United States. *In Proceedings of the 74th Annual Meeting of U. S. Animal Health Association 1970.* Warwick Hotel, Philadelphia, Pennsylvania, pp. 323–335.

Gough, R.E. 1984. Laboratory confirmed outbreaks of duck virus enteritis (duck plague) in the United Kingdom from 1977 to 1982. *Veterinary Record* 114:262–265.

Gough, R.E. 1997. Goose parvovirus. In *Diseases of Poultry,* B.W. Calnek, H.J. Barnes, C.W. Beard, L.R. McDougald, and Y.M. Saif (eds.). Iowa State University Press, Ames, Iowa, pp. 777–783.

Gough, R.E., and D.J. Alexander. 1990. Duck virus enteritis in Great Britain, 1980 to 1989. *Veterinary Record* 126:595–597.

Gough, R.E., E.D. Borland, I.F. Keymer, and J.C. Stuart. 1987. An outbreak of duck virus enteritis in commercial ducks and geese in East Anglia. *Veterinary Record* 121:85.

Gough, R.E., and W.R. Hansen. 2000. Characterization of a herpesvirus isolated from domestic geese in Australia. *Avian Pathology* 29:417–422.

Gunther, B.M.F., B.G. Klupp, M. Gravendyck, J.E. Lohr, T.C. Mettenleiter, and E.F. Kaleta. 1997. Comparison of the genomes of 15 avian herpesvirus isolates by restriction endonuclease analysis. *Avian Pathology* 26:305–316.

Hall, S.A., and J.R. Simmons. 1972. Duck plague (duck virus enteritis) in Britain. *Veterinary Record* 90:691.

Hansen, W.R., S.E. Brown, S.W. Nashold, and D.L. Knudson. 1999. Identification of duck plague virus by polymerase chain reaction. *Avian Diseases* 43:106–115.

Hansen, W.R., S.W. Nashold, D.E. Docherty, S.E. Brown, and D.L. Knudson. 2000. Diagnosis of duck plague in waterfowl by polymerase chain reaction. *Avian Diseases* 44:266–274.

Hanson, J.A., and N.G. Willis. 1976. An outbreak of duck virus enteritis (duck plague) in Alberta. *Journal of Wildlife Diseases* 12:258–262.

Hess, W.R., and A.H. Dardiri. 1968. Some properties of the virus of duck plague. *Archiv fur die Gesamte Virusforschung* 24:148–153.

Hossain, M.T., M.A. Islam, S. Akter, M. Sadekuzzaman, M.A. Islam, M.M. Amin. 2004. Effect of dose and time of vaccination on immune response of duck plague vaccine in ducks. *Bangladesh Journal of Veterinary Medicine* 2:117–119.

Islam, M.R., and M.A.H.N.A. Khan. 1995. An immunocytochemical study on the sequential tissue distribution of duck plague virus. *Avian Pathology* 24:189–194.

Jacobsen, G.S., J.E. Pearson, and T.M. Yuill. 1976. An epornitic of duck plague on a Wisconsin game farm. *Journal of Wildlife Diseases* 12:20–26.

Jansen, J. 1961. Duck plague. *British Veterinary Journal* 117:349–356.

Jansen, J. 1964. The interference phenomenon in the development of resistance against duck plague. *Journal of Comparative Pathology* 74:3–7.

Jansen, J. 1968. Duck plague. *Journal of the American Veterinary Medical Association* 152:1009–1016.

Jansen, J., and H. Kunst. 1949. Is eendepest verwant aan hoender pest of pseudohoenderpest? = Is duck plague related to Newcastle disease or to fowl plague? *Tijdschrift voor Diergeneeskunde* 74:705–707.

Jansen, J., and H. Kunst. 1964a. The reported incidence of duck plague in Europe and Asia. *Tijdschrift voor Diergeneeskunde* 89:765–769.

Jansen, J., and H. Kunst. 1964b. Scheiden geente eendekuikens het entvirus uit? = Do vaccinated ducklings excrete the vaccine? *Tijdschrift voor Diergeneeskunde* 89:1534–1535.

Jansen, J., and H. Kunst. 1964c. Vaccination of ducklings against duck plague by the addition of attenuated virus to the drinking water. *Tijdschrift voor Diergeneeskunde* 89:1234–1235.

Jansen, J., and H. Kunst. 1967a. Een vergelijkend onderzoek van de Nederlandse en de Amerikaanse eendepest. = A comparative research between Dutch and American duck plague. *Tijdschrift voor Diergeneeskunde* 92:1454–1458.

Jansen, J., and H. Kunst. 1967b. Kan de avirulente kippeei-entstof tegen eendepest virulent worden? = Can the avirulent ckicken egg–adapted vaccine strain against duck plague regain its natural virulence? *Tijdschrift voor Diergeneeskunde* 92:646–647.

Jansen, J., H. Kunst, and R. Wemmenhove. 1963. The active immunization of ducks against duck plague. *Tijdschrift voor Diergeneeskunde* 88:927–932.

Jansen, J., and R. Wemmenhove. 1966. De immuniteit ruim een jaar na enting tegen eendepest. = The immunity, a good year after vaccination against duck plague. *Tijdschrift voor Diergeneeskunde* 91: 838–841.

Kaleta, E.F. 1998. Herpesviruses of free-living and pet birds. In *A Laboratory Manual for the Isolation and Identification of Avian Pathogens,* D.E. Swayne, J.R. Glisson, M.W. Jackson, J.E. Pearson, and W.M. Reed (eds.). American Association of Avian Pathologists, University of Pennsylvania, Kennett Square, Pennsylvania, pp. 129–136.

Kaschula, V.R. 1950. A new virus disease of the Muscovy duck [*Cairina moschata* (Linn)] present in Natal. *Journal of the South African Veterinary Medical Association* 21:18–26.

Ketterer, P.J., B.J. Rodwell, H.A. Wesbury, P.T. Hooper, A.R. Mackenzie, J.G. Dingles, and H.C. Prior. 1990. Disease of geese caused by a new herpesvirus. *Australian Veterinary Journal* 67:446–448.

Keymer, I.F., and R.E. Gough. 1986. Duck virus enteritis (anatid herpesvirus infection) in mute swans (*Cygnus olor*). *Avian Pathology* 15:161–170.

Kocan, R.M. 1976. Duck plague virus replication in muscovy duck fibroblast cells. *Avian Diseases* 20:574–580.

Kulkarni, D.D., P.C. James, and S. Sulochana. 1998. Assessment of the immune response to duck plague vaccinations. *Research in Veterinary Science* 64:199–204.

Kumar, N.V., Y.N. Reddy, and M.V.S. Rao. 2004a. Development of enzyme linked immunosorbent assay for the detection of antibodies to duck plague virus. *Indian Veterinary Journal* 81:363–365.

Kumar, N.V., Y.N. Reddy, and M.V.S. Rao. 2004b. Enzyme linked immunosorbent assay for detection of duck plague virus. *Indian Veterinary Journal* 81:481–483.

Kumar, N.V., Y.N. Reddy, and M.V.S. Rao. 2005. Dot immunobinding assay for the detection of duck plague virus. *Indian Veterinary Journal* 82:361–364.

Kunst, H. 1968. Klassifikatie van het eendepestvirus. = Classification of the duck plague virus. *Tijdschrift voor Diergeneeskunde* 93:1025–1027.

Leibovitz, L. 1969. The comparative pathology of duck plague in wild anseriformes. *Journal of Wildlife Management* 33:275–290.

Leibovitz, L. 1971. Gross and histopathologic changes of duck plague (duck virus enteritis). *American Journal of Veterinary Research* 32:275–290.

Leibovitz, L., and J. Hwang. 1968. Duck plague on the American continent. *Avian Diseases* 12:361–378.

Lin, W., K.M. Lam, and W.E. Clark. 1984. Active and passive immunization of ducks against duck viral enteritis. *Avian Diseases* 28:968–973.

Lucam, F. 1949. La peste aviaire en France. *Report to the 14th* International Veterinary Congress 2:380–382.

Montali, R.J., M. Bush, and G.A. Greenwell. 1976. An epornitic of duck viral enteritis in a zoological park. *Journal of the American Veterinary Medical Association* 169:954–958.

Morrissy, C.J., P.W. Daniels, S.L. Lowther, W. Goff, I. Pritchard, T.D. Tu, K.V. Phuc, D. Hung, N.T.T. Hong, N.T. Trung, P.B. Spradbrow, and H.A. Westbury. 2004. Duck plague in Vietnam and the development of diagnostic capability. In *Proceedings of the 2003 Control of Newcastle Disease and Duck Plague in Village Poultry Workshop,* No. 117, J. Meers, P. B. Spradbrow, and T.D. Tu (eds.). Australian Center for International Agricultural Research, Canberra, Australia, pp. 25–29.

Mukerji, A., M.S. Das, B.B. Ghosh, and J.L. Ganguly. 1963. Duck plague in West Bengal—part I. *Indian Veterinary Journal* 40:457–462.

Newcomb, S.S. 1968. Duck virus enteritis (duck plague) epizootiology and related investigations. *Journal of the American Veterinary Medical Association* 153:1897–1902.

Pearson, G.L., and D.R. Cassidy. 1997. Perspectives on the diagnosis, epizootiology, and control of the 1973 duck plague epizootic in wild waterfowl at Lake Andes, South Dakota. *Journal of Wildlife Diseases* 33:681–705.

Phuc, K.V., D. Hung, N.T.L. Huong, T.D. Tu, N.T. Trung, C.J. Morrissy, and L.I. Pritchard. 2004. Application of the polymerase chain reaction (PCR) for the detection of duck plague virus in Vietnam. *In Proceedings of the 2003 Control of Newcastle Disease and Duck Plague in Village Poultry Workshop,* No. 117, J. Meers, P.B. Spradbrow, and T.D. Tu (eds.). Australian Center for International Agricultural Research, Canberra, Australia, pp. 40–46.

Plummer, P.J., T. Alefantis, S. Kaplan, P. O'Connell, S. Shawky, and K.A. Schat. 1998. Detection of duck enteritis virus by polymerase chain reaction. *Avian Diseases* 42:554–564.

Pritchard, L.I., C. Morrissy, K. Van Phuc, P.W. Daniels, and H.A. Westbury. 1999. Development of a polymerase chain reaction to detect Vietnamese isolates of duck virus enteritis. *Veterinary Microbiology* 68:149–156.

ProMed Mail. 2005, June 2, Archive Number 20050602.1537. International Society for Infectious Diseases. [Online] Retrieved from the World Wide Web:www.promedmail.org.

Reece, R.L., D.A. Barr, R.T.H.J. Badman, and S. McOrist. 1987. Diseases of anseriformes associated with intranuclear inclusion bodies in epithelial cells. *Australian Veterinary Journal* 64:290–291.

Richter, J.H.M., and M.C. Horzinek. 1993. Duck plague. In *Virus Infections of Birds,* J.B. McFerran and M.S. McNulty (eds.). Elsevier Science Publishers, Amsterdam, Netherlands, pp. 77–90.

Roizman, B., A. Bartha, P.M. Biggs, L.E. Carmichael, A. Granoff, B. Hampar, A.S. Kaplan, L.V. Melendez, K. Munk, A. Nahmias, G. Plummer, J. Rajcani, F. Rapp, M. Terni, G. de The, D.H. Watson, and P. Wildy. 1973. Provisional labels for herpesviruses. *Journal of General Virology* 20:417–419.

Roizman, B., R.C. Desroslers, B. Fleckenstein, C. Lopez, A.C. Minson, and M.J. Studdert. 1992. The family Herpesviridae:an update. *Archives of Virology* 123:243–449.

Salguero, F.J., P.J. Sanchez-Cordon, A. Nunez, and J.C. Gomez-Villamandos. 2002. Histological and ultrastructural changes associated with herpesvirus infection in waterfowl. *Avian Pathology* 31:133–140.

Sandhu, T.S., and L. Leibovitz. 1997. Duck virus enteritis (duck plague). In *Diseases of Poultry,* B.W. Calnek, H.J. Barnes, C W. Beard, L.R. McDougald, and Y.M. Saif (eds.). Iowa State University Press, Ames, Iowa, pp. 675–683.

Schat, K.A., and H.G. Purchase. 1998. Cell culture methods. In *A Laboratory Manual for the Isolation and Identification of Avian Pathogens,* D.E. Swayne, J.R. Glisson, M.W. Jackwood, J.E. Pearson, and W.M. Reed (eds.). American Association of Avian Pathologists, University of Pennsylvania, Kennett Square, Pennsylvania, pp. 125–128.

Shawkey, S.A., and T.S. Sandhu. 1997. Inactivated vaccine for protection against duck virus enteritis. *Avian Diseases* 41:461–468.

Shawky, S., and K.A. Schat. 2002. Latency sites and reactivation of duck enteritis virus. *Avian Diseases* 46:308–313.

Snyder, S.B., J.G. Fox, L.H. Campbell, K.F. Tam, and O.A. Soave. 1973. An epornitic of duck virus enteritis (duck plague) in California. *Journal of the American Veterinary Medical Association* 163:647–652.

Spieker, J.O. 1978. Virulence assay and other studies of six North American strains of duck. Ph.D. Thesis. University of Wisconsin, Madison, Wisconsin, 110 pp.

Spieker, J.O., T.M. Yuill, and E.C. Burgess. 1996. Virulence of six strains of duck plague virus in eight waterfowl species. *Journal of Wildlife Diseases* 32:453–460.

Stanton III, J.D., E.C. Soutiere, and R.A. Lancia. 1992. Survival and reproduction of game-farm female mallards at remington farms, Maryland. *Wildlife Society Bulletin* 20:182–188.

Suwathanaviroj, V., U. Tantaswasdi, S. Kuhawanta, R. Rattanarajchtikul, and N. Chaimongkol. 1977. The first outbreak of duck plague in Thailand. *Journal of the Thai Veterinary Medical Association* 28:61–79.

Toth, T.E. 1970. Active immunization of White Pekin ducks against duck virus enteritis (duck plague) with modified-live-virus vaccine:immunization of ducklings. *American Journal of Veterinary Research* 31:1275–1281.

Toth, T.E. 1971a. Active immunization of White Pekin ducks against Duck virus enteritis (duck plague) with modified-live-virus vaccine:serologic and immunologic response of breeder ducks. *American Journal of Veterinary Research* 32:75–81.

Toth, T.E. 1971b. Two aspects of duck virus enteritis:parental immunity, and persistence/excretion of virulent virus. In *Proceedings 74th Annual Meeting of the United States Animal Health Association 1970.* Philadelphia, Pennsylvania, pp. 304–314.

Trung, N.T., N.T.T. Hong, K.V. Phuc, D. Hung, N.T. Ha, D.V. Dung, B.T.T. Trinh, H.H. Mai, D.V. Tien, N.V. Cuong, D.X. Trach, and P. Daniels. 2004. Field trials of a cell culture adapted duck plague vaccine. *In Proceedings of the 2003 Control of Newcastle Disease and Duck Plague in Village Poultry Workshop,* No. 117, J. Meers, P.B. Spradbrow, and T.D. Tu (eds.). Australian Center for International Agricultural Research, Canberra, Australia, pp. 66–70.

Tu, T.D., K.V. Phuc, N.T.L. Huong, L. Nind, D. Hung, T.D. Minh, D.T.N. Thao, and P. Spradbrow. 2004. Isolation and identification of duck plague viruses from naturally infected ducks in southern Vietnam. *In Proceedings of the 2003 Control of Newcastle Disease and Duck plague in Village Poultry Workshop,* No. 117, J. Meers, P.B. Spradbrow, and T.D. Tu (eds.). Australian Center for International Agricultural Research, Canberra, Australia, pp. 30–34.

Van Dorssen, C.A., and H. Kunst. 1955. Over de gevoeligheid van eenden en diverse andere watervogels voor eendenpest. = Susceptibility of ducks and various waterfowl to duck plague virus. *Tijdschrift voor Diergeneeskunde* 80:1286–1295.

Vijaysri, S., S. Sulochana, and K.T. Punnoose. 1997. Restriction endonuclease analysis of duck plague viral DNA. *Journal of Veterinary and Animal Sciences* 28:86–91.

Walker, J.W., C.J. Pfow, S.S. Newcomb, W.D. Urban, H.E. Nadler, and L.N. Locke. 1970. Status of duck virus enteritis (duck plague) in the United States. *In Proceedings 73rd Annual Meeting of U.S. Animal Health Association* 1969. Sheraton-Schroeder Hotel, Milwaukee, Wisconsin, pp. 254–279.

Wobeser, G. 1987. Experimental duck plague in blue-winged teal and Canada geese. *Journal of Wildlife Diseases* 23:368–375.

Wobeser, G. 1997. *Diseases of wild waterfowl,* 2nd ed. Plenum Press, New York, New York, 324 pp.

Wobeser, G., and D.E. Docherty. 1987. A solitary case of duck plague in a wild mallard. *Journal of Wildlife Diseases* 23:479–482.

Wolf, K., and C.N. Burke. 1982. Survival of duck plague virus in water from Lake Andes National Wildlife Refuge, South Dakota. *Journal of Wildlife Diseases* 18:437–440.

Woolcock, P.R. 1998. Duck virus enteritis. In *A laboratory manual for the isolation and identification of avian pathogens,* D.E. Swayne, J.R. Glisson, M.W. Jackson, J.E. Pearson, and W.M. Reed (eds.). American Association of Avian Pathologists, University of Pennsylvania, Kennett Square, Pennsylvania, pp. 125–128.

Woolcock, P.R. 2004. Duck virus enteritis. In *OIE Manual of Diagnostic Tests and Vaccines for Terrestrial Animals,* Vol. 2, OIE Biological Standards Commission (eds.). World Organization for Animal Health, Office International des Epizooties, Paris, France, pp. 913–920.

Woolcock, P.R., and J. Fabricant. 1997. Duck hepatitis. In *Diseases of Poultry,* B. W. Calnek, H. J. Barnes, C.W. Beard, L.R. McDougald, and Y.M. Saif (eds.). Iowa State University Press, Ames, Iowa, pp. 661–673.

XiaoYan, Y., L. Wei, and Q. XueFeng. 2004. Detection of distribution of virulent duck plague virus in adult ducks by PCR. *Chinese Journal of Veterinary Science and Technology* 34:66–69.

Yuan, G., A. Cheng, M. Wang, F. Liu, X. Han, Y. Liao, and C. Xu. 2005. Electron microscope studies of the morphogenesis of duck enteritis virus. *Avian Diseases* 49:50–55.

5
Avian Influenza

David E. Stallknecht, Eva Nagy, D. Bruce Hunter, Richard D. Slemons

INTRODUCTION

Influenza viruses are RNA viruses belonging to the family Orthomyxoviridae. They have been isolated from many species of mammals including humans, pigs, horses, mink, stone marten, felids, marine mammals, and a wide range of domestic and wild birds. Aquatic birds are thought to be the source of all influenza A viruses in other animal species (Webster et al. 1992). Prior to 2002, the occurrence of sporadic avian influenza outbreaks (overt clinical illness) caused by low pathogenic (LP) or high pathogenic (HP) avian-origin influenza viruses (AIVs) were almost exclusively documented in domestic poultry and captive birds in Europe, Asia, Australia, North America, and Africa. Historically, the outbreaks caused by the HP AIVs were referred to as "fowl plague." Today these outbreaks, which are associated with significant economic losses and animal suffering, are most commonly referred to as "high pathogenic avian influenza" or "HPAI." Interestingly, around the world, subclinical AIV infections in wild birds, especially waterfowl, gulls, and shore birds were documented far more frequently than AIV infections in domestic birds, yet reports of disease in individual wild birds and/or outbreaks in wild birds associated with these infections were a rarity. In fact, prior to 2002, only one outbreak of AI had been documented in wild birds (Common Terns; *Sterna hirundo*) along the coast of South Africa in 1961 (Becker 1966). In that situation the highly pathogenic A/tern/South Africa/1961 (H5N3) virus disappeared as rapidly as it had appeared, and over the years there was general growing consensus that although AIV infections were a significant threat to poultry, they had little or no impact on wild bird populations.

The first indication of potential change occurred in 2002. Lineages of the Asian HP H5N1 AIV, first reported in Asia in 1997 and believed by many to be endemic in poultry in some areas of Asia, were found to be responsible for the death of captive exotic and local wild birds in two parks and two distantly located Gray Herons (*Ardea cinerea*) and one Black-headed Gull (*Larus ridibundus*) in Hong Kong (Ellis et al. 2004). The sources of these viruses were never confirmed but both wild birds and virus spillover from infected domestic poultry were proposed as possible sources. The two outbreaks and individual cases were considered to be unusual events. During 2003 and 2004, the first and second waves of the Asian HP H5N1 AI epizootic in poultry became apparent as reports surfaced from most Southeast Asian countries, China, South Korea, and Japan. There were also reports of sporadic fatal cases of AI in single or a few wild birds, usually scavengers and raptors. The third wave of the Asian HP H5N1 AI epizootic in poultry arrived with new reports from Southeast Asia in December 2004. Then scattered sporadic cases of fatal AI infections and AI outbreaks in poultry and wild birds began to increase at other locations; in China in May 2005 more than 6000 wild water birds—Bar-headed Geese (*Anser indicus*), Great Cormorant (*Phalacrocorax carbo*), Great Black-headed Gull (*Larus ichthyaetus*), Brown-headed Gull (*Larus brunnicephalus*), Ruddy Shell Duck (*Tadorna ferruginea*), and Tufted Duck (*Aythya fuligula*)—died on Qinghai Lake (Lui et al. 2005), and then in western Siberia, Kazakhstan, and Mongolia in late July to early August, and then from the areas around the Caspian Sea and Black Sea, the mideast, eastern Europe, India, and into central Europe by February 2006 and Scotland in March 2006. At the time of writing this manuscript, the Asian HP H5N1 AI outbreaks have been reported in poultry but not yet wild birds in multiple countries in both western and eastern Africa.

The mechanism or mechanisms responsible for this apparent rapid geographic spread of the Asian HP H5N1 AIV have not been determined. Circumstantial evidence appears to increasingly incriminate wild birds as playing a role, but this has not been definitively confirmed. On the other hand, there is direct evidence that the virus has been spread between countries and continents by the movement of infected captive birds and imported poultry and poultry products containing the virus. Will wild birds become a maintenance host for the Asian lineage of high pathogenic H5N1 AIVs, and what impact will these viruses have on wild bird populations? These are critical, unanswered questions and the final outcome might have important implications for wild bird populations in the future.

Today most significance given to type A influenza infections in wild, free-ranging birds stems from analysis of epidemiological and virological data that incriminates low pathogenic AIVs from wild birds as the viral ancestors, or genetic pool, from which influenza A viruses infecting domestic birds, lower mammals, and humans ultimately originated. In 2005, researchers provided evidence that the 1918 human pandemic influenza A virus was a virus that originated from birds and crossed the avian-human species barrier *in toto,* resulting in the infamous 1918 pandemic (Taubenberger et al. 2005). There is now convincing evidence that all three human pandemic influenza A viruses of the twentieth century appear to have come totally or in part from type A influenza viruses that originated from birds.

The increased awareness of the interspecies transmission and adaptive capabilities of type A influenza viruses of avian origin has resulted in renewed interest in the large pool of antigenic and genetically diverse populations of type A influenza viruses maintained in wild birds. These viruses, and especially the status of the Asian lineages of the HP H5N1 AIV, have now become a source of extensive concern for wildlife-, domestic animal–, and human-health experts around the world. If the concerns prove to be warranted, current efforts to define the biological mechanisms responsible for interspecies transmission, adaptation to new hosts, and the emergence of new type A influenza viruses will prove well justified.

SYNONYMS

Fowl plague, fowl pest, avian flu, bird flu, type A influenza, influenza A.

HISTORY

The name for influenza viruses comes from the Latin *influentia* "epidemic," originally used because epidemics were thought to be due to astrological or other occult "influences." Although the history of avian influenza probably dates back thousands of years, the first written document goes back only to the nineteenth century. The history of avian influenza in domestic fowl has been extensively reviewed (Easterday 1975; Wilkinson and Waterson 1975; Alexander 1982; 1986a; Webster and Kawaoka 1988). AI, first described as *peste aviare* (fowl plague) in Italy in 1878, is now considered the beginning of the disease (Stubbs 1948). Although originally described as "fowl plague," this disease may have been confused with Newcastle Disease (ND). The two diseases were differentiated in 1927 when Doyle described ND as a distinct disease. AI was again reported in Germany in 1890 and the United States in 1924–1925. By 1930, outbreaks of fowl plague in domestic poultry had been reported in England, Austria, Hungary, Switzerland, France, Belgium, Holland, Egypt, China, Japan, Argentina, and Brazil.

During 1901, the discovery that fowl plague was caused by a filterable agent was reported independently by Centanni and Sevonuzzi (1901), Maggiora and Valinti (1901), and Lode and Gruber (1901) (cited in Wilkinson and Waterson 1975). The agent was propagated in eggs in 1934 (Burnett and Ferry 1934) and shown to be an influenza A virus by Schafer and colleagues based on comparative seroimmunological studies and shared chemical, physical, and biological properties (cited by Wilkinson and Waterson 1975). The demonstration of hemagglutinating properties of influenza viruses led to increased surveillance and isolation of animal influenza viruses, especially from avian species (Easterday 1975).

A chronology of recovery and identification of avian influenza viruses from 1927 to 1970 was published by Easterday and Tumova (1972). Significant events during this period included the isolation of antigenically distinct AIVs from domestic ducks (Roberts 1964; Easterday 1975); the isolation of A/chicken/Scotland/59 (H5N1) and A/turkey/Ontario/7732/66 (H5N9), which represented HP AIVs that were antigenically distinct from the traditional H7N7 fowl plague viruses (Pereira et al. 1965; Easterday 1975); and the recognition of low pathogenic (LP) H5 and H7 AIVs present in domestic fowl (Beard and Easterday 1973; Alexander 1982; Hinshaw and Webster 1982; Swayne 2003).

During 1961, A/tern/South Africa/61 (H5N3) was isolated from Common Terns in South Africa (Becker 1966); this is the first reported AIV isolation from a wild bird. The subsequent detection of AIV antibodies in 21 species of free-living birds from 1968 to 1972 suggested that AIV was present in a diversity of wild avian species (Easterday et al. 1968; Asplin 1970; Laver and Webster 1972; Winkler et al. 1972). In 1971 this was confirmed by the recovery of an AIV from one of 201 tracheal swabs collected from Wedge-tailed Shearwaters (*Puffinus pacificus*) in Australia (Downie and Laver, 1973). In 1972, 41 antigenically diverse AIV isolates were recovered from approximately 2,000 cloacal swabs taken from wild, free-ranging ducks representing eight species sampled at five locations in southern California, the Pacific Migratory Bird Flyway (Slemons et al. 1974), and two

AIV isolates were recovered from cloacal swabs collected from exotic birds being imported into the United States (Slemons et al. 1973). In 1973 the recovery of four AIV isolates from cloacal swabs collected from ducks and geese in Delaware, located in the Atlantic Migratory Bird Flyway, confirmed the findings from California and pointed out the importance of collecting cloacal swabs when conducting AIV surveillance in wild birds (Rosenberger et al. 1974). These papers also called attention to the critical enteric component in the maintenance of influenza A viruses in wild birds. From 1970 to 1988 there were more than 50 published reports of AIVs from free-living species (Stallknecht and Shane 1988).

DISTRIBUTION

Avian influenza viruses have a global distribution and are likely found everywhere that competent host species are present (Olsen et al. 2006). AIVs have been isolated from wild birds on all continents except Antarctica, and there is serological evidence that AIVs occasionally circulate there as well (Austin and Webster 1993). However, most isolations and host records, to date, have come from North America and Europe. This relates to surveillance efforts and probably does not reflect differences in AIV prevalence. It was not until 2006 that the first isolation was reported from wild birds in South America (Spackman et al. 2006).

HOST RANGE

Wild birds are reservoirs for all known HA and NA subtypes of influenza A viruses (Hinshaw et al. 1980; Hinshaw et al. 1982; Suss et al. 1994), and several reviews of AIV host range in free-living bird populations are available (Stallknecht and Shane 1988; Hanson 2002; Olsen et al. 2006). Naturally occurring infections with AIV have been reported in free-living birds representing more than 100 species in 13 avian orders (Table 5.1). Most of the species are associated with aquatic habitats, and at present, there are two avian groups that are considered to be the most important reservoirs of AIV: the Anseriformes (ducks, geese, and swans) and the Charadriiformes (gulls, terns, and shorebirds).

Species within the family Anatidae of the order Anseriformes have accounted for most of the AIV isolations reported to date, and AIVs have been isolated from more than 30 of the 158 species of ducks and geese worldwide. Most of these isolates have been reported from species within the subfamily Anatinae, which includes the dabbling and diving ducks, and more isolations of AIV have been reported from Mallard (*Anas platyrhyncos*) than any other species. Within the Charadriiformes, AIVs have been isolated from three families (Charadriidae, Laridae, and Alcida), but most AIV isolations have been reported from one species, the Ruddy Turnstone (*Arenaria interpres*). There is a significant number of negative isolation results reported from other species in this family (Stallknecht 1998; Olsen et al. 2006). Isolations have been reported from seven additional avian orders, which include species commonly associated with aquatic habitats (Ciconiiformes, Gaviiformes, Gruiformes, Pelecaniformes, Podicipediformes, and Procellariiformes). Collectively, AIV has been isolated from few species in these groups, but with few reports of surveillance in which they have been included, it is difficult to evaluate their potential reservoir status. Although there are reports of AIV from birds commonly associated with more terrestrial habitats (species included in the Columbiformes, Piciformes, and Passeriformes), most AIV isolation attempts associated with species not associated with aquatic habitats have been unsuccessful (Deibel et al. 1985; Hinshaw and Webster 1982; Nettles et al. 1985), and these groups are not currently considered as important AIV reservoirs.

Prior to 2002, there was only a single report of an HP AIV isolation from wild birds that were not known to be associated with infected domestic fowl. This virus (an H5N3) was isolated from Common Terns during a mortality event in South Africa (Becker 1966) and is the only isolation cited in Table 5.1 that represents an HPAI virus. The host range for AIV, however, has recently increased with the HP H5N1 AI outbreak in Eurasia. In 2002 and 2003, Asian lineages of HP H5N1 AIVs were isolated from both captive and free-living birds in Hong Kong (Ellis et al. 2004). These outbreaks were significant because they represented the first case of AIV induced mortality in free-living wild bird species since the South African event. Isolations of the Asian lineages of HP H5N1 AIVs have been reported since 2002 in more than 60 species of wild birds in both Asia and Eastern Europe (USGS 2006a; USGS 2006b) and it appears that these viruses may have been transported throughout Eurasia during migration in 2005. Reports of Asian HP H5N1 AI in free-living wild birds include isolations from Bar-headed Goose, White-fronted Goose (*Anser albifrons*), Red-breasted Goose (*Branta ruficollis*), Whooper Swan (*Cygnus cygnus*), Mute Swan (*Cygnus olor*), Gadwall (*Anas strepera*), Ruddy Shelduck, Tufted Duck, Common Pochard (*Aythya ferina*), Smew (*Mergellus albellus*), Green Sandpiper (*Tringa ochropus*), Brown-headed Gull, Great Black-backed Gull, Black-headed Gull, Gray Heron, Chinese Pond Heron (*Ardeola bacchus*), Little Egret (*Egretta garzetta*), Asian Open-billed Stork (*Anastomus oscitans*), Rock Pigeon (*Columba livia*), Red Turtle Dove (*Streptopelia tranquebarica*), Peregrine Falcon (*Falco

Table 5.1. Reports of avian influenza virus isolations from free-living wild birds.

ANSERIFORMES		
FAMILY: ANATIDAE		
SUBFAMILY: ANATINAE		
American Black Duck	(*Anas rubripes*)	Rosenberger et al. 1974; Boudreault et al. 1980; Deibel et al. 1985; Hinshaw et al. 1986b; Slemons et al. 1991
American Wigeon	(*Anas americana*)	Slemons and Easterday, 1975; Boudreault et al. 1980; Hinshaw et al. 1980; Kocan et al. 1980; Slemons et al., 1991; Alfonso et al. 1995
Australian Shelduck	(*Tadorna tadornoides*)	Mackenzie et al. 1984
Blue-winged Teal	(*Anas discors*)	Slemons et al. 1974; 1991; Slemons and Easterday 1975; Hinshaw et al. 1978; 1980; 1986; Boudreault et al. 1980; Deibel et al. 1985; Stallknecht et al. 1990a; Hanson et al. 2005
Bufflehead	(*Bucephala albeola*)	Hinshaw et al. 1980; Slemons et al. 1991
Canvasback	(*Aytha valisineria*)	Hinshaw et al. 1978; 1980
Cinnamon Teal	(*Anas cyanoptera*)	Slemons et al., 1974; Hanson et al. 2005
Eurasian Wigeon	(*Anas penelope*)	Hannoun et al., 1980; Fouchier et al. 2003*
Falcated Teal	(*Anas falcata*)	Isachenko et al. 1974
Gadwall	(*Anas strepera*)	Slemons et al. 1974; Thorsen et al. 1980; Hinshaw et al. 1980; Ottis et al. 1983; Nettles et al. 1985; Stallknecht et al. 1990a
Garganey Teal	(*Anas querquedula*)	Iftimovici et al. 1980
Common Teal	(*Anas crecca*)	Slemons et al. 1974;1991; Slemons and Easterday 1975; Kida et al. 1979; Boudreault et al. 1980; Hannoun et al. 1980; Hinshaw et al. 1980; Kocan et al. 1980; Webster et al. 1981; Abenes et al. 1982; Sinnecker et al. 1983; Mikami et al. 1987; Stallknecht et al. 1990a; Hanson et al. 2005
Gray Teal	(*Anas gibberifrons*)	Mackenzie et al. 1984
Long-tailed Duck	(*Clangula hyemalis*)	Sinnecker et al. 1983
Mallard	(*Anas platyrhynchos*)	Isachenko et al. 1974, Rosenberger et al. 1974; Roslaya et al. 1974; Slemons et al. 1974; 1975; 1991; Bahl et al. 1975; 1977; Romvary et al. 1976a; Webster et al. 1976; Hannoun 1977; 1980; Gresikova et al. 1978; Hinshaw et al. 1978; 1980; 1985; 1986b; Yamane et al. 1979; Boudreault et al. 1980; Kocan et al., 1980; Ottis and

(*Continued*)

Table 5.1. *(Continued)*

		Bachmann. 1980; 1983; Stunzner et al. 1980; Thorsen et al. 1980; Lipkind et al. 1981; Smitka et al. 1981; Turek et al. 1983; Sinnecker et al. 1983; Deibel et al. 1985; Nettles et al. 1985, Mikami et al. 1987; Alfonso et al., 1995, Stanislawek et al. 2002; DeMarco et al. 2003; Fouchier et al. 2003*; Hanson et al. 2003; Hua et al., 2005; Munster et al. 2005
Mottled Duck	(*Anas fulvigula*)	Stallknecht et al. 1990a
Northern Pintail	(*Anas acuta*)	Slemons et al. 1974; 1991; Hinshaw et al. 1978;1979; 1980; Yamane et al. 1978; Kida et al., 1979; Boudreault et al. 1980; Hannoun et al. 1980; Lipkind et al. 1981; Deibel et al. 1985; Hanson et al. 2003; 2005
Northern Shoveler	(*Anas clypeata*)	Slemons et al., 1974; 1991; Boudreault et al. 1980; Mikami et al. 1987; Fouchier et al. 2003*
Australian Black Duck	(*Anas superciliosa*)	Mackenzie et al. 1984
Redhead	(*Aythya americana*)	Slemons et al. 1975; Hinshaw et al. 1980
Ring-necked Duck	(*Athya collaris*)	Slemons et al. 1975; Boudreault et al. 1980
Ruddy Duck	(*Oxyura jamaicensis*)	Slemons et al. 1974; Hinshaw et al. 1980
Spotbill Duck	(*Anas poecilorhyncha*)	Yamane et al. 1978; 1979; Abenes et al. 1982
Tufted Duck	(*Aythya fuligula*)	Tsubokura et al. 1981a, b; Ottis and Bachmann. 1983
White-winged Scoter	(*Melanitta deglandi*)	Sinnecker et al. 1983
Wood Duck	(*Aix sponsa*)	Boudreault et al. 1980; Deibel et al. 1985
Yellowbill Duck	(*Anas undulata*)	Pfitzer et al. 2000
SUBFAMILY: ANSERINAE		
Brant Goose	(*Branta bernicia*)	Fanning et al. 2002*; Fouchier et al. 2003*
Canada Goose	(*Branta canadensis*)	Rosenberger et al. 1974; Boudreault et al. 1980, Hinshaw et al. 1986b; Ito et al. 1995
Egyptian Goose	(*Alopochen aegyptiacus*)	Pfitzer et al. 2000
Graylag Goose	(*Anser anser*)	Sinnecker et al. 1983; Suss et al. 1994; Fouchier et al. 2003*
White-fronted Goose	(*Anser albifrons*)	Slemons et al. 1975
Mute Swan	(*Cygnus olor*)	Sinnecker et al. 1983; Graves 1992; Suss et al. 1994
Whistling Swan	(*Cygnus columbianus*)	Tsubokura et al. 1981a; Otsuki et al. 1984; 1987

Table 5.1. *(Continued)*

SUBFAMILY: TADORINAE		
Common Shelduck	(*Tadorna tadorna*)	Hannoun et al. 1977; 1980
Cape Shelduck	(*Tadorna cana*)	Pfitzer et al. 2000
CHARADRIIFORMES		
FAMILY: CHARADRIIDAE		
Dunlin	(*Calidris alpina*)	Honda et al. 1981
Eurasian Woodcock	(*Scolopax rusticola*)	Isachenko et al. 1974; Roslaya et al. 1974
Least Sandpiper	(*Calidris minutilla*)	Hanson 2003
Red Knot	(*Calidris canutus*)	Hanson 2003
Ruddy turnstone	(*Arenaria interpres*)	Kawaoka et al. 1988; Saito et al. 1994; Hanson 2003
Sanderling	(*Calidris alba*)	Kawaoka et al. 1988
Semipalmated Sandpiper	(*Calidris pusilla*)	Hanson 2003
Spur-winged Lapwing	(*Vanellus spinosus*)	Manjunath et al. 1981
Temmick's Stint	(*Calidris temminckii*)	Zakstelskaya et al. 1975
FAMILY: LARIDAE		
Arctic Tern	(*Sterna paradisaea*)	Zakstelskaya et al. 1975; Sinnecker et al. 1983
Black-headed Gull	(*Larus ridibundus*)	Sinnecker et al. 1983; Fouchier et al. 2003*
Black-tailed Gull	(*Larus crassirostris*)	Tsubokura et al. 1981a
Common Tern	(*Sterna hirundo*)	Becker 1966; Zakstelskaya et al. 1974; L'vov 1978
Franklin's Gull	(*Larus pipixcan*)	Hinshaw et al. 1982
Greater Black-backed Gull	(*Larus marinus*)	Hinshaw et al. 1982
Herring Gull	(*Larus argentatus*)	Zakstelskaya et al. 1975; Hinshaw et al. 1982; Kawaoka et al. 1988
Laughing Gull	(*Larus atricilla*)	Kawaoka et al. 1988
Lesser Noddy	(*Anous tenuirostris*)	Mackenzie et al. 1984
Ring-billed Gull	(*Larus delawarensis*)	Hinshaw et al. 1982; Nettles et al. 1985; Graves 1992; Campbell 1999
Sandwich Tern	(*Sterna sandvicensis*)	Sinnecker et al. 1983
Slender-billed Gull	(*Larus genei*)	L'vov 1978
Sooty Tern	(*Sterna fuscata*)	Mackenzie et al. 1984
White-winged Black Tern	(*Cihldonias leucoptera*)	Roslaya et al. 1974
FAMILY: ALCIDAE		
Common Murre	(*Uria aalge*)	Sazonov et al. 1977
Guillemot	(*Cepphus spp.*)	Fouchier et al. 2003*
CICONIIFORMES		
Glossy Ibis	(*Plegadis falcinellus*)	Iftimovici et al. 1980
Gray Heron	(*Ardea cinerea*)	Iftimovici et al. 1980; Roslaya et al. 1974; 1975
Hadada Ibis	(*Hagedashia hagedash*)	Pfitzer et al. 2000
Squacco Heron	(*Ardeola ralloides*)	Iftimovici et al. 1980
COLUMBIFORMES		
Collard Dove	(*Streptopelia decaocto*)	Romvary et al. 1975

(Continued)

Table 5.1. *(Continued)*

GALLIFORMES		
Ring-necked Pheasant	(*Phasianus colchicus*)	Romvary et al. 1976a
Rock Partridge	(*Alectoris graeca*)	Lipkind et al. 1981
GAVIIFORMES		
Arctic Loon	(*Gavia arctica*)	Iftimovici et al. 1980
Red-throated Loon	(*Gavia stellata*)	Zakstelskaya et al. 1975
GRUIFORMES		
American Coot	(*Fulica americana*)	Slemons et al. 1975; Boudreault et al. 1980
Eurasian Coot	(*Fulica atra*)	Romvary et al. 1976a; Lipkind et al. 1981; Ottis et al. 1983; Mackenzie et al. 1984; Suss et al. 1994
PASSERIFORMES		
American Redstart	(*Setophaga ruticilla*)	Boudreault et al. 1980
Barn Swallow	(*Hirundo rustica*)	Amin et al. 1980
Black-faced Bunting	(*Emberiza spodocephala*)	Roslaya et al. 1974
Carrion Crow	(*Corvus corone*)	Isachenko et al. 1974
Common Jackdaw	(*Corvus monedula*)	Isachenko et al. 1974
Common Redstart	(*Phoenicurus phoenicurus*)	Amin et al. 1980
Common Whitethroat	(*Sylvia communis*)	Amin et al. 1980
Dark-eyed Junco	(*Junco hyemalis*)	Boudreault et al. 1980
Common Starling	(*Sturnus vulgaris*)	Lipkind et al. 1979
Garden Warbler	(*Sylvia borin*)	Amin et al. 1980
Hermit Thrush	(*Catharus guttatus*)	Boudreault et al. 1980
House Sparrow	(*Passer domesticus*)	Romvary et al. 1976b
Icterine Warbler	(*Hippolais icterina*)	Amin et al. 1980
Purple Finch	(*Carpodacus purpureus*)	Boudreault et al. 1980
Red-backed Shrike	(*Lanius collurio*)	Amin et al. 1980
Song Sparrow	(*Melospiza melodia*)	Boudreault et al. 1980
Spotted Flycatcher	(*Musicapa striata*)	Isachenko et al. 1974
Swainson's Thrush	(*Catharus ustulatus*)	Boudreault et al. 1980
Tennessee Warbler	(*Vermivora peregrina*)	Boudreault et al. 1980
Willow Flycatcher	(*Empidonax traillii*)	Boudreault et al. 1980
Willow Warbler	(*Phylloscopus trochilus*)	Amin et al. 1980
Yellow vented Bulbul	(*Pycnonotus goiaver personatus*)	Ibrahim et al. 1990
Yellow Wagtail	(*Motacilla flava*)	Amin et al. 1980
Yellow Warbler	(*Dendroica petechia*)	Boudreault et al. 1980
Yellow-breasted Bunting	(*Emberiza aureola*)	Roslaya et al. 1974
Yellow-rumped Warbler	(*Dendroica coronata*)	Boudreault et al. 1980
Yellow-throated Warbler	(*Dendroica dominica*)	Boudreault et al. 1980
PELECANIFORMES		
Great Cormorant	(*Phalacrocorax carbo*)	Iftimovici et al. 1980; Suss et al. 1994
PICIFORMES		
Great-spotted Woodpecker	(*Dendrocopos major*)	Roslaya et al. 1974
PODICIPEDIFORMES		
Pied-billed Grebe	(*Podilymbus podiceps*)	Boudreault et al. 1980
PROCELLARIIFORMES		
Wedge-tailed Shearwater	(*Puffinus pacificus*)	Downie et al. 1973; 1977; Mackenzie et al. 1984

* PCR positive for AIV

peregrinus), Mountain Hawk-eagle (*Spizaetus nipalensis*), Northern Goshawk (*Accipiter gentiles*), Common Buzzard (*Buteo buteo*), Common Gallinule (*Gallinula chloropus*), Common Coot (*Fulica atra*), Purple Swamphen (*Porphyrio porphyrio*), Brown Crake (*Amaurornis akool*), Large-billed Crow (*Corvus macrorhynchos*), House Crow (*Corvus splendens*), Korean Magpie (*Pica pica, sericea*), Black Drongo (*Dicrurus macrocercus*), Black-naped Oriole (*Oriolus chinensis*),White-rumped Munia (*Lonchura stiata*), House Sparrow (*Passer domesticus*), Japanese White-eye (*Zosterops japonicus*), Kalij Pheasant (*Lophura leucomelanos*), Common Peafowl (*Pavo cristatus*), Great Cormorant, Little Cormorant (*Halietor niger*), and Great Crested Grebe (*Podiceps cristatus*) (Ellis et al. 2004; Chen et al. 2005; Liu et al. 2005, Kwon et al. 2005; Mase et al. 2005; USGS 2006a). The USGS Web site (USGS 2006b) maintains an updated inventory of species affected by the Asian H5N1 AIV.

These results reflect a wide host range for the Eurasian HP H5N1 AIVs but at present offer little insight into potential wildlife reservoirs for these viruses. In evaluating these and other host reports, it is important to understand the difference between a susceptible host and a reservoir host. There have been numerous reported AIV isolations (including HP AIVs) from birds associated with AIV-infected poultry flocks (Cross 1987), from captive birds in zoological collections (Ellis et al. 2004), and from wild birds imported for the pet trade (Alexander 2000). Although these isolations provide evidence of AIV susceptibility and provide evidence of anthropogenic activities potentially affecting wildlife, they have limited relevance to understanding the natural history of these viruses in free-living populations. However, it is interesting that most of the wild birds from which HP H5N1 AIV has been reported fall into two categories. The first involves aquatic birds, and this group is predominated by members of the Anseriformes, which is consistent with the known natural history of AIV. The second group includes raptors and other species (for example, crows), which potentially either predate or scavenge other birds (wild or domestic). This is not known to occur with naturally occurring AIVs in wild birds. This difference may not reflect differences in host range but rather increased exposure to the HP H5N1 AI viruses through infected domestic fowl and increased detection due to resulting mortality.

ETIOLOGY AND PATHOGENESIS

Name, Origin and Classification

Influenza viruses are classified into the family Orthomyxoviridae. There are five genera in the family Orthomyxoviridae; among them are genus Influenza A virus, genus Influenza B virus, and genus Influenza C virus (Kawaoka et al. 2005). Influenza A, B, and C viruses are distinguished on the basis of the antigenic properties of their group-specific nucleocapsid and matrix proteins, which are located inside the lipid envelope of the virion (Webster and Kawaoka 1988). Birds are naturally infected with Influenza A viruses only, therefore only these viruses are described.

By convention, influenza virus isolates are identified or named based on their serotype / host species of origin / site of origin specimen collection / laboratory strain designation / year of specimen collection and (hemagglutinin [HA] and neuraminidase [NA] subtype); for example: A/tern/South Africa/1/61/ (H5N3) (WHO 1980).

Influenza virions are generally spherical or pleomorphic; however, filamentous forms occur. They are 80–120 nm diameter, enveloped, and the envelope is derived from the cell membrane lipids. The viral nucleocapsid is segmented with helical symmetry and consists of different sizes from 30 to 120 nm in length (Noda et al. 2006).

The nucleic acid of influenza viruses is linear, negative sense single stranded (ss) RNA. The length of the 8 segments ranges from 874 nucleotides (nt) to 2396 nts, and the size of the genome varies from 10.0 to 14.5 kb (Lai et al. 1980).

AIVs have two main surface proteins: the trimeric rod-shaped hemagglutinin (HA) protein that is most abundant, and the tetrameric mushroom-shaped neuraminidase (NA) protein. The hydrophobic ends of these proteins are embedded in the lipid membrane, and the balance of the proteins project out from the lipid envelope. The envelope also contains a small number of M_2 membrane ion channel proteins. The internal proteins are the M_1 membrane (matrix) protein and the viral ribonucleoproteins (RNP) consisting of the nucleocapsid (NP) protein and 3 polypeptides forming the RdRp (polymerase proteins: PA, PB_1 and PB_2). NS_2 is also present in the virion.

Based on antigenicity, 16 subtypes of HA (H1-H16) and nine subtypes of NA (N1-N9) of influenza A viruses are recognized. In addition, antigenic variation within subtypes can occur. The HA protein is involved in virus attachment and fusion of the viral envelope with the cell membrane and is the target of subtype specific neutralization antibodies that are responsible for host protection. The NA protein cleaves sialic acid from glycoproteins, but its actual role in the replication cycle is unclear. The virions are sensitive to heat, lipid solvents, non-ionic detergents, formaldehyde, irradiation, and oxidizing agents.

The basic replication cycle of influenza A viruses involves the attachment of the viral HA to the host cell sialic acid-containing receptors, virus entry into the cell by receptor-mediated endocytosis followed by fusion between the viral and host cell endosomal membranes, followed by release of the nucleocapsid into the cytoplasm and transportation to the nucleus of the cell. The fusion event depends on prior posttranslational cleavage of the precursor hemagglutinin molecule, H0, into H_1 and H_2, hemagglutinin subunits by host cell proteases. The susceptibility of the H0 precursor molecule to host proteases is an important factor in determining the virulence of the virus. Generally RNA viruses replicate in the cytoplasm, but the transcription and replication of the RNA genome of influenza viruses takes place in the nucleus of the infected cell. Viral protein synthesis takes place in the cytoplasm using the cellular translation machinery. The proteins associated with the genomic RNA are transported to the nucleus and then migrate to the cytoplasm. Envelope proteins are inserted into the plasma membranes, and virions are formed by budding, incorporating the matrix (M) protein and nucleocapsids that have aligned below the membrane patches of the HA and NA.

Most AIVs will replicate in the allantoic and amniotic cavities of nine- to 11-day-old embryonating chicken eggs. This is the most common protocol of isolating AIVs, especially from wild birds. Primary chicken kidney and fibroblast cells will also support the replication of many AIV isolates, but replication efficiency can be variable and dependent upon strain of the virus. The *in vitro* host range of AIVs can be extended by the addition of trypsin to the growth medium so that multiple cycles of replication can occur in certain primary chicken cell cultures and cell lines, for example, Madin Darby canine kidney cells.

Biological Characteristics of Influenza Viruses

There is a great deal of biological variation among avian influenza viruses. All HA (H1-16) and NA (N1-9) subtypes of type A influenza viruses have been recovered from avian species, though not all have been recovered from any single avian species (Figure 5.1). The HA-NA combination distributions in avian species have not been fully evaluated. This is in contrast to antigenic diversity among influenza A viruses maintained in single mammalian species. Currently H3N3 influenza A viruses are known to be maintained in horses, and the A/equine-1 (H7N7) virus lineage may not be present in horses. The H1N1, H3N2, and H1N2 are currently being maintained in swine in North America, although swine have been infected with other subtypes including influenza A viruses possessing the H4 and H9 subtypes. H1N1, H2N2, and H3N2 HA-NA combinations are, or were, maintained in humans, although humans have also been infected with H5, H7, H9, and H10 avian-origin influenza viruses, which have not established a new maintenance cycle in humans.

New subtypes, in other words new combinations of HA and NA genes (proteins), can emerge by reassortment if a single cell of an animal is infected with two different subtypes simultaneously. Reassortment of

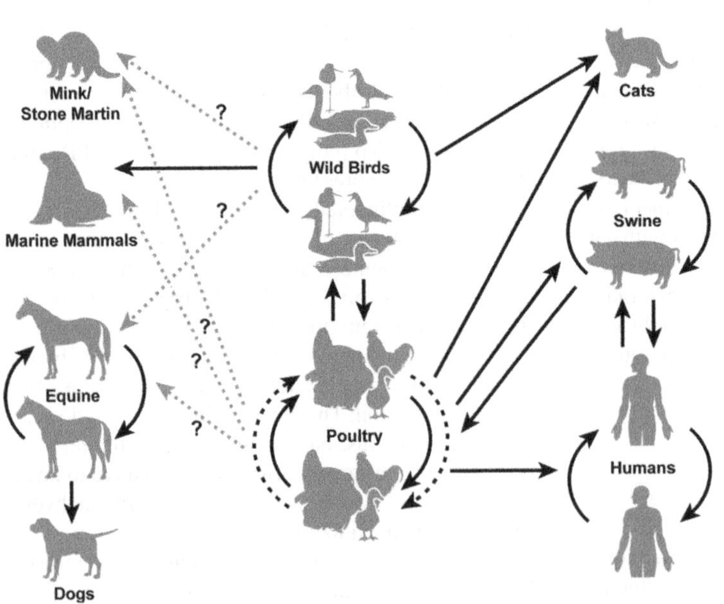

Figure 5.1. Known and suspected routes of interspecies transmission of AIV. All type A influenza viruses infecting domestic bird and mammalian species (including humans) originated from the wild bird reservoir. However, these viruses, when adapted to these new hosts (domestic poultry, equine, swine, and human), are self sustaining; they have essentially evolved into "new" viruses that are genetically distinct from their avian precursors. These routes of transmission also represent the potential paths for recombination events between viruses associated with these host systems.

influenza viruses is common in wild bird populations and represents a potentially important mechanism for inserting genes of AIV subtypes (including new HA subtypes) into existing viruses associated with domestic animals and humans. This process of reassortment is called "antigenic shift."

Influenza viruses are also susceptible to minor spontaneous genetic mutations of the HA and NA protein sequences that may result in minor antigenic changes of these surface proteins, a process called "antigenic drift." The mutants are less rapidly neutralized by antibodies generated against the prototype strains of the same subtype. Differences in the RNA and protein composition of the variants have been shown (Webster et al. 1992).

There are limited genetic studies focusing exclusively on wild bird isolates, and most phylogenetic studies have involved comparisons of wild bird viruses with viruses derived from domestic animals (Spackman et al. 2005). Although it has been proposed that these viruses are in a state of evolutionary stasis due to a lack of selective pressure (Gorman et al. 1992), recent studies have clearly demonstrated a high degree of recombination (Hatchette et al. 2004), a high level of nucleotide variation within multiple genes (Widjaja et al. 2004; Spackman et al. 2005), and the existence of multiple lineages of AIV within individual wild bird populations (Spackman et al. 2005). Based on genetic sequence differences observed in the M, NS, NP, and the HA (H4, H5, and H7) proteins, AIV from free-living birds are broadly grouped into North American and Eurasian lineages (Donis et al. 1986; Gorman et al. 1990; Schafer et al. 1993; Spackman et al. 2005), and there is evidence of limited genetic flow between these continents (Mararova et al. 1999; Spackman et al. 2005).

Host Restriction and Adaptation of Avian Influenza Viruses

To gain entry to a host cell, the hemagglutinin molecules on the surface of the AIV bind to complex glycans-carbohydrate cell receptors on the host cell that contain terminal sialic acids. Avian influenza viruses bind preferentially to α2-3–linked sialic acids on receptors found mainly in the intestinal tract of birds, whereas human strains of influenza viruses preferentially target SAα2-6-Gal-terminated saccharides found in epithelial cells of the human upper respiratory tract. The α2-3–linked sialic acid receptors are also present in the human respiratory tract, but they tend to be less accessible because they are located deeper in the lower airways, which may explain why replication of avian viruses in humans is generally restricted (Shinya et al. 2006). Swine cells contain both types of receptors, so they can be readily infected with both avian and human influenza viruses, and if a cell is infected simultaneously with the two viruses, new "reassorted" viruses can emerge, potentially capable of infecting humans. Therefore pigs are considered the "mixing vessel" for influenza viruses (Ito et al. 1998). Although it has been recorded that avian influenza viruses can infect humans and cause fatal disease due to massive infection with highly pathogenic avian H5N1 viruses, no significant human-to-human transmission has yet been reported. The switch from α2-3 to α2-6 receptor specificity is a critical step in the adaptation of avian viruses to a human host, and it seems to be one of the reasons that most avian influenza viruses are not easily transmitted from human to human. However, the adaptation of the avian virus to a new host may occur by optimizing the specificity of the HA to the new host (Kuiken et al. 2006).

Pathogenicity of Avian Influenza Viruses

Different subtypes, and strains within a subtype, vary greatly in pathogenicity. Viruses are classified as HP or LP strains based on the outcome of intravenous pathogenicity index (IVPI) assays in chickens and/or the amino acid sequence at the cleavage site of the hemagglutinin, and/or the ability of the virus to cause cytopathic effect in cell culture in the absence of trypsin (Alexander 1986b; Webster and Rott 1997; Swayne et al. 1998). Highly pathogenic strains have historically been restricted to the H5 and H7 subtypes, but most H5 and H7 viruses possess low pathogenic properties. The cleavage of the hemagglutinin protein is of paramount importance in determining the virulence, but the combination of genes, including the nucleoprotein and polymerase genes, also contributes. Whether the infection is localized or becomes systemic depends on the amino acid sequence at the cleavage site of the precursor hemagglutinin. Cleavage is necessary for the hemagglutinin to become fully functional (Kuiken et al. 2006). In LPAI viruses, cleavage is catalyzed by trypsin and trypsin-like enzymes (proteases) limited to the respiratory and intestinal tracts.

HPAI influenza viruses have changes in the cleavage site that allow the precursor hemagglutinin to be processed by a variety of ubiquitous intracellular proteases found in many body tissues, resulting in the potential for systemic, multi-organ infections. HPAI viruses are not normally present in bird populations but arise from LPAI viruses. The main mechanisms of change of LPAI viruses to HPAI viruses are an insertion of extra basic amino acids in the cleavage site and substitutions of nonbasic amino acid with basic amino acids (Perdue et al. 1996). Loss of a sugar group on the site that covers the cleavage area, and insertion of extraneous genetic information and recombination, have also been reported as causes of change in virulence (Pasick et al. 2005).

EPIZOOTIOLOGY

Subtype Diversity

Avian influenza virus subtypes are not equally represented among wild bird populations. This variation can occur between hosts, locations, and years. Most of the AIVs isolated from ducks are represented by viruses in the H3, H4, and H6 subtypes (Stallknecht 1990a; Sharp et al. 1993; Krauss et al. 2004). The H11 subtype also is common in duck populations (Ottis and Bachman 1983; Stallknecht 1990a; Slemons et al. 1991). Viruses representing the H5, H7, and H9 are generally reported at low prevalence rates from ducks (Stallknecht and Shane 1988; Krauss et al. 2004), but these virus subtypes can be more common at specific locations and times (Hanson et al. 2003; Munster et al. 2005). The H8 subtype is extremely rare in ducks, with only five isolations reported to date (Stallknecht et al. 1990a; Krauss et al. 2004; Hanson et al. 2005). Subtype diversity is not constant between years, and predominant subtypes, such as the H3, H4, and H6, are reported to follow a two-year cycle (Krauss et al. 2004).

In shorebirds and gulls, subtype diversity is not as well understood, but it is apparent that differences exist in the AIV subtype diversity observed in species of Charadriiforme as compared to ducks (Kawaoka et al. 1988; Hanson 2002; Krauss et al. 2004). To date, nine subtypes of AIVs have been shown to occur more often in shorebirds than ducks, including the H5, H7, H9, and H13 AIVs (Krauss et al. 2004). It is important to understand that existing data on subtype diversity in shorebirds is limited in scope, with most isolates recovered from one species (Ruddy Turnstone) at one location (Delaware Bay, U.S.A.). Recently a new subtype (H16), genetically related to the H13 of gulls, was isolated from Black-backed gulls in Sweden (Fouchier et al. 2005).

Transmission and maintenance in wild birds

Replication of AIV in ducks occurs primarily in the intestinal tract (Slemons and Easterday 1977) with high concentrations of infectious virus shed in feces (Hinshaw et al. 1982; Webster et al. 1978). Therefore maintenance of AIV in wild bird populations is believed to be primarily by fecal/oral transmission (Hinshaw et al. 1979; Sandu and Hinshaw 1981; Sinnecker et al. 1983). Webster et al. (1978) reported that experimentally infected Muscovy Ducks (*Cairina moschata*) shed 6.4 grams of fecal material per hour, with an infectivity of $1 \times 10^{7.8}$ EID_{50}. These birds shed an estimated 1×10^{10} EID_{50} of AIV over a 24-hour period. In addition to a high level of viral shedding, the duration of viral shedding in ducks can be prolonged. Hinshaw et al. (1980) demonstrated that infected Pekin ducks were capable of shedding A/duck/Alberta/35/76 for more than 28 days.

Avian influenza viruses have been isolated from surface water in Canada (Hinshaw et al. 1980), Minnesota (Halvorson et al. 1983), and Alaska (Ito et al. 1995), but always in association with ducks (Hinshaw 1986a). Existing data on AIV persistence in water is limited. Experimental environmental persistence of AIV was investigated by Webster et al. (1978) using A/Duck/Memphis/546/74 (H3N2) in both fecal material and nonchlorinated river water. An initial dose of $10^{6.8}$ EID_{50} (feces) and $10^{8.1}$ EID_{50} (water) remained infective for at least 32 days when the experiment ended. Only two other studies (Stallknecht et al. 1990b, c) have evaluated the persistence of wild types of AIV in water. These studies demonstrated that AIVs can persist for extended periods of time in water at 4°C, 17°C, and 28°C and that water pH and salinity, within ranges normally encountered in the field, can greatly affect AIV persistence. Contaminated surface and ground water used by waterfowl have been suggested as long- and short-term sources of AIV for domestic turkeys (Halvorson et al. 1985). Dabbling ducks (genus *Anas*) are more frequently infected with AIV than other genera. Olsen et al. (2006) suggested that dabbling ducks may encounter greater exposure to AIV from contaminated surface or pond water than diving ducks, possibly because of their surface feeding behavior. AIVs are likely maintained in nature by the combined effects of continual bird-to-bird transmission and environmental persistence. In ducks, transmission reaches a peak during the late summer and early fall, coinciding with staging and a high population of young, susceptible birds. AIV infections can occur on wintering areas, and virus transmission has been demonstrated on wintering areas by the isolation of AIV from resident Mottled Duck (*Anas fuvigula*) in the U.S.A. (Stallknecht et al. 1990a) and by seroconversions in ducks wintering in Italy (DeMarco et al. 2003). It has been suggested that different host species may provide unique but connected roles in AIV maintenance. For example, Blue-winged Teal (*Anas discors*) are early migrants that are not present in northern areas when the AIV prevalence rates peak in other duck species (Stallknecht et al. 1990a). This migratory behavior may result in a susceptible population for virus maintenance on wintering grounds. AIVs have been detected in Blue-winged Teal and other duck species into the late winter and early spring (Hanson et al. 2005), indicating that AIVs are present in duck populations prior to spring migration. A very low prevalence of AIV (0.3%) also has been reported from ducks on breeding grounds in April (Sharp et al. 1993). A similar multispecies relationship may exist with ducks and shorebirds, which share susceptibility to some AIVs (Kawaoka et al. 1988); each group may play a related but different role in the movement and maintenance of these viruses (Krauss et al. 2004).

The isolation of these viruses from unconcentrated lake water and the demonstration of very long-term persistence of AIVs in water under experimental conditions provide the basis for the hypothesis that environmental persistence contributes to AIV maintenance in wild birds. Although it is possible that this is a contributory factor, additional study is required to understand its potential importance.

Temporo-Spatial Patterns

In duck populations, the prevalence of AIV infections peaks in late summer/early fall and is associated with premigration staging (Hinshaw et al. 1985). This is attributable to increased concentrations of susceptible hatching-year birds at this time, and this is supported by AIV infection rates that can exceed 30% in this age group. For this reason, AIV surveillance can be greatly enhanced by concentrating on juvenile birds during this time period. Temporal patterns for species of Charadriiformes are less understood but it has been reported that peak prevalence occurs in the spring and a lesser peak occurs in the fall (Kawaoka et al. 1988). This seasonality, however, is largely based on observations at Delaware Bay.

The temporal patterns observed in ducks correspond to consistent spatial patterns. In general, AIV prevalence in North America is highest in waterfowl staging areas in Canada and the northern United States and can exceed 30% in juvenile ducks (Hinshaw et al. 1985). During fall migration, prevalence rapidly decreases and may be less than 1–2% on wintering areas (Stallknecht and Shane 1988). Low AIV prevalence estimates have also been reported in ducks on wintering areas in Europe (Fouchier et al. 2003; Olsen et al. 2006).

Spatial patterns, as with temporal patterns, in Charadriiformes are more difficult to understand, but a strong spatial relationship has been observed with Ruddy Turnstones during spring migration stopovers at Delaware Bay (Kawaoka et al. 1988; Hanson 2002; Krauss et al. 2004). This is the only site, worldwide, where consistent AIV isolations from shorebirds have been reported, and in general, reported prevalence rates from these species are either very low or negative (Stallknecht et al. 1998; Hanson 2002; Fouchier et al. 2003).

CLINICAL SIGNS

Wild birds infected with LP AIV generally show no clinical signs. However, clinical disease has been reported in wild birds infected with certain strains of HP AIV (Asian lineages of H5N1 and the A/tern/South Africa/1/61/ H5N3). In these cases, clinical signs can range from unapparent to mortality. In chickens, clinical signs associated with HP AIV include tremors of the head and neck, torticollis, opisthotonus, and depression (Swayne 2003). Respiratory signs such as rales, sneezing, and coughing may be present. Some birds die very quickly without clinical signs. Neurological signs similar to those in chickens have been observed in free-flying wild birds infected with HP H5N1 AIV (Lui et al. 2006) and in experimentally infected wild bird species (Wood Duck [*Aix sponsa*] and Laughing Gull) (Figure 5.2). Experimentally infected birds died two to three days after onset of clinical signs; however, some affected birds did recover. Other species such as Blue-winged Teal were infected but demonstrated no clinical signs (SCWDS unpublished data).

PATHOLOGY

There are no pathognomonic lesions for avian influenza in birds, and lesion distribution and severity are dependent on the pathogenicity of the virus and

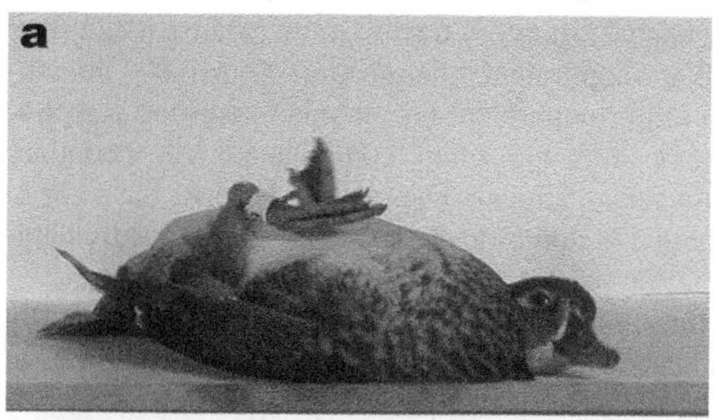

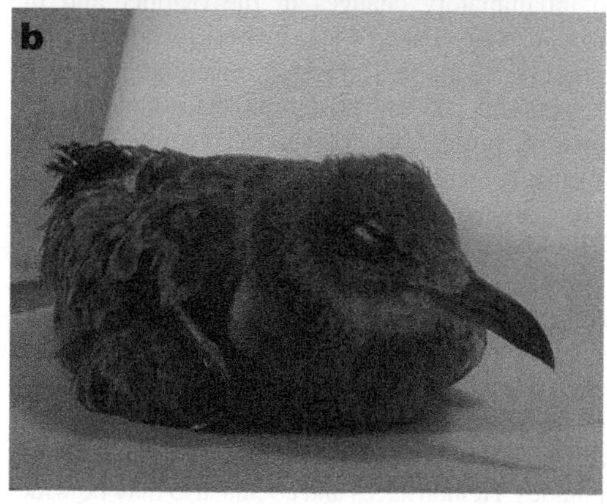

Figure 5.2. Neurological signs associated with HP H5N1 AIV in a) a Wood Duck (*Aix sponsa*) and b) Laughing Gull (*Larus atricilla*). Clinical signs persisted for 2–3 days prior to death. In two cases, birds (one wood duck and one gull) recovered.

many host factors including species, age, immune status, and the time the bird was examined post infection (PI). Prior to the late 1990s, with the exception of the die-off of Common Terns in South Africa there were no reports of mortality events caused by avian influenza in wild birds or descriptions of pathology. The emergence of the H5N1 virus in Asia changed this situation as numerous reports of mortality in wild or free-flying birds flowed over the World Wide Web, but few of these documented pathological changes in the affected birds. The pathology of avian influenza in commercial poultry is well described (Hooper and Selleck 1998; Swayne and Suarez 2000; Swayne and Halverson 2003; and others) but at the time of the writing of this chapter, descriptions of pathology caused by AIVs in nonpoultry species are mainly limited to experimental infections rather than naturally occurring disease.

In general, LP AIVs produce mild to moderate and occasionally severe respiratory lesions in gallinaceous species including edema of the eyelids, conjunctivitis, catarrhal to fibrinopurulent rhinitis, sinusitis, and tracheitis. Microscopic lesions range from mild edema and mononuclear cell infiltrates in the submucosa of the upper respiratory tract to more extensive catarrhal and fibrinopurulent inflammation. Sometimes interstitial to fibrinopurulent pneumonia is present. Respiratory lesions are often complicated by secondary pathogens. Similar respiratory lesions have been reported in domestic ducks infected with mildly pathogenic avian influenza viruses.

In commercial turkey hens and chickens, mildly pathogenic avian influenza viruses may cause drops in egg production accompanied by regression of ovaries and inflammatory changes in the oviduct and the coelomic cavity. Pancreatic acinar necrosis is reported in turkeys. Lymphoid changes including apoptosis, necrosis, and generalized lymphocyte depletion are commonly present in gut associated lymphoid tissues as well as spleen, thymus, and bursa of Fabricius.

HP AIVs may cause lesions ranging from few or no visible macroscopic changes in peracute infections to severe multi-organ involvement. The lesion distribution and the lesion character change with time PI. During the initial phase of acute infection in gallinaceous species, birds may die with severe pulmonary congestion, edema, and hemorrhage, and microscopically there are numerous micro-thrombi in pulmonary air capillaries. Hemorrhages and edema also may be widespread in other organs, including brain, wattles, eyelids, subcutaneous tissues of the hocks, shanks, feet and over virtually any or all serosal surfaces. Early in the infection, virus localizes in pulmonary and other endothelial cells and in monocyte/macrophages, and it has been suggested that cytokine release such as tumor necrosis factor (TFN-α) a mediator of vascular permeability and apoptosis, may trigger these dramatic vascular changes (Perkins and Swayne 2001). In chickens there is evidence that cytokine release may alter coagulation pathways contributing to the acute vascular phase (Muramoto et al. 2006).

After two to three days (PI) in experimental studies, the HP AIV is disseminated throughout the body and viral antigen can be detected in most organs, resulting in multi-organ necrosis and inflammation. The distribution of lesions is dependent very much on the strain of the virus and host species.

Pulmonary involvement is common in gallinaceous birds, as characterized by submucosal edema, loss of cilia from epithelial surfaces, exudative interstitial pneumonia with congestion and hemorrhage, and fibrinous microthrombi in capillaries. Upper respiratory involvement is variable. Respiratory lesions have been reported in experimentally infected domestic ducks.

In systemic infections, hemorrhage, apoptosis, and cell necrosis and inflammation may occur in any parenchymal organ, but most frequently involves heart, brain, spleen, pancreas, and adrenal glands. Hemorrhage, apoptosis, and necrosis may be present in enteric lymphoid areas such as the esophageal-proventricular junction, Peyers patches, and cecal tonsils. Brain lesions are variable and include endothelial cell hypertrophy accompanied by perivascular edema, randomly disseminated foci of neuronal necrosis, and occasional involvement of ependymal cells and the choroid plexus. In birds that survive a few days, there may be glial cell infiltration and perivascular cuffing with mononuclear cells.

There is marked variation in the susceptibility of different bird species (even within the same order) to a single isolate of avian influenza virus. Perkins and Swayne published several papers describing experimental intranasal infection of a variety of species using the A/chicken/Hong Kong/220/97 (H5N1) isolate. This virus produced respiratory lesions in seven gallinaceous species: white leghorn chickens (*Gallus domesticus*), broad-breasted white turkeys (*Meleagris gallopavo*), Japanese Quail (*Coturnix japonicus*), Northern Bobwhite (*Colinus virginianus*), Helmeted Guineafowl (*Numida meleagris*), Ring-necked Pheasants (*Phasianus colchicus*) and Chukar (*Alectoris chukar*) (Perkins and Swayne 2001). There was a gradation of lesions among these species and they were generally most pronounced in chickens, Japanese quail, and Guinea fowl and less frequent and less severe in Northern Bobwhite, Ring-necked Pheasants, and Chukar. All of these species developed splenomegaly, renomegaly with parenchymal pallor and often urate retention, multifocal hepatocyte necrosis, pancreatic acinar necrosis, and bone marrow depletion (both erythroid and myeloid cell lines). Brain lesions also occurred and were characterized by endothelial cell hypertrophy accompanied by perivascular edema and mild to moderate randomly disseminated foci of neuronal necrosis. Microgliosis and the formation of glial nodules progressed in severity with time post infection.

In contrast, several passerine species infected with the same virus had a different distribution pattern of lesions (Perkins and Swayne 2003). Zebra Finch (*Poephila guttata*) had high mortality and virus was present in multiple organs but the pancreas was most severely affected with confluent pancreatic acinar necrosis. The House Finch (*Carpodacus mexicanus*) and Budgerigar (*Melopsittacus undulatus*) had lower mortality and by day six to 14 PI developed mild splenomegaly, pancreatic lesions, and perivascular edema and necrosis in the brain. House Sparrows (*Passer domesticus*) did not become ill or develop gross lesions but viral antigen was detected in heart and testicle of a few birds. The Common Starling (*Sternus vulgaris*) appeared completely refractory to this virus.

Domestic geese and Emu (*Dramaius novaehollandiae*) infected with the same A/chicken/Hong Kong/220/97 (H5N1) isolate developed pancreatitis and meningoencephalitis. Domestic ducks developed very mild lesions in the respiratory tract, and mild splenic enlargement and virus was isolated PI from oropharyngeal swabs and lungs. The Rock Pigeon was completely refractory to infection and no virus was recovered or viral antigen detected PI (Perkins and Swayne 2002a). Laughing Gulls infected with this virus developed only mild conjunctival edema and mild respiratory lesions (Perkins and Swayne 2002b). In contrast, Laughing Gulls infected with A/tern/ South Africa/61 (H5N3) virus developed systemic disease including hepatitis and necrotizing pancreatitis (Perkins and Swayne 2002b).

Lee et al. (2005) also carried out comparative studies in domestic chickens, Japanese Quail, and Pekin Ducks using a Korean avian influenza virus isolate A/chicken/Korea/ES/03 (H5N1). The chickens developed high mortality, acute pulmonary lesions, and myocardial and splenic necrosis. The quail developed pancreatic necrosis, neuronal necrosis, and myocyte degeneration. The Pekin Ducks had lower mortality, lower titers of virus in tissues, and fewer lesions restricted primarily in the respiratory tract (heterophilic sinusitis, rhinitis, and airsacculitis).

Highly pathogenic avian influenza was diagnosed in a mortality event in wild Korean Magpie in South Korea (Kwon et al. 2005). These birds had widespread multifocal to confluent necrosis of multiple organs, particularly pancreas, spleen, adrenal gland, testicle, and brain. Viral antigen was present in multiple locations including respiratory endothelium.

Lui et al. (2006) reported naturally occurring mortality on Lake Qinghai in Qinghai Province western China involving Bar-headed Goose, Great Black-headed Gulls, and Brown-headed Gulls. These birds had clinical neurological signs (tremors and opisthotonus) and diarrhea and at necropsy had pancreatic necrosis, brain lesions including glial cell infiltration, and mononuclear perivascular cuffing and nephropathy.

Significant antigenic variation has occurred in avian H5N1 viruses from Asia between 1997 and 2002 (Sturm-Ramirez et al. 2004) and these viruses appear to be progressively becoming better adapted and more pathogenic for waterfowl. Experimental infection of Mallards with H5N1 viruses isolated pre-2002 produced little or no disease. Experimental infection with A/chicken/Hong Kong/220/97 (H5N1) isolates in ducks produced only mild respiratory lesions (Perkins and Swayne 2002b). Isolates from 2002 (Teal/HK/2978.1/02, RBPochard/HK/821/02, and Gs/HK/739.2/02) caused significant mortality, clinical neurological signs (balance problems, tremors, and incoordination), and multisystemic involvement including multifocal encephalitis and lymphoid depletion in spleen and bursa of Fabricius (Sturm-Ramirez et al. 2004).

DIAGNOSIS

Clinical signs and lesions (macroscopic and/or microscopic) observed in live or dead wild birds may be suggestive of avian influenza but the diagnosis must be confirmed by isolating virus or demonstrating AIV nucleic acid or antigen within infected tissues or by demonstrating seroconversion in live birds using acute and convalescent serum samples. In an outbreak or epizootic situation, after the etiology is confirmed other direct diagnostic tests, such as rapid antigen and RNA detection and characterization, can be validated. These rapid diagnostic tests become invaluable for prevention, control, and eradication programs. It is critical to remember that because of the wide range of healthy wild birds that may harbor LP AIVs (even AIV possessing the H5N1 HA-NA combination and the H7) in nature, the isolation of AIVs from a wild bird or single positive serological titer confirms viral exposure but does not confirm a disease state or represent a crisis situation.

Serologic Testing

Although serologic testing has potential application for wildlife studies, there are many unknowns related to test sensitivity and specificity, the duration of a detectable antibody response, and species differences.

Serologic testing of wild birds has not been routinely used for AIV surveillance. Available serologic tests include agar gel immunodiffusion (AGID), hemagglutination inhibition (HI), and competitive ELISA. The AGID test, which measures antibodies to the NP, have the advantage of being influenza-A specific, but results have proven inconsistent when applied to ducks (Slemons and Easterday 1972) and are generally not recommended for wild birds. Results from HI testing also have proven inconsistent; antibodies are often not detectable against killed intact virus (Kida 1980); nonspecific inhibitors may be present in serum samples; and serum may cause nonspecific agglutination of chicken erythrocytes. Some of these problems can be avoided by treatment of serum with receptor-destroying enzyme and potassium periodate, matching erythrocytes with the species being tested, or through pretreatment of the serum with chicken erythrocytes (Swayne 2003).

The HI test has the advantage of measuring subtype-specific antibodies. Competitive ELISA tests directed at antibodies to the NP have been developed (Shafer et al. 1998) and have been used for wildlife surveillance (De Marco et al. 2003). These tests have the advantage of increased sensitivity and unlike traditional ELISA formats are not species specific.

Virus Isolation/Antigen and Nucleic Acid Detection

Virus isolation in nine- to 11-day-old embryonating chicken eggs is the gold standard for the diagnosis of AI infections in wild birds. The isolation of an AIV in this system may or may not result in embryo death. Viruses are detected through hemagglutination of chicken erythrocytes by harvested allantoic fluid. Viruses can be detected in allantoic fluid within the first 24 hours but generally the fluid is harvested and tested at 72 to 96 hours post inoculation. Viruses can be identified as type A influenza by AGID, and more rapidly using polymerase chain reaction (PCR) methods, or through commercially available antigen capture tests. Viruses are subtyped through hemagglutination and neuraminidase inhibition (Pearson and Senne 1986), with testing being generally deferred to national or international AIV reference laboratories.

For antigen detection, immunohistochemistry directed at the NP has proven effective for detection of AIV antigen in microscopic tissue sections. An antigen capture technique also has been described (Kobayashi et al. 1993) for use in infected poultry but has not been applied to wild bird diagnostics or surveillance. Several commercial rapid antigen detection tests for type A influenza were designed for human diagnostics and may have some utility for wild bird testing. Although these tests appear to be specific, they often lack sensitivity.

PCR techniques are of growing importance in AIV diagnosis and surveillance and can be directed at specific HA subtypes or to type A influenza virus. Real time RT-PCR (rtRT-PCR) has been used successfully for the surveillance of wild birds in Europe (Fouchier et al. 2000) and is being utilized for HP H5N1 AI virus in the United States. These tests have the advantage of speed (which can be greatly increased with the use of robotics) and increased sensitivity; however, some reduction of sensitivity may occur due to PCR inhibitors in cloacal swabs.

IMMUNITY

There is little information on immunity to AIV infection in wild birds. The immune response of domestic avian species to infection with AIV has been reviewed by Suarez and Schultz (2000). The response includes an early (within five days of infection) IgM response followed by an IgG response. Neutralizing antibodies are produced against both the HA and NA and these antibodies are protective against challenge by the same subtype. The antibody response can vary among species, and in ducks it is generally poor. Little is known about avian mucosal antibody production or the cell-mediated immune response. Vaccination with inactivated, vectored, and DNA vaccines have proven effective in reducing or eliminating morbidity and mortality associated with AIV infection in domestic birds including domestic ducks. Although many of these vaccines do not totally eliminate virus shedding, they may reduce AIV transmission.

PUBLIC HEALTH CONCERNS

Humans can be infected with both LP and HP AIVs. Human illness due to infection with LP AIVs (including H7N7, H9N2, and H7N2) has ranged from very mild symptoms (for example, conjunctivitis) to generalized influenza-like illness. Illness from HP AIV has ranged from mild (H7N3, H7N7) to severe or fatal (H7N7, H5N1). Human infections have been linked to exposure to infected commercial poultry, but to date there has never been a documented case of direct transmission of AIVs from a wild bird to a human.

Reported infections of humans with HPAI H5N1 (Subbarao et al. 1998), H7 (Fouchier et al. 2004), and H9 (Lin et al. 2000) avian viruses, as well as the recent evidence that the 1918 H1N1 pandemic influenza viruses were derived from avian sources shortly before the pandemic (Taubenberger et al. 2005), have added an additional dimension to this potential problem. At the present time, despite the 200-plus diagnosed cases and the high case fatality rate in people, the Asian HP H5N1 virus is not very efficient at infecting humans, and sustained human-to-human transmission has not been documented. Should efficient human-to-human transmission occur, exposure to HP H5N1 AIV infected wild birds would probably not be a significant issue.

Wildlife biologists or other individuals who handle wild birds should be aware of possible AIV transmission when handling waterfowl or other potentially infected birds. There are no data available to estimate the risk of such an event and no historic information to support such a possibility, but it cannot be discounted. Because this would probably relate to fecal/oral or fecal/mucous membrane contact rather than aerosol, standard precautions, such as gloves and hand washing, should eliminate or greatly reduce this possibility.

DOMESTIC ANIMAL CONCERNS

AIVs, especially HPAI viruses, are a recurring problem in domestic poultry worldwide and their impact can be extreme in terms of direct mortality and economic losses associated with control, eradication, and loss of international markets. There is good evidence that most HPAI outbreaks in commercial poultry originated from LPAI viruses and that these LPAI viruses originate from wild birds. The significance of the HPAI H5N1 viruses in wild birds is currently unclear. They can be infected and there is good evidence of the wild bird involvement in the movement of these viruses. However, it is currently unknown whether these viruses will persist in these populations or which species are or could be involved in virus transmission and maintenance.

The transmission of any AIV from wild birds to domestic birds can be prevented through biosecurity and the prevention of direct or indirect contact. There also is potential in some cases to limit the probability of transmission through vaccination of domestic flocks. However, worldwide there are economic limitations to such actions.

WILDLIFE POPULATION IMPACTS AND MANAGEMENT IMPLICATIONS

Historically there has been no known negative impact on wild bird populations associated with LP AIVs despite evidence that AIV infections are widespread, involve many species, and may have very high prevalence rates in certain species. The Asian lineage H5N1 HPAIVs potentially could change this scenario if indeed they become established, maintained, and are spread within wild bird populations. Mortality from infection with this virus has been reported in >60 species of wild birds and significant losses reported in certain susceptible species. The outbreak in waterfowl on Qinghai Lake, China, killed an estimated 10% of the global Bar-headed Geese population (Olsen et al. 2006), demonstrating the potential for loss in a local or susceptible species.

It is unknown what effects (short or long term) that HP H5N1 AIV may have if it becomes established in wild bird populations, and it is important to understand that establishment is not guaranteed. There is currently no evidence of widespread infection in wild birds in Asia, Africa, or Europe, and only additional time will reveal the full scope of this potential problem. Potential problems relate not only to direct impacts associated with wild bird mortality but also to indirect impacts associated with "fear." These indirect impacts could range from closure of recreation areas, loss of support for natural resource management, and an overall perception by the public that birds represent a public or animal health threat rather than an important and irreplaceable resource.

TREATMENT AND CONTROL

There are no options for treatment or control of infection or disease (HP H5N1 AI) in wild birds other than prevention. With regard to HP H5N1 AI, vaccination of high-risk endangered species may prove effective, but information on vaccine efficacy in wild species is not available.

LITERATURE CITED

Abenes, G.B., K. Okazaki, H. Fukushi, H. Kida, E. Honda, K. Yagyu, M. Tsuji, H. Sato, E. Ono, R. Yanagawa, and N. Yamauchi. 1982. Isolation of orthomyxoviruses and paramyxoviruses from feral birds in Hokkaido, Japan 1980 and 1981. *Japanese Journal of Veterinary Science* 44:703–708.

Alexander, D.J. 1982. Avian influenza-recent developments. *Veterinary Bulletin* 52:341–359.

Alexander, D.J. 1986a. Avian influenza-historical aspects. In *Proceedings 2nd International Symposium on Avian Influenza*. Athens, Georgia, U.S.A., pp. 4–13.

Alexander, D.J. 1986b. Criteria for the definition of pathogenicity of avian influenza viruses. In *Proceedings 2nd International Symposium on Avian Influenza*. Athens, Georgia, U.S.A., pp. 228–245.

Alexander, D.J. 2000. A review of avian influenza in different bird species. *Veterinary Microbiology* 74:3–13.

Alfonso, C.P., B.S. Cowen, and H. Van Campen. 1995. Influenza A viruses isolated from waterfowl in two wildlife management areas of Pennsylvania. *Journal of Wildlife Diseases* 31:179–185.

Amin, A., M.A. Shalaby, and I.Z. Imam. 1980. Studies on influenza virus isolated from migrating birds in Egypt. *Comparative Immunology Microbiology and Infectious Diseases* 3:241–246.

Asplin, F.D. 1970. Examination of sera from wildfowl for antibodies against the viruses of duck plague, duck hepatitis, and duck influenza. *Veterinary Record* 87:182–183.

Austin, J.F., and R.G. Webster. 1993. Evidence of Ortho- and Paramyxoviruses in fauna from Antartica. *Journal of Wildlife Diseases* 29:568–571.

Bahl, A.K., B.S. Pomeroy, B.C. Easterday, and S. Mamgundimedjo. 1975. Isolation of type A influenza viruses from migratory waterfowl along the Mississippi flyway. *Journal of Wildlife Diseases* 11:360–363.

Bahl, A.K., B.S. Pomeroy, S. Mangundimedjo, and B.C. Easterday. 1977. Isolation of type A influenza and Newcastle Disease viruses from migratory water-fowl in Mississippi flyway. *Journal of the American Veterinary Medical Association* 171:949–951.

Beard, C.W., M. Brugh, and D. Johnson. 1984. Laboratory studies with the Pennsylvanian avian influenza virus (H5N2). In *Proceedings 88th Annual Conference of the United States Animal Health Association,* pp. 462–473.

Beard, C.W., and B.C. Easterday. 1973. A/turkey/Oregon/71, an avirulent influenza isolate with the hemagglutinin of fowl plague virus. *Avian Diseases* 17:173–178.

Becker, W.B. 1966. Isolation and classification of tern virus:Influenza Virus A/Tern/South Africa/1961. *Journal of Hygiene* 64:309–320.

Boudreault, A., J. Lecomte, and V.S. Hinshaw. 1980. Antigenic characterization of influenza A viruses isolated from avian species in Ontario, Quebec and Maritimes during the 1977 season. *Revue Canadienne De Biologie* 39:107–114.

Burnet, F.M., and J.D. Ferry. 1934. The differentiation of the viruses of fowl plague and Newcastle Disease, experiments using the technique of chorioallantoic membrane inoculation of the developing egg. *British Journal of Experimental Pathology* 15:56–64.

Campbell, D.G. 1999. Gull mortality—Kitchener. *Wildlife Health Centre Newsletter* 6:8–9.

Chen, H., G.J.D. Smith, S.Y. Zhang, K. Oin, J. Wang, K.S. Li, R.G. Webster, and K. Yu. 2005. H5N1 outbreak in migratory waterfowl:Nature online. Retrived from the World Wide Web:http:/www.nature.com/nature/journal/vaop/ncurrent/full/natureo3974.

Cross, G.M. 1987. The status of avian influenza in poultry in Australia. *Proceedings 2nd International Symposium on Avian Influenza.* Athens, Georgia, U.S.A., pp. 96–103.

Crawford, P.C., E.J. Dubovi, W.L. Castleman, I. Stephenson, E.P. Gibbs, C. Smith, R.C. Hill, P.P. Rerro, J. Pompey, R.A. Bright, M.J. Medina, C.M. Johnson, C.W. Olsen, N.J. Cox, A.I. Klimov, J.M. Katz, and R.O. Donis. 2005. Transmission of equine influenza in dogs. *Science* 310:482–485.

De Marco, M.A., G.E. Foni, L. Campitelli, E. Raffini, L. Di Trani, M. Delogu, V. Guberti, G. Barigazzi, and W. Di Donatelli. 2003. Circulation of influenza viruses in wild waterfowl wintering in Italy during the 1993–99 period:Evidence of virus shedding and seroconversion in wild ducks. *Avian Diseases* 47:861–866.

De Marco, M.A., L. Campitelli, E. Foni, E. Raffini, G. Barigazzi, M. Delongu, V. Guberti, L. Di Trani, M. Trollis, and I. Donatelli. 2004. Influenza surveillance in birds in Italian wetlands (1992–1998):is there a host-restricted circulation of influenza viruses in sympatric ducks and coots? *Veterinary Microbiology* 98:197–208.

Deibel, R., D.E. Emord, W. Dukelow, V.S. Hinshaw, and J. M. Wood. 1985. Influenza viruses and paramyxoviruses in ducks in the Atlantic Flyway, 1977–1983, including an H5N2 isolate related to the virulent chicken virus. *Avian Diseases* 29:970–985.

Donis, R.O., W.J. Bean, Y. Kawaoka, and R.G. Webster. 1989. Distinct lineages of influenza virus H4 hemagglutinin genes in different regions of the world. *Virology* 169:408–417.

Downie, J.C., and W.G. Laver. 1973. Isolation of a Type A influenza virus from an Australian pelagic bird. *Virology* 51:259–269.

Downie, J.C., V. Hinshaw, and W.G. Laver. 1977. Ecology of Influenza—Isolation of type A influenza viruses from Australian pelagic birds. *Australian Journal of Experimental Biology and Medical Science* 55:635–643.

Easterday, B.C. 1975. Animal influenza. In *The Influenza Viruses and Influenza,* E. D. Kilbourne (ed.). New York:Academic Press, pp. 449–481.

Easterday, B.C., and B. Tumova. 1972. Avian influenza. In *Diseases of Poultry,* 6th Ed., M.S. Hofstad, and H.E. Biester (eds.). Iowa State University Press, Ames, IA, U.S.A., pp. 482–496.

Easterday, B.C., D.O. Trainer, B. Tumova, and H.G. Pereira. 1968. Evidence of infection with influenza viruses in migratory waterfowl. *Nature* 219:523–524.

Ellis, T.M., R.B. Bousfield, L.A. Bisset, K.C. Dyrting, G. Luk, S.T. Tsim, K. Sturm-Ramirez, R.G. Webster, Y. Guan, and J.S. Peiris. 2004. Investigation of outbreaks of highly pathogenic H5N1 avian influenza in waterfowl and wild birds in Hong Kong in late 2002. *Avian Pathology* 33:492–505.

Fouchier, R.A., T.M. Bestebroer, S. Herfst, L. Van Der Kemp, G.F. Rimmelzwaan, and A.D. Osterhaus. 2000. Detection of influenza A viruses from different species by PCR amplification of the conserved sequences in the matrix gene. *Journal of Clinical Microbiology* 38:4096–4101.

Fouchier, R.A., B. Olsen, S. Bestebroer, S. Herfst, L. Van der Kemp, G.F. Rimmelzwaan, and A.D. Osterhaus. 2003. Influenza A virus surveillance in wild birds in northern Europe in 1999 and 2000. *Avian Diseases* 47:857–860.

Fouchier, R.A., P.M. Schneeberger, F. W. Rozendaal, J.M. Broekman, S.A. Kemink, V. Munster, T. Kuiken, G.F. Rimmelzwaan, M. Schutten, G.J Van Doornum, G. Koch, A. Bosman, M. Koopmans, and A.D. Osterhaus. 2004. Avian influenza A virus (H7N7) associated with human conjunctivitis and a fatal case of acute respiratory distress syndrome. In *Proceedings National Academy of Science,* U.S.A. 101:1356–1361.

Fouchier, R.A., V. Munster, A. Wallensten, T.M. Bestebroer, S. Herfst, D. Smith, G.F. Rimmelzwaan, B. Olsen, and A.D. Osterhaus. 2005. Characterization of a novel influenza A virus hemagglutinin subtype (H16) obtained from black-headed gulls. *Journal of Virology* 79:2814–2822.

Gorman, O.T., W.J. Bean, Y. Kawaoka, and R.G. Webster. 1990. Evolution of the nucleoprotein gene of influenza A virus. *Journal of Virology* 64:1487–1497.

Gorman, O.T., W.J. Bean, and R.G. Webster. 1992. Evolutionary processes in influenza viruses:divergence, rapid evolution, and stasis. *Current Topics Microbiology and Immunology* 176:75–97.

Graves, I.L. 1992. Influenza viruses in birds of the Atlantic flyway. *Avian Diseases* 36:1–10.

Gresujiva, M., B. Tumova, A. Stumpa, and M. Sekeyova. 1978. Isolation of Influenza Virus from Wild Ducks (*Anas platyrhynchos*). *Acta Virologica* 22:296–301.

Halvorson, D.A., D. Karunakaran, D. Senne, C. Kelleher, C. Bailey, A. Abraham, V. Hinshaw, and J. Newman. 1983. Simultaneous monitoring of sentinel ducks and turkeys in Minnesota. *Avian Diseases* 27:77–85.

Halvorson, D.A., C.J. Kelleher, and D.A. Senne. 1985. Epizootiology of avian influenza: Effect of season on incidence in sentinel ducks and domestic turkeys in Minnesota. *Applied and Environmental Microbiology* 49:914–919.

Hannoun, C. 1977. Isolation from birds of influenza viruses with human neuraminidase. In *Proceedings of the International Symposium on Influenza Immunization (II), Develop. Biol. Standard.* Geneva, Switzerland, pp. 469–472.

Hannoun, C., and J.M. Devayx. 1980. Circulation of influenza viruses in the bay of the Somme River. *Comparative Immunology Microbiology and Infectious Diseases* 3:177–183.

Hanson, B.A. 2002. Temporal, spatial and species patterns of avian influenza viruses among wild birds. MS Dissertation, The University of Georgia, Athens, Georgia, 95 pp.

Hanson, B.A., D.E. Stallknecht, D.E. Swayne, L.A. Lewis, and D.A. Senne. 2003. Avian influenza viruses in Minnesota ducks during 1998–2000. *Avian Diseases* 47:867–871.

Hanson, B., D.E. Swayne, D.A. Senne, D.S. Lobpries, J. Hurst, and D.E. Stallknecht. 2005. Avian influenza and paramyxoviruses in wintering and resident ducks in Texas. *Journal of Wildlife Diseases* 41:624–629.

Hatchette, T.F., D. Walker, C. Johnson, A. Backer, S.P. Pryor, and R.G. Webster. 2004. Influenza A viruses in feral Canadian ducks; extensive reassortment in nature. *Journal of General Virology* 85:2327–2337.

Hinshaw, V.S. 1986. The nature of avian influenza in migratory waterfowl including interspecies transmission. In *Proceedings 2nd International Symposium on Avian Influenza.* Athens, GA, U.S.A., pp.133–141.

Hinshaw, V.S., and R.G. Webster. 1982. The natural history of influenza A viruses. In *Basic and Applied Influenza Research,* A. S. Beare (ed.). CRC Press Inc., Boca Raton, FL, U.S.A., pp. 79–104.

Hinshaw, V.S., R.G. Webster, and B. Turner. 1979. Waterborne transmission of influenza A viruses. *Intervirology* 11:66–69.

Hinshaw, V.S., R.G. Webster, and B. Turner. 1978. Novel influenza A viruses isolated from Canadian feral ducks:Including strains antigenically related to swine influenza (Hsw1N1) viruses. *Journal of General Virology* 41:115–127.

Hinshaw, V.S., R.G. Webster, and B. Turner. 1980. The perpetuation of orthomyxoviruses and paramyxoviruses in Canadian waterfowl. *Canadian Journal of Microbiology* 26:622–629.

Hinshaw, V.S., G.M. Air, A.J. Gibbs, L. Graves, B. Prescott, and D. Karunakaran. 1982. Antigenic and genetic characterization of a novel hemagglutinin subtype of influenza A viruses from gulls. *Journal of Virology* 42:865–872.

Hinshaw, V.S., J.M. Wood, R.G. Webster, R. Deibel, and B. Turner. 1985. Circulation of influenza viruses and paramyxoviruses in waterfowl originating from two different areas of North America. *Bulletin of the World Health Organization* 63:711–719.

Hinshaw, V.S., V.F. Nettles, L. F. Schorr, J.M. Wood, and R.G. Webster. 1986. Influenza virus surveillance in waterfowl in Pennsylvania after the H5N2 avian outbreak. *Avian Diseases* 30:207–212.

Honda, E., H. Kida, R. Yanagawa, Y. Matsuura, K. Yagyu, M. Tsuji, K. Ueno, N. Yamauchi, S. Mishima, H. Ogi, and K. Shimazaki. 1981. Survey of influenza viruses in feral birds in 1979 and isolation of a strain possessing Hav6Nav5 from cloaca of an Eastern Dunlin. *Japanese Journal of Veterinary Research* 29:83–87.

Hooper P., and P. Selleck. 1998. Pathology of low and

high virulent influenza virus infections. In *Proceedings 4th International Symposium on Avian Influenza.* Athens, GA, U.S.A., pp. 134–141.

Hua, Y.-P., H.-L. Chai, S.-Y. Y and, X.-W. Zeng, and Y. Sun. 2005. Primary survey of avian influenza virus and Newcastle disease virus infection in wild birds in some areas of Heilongjiang Province, China. *Journal of Veterinary Science* 6:311–315.

Ibrahim, H.M., I.P.R. Awamg, D.J. Alexander, R.J. Manvell, I. Aini, and A. L. Ibrahim. 1990. Isolations of influenza A viruses from passerine birds in Malaysia. *Veterinary Record* 127:528–528.

Iftimovici, R., V. Iacobescu, A. L. Petrescu, A. Mutiu, and M. Chelaru. 1980. Isolation of influenza virus A/USSR 90/77 (H1N1) from wild birds. *Reviews Roumanian Medical Virology* 31:243.

Isachenko, V.A., L.Y. Zakstelskaya, I.G. Roslaya, L.D. Odinok, E.V. Molibog, and D.K. Lvov. 1974. Strains similar to Hong-Kong variant of influenza virus isolated from synanthropic and wild migrating birds. (In Russian.) *Ivanovsky Institute Virology* 2:156–165.

Ito, T., K. Okazaki, Y. Kawaoka, A. Takada, R.G. Webster, and H. Kida. 1995. Perpetuation of influenza A viruses in Alaskan waterfowl reservoirs. *Archives of Virology* 140:1163–1172.

Ito, T., J.N. Couceiro, S. Kelm, L.G. Baum, S. Krauss, M.R. Castrucci, I. Donatelli, H. Kida, J.C. Paulson, R.G. Webster, and Y. Kawaoka. 1998. Molecular basis for the generation in pigs of influenza A viruses with pandemic potential. *Journal of Virology* 72:7367–7373.

Kawaoka, Y., T. M. Chambers, W.L. Sladen, and R.G. Webster. 1988. Is the gene pool of influenza viruses in shorebirds and gulls different from that in wild ducks? *Virology* 163:247–250.

Kawaoka, Y., N. J. Cox, O. Haller, S. Hongo, N. Kaverin, H.-D. Klenk, R.A. Lamb, J. McCauley, P. Palese, E. Rimstad, and R.G. Webster. 2005. Orthomyxoviridae. In *Virus Taxonomy:Eighth Report of the International Committee on Taxonomy of Viruses.* C. M. Fauquet, M.A. Mayo, J. Maniloff, U. Desselberger, and L.A. Ball (eds.). Academic Press, San Diego, CA, U.S.A., pp. 681–693.

Keawcharoen, J., K. Oraveerakul, T. Kuiken, R.A. Fouchier, A. Amonisin, S. Payungporn, S. Noppornpanth, S. Wattandodorn, A. Theamboonlers, A. Tantilertcharoen, R. Pattanarangsan, N. Arya, P. Ratanakorn, A.D. Osterhaus, and Y. Poovorawan. 2004. Avian influenza H5N1 in tigers and leopards. *Emerging Infectious Diseases* 10:2198–2191.

Kida, H., and R. Yanagawa. 1979. Isolation and characterization of influenza A viruses from wild free-flying ducks in Hokkaido, Japan. *Zentralblatt Fur Bakteriologie Mikrobiologie Und Hygiene. Series A, Medical Microbiology Infectious Diseases Virology Parasitology* 244:135–143.

Klenk, H-D., and W. Garten. 1994. Host cell proteases controlling virus pathogenicity. *Trends Microbiology* 2:39–43.

Kida, H. R., R. Yanagawa, and Y. Matsuoka. 1980. Duck influenza lacking evidence of disease signs and immune response. *Infection and Immunity* 30:547–553.

Kobayashi, S., V. Sivanandan, K.V. Nagaraja, S.M. Goyal, and D.A. Halvorson. 1994. Antigen-capture enzyme-immunoassay for detection of avian influenza-virus in turkeys. *American Journal of Veterinary Research* 54:1385–1390.

Kocan, A.A., V.S. Hinshaw, and G.A. Daubney. 1980. Influenza A viruses isolated from migrating ducks in Oklahoma. *Journal of Wildlife Diseases* 16:281–285.

Kwon, Y-K., S-J. Joh, M-C. Kim, Y-J. Lee, J-G. Choi,. E-K. Lee, S-H. Wee, H-W. Sung, J-H. Kwon, M-I. Kang, and J-H. Kim. Highly pathogenic avian influenza in magpies (*Pica pica sericea*) in South Korea. 2005. *Journal of Wildlife Diseases* 41:618–623.

Krauss, S., D. Walker, S. Paul-Pryor, L. Niles, L. Chenghong, V.S. Hinshaw, and R.G. Webster. 2004. Influenza A viruses in migrating wild aquatic birds in North America. *Vector-Borne and Zoonotic Diseases* 4:177–189.

Kuiken, T., G. Rimmelzwaan, D. van Riel, G. Van Amerongen, M. Baars, R. Fouchier, and A. Osterhaus. 2004. Avian influenza in cats. *Science* 306:241.

Kuiken, T., E.C. Holmes, J. McCauley, G. F. Rimmelzwaan, C.S. Williams, and B.J. Grenfell. 2006. Host species barriers to influenza virus infections. *Science* 312:394–397.

Lai, C.J., L.J. Markoff, S. Zimmerman, B. Cohen, J.A. Berndt, and R.M. Chanock. 1980. In *Proceedings National Academy of Science,* U.S.A., 77:210–214.

Laver, W.G., and R.G. Webster. 1972. Antibodies to human influenza virus neurominidase (the A/Asian/57 H2N2 Strain) in sera from Australian pelagic birds. *Bulletin World Health Organization* 47:535–541.

Lee, C-W., D.L. Suarez, T.M. Tumpey, H-W. Sung, Y-K. Kwon, Y-J. Lee, J-G. Choi, S-J. Joh, M-C. Kim, E-K. Lee, J-M. Park, X. Lu, J. M. Katz, E. Spackman, D.E. Swayne, and J-H. Kim. 2005. Characterization of highly pathogenic H5N1 avian influenza A viruses isolated from South Korea. *Journal of Virology* 79:3692–3701.

Lin, Y. P., M. Shaw, V. Gregory, K. Cameron, W. Lim, A. Klimov, K. Subbarao, Y. Guan, S. Krauss, S. Shortridge, R.G. Webster, N. Cox, and A. Hay. 2000. Avian-to-human transmission of H9N2 subtype influenza A viruses:relationship between H9N2 and H5N1 human isolates. In *Proceedings National Academy of Science,* U.S.A. 97:9654–9658.

Lipkind, M., Y. Weisman, E. Shihmanter, and D. Shoham. 1981. Review of the three-year studies on the ecology of avian influenza viruses in Israel. In *Proceedings 1st International Conference on Avian Influenza.* Beltsville, MD, U.S.A., pp. 68–78.

Lipkind, M.A., Y. Weisman, E. Shihmanter, and D. Shoham. 1979. The first isolation of animal influenza virus in Israel. *Veterinary Record* 105:510–511.

Liu, J., H. Xiao, F. Lei, Q. Zhu, K. Qin, X. Zhang,, D. Zhao, G. Wang, Y. Reng, J. Ma, W. Liu, J. Wang, and F. Gao. 2005. Highly pathogenic H5N1 influenza virus infection in migratory birds. Science online, Retrieved from the World Wide Web:www.science.org /cgi/content/full/1115273/DCI.

L'vov, D. K. 1978. Circulation of influenza viruses in natural biocoenosis. In *Viruses and Environment.* E. Kurstak and K. Marmorosch (eds.). Academic Press, New York, NY, U.S.A., pp. 351–380.

Lu, H., A.E. Castro, K. Pennick, J. Liu, Q. Yang, P. Dunn, D. Weinstock, and D. Henzler. 2003. Survival of avian influenza virus H7N2 in SPF chickens and their environments. *Avian Diseases* 47:1015–1021.

Lui, J., H. Xiao, F. Lei, Q. Zhu, K. Qin, X.-W. Zhang, X.-L. Zhang, D. Zhao, G. Wang, Y. Feng, J. Ma, W. Liu, J. Wang, and G.F. Gao. 2005. Highly pathogenic H5N1 influenza virus infection in migratory birds. *Science* 309:1206.

Mackenzie, J.S., E.C. Edwards, R.M. Holmes, and V.S. Hinshaw. 1984. Isolation of orthoviruses and paramyxovirus from wild birds in Western Australia and the characterization of novel influenza A viruses. *Australian Journal of Experimental Biology and Medical Science* 62:89–99.

Manjunath, L.H., and B.B. Mallick. 1981. Prevalence of myxo- and paramyxoviruses in birds of Himalayan region. *Indian Journal of Animal Sciences* 51:1139–1143.

Makarova, N.V., N.V. Kaverin, S. Krauss, D. Senne, and R.G. Webster. 1999. Transmission of Eurasian avian H2 influenza virus to shorebirds in North America. Journal of General Virology 80:3167–3171.

Mase, M., K. Tsukamoto, T. Imada, K. Imai, N. Tanimura, K. Nakamura, Y. Yamoto, T. Hitomi, T. Kira, T, Nakai, M. Hrimoto, Y. Kawaoka, and S. Yamaguchi. 2005. Characterization of H5N1 highly pathogenic influenza viruses isolated during the 2003–2004 influenza outbreak in Japan. *Virology* 332:167–176.

Mikami, T., M. Kawamura, T. Kondo, T. Murai, M. Horiuchi, H. Kodama, H. Izawa, and H. Kida. 1987. Isolation of ortho- and paramyxoviruses from migrating feral ducks in Japan. *Veterinary Record* 120:417–418.

Munster, V.J., A. Wallensten, C. Baas, G. F. Rimmelzaann, M. Schutten, B. Olsen, A.D. Osterhaus, and R.A. Fouchier. 2005. Mallards and highly pathogenic avian influenza ancestral viruses, Northern Europe. Emerging Infectious Diseases 11:1545–1551.

Muramoto, Y., H. Ozaki, A. Takada, C-H. Park, Y. Sunden, T. Umemura, Y. Kawaoka, H. Matsuda, and H. Kida. 2006. Highly pathogenic H5N1 influenza virus causes coagulopathy in chickens. *Microbiology and Immunology* 50:73–81.

Nettles, V.F., J.M. Wood, and R.G. Webster. 1985. Wildlife surveillance associated with an outbreak of lethal H5N2 avian influenza in domestic poultry. *Avian Diseases* 29:733–741.

Noda, T., H. Sagara, A. Yen, A. Takada, H. Kida, R.H. Cheng, and Y. Kawaoka. 2006. Architecture of ribonucleoprotein complexes in influenza A virus particles. *Nature* 439:490–492.

Olsen, C.W. 2002. The emergence of novel swine influenza viruses in North America. *Virus Research* 85:199–210.

Olsen, B., V.J. Munster, A. Wallensten, J. Waldenstrom, A.D. Osterhaus, and R.A. Fouchier. 2006. Global patterns of influenza A virus in wild birds. *Science* 312:384–388.

Otsuki, K., O. Takemoto, R. Fujimoto, K. Yamazaki, N. Kubota, H. Hosaki, Y. Kawaoka, and M. Tsubokura. 1987. Isolation of influenza A viruses from migratory waterfowls in San-in District, Western Japan, in the winter of 1982–1983. *Acta Virologica* 31:439–442.

Otsuki, K., O. Takemoto, R. Fujimoto, K. Yamazaki, T. Kubota, H. Hosaki, T. Mitani, Y. Kawaoka, and M. Tsubokura. 1984. Isolation of H5 Influenza Viruses from Whistling Swans in Western Japan in November 1983. *Acta Virologica* 28:524.

Ottis, K., and P. A. Bachmann. 1980. Occurrence of Hsw1N1 subtype influenza A viruses in wild ducks in Europe. *Archives Virology* 63:185–190.

Ottis, K., and P. A. Bachmann. 1983. Isolation and characterization of ortho- and paramyxoviruses from feral birds in Europe. Zentralblatt fur Veterinarmedizin B 30:22–35.

Pasick, J., K. Handel, J. Robinson, J. Coops, D. Ridd, K. Hills, H. Kehler, C. Cottam-Birt, J. Neufeld, Y. Berhane, and S. Czub. 2005. Intersegmental recombination between the haemagglutinin and matrix genes was responsible for the emergence of a highly pathogenic H7N3 avian influenza virus in British Columbia. *Journal of General Virology* 86:727–731.

Pearson, J. E., and D. A. Senne. 1986. Diagnostic procedures for avian influenza. In *Proceedings 2nd International Symposium on Avian Influenza.* Athens, GA, U.S.A., pp. 222–227.

Perdue, M. L., M. Garcia, J. Beck, M. Brugh, and D. E. Swayne. 1996. An Arg-Lys insertion at the hemagglutinin cleavage site of an H5N2 avian influenza isolate. *Virus Genes* 12:77–84.

Pereira, H.G., B. Tumova, and V.G. Low. 1965. Avian influenza A viruses. *Bulletin World Health Organization* 32:855–860.

Perkins, L.E.L., and D.E. Swayne. 2001. Pathogenicity of A/Chicken/Hong Kong/220/97 (H5N1) avian influenza virus in seven gallinaceous species. *Veterinary Pathology* 38:149–164.

Perkins L.E.L., and D.E. Swayne. 2002. Pathogenicity of a Hong Kong–origin H5N1 highly pathogenic avian influenza virus for emus, geese, ducks, and pigeons. *Avian Diseases* 46:53–63.

Perkins L.E.L., and D. E. Swayne. 2002. Susceptibility of Laughing Gulls (*Larus atricilla*) to H5N1 and H5N3 highly pathogenic avian influenza viruses. *Avian Diseases* 46:877–885.

Perkins L. E. L., and D. E. Swayne. 2003. Varied pathogenicity of a Hong Kong–origin H5N1 avian influenza virus in four passerine species and budgerigars. *Veterinary Pathology* 40:14–24.

Pfitzer, S., D.J. Verwoerd, G.H. Gerdes, A.E. Labuschagne, A. Erasmus, R. J. Manvell, and C. Grund. 2000. Newcastle disease and avian influenza A virus in wild waterfowl in South Africa. *Avian Diseases* 44:655–660.

Roberts, D.H. 1964. The isolation of influenza A virus and Mycoplasma associated with duck sinusitis. *Veterinary Record* 76:470–473.

Romvary, J., and J. Tanyi. 1975. Occurrence of Hong Kong influenza A (H3N2) virus infection in Budapest Zoo. *Acta Veterinaria Academiae Scientiarum Hungaricae* 25:251–254.

Romvary, J., J. Meszaros, J. Tanyi, J. Rozsa, and L. Fabian. 1976a. Influenza infectedness of captured and shot wild birds on northeastern and southeastern parts of Hungary. *Acta Veterinaria Academiae Scientiarum Hungaricae* 26:363–368.

Romvary, J., J. Meszaros, J. Tanyi, J. Rozsa, and L. Fabian. 1976b. Spreading of virus infection among wild birds and monkeys during influenza epidemic caused by Victoria(3)75 variant of a (H3N2) virus. *Acta Veterinaria Academiae Scientiarum Hungaricae* 26:369–376.

Rogers, G.N., and J.C. Paulson. 1983. Receptor determinants of human and animal influenza virus isolates. Differences in receptor specificity of the H3 hemagglutinin based on species of origin. *Virology* 127:361–373.

Rosenberger, J. K., W.C. Krauss, and R.D. Slemons. 1974. Isolation of Newcastle disease and type-A influenza viruses from migratory waterfowl in Atlantic Flyway. Avian Diseases 18:610–613.

Roslaya, I.G., G.E. Roslyakov, and D.K. L'vov. 1975. Isolation of influenza A viruses and detection of antibodies in common herons (*Ardea cinera*) nesting in the lower Amur. *Ekologiia Virusov* 3:138–142.

Roslaya, I.G., G.E. Roslyakov, D.K. L'vov, V. A. Isacenko, L.Y. Zakstelskaya, L. Ya, and I. T. Trop. 1974. Circulation of arbo- and myxoviruses in populations of waterfowl and shore birds of the lower Amur. (In Russian.) *Ivanovsky Institute of Virology* 2:148–156.

Saito, T., T. Horimoto, Y. Kakaoka, D.A. Senne, and R.G. Webster. 1994. Emergence of a potentially pathogenic H5N2 influenza virus in chickens. *Virology* 201:277–284.

Sandu, T., and V.S. Hinshaw. 1981. Influenza A virus infection in domestic ducks. In *Proceedings 1st International Symposium on Avian Influenza.* Beltsville, MD, U.S.A., pp. 222–227.

Sazonov, A.A., D.K. L'vov, R.G. Webster, T.V. Sokolova, N.A. Braude, and N.V. Portyanko. 1977. Isolation of an influenza virus, similar to A/Port Chalmers/1/73 (H3N2) from a common murre at Sakhalin Island in U.S.S.R (Strain A/CommonMurre/Sakhalin/1/74). *Archives Virology* 53:1–7.

Schafer, J.R., Y. Kawaoka, W.J. Bean, J. Suss, D. Senne, and R.G. Webster. 1993. Origin of the pandemic 1957 H2 influenza A virus and the persistence of its possible progenitors in the avian reservoir. *Virology* 194:781–788.

Sharp, G.B., Y. Kawaoka, S.M. Wright, B. Turner, V. Hinshaw, and R.G. Webster. 1993. Wild ducks are the reservoir for only a limited number of influenza A subtypes. *Epidemiology and Infection* 110:161–176.

Shafer, A.L., J.B. Katz, and KA. Eernisee. 1998. Development and validation of a competitive enzyme-linked immunosorbent assay for detection of type A influenza antibodies in avian sera. *Avian Diseases* 42:28–34.

Shinya, K., M. Ebina, S. Yamada, M. Ono, N. Kasai, and Y. Kawaoka. 2006. Avian flu:influenza virus receptors in the human airway. *Nature* 440:435–436.

Sinnecker, R., H. Sinnecker, E. Zilske, and D. Kohler. 1983. Surveillance of pelagic birds for influenza A viruses. *Acta Virologica* 27:75–79.

Slemons, R.D., and B.C. Easterday. 1972. Host response differences among five avian species to influenza virus A/turkey/Ontario/7732/66 (Hav5N). *Bulletin World Health Organization* 47:521–525.

Slemons, R.D., D.C. Johnson, and T.G. Malone. 1973. Influenza type A isolated from imported exotic birds. *Avian Diseases* 17:458–459.

Slemons, R.D., D.C. Johnson, J.S. Osborn, and F. Hayes. 1974. Type A influenza viruses isolated from wild free-flying ducks in California. *Avian Diseases* 18:119–124.

Slemons, R.D., and B.C. Easterday. 1975. The natural history of type A influenza viruses in wild waterfowl. In *Proceedings 3rd International Wildlife Disease Conference, Munich, Germany.* L.A. Page (ed.). Plenum Press, New York. NY, U.S.A., pp. 215–224.

Slemons, R.D., and B.C. Easterday. 1977. Type-A influenza viruses in feces of migratory waterfowl. *Journal American Veterinary Medicine Association* 171:947–948.

Slemons, R.D., and B.C. Easterday. 1978. Virus replication in the digestive track of ducks exposed by aerosol to type-A influenza virus. *Avian Diseases* 22:367–377.

Slemons, R.D., M.C. Shieldcastle, L.D. Heyman, K.E. Bednarik and D.A. Senne. 1991. Type A influenza viruses in waterfowl in Ohio and implications for domestic turkeys. *Avian Diseases* 35:165–173.

Smitka, C.W., and H.F. Massab. 1981. Ortho- and paramyxoviruses in the migratory waterfowl of Michigan. *Journal of Wildlife Diseases* 17:147–151.

Songserm, T., F. Jam-on, N. S. Heng, and N. Meemak. 2005. A study on the stability and survival of avian influenza virus H5N1 in different conditions and sensitivity to disinfectants. Abstract of the OIE/FAO International Conference on Avian Influenza, Paris, France.

Spackman, E., D.E. Stallknecht, R.D. Slemons, K. Winker, D. L. Suarez, M. Scott, and D.E. Swayne. 2005. Phylogenetic analysis of type A influenza genes in natural reservoir species in North America reveals genetic variation. *Virus Research* 114:89–100.

Spackman, E., K. Winker, K. McCracken, and D.E. Swayne. 2006. An avian influenza virus from waterfowl in South America contains genes from North American Avian and Equine lineages. *Avian Disease* (in press).

Stallknecht, D.E., and S.M. Shane. 1988. Host range of avian influenza virus in free-living birds. *Veterinary Research Communications* 12:125–141.

Stallknecht, D.E. 1998. Ecology and epidemiology of avian influenza viruses in wild bird populations:Waterfowl, shorebirds, pelicans, cormorants, etc. In *Proceedings 4th International Symposium on Avian Influenza.* Athens, GA, U.S.A., pp. 61–69.

Stallknecht, D.E., S.M. Shane, P.J. Zwank, D.A. Senne, and M.T. Kearney. 1990a. Avian influenza viruses from migratory and resident ducks of coastal Louisiana. *Avian Diseases* 34:398–405.

Stallknecht, D.E., S.M. Shane, M.T. Kearney, and P.J. Zwank. 1990b. Persistence of avian influenza virus in water. *Avian Diseases* 34:406–411.

Stallknecht, D.E., M.T. Kearney, S.M. Shane, and P.J. Zwank. 1990c. Effects of pH, temperature, and salinity on persistence of avian influenza viruses in water. *Avian Diseases* 34:412–418.

Stanislawek, W. L., C. R. Wilks, J. Meers, G. W. Horner, D.J. Alexander, R. J. Manvell, J. A. Kattenbelt, and A. R. Gould. 2002. Avian paramyxoviruses and influenza viruses isolated from mallard ducks (*Anas platyrhynchos*) in New Zealand. *Archives of Virology* 147:1287–1302.

Stubbs, E.L. 1948. Fowl Pest. In *Diseases of Poultry,* 2nd Ed., H.E. Biester and L.H. Schwarte (eds.). Iowa State University Press, Ames, IA, U.S.A., pp. 603–614.

Stunzner, D., W. Thiel, F. Potsch, and W. Sixl. 1980. Isolation of influenza viruses from exotic and central European birds. *Zentralblatt Fur Bakteriologie Mikrobiologie Und Hygiene Series A, Medical Microbiology Infectious Diseases Virology Parasitology* 247:8–17.

Sturm-Ramirez, K.M., T. Ellis, B. Bousfield, L. Bissett, K. Dyrting, J.E. Rehg, L. Poon, Y. Guan, M. Peiris, and R.G. Webster. 2004. Reemerging H5N1 influenza viruses in Hong Kong in 2002 are highly pathogenic to ducks. *Journal of Virology* 78:4892–4901.

Subbarao, K., A. Klimov, J. Katz, H. Regnery, W. Lim, H. Hall, M. Perdue, D.E. Swayne, C. Bender, J. Huang, M. Hemphill, T. Rowe, M. Shaw, S. Xu, K. Fukuda, and N. Cox. Characterization of an avian influenza A (H5N1) virus isolated from a child with a fatal respiratory illness. *Science* 279:363–396.

Suss, J., J. Schafer, H. Sinnecker, and R.G. Webster. 1994. Influenza virus subtypes in aquatic birds of eastern Germany. *Archives of Virology* 135:101–114.

Suarez, D.L., and C.S. Schultz. 2000. Immunology of avian influenza virus. A review. *Developmental and Comparative Immunology* 24:269–283.

Swayne, D.E., J.R. Beck, M. Garcia, M.L. Perdue, and M. Brugh. 1998. Pathogenicity shifts in experimental avian influenza infections in chickens. In *Proceedings 4th International Symposium on Avian Influenza.* Athens, GA, U.S.A., pp. 171–181.

Swayne, D.E., and D.A. Halvorson. 2003. Influenza. In *Diseases of Poultry,* 11th Ed., Y.M. Saif (ed.). Iowa State Press, Ames, IA, U.S.A., pp. 135–161.

Swayne, D.E., and D.L. Suarez. 2000. Highly pathogenic avian influenza. *Review Scientific and Technical Office International des épizooties* 19:463–482.

Taubenberger, J.K., A.H. Reid, R.M. Lournes, R. Wang, G. Jin, and T.G. Fanning. 2005. Characterization of the 1918 influenza virus polymerase genes. *Nature* 437:889–893.

Thorsen, J., I.K. Barker, and V.S. Hinshaw. 1980. Influenza viruses isolated from waterfowl in southern Ontario, 1976–1978. *Canadian Journal of Microbiology* 26:1511–1514.

Timoney, P.J. 1996. Equine influenza. *Comparative Immunology, Microbiology and Infectious Diseases* 19:205–211.

Tsubokura, M., K. Otsuki, Y. Kawaoka, and R. Yanagawa. 1981a. Isolation of influenza A viruses from migratory waterfowls in San-in District, Western Japan in 1979–1980. *Zentralblatt Fur Bakteriologie Mikrobiologie Und Hygiene Serie B-Umwelthygiene Krankenhaushygiene Arbeitshygiene Praventive Medizin* 173:494–500.

Tsubokura, M., K. Otsuki, H. Yamamoto, Y. Kawaoka, and K. Nerome. 1981b. Isolation of an Hswl Nav4 Influenza Virus from a Tufted Duck (*Aythya fuligula*) in Japan. *Microbiology and Immunology* 25:819–825.

Turek, R., B. Tumova, V. Mucha, and A. Stumpa. 1983. Type A influenza virus strains isolated from free-living ducks in Czechoslovakia during 1978–1981. *Acta Virologica* 27:523–527.

USGS. 2006a. Referenced reports of highly pathogenic avian influenza H5N1 in wildlife and domestic animals. [Online.] Retrieved from World Wide

Web:www.nwhc.usgs.gov/research/avian_influenza/a vian_influenza_text/htm. Accessed April 2006.

USGS. 2006b. List of species affected by H5N1 (avian influenza). National Wildlife Health Center Web site. [Online.] Retrieved from the World Wide Web:www.nwhc.usgs.gov/disease_information/avian _influenza/affected_species_chart.jsp.

Webster, R.G., M. Morita, C. Pridgen, and B. Tumova. 1976. Ortho- and paramyxoviruses from migrating feral ducks:characterization of a new group of influenza A viruses. *Journal of General Virology* 32:217–225.

Webster, R.G., M. Yakhno, V. S. Hinshaw, W.R. Bean Jr., and K.G. Murti. 1978. Intestinal influenza:replication and characterization of influenza viruses in ducks. *Virology* 84:268–278.

Webster, R.G., W.G. Laver, G.M. Air, and G.C. Schild. 1982. Molecular mechanism of variation in influenza viruses. *Nature* (London) 296:115–121.

Webster, R.G., and Y. Kawaoka. 1988. Avian influenza. *CRC Critical Reviews Poultry Biology* 1:211–246.

Webster, R.G., and R. Rott. 1988. Influenza virus A pathogenicity:the pivotal role of the hemagglutinin. *Cell* 50:665–666.

Webster, R.G., W. J. Bean, O.T. Gorman, T.M. Chambers, and Y. Kawaoka. 1992. Evolution and ecology of influenza viruses. *Microbiological Reviews* 56: 152–179.

Webster, R.G., and Y. Kawaoka. 1994. Influenza:an emerging and reemerging disease. *Seminars in Virology* 5:103–111.

Widjaja, L., S.L. Krauss, R.J. Webby, T. Xie, and R.G. Webster. 2004. Matrix gene of influenza A viruses from wild aquatic birds:ecology and emergence of influenza viruses. *Journal of Virology* 78:8771–8779.

Wilkinson, L., and A.P. Waterson. 1975. The development of the virus concept as reflected in corpora of studies on individual pathogens 2. The agent of fowl plague-A model virus? *Medical History* 19:52–71.

Winkler, W.G., D.O. Trainer, and B.C. Easterday. 1972. Influenza in Canada geese. *Bulletin World Health Organization* 47:507–513.

WHO. 1980. A revision of the system of nomenclature for influenza viruses:a WHO memorandum. *Bulletin World Health Organization* 58:585–591.

Yamane, N., T. Odagiri, J. Arikawa, H. Morita, N. Sukeno, and N. Ishida. 1978. Isolation of orthomyxovirus from migrating and domestic ducks in northern Japan in 1976–1977. *Japanese Journal of Medical Science & Biology* 31:407–415.

Yamane, N., T. Odagiri, J. Arikawa, and N. Ishida. 1979. Isolation and characterization of influenza A viruses from wild ducks in northern Japan:appearance of Hsw1 antigens in the Japanese duck population. *Acta Virologica* 23:375–384.

Zakstelskaya, L.Y., M.A. Yakhno, V.A. Isachenko, S.M. Klimenko, E.V. Molibog, V.P. Andreev, D.K. L'vov, and S.S. Yamnikova. 1974. Isolation and peculiarities of influenza virus (tern) (Turkmenistan 18) 73. Virologiia Virusov. 2:93–98.

Zakstelskaya, L.Y., C.C. Timofeeva, M.A. Yakhno, E.V. Molibog, V.A. Isachenko, and D.K. Lvov. 1975. Isolation of influenza A viruses from wild migratory waterfowl in the north of European part of the USSR. *Ekologiia Virusov* 3.

6
Avian Pox

Charles van Riper III and Donald J. Forrester

INTRODUCTION

Avian pox, a viral disease of birds, is caused by one of the larger viruses of the poxvirus group. This relatively slow-developing disease is characterized in birds by discrete, proliferative lesions on the skin of the toes, legs, or head, and/or mucous membranes of the mouth and upper respiratory tract. Systemic infections may also occur (Tripathy and Reed 2003). It is comparable to the pox infections of wild mammals (see Robinson and Kerr 2001), of domestic mammals (for example, sheep sore-mouth, swine poxes; see Tripathy et al. 1981), and those of man (smallpox). This subgroup of avipoxviruses contains a number of species and strains that vary in their pathogenicity and host specificity.

This widespread avian disease has been found in a large number of bird families, with some (for example, Phasianidae, Emberizidae) seeming more susceptible than others. In most birds avian pox infections are mild and rarely result in death. However, when lesions are on the eyelids or mucous membranes of the oral and/or respiratory cavities, mortality can be high. Those avian populations that have been isolated on islands (for example, Canary Islands, Hawaiian island chain, Galapagos Islands) are more greatly impacted than are birds in continental situations where the hosts, vectors, and viruses have had a longer co-evolutionary history (Vargas 1987; van Riper et al. 2002).

As with many other diseases that are density dependent, avian pox transmission is enhanced with increasing vector and/or host densities. Therefore, this disease is found to have a greater significance in captive situations such as zoos (Fowler 1981), bird rehabilitation centers (Wheeldon et al. 1985), and game farms (Karstad 1965), where birds occur in much higher densities than in the wild. In the wild, the warmer and mesic regions of the world support more potential vectors, thus in these areas the prevalence of avian pox is higher, particularly in flocking wild birds (Annuar et al. 1983; Forrester 1991).

SYNONYMS

Avian pox, pox, bird pox, poxvirus infection, fowl pox, avian diphtheria, contagious epithelioma, molluscum contagiosum, Gefluegelpocken (German), viruela aviar (Spanish), variole aviaire (French), bouba (Portuguese).

HISTORY

Avian pox infections were among the earliest described avian diseases (for example, Heusinger 1844) because of the ease in identification of the obvious external lesions. Bollinger (1873) and Borrel (1904) were the first to demonstrate a relationship between histologic lesions and structure of inclusion bodies, setting the stage for histopathologic techniques being employed to confirm visual diagnoses. Evidence that avian poxvirus was associated with the inclusion bodies and was the etiological agent was conclusively demonstrated by Woodruff and Goodpasture (1930).

During the mid-twentieth century, pox virus identification focused on virus culture on the ectodermal chorioallantoic membrane (CAM) of embryonated chicken eggs (Cunningham 1966) and remains today one of the identification tools of choice. Later during the 1950s, electron microscopy gained importance as a diagnostic tool. Today, identification of avian pox strains has moved into the molecular arena, with the use of Gel-electrophoresis and PCR (Polymerase chain reaction) analyses of mitochondrial DNA sequences (Schnitzlein et al. 1988).

The literature on avian pox in wild birds was summarized by Kirmse (1967a), Karstad (1971), and then Bolte et al. (1999). Over the past half-century, the majority of scientific papers on avian pox infections in wild birds have come from case reports of usually singly infected individuals (for example, Simpson et al. 1975; Fitzner et al. 1985). There have been a smaller number of studies (for example, Davidson et al. 1980; Tikasingh et al. 1982; McClure 1989; Forrester 1991, 1992; van Riper et al. 2002; Atkinson et al. 2005, Smits et al. 2005) directed toward questions at the overall host and community population levels. The more recent work on avian pox has focused on areas of molecular structure within wild bird strains when compared to fowlpox virus (for example, Tripathy et al. 2000; Tripathy and Reed 2003), the influence of avian pox on House Finch (*Carpodacus mexicanus*) plumage coloration (for example, Zahn and Rothstein, 1999), and the continued impact on native island birds (Medina et al. 2004; Atkinson et al. 2005).

DISTRIBUTION

The geographic distribution of avian poxviruses is worldwide, with the exception that there are no published records from wild birds with this disease in the Arctic or Antarctic, or some of the more remote regions of the world (Figure 6.1). Published information is greatly skewed geographically to those localities where scientists have been actively working on this disease (for example, North America, Australia, Europe, Asia), thus the few existing published reports from wild birds throughout much of Africa and South America. The current state of our knowledge on avian pox in wild bird populations generally reveals a higher prevalence in temperate and warmer areas of the globe.

Even within continents, avian pox distributions tend to be confined to localized regions. For example, Forrester (1991) examined the distribution of avian pox in Wild Turkeys (*Meleagris gallopavo*) over North America and found the disease concentrated in the moister and warmer southeastern United States, even though Wild Turkeys occur in every state except Alaska. Where avian pox has been introduced to remote islands (for example, Hawaii, Galapagos, Canary Islands), the disease rapidly spreads, resulting in much higher prevalences in the native avifauna than occurs among the introduced avian species (Warner 1968; Vargas 1987; VanderWerf 2001; van Riper et al. 2002; Atkinson et al. 2005, Smits et al. 2005).

HOST RANGE

There are now recognized approximately 183 families and 9,800 species of birds (Clements 2000). Most avian species, if adequately exposed, are susceptible to one or more of the avian poxvirus strains and/or species. Kirmse (1967a) reported naturally occurring avian pox infections in 60 species of wild birds, comprising 20 families. Bolte et al. (1999) has provided a more recent update, of which they found about 20 orders recorded with *Avipoxvirus* infections. We have found records of poxvirus infections in 278 bird species from 70 families and 20 orders (see Table 6.1, at the end of this chapter). It is interesting that avian pox has never been reported from the Tinamous (Tinamiformes), Loons (Gaviiformes), Nightjars (Caprimulgiformes), and Kingfishers (Coraciiformes). It has been only recently that avian pox has been regularly observed in wild waterfowl (Morton and Dietrich 1979; Cox 1980), although it has long been known that domestic ducks and geese are susceptible

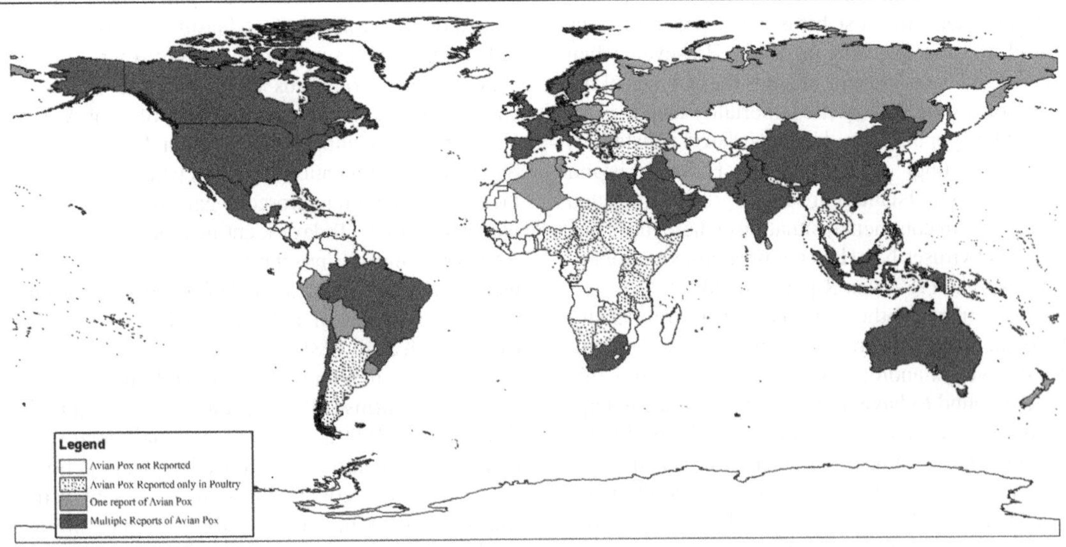

Figure 6.1. Distribution of countries throughout the world in which avian pox has been reported in birds. Those countries with heavy stippling are ones in which avian pox has been reported from multiple bird families; moderate stippling indicates reporting from a single record; and the absence of stippling indicates that avian pox has not positively been identified in those countries.

(Kirmse 1967b). This same pattern holds true for the Falconiformes, Columbiformes, and Psittaciformes (Cooper 1978; Hitchner and Clubb 1980; Petrak 1982), where infections are now being reported from wild birds when, heretofore, earlier cases were reported only infrequently from captive situations.

ETIOLOGY

Avian pox is caused by viruses of the genus *Avipoxvirus* in the family Poxviridae (Murphy et al. 1999). The source and reservoir of avian pox is primarily infected birds but also can be related to viable viruses present on exfoliated scabs and contaminated objects (for example, perches) in the environment or aviary. The virus particle is large, about 150 to 250 nm by 265 to 350 nm in size, and is oval or brick-shaped and covered with irregularly spaced surface knobs (Wilner 1969). Coupar et al. (1990) identified the genome of the avian poxvirus as composed of a single double-stranded, 300 Kb DNA molecule. This DNA-containing, enveloped virus develops in the cytoplasm of infected avian epithelial cells. Infected cells characteristically contain large acidophilic intracytoplasmic inclusions (Bollinger bodies). Electron microscopy of avian pox inclusions reveals viral particles embedded in a rather homogeneous matrix, typical of poxviruses in general (Figure 6.2).

Avian poxviruses can withstand extreme environmental conditions, particularly desiccation, sometimes surviving on perches and in dried scabs for months and years (Tripathy 1993). Much of this can be attributed to the very large size of the virus. The virus is resistant to ether, with the pigeonpox virus being resistant to both chloroform and ether (Tantwai et al. 1979). Andrews et al. (1978) demonstrated that the virus can withstand 1% phenol and 1:1,000 formalin for nine days, but that 1% potassium hydroxide or heating to 50°C for 30 minutes (or 60°C for eight minutes) inactivated the virus.

Avian poxviruses have been classified according to their hosts of origin (Cunningham 1972). Tripathy (1993) listed 13 recognized species. Based on host specificity, poxvirus strains have been identified and classified as mono-, bi-, or tri-pathogenic. A Northern Flicker *(Colaptes auratus)* strain is a good example of a monopathogenic strain because among 19 species of inoculated wild and domestic birds, only the Northern Flicker was found susceptible to infection (Kirmse

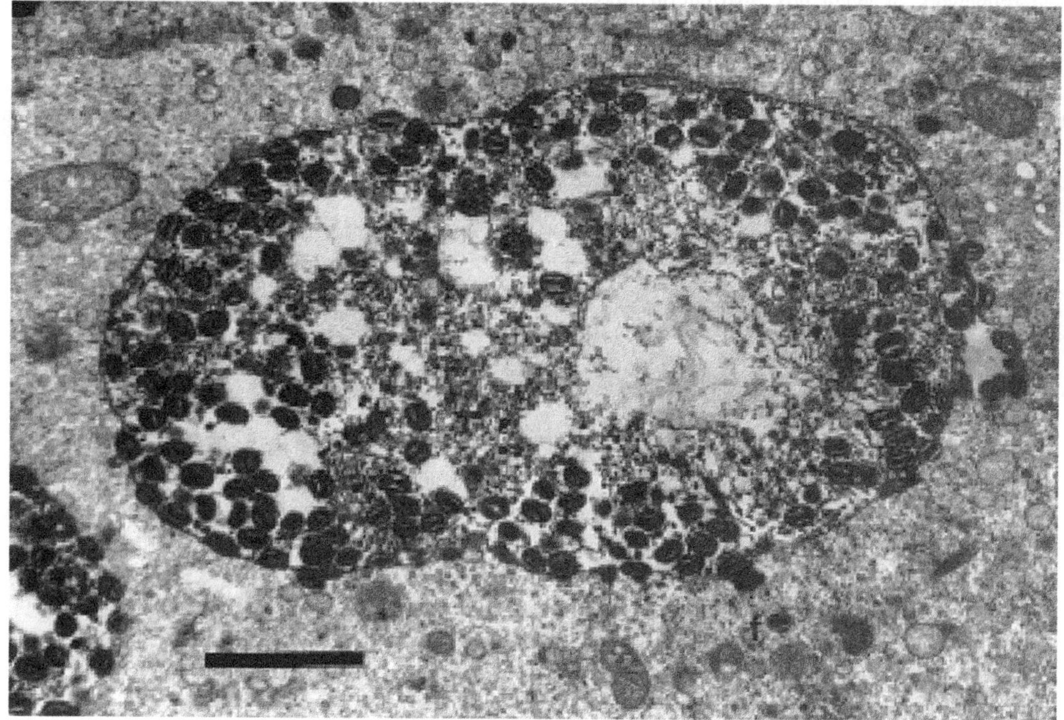

Figure 6.2. An electron micrograph of an avian poxvirus inclusion body in an Imperial Eagle (*Aquila heliaca*), with numerous viral particles. (Figure published in Hernandez et al. [2001] and reprinted with permission of the author and *Journal of Avian Pathology.*) 7,000x

1966). More often, avian pox strains are pathogenic for several species (for example, Tripathy et al. 2000).

Karstad (1971) argued that strains adapted to various avian hosts were not different enough to consider them valid poxvirus species because their basic virus characteristics appeared to be identical. Utilizing recent increases in the sophistication of molecular research, Francki et al. (1991) listed fowlpox, turkeypox, canarypox, pigeonpox, quailpox, sparrowpox, starlingpox, juncopox, and psittine poxviruses as valid species. To this species list, Tripathy (1993) added peacockpox, penguinpox, mynahpox, and albatrosspox viruses. Even with this extensive list of avian pox species, the majority of our information on this disease is the result of studies that have come from research on fowlpox in domestic poultry, principally chickens (*Gallus gallus*).

EPIZOOTIOLOGY

There are a number of biotic and abiotic factors that affect the distribution and prevalence of avian pox. Weather (for example, temperature, moisture) conditions (van Riper et al. 2002), vector numbers (Akey et al. 1981), host densities (Forrester and Spalding 2003), and numbers of poxviruses that are present all interact in a synergistic fashion to mold the epizootiological framework of avian pox distribution among bird species and their populations. These four factors also determine in a large part the character and primary causes of an avian pox outbreak. The most important factors influencing avian pox epizootiology are host density, host susceptibility, and numbers of vectors that occur within a certain space and time of the environment (Forrester 1991; van Riper et al. 2002).

Avian pox can occur at any time of the year in wild birds. In temperate regions, where vectors are not active during the winter period, infections occur primarily in the summer (Arnall and Keymer 1975) and early fall (Tripathy 1993). In warmer regions of the world, avian pox is reported throughout the entire year, but most often during fall and winter months. It is at this time that host densities are highest because young-of-the-year are present, complemented by the post breeding flocking behavior of many bird species (van Tyne and Berger 1976; Pettingill 1985). In addition, those vectors that are specific to poxvirus transmission are usually most abundant during the fall and early winter period (Akey et al. 1981; LaPointe 2000). For example, McClure (1989) reported avian pox throughout the year in a population of House Finches from California, but highest prevalence was during the fall and winter. Forrester (1991) found fall peaks of infection in Wild Turkeys from Florida that occurred subsequently to peak mosquito activities (Figure 6.3). In Hawaii, van Riper et al. (2002) found fall and early winter peak infections. In temperate regions of North America, during the fall and early winter the cutaneous form of avian pox is most common, whereas late in the winter the diphtheritic form predominates (Cunningham 1972).

Poxviruses can be transmitted in a number of different ways. Even though they are unable to penetrate unbroken skin, small abrasions are sufficient to permit

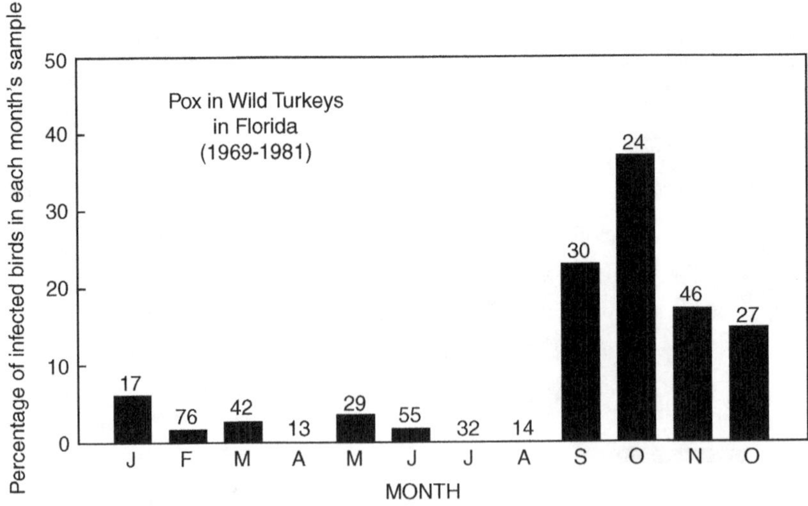

Figure 6.3. Seasonal occurrence of avian pox in Wild Turkeys from 12 counties in Florida, 1969–1981. The numbers on top of each bar indicate sample size. (From Forrester [1991] and reprinted with permission of Bulletin of the Society of Vector Ecology.)

infection. The most common method of transmission is by means of biting insects such as mosquitoes, mites, midges, and/or flies. At the time of year when vectors are at the highest numbers, avian pox transmission is greatest (Akey et al. 1981; Forrester 1991). Many biting insects have been shown to be mechanical vectors only, transferring virus from infected to susceptible birds by contamination of their skin-piercing mouthparts (Locke et al. 1965; Shirinov et al. 1972; Akey et al. 1981; Sileo et al. 1990). Transmission can also occur directly by contact between infected and susceptible birds or by contact with contaminated objects, such as bird-feeder perches (Bleitz 1958; Rosen 1959). Aerosol transmission, although rare, can occur from viruses being carried along with dust, particularly in confined situations (that is, aviaries). Burnet (in Kirmse 1967a) found that lesions developed at sites of minor experimental skin injury in birds inoculated intravenously.

Susceptibility of the avian host species is a large factor in the epizootiology of avian pox. In continental regions, where avian pox and its hosts have had a long co-evolutionary history, the most commonly reported (modal) avian pox prevalence of lesions on wild birds is quite low and varies between 0.5 and 1.5%. In more susceptible avian hosts, avian pox prevalence can reach 25% (for example, House Finches in California–[McClure 1989]) and in some populations up to 50% of the birds are supporting active lesions (for example, Northern Bobwhites [*Colinus virginianus*] in Georgia and Florida; Davidson et al. 1980). Overall, on remote islands avian pox prevalences tend to be generally higher (for example, Galapagos 28% [Vargas 1987]; Volcano, Hawaii 35% [van Riper et al. 2002]; Kona, Hawaii 10% [Atkinson et al. 2005]; New Zealand >10% [Westerkof 1953]). A recent paper by Medina et al. (2004) identified the first avian pox case in the Canary Islands, and this could well be the beginning of an epizootic for birds of that island (Smits et al. 2005).

CLINICAL SIGNS

Avian pox occurs primarily in two different forms: (1) the more common skin form, in which discrete, wart-like, proliferative lesions develop on the skin (Figures 6.4 and 6.5); and (2) the less common diphtheritic form in which moist, necrotic lesions develop on the mucous membranes of the mouth and upper respiratory tract (Figure 6.6). A third form, systemic infection, is rarely found in wild birds (Tripathy and Reed 2003). Lesions are most common on the unfeathered parts of the body—the legs, feet, eyelids, base of the beak, and the comb and wattles of gallinaceous birds. For example, in Hawaii, van Riper et al. (2002) demonstrated that most lesions in wild birds occur on one toe, with half that number on two toes and the leg. Often the lesions are few in number, appearing as innocuous warty growths on one or two toes, at the base of the bill, or on an eyelid. However, a preponderance of lesions on the eyelids may cause mortality, as has been reported in granivorous birds, such as pheasants, quail, and turkeys that have become unable to see and cannot find food (for example, Forrester and Spalding 2003).

In wild birds that have webbed feet, pox lesions appear along the ramifications of blood vessels in the foot webs, much like the distribution of leaves on branches of a tree. Focal epithelial proliferation and later necrosis and sloughing occur mainly on the plantar surfaces of the webs and toes. When fully developed, these lesions appear as circular pocks, 3 to 5 mm in diameter, with central areas of necrosis, bordered by zones of erythema. In perching wild birds, lesions start as a swelling on the toe, leg, or facial region. The swelling appears

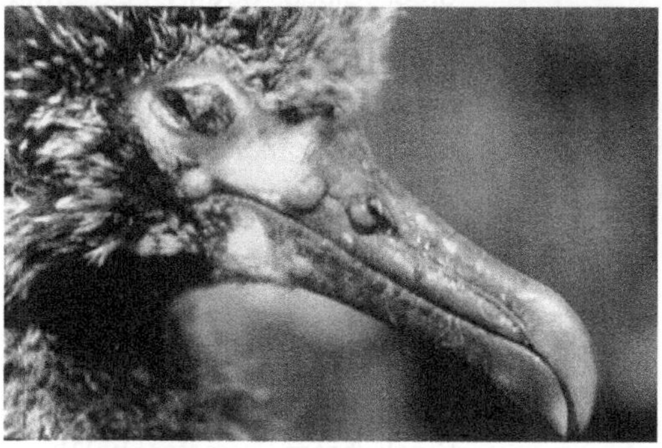

Figure 6.4. Facial avian pox lesions on a young Laysan Albatross (*Diomedea immutabilis*). (From Friend and Franson [1999] with permission of the U.S. Geological Survey.)

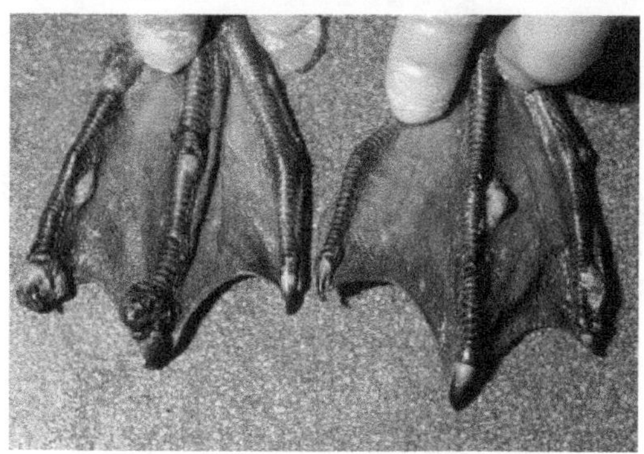

Figure 6.5. Avian pox lesions on the feet of a young Laysan Albatross (*Diomedea immutabilis*). (From Friend and Franson [1999] with permission of the U.S. Geological Survey.)

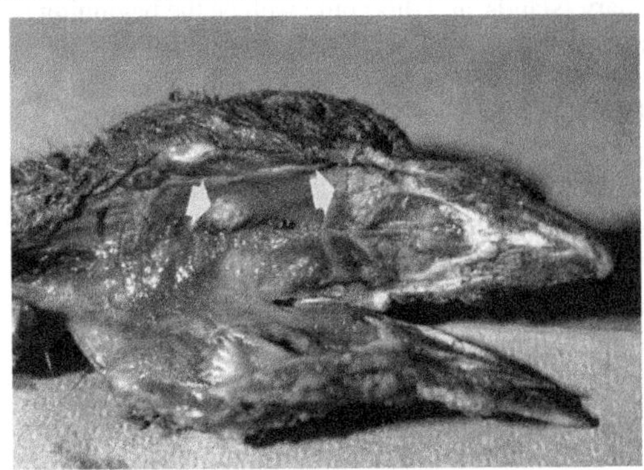

Figure 6.6. Diphtheritic avian pox lesions (arrows) in the oral cavity of a Wild Turkey (*Meleagris gallopavo*). The bird was from Hendry County, Florida and died in 1991. (From Forrester and Spalding [2003], with photo courtesy of Garry W. Foster and permission from the University Press of Florida.)

smooth, reddish, and dome shaped. Eventually the swelling cracks or bursts and lesions begin to form.

Avian pox lesions heal, following degeneration and sloughing of the abnormally proliferated epithelium. In some instances, toes and whole feet can be lost (van Riper et al. 2002). Following infection with avian poxvirus, many birds recover, but young birds are usually more severely affected than are adults. Individual birds that acquire avian pox infections lose digits and can also become permanently blinded. For example, Forrester (1991) followed the development of cutaneous lesions on a sentinel domestic turkey in Florida (Figure 6.7A–D). On day six post-exposure, small areas of swelling were present; by day eight, small lesions had appeared; by day 15, the lesions had grown considerably by day 29, lesions began to cover the eye; and after 50 days the turkey was blind. When birds are blinded in the wild, emaciation follows and birds quickly succumb because of the inability to procure food or due to predation (for example, Jenkins et al. 1989; Forrester and Spalding 2003).

In some advanced cases, lesions are present on both mucous membranes and skin. Lesions of the mucous membranes, particularly of the mouth and upper air passages, most often result in high mortality (Davidson et al. 1980). In chickens that had the diphtheritic form of pox, mortality rates were higher than in birds with cutaneous pox (Cunningham 1972). In canaries, acute systemic infections are commonly associated with many deaths (Stroud 1933; Arnall and Keymer 1975). In the wild, birds are rarely found alive with advanced avian pox infections because they usually die or are preyed upon prior to reaching this level of intensity.

PATHOGENESIS

Upon successful entry of the poxvirus into avian host epithelium, within one hour the virus penetrates cell

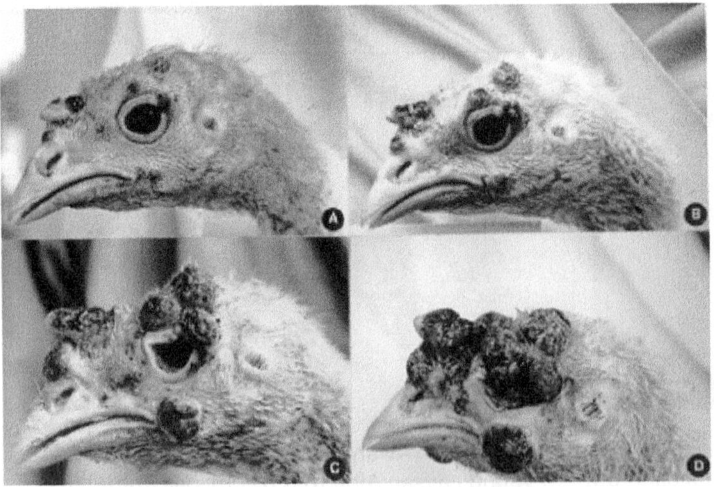

Figure 6.7. Development of cutaneous avian pox lesions on the head of a sentinel domestic turkey that had been infected naturally by vectors at Fisheating Creek (Glades County, FL) during September 1978. After being exposed as a sentinel for two weeks, the turkey was kept in an isolation room at the University of Florida, Gainesville, and observed for the development of lesions. The photographs were taken at eight days (A), 11 days (B), 15 days (C), and 29 days (D) after the bird was removed from the sentinel cage at Fisheating Creek. (From Forrester [1991]; photographs courtesy of Garry W. Foster and by permission of *Bulletin of the Society of Vector Ecology*.)

membranes and then uncoats prior to synthesis of a new virus from precursor material (Arhelger et al. 1962). In the host dermal epithelium, biosynthesis involves two distinct phases, the first being host response during the first 72 hours, followed by synthesis of infectious virus from 72 to 96 hours (Cheever et al. 1968). Beginning at 36 to 48 hours, synthesis of host DNA is accompanied by epithelial hyperplasia, with host DNA declining abruptly at 60 hours. Arhelger and Randall (1964) and Tajima and Ushijima (1966) demonstrated that the replication of viral DNA in the avian host begins between 12 to 24 hours, followed by an exponential rate of synthesis between 60 to 72 hours. Hyperplasia ends at 72 hours with a 2.5-fold increase in cell numbers (Cunningham 1972). The ratio of viral to host DNA increases up to 2:1 at 100 hours, with the maximum titer of virus attained following cell proliferation. There is also, during morphogenesis of the virus, incomplete, intermediate, or developmental forms in transition stages, leading to mature forms or virions.

The next phase consists of a relatively long latent period, with areas of viroplasm within the cytoplasm surrounded by incomplete membranes. The viroplasmic particles condense and acquire an additional outer membrane to become incomplete virions. These virions migrate to vacuoles of the inclusion bodies and thus acquire a membrane coat (Cheville 1966). The virus then emerges from the cells by a budding process, resulting in an additional outer membrane that is obtained from the cell membrane (Arheleger and Randall 1964; Kreuder et al. 1999; Hernandez et al. 2001). This process produces the classical inclusion body (Bollinger body) that is observable via light microscopy. Cunningham (1966) argued that the Bollinger body is not always a structure indispensable for the development and maturation of avian pox in wild birds and that infectious virus may be produced by cells in which matrix inclusion bodies only are present.

Following entry into an avian host, the overall initial incubation period described above varies with the poxvirus strain and host species. Tripathy and Reed (2003) suggested a period from four to 10 days in chickens, turkeys, and pigeons, and Kirmse (1969) found in wild birds incubation periods up to one month. Duration of the disease is equally variable, with avian pox in chickens persisting for about four weeks. Many studies of avian pox in wild birds show a long incubation period duration, with up to several months in Chipping Sparrows *(Spizella passerina)* (Musselman 1928), 82 days in a Mourning Dove *(Zenaida macroura)* (Kossack and Hanson 1954), more than 81 days in a Dark-eyed Junco (*Junco hyemalis*), 13 months in a Northern Flicker (Kirmse 1969), more than 109 days in a Dark-eyed Junco (Hood, pers. com. as cited in Karstad 1971), and 90 to 150 days in the House Finch (McClure 1989).

In chickens, cutaneous lesions become inflamed and hemorrhagic just prior to regression (Cunningham 1966). Desiccation and scab formation then follows, with eventual sloughing and replacement by normal skin. This same pattern occurs in wild birds, but cutaneous lesions may be few, sometimes only one or two, and the whole process of development, regression, and healing of lesions may be much prolonged (Karstad 1971). Perhaps the fewer number of lesions in wild birds occurs because of a high natural resistance to infection, combined with minimal host response. Whatever the reasons, it is obvious that a rather good host-parasite relationship exists in such infections and that it is beneficial to survival of the virus for it to be carried for a long period of time by an individual host.

PATHOLOGY

Avian pox infections cause localized proliferations of epithelial cells. Affected cells become hyperplastic and hypertrophic as the increased rate of multiplication occurs in the basal germinal layer of cells within the epithelium. Hypertrophy and large granular acidophilic intracytoplasmic inclusions appear as the cells mature in layers of epithelium above the stratum germinativum (Figure 6.8). The "stacking" of infected epithelial cells to form "pocks" occurs at variable rates, and lesions may persist for different lengths of time in various species (Karstad 1971).

Diphtheritic lesions are infrequently detected in wild bird avian pox infections. Cunningham (1972) described lesions on the mucous membranes of chickens as white, opaque, slightly elevated nodules that rapidly increase in size, often coalescing to form a yellowish, cheesy, necrotic material that has the appearance of a pseudomembrane. He said that the condition is aggravated by invasion of contaminating bacteria and that it may extend to involve the sinuses and pharynx, causing respiratory distress. Wobeser (1997) cites only one known case in waterfowl. In a compilation of physical locations where avian pox has been found on birds throughout the world, we found 25 reports of diphtheritic lesions (Table 6.2). This information is based on the references cited by Kirmse (1967a), Bolte et al. (1999), and subsequent published reports.

In the later stages of development, large persistent avian pox lesions may be subject to trauma, resulting in hemorrhage, necrosis, and portals of entry for bacteria and fungi. This was the case with a juvenile Reddish Egret (*Egretta rufescens*) that Conti et al. (1986) and Forrester and Spalding (2003) found in

A
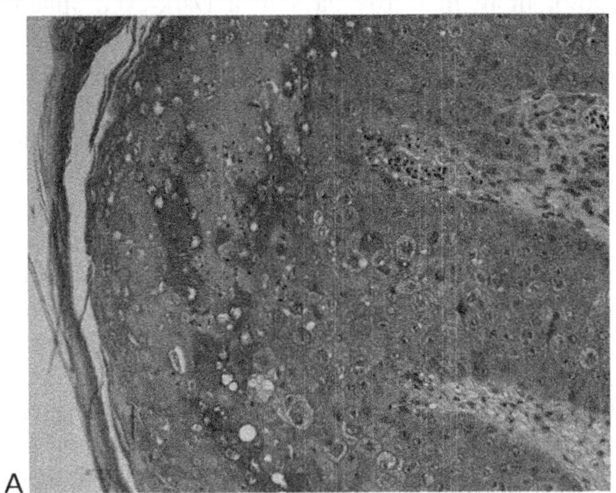

B
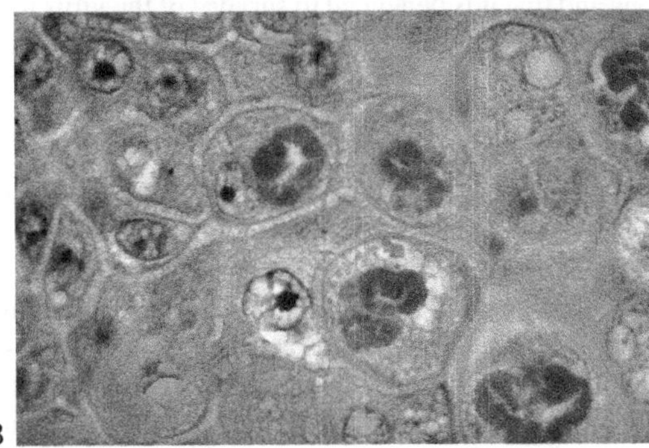

Figure 6.8. (a) Histologic section of avian poxvirus infection of skin from the toe region of a naturally infected domestic chicken (*Gallus gallus*) collected in Volcano Village, Island of Hawaii. Note the marked epithelial hyperplasia and intracytoplasmic inclusion bodies. H&E stain X 100x. (b) High magnification view of the same lesion showing the ballooning of epithelial cells and the large "Bollinger bodies" in the cytoplasm. 1000x.

Florida. Locke et al. (1965) described mortality in Red-tailed Tropicbirds *(Phaethon rubricauda)* in which avian pox was complicated by secondary mycotic infections. Histologic sections of cutaneous avian pox lesions usually reveal areas of necrosis on or near the surface, in which masses of bacteria or fungi are found. There are usually no obvious systemic effects of these secondary bacterial or mycotic infections.

Secondary infections with bacteria and fungi often occur in wild birds following inflammation of the epithelial cells by the poxvirus. These infections have nothing specific about them, occurring as they would in any skin surface where abrasion and contamination occur (Karstad 1971). Elevated avian pox lesions predispose the skin surfaces to trauma. Bird-banders often find that birds with avian pox lesions become entangled in mist nets in such a way that the warty lesions are injured and bleed (Bleitz 1958). However, in most bird species avian poxvirus infections are mild and self-limiting (Simpson et al. 1975), and the lesions slough off without subsequent secondary bacterial and fungal infections.

The lesions of avian pox in canaries and other more susceptible birds (for example, Hawaiian honeycreepers) are sometimes quite different. Lesions frequently seen are fibrinous inflammation of serous membranes; liver degeneration or necrosis also occurs, with edema and hyperemia of the lungs, and fibrinous pneumonitis often results (van Riper et al. 2002). Such lesions are seen in canaries with the acute systemic form of the disease. In other cases, cutaneous lesions or diphtheritic lesions may predominate. Canaries and honeycreepers may have cutaneous lesions on not only exposed skin areas but also the feathered portions of the body (van Riper and van Riper 1985).

Goodpasture and Anderson (1962) described strains of avian pox isolated from the Dark-eyed Junco and from a Wood Thrush (*Hylocichla mustelina*) that were characterized by the development of intranuclear as well as intracytoplasmic inclusions. Both types of inclusions occurred in the original junco host as well as in chickens infected with the junco strain. In avian pox–infected Dark-eyed Juncos, Karstad (1971) found that one of four had intranuclear as well as typical intracytoplasmic inclusions. He also found typical avian pox intranuclear and intracytoplasmic inclusions in hypertrophied epithelial cells in a cutaneous lesion from a Northern Mockingbird *(Mimus polyglottos)*. Furthermore, one of six Northern Flickers with cutaneous avian pox lesions had small, eosinophilic, rod-shaped inclusions in the nuclei of cells that also contained typical Bollinger bodies. Histologic examination of an avian pox lesion from a Savannah Sparrow *(Passerculus sandwichensis)* revealed rod- or brick-shaped inclusions in the cytoplasm of hypertrophic epithelial cells that bore typical Bollinger bodies. In the Imperial Eagle (*Aquila heliaca*), Hernandez et al. (2001) demonstrated more typical inclusion bodies (Figure 6.2).

DIAGNOSIS

The visual observation of lesions on a wild bird does not represent a definitive diagnosis of avian pox infection. In the past, many authors have assumed that because they observed pox-like skin lesions on birds, they were dealing with avian pox (for example, Power and Human 1976). There are a number of avian

Table 6.2. Locations of avian pox lesions found on selected wild bird hosts. This table provides a snapshot of pox intensity by physical location on the bird. By examining the table, one can obtain a general index of where one might expect to find lesions at different physical locations on a sample of infected birds.

	Lesion Location		
ORDER	Feet & Legs	Face & Head	Diphtheritic (Oral cavity)
Struthioniformes	3	1	1
Tinamiformes	–	–	–
Sphenisciformes	1	0	0
Gaviiformes	–	–	–
Podicipediformes	1	0	0
Procellariiformes	2	1	0
Pelecaniformes	2	1	1
Ciconiiformes	2	1	0
Phoenicopteriformes	1	1	0
Anseriformes	28	4	5
Falconiformes	26	6	1
Galliformes	53	11	5
Opisthocomiformes	–	–	–
Gruiformes	2	2	0
Charadriiformes	4	2	0
Pterocliformes	–	–	–
Columbiformes	13	4	2
Psittaciformes	11	1	7
Cuculiformes	1	0	0
Strigiformes	4	3	1
Caprimulgiformes	–	–	–
Apodiformes	2	1	0
Coliiformes	–	–	–
Trogoniformes	–	–	–
Coraciiformes	1	0	0
Piciformes	2	1	0
Passeriformes	217	9	2
TOTAL	377	49	25

diseases that have similar lesions to those of poxvirus infections. Mites and bacteria will sometimes cause lesions on the legs that look very similar to avian pox lesions. Candidiasis, capillariasis, and trichomoniasis all cause lesions in the oral cavity that look similar to the diphtheritic form of avian pox.

Whenever possible, isolation via the propagation of virus on chorioallantoic membranes of chicken embryos should be used as the definitive diagnosis of choice (Hansen 1987). Some strains of avian poxvirus in wild birds do not grow readily in chicken embryos. Krone et al. (2004) were unable to culture poxviruses from a Peregrine Falcon (*Falco peregrinus*) on chicken egg CAM, so they attempted culture in Peregrine Falcon eggs, and van Riper et al. (2002) cultured the Hawaiian avian poxvirus from Hawaii Amakihi (*Hemignathus virens*), Apapane (*Himatione sanguinea*), Laysan Finch (*Telespiza cantans*), and Iiwi (*Vestiaria coccinea*) in House Finch eggs.

At a minimum, for a positive demonstration of an avian pox infection there needs to be at least a histological examination of infected tissue that shows *avian poxvirus* intracytoplasmic inclusion (Bollinger) bodies (Kirmse 1966). Demonstration of typical avian poxvirus particles by electron microscopy would also provide a positive confirmation of an avian pox infection (Figure 6.2). Beaver and Cheatham (1963) studied the cytopathology of a Dark-eyed Junco poxvirus strain by electron microscopy, and the nuclear inclusion was seen to be devoid of viral particles, being composed of a loose array of irregularly branching filaments. In an avian pox outbreak in the Peregrine Falcon in Germany, Krone et al. (2004) found much the same pattern after negative staining on an electron micrograph.

Recent advances in molecular techniques now provide an opportunity for a more detailed and rapid diagnosis of avian pox infections. These techniques have been discussed by Tripathy (2000) and Tripathy and Reed (2003) and include restriction fragment length polymorphism (RFLP) analysis, use of genomic fragments as probes, and polymerase chain reaction (PCR) tests.

IMMUNITY

Birds that have recovered from avian pox infections, or that have been vaccinated, are usually immune to reinfection with that virus strain. This immunity is largely cell mediated, although antibodies can play a role (Fenner 1968). Transovarial transmission of immunity for avian pox has not been demonstrated. Strains isolated from a single host species may vary in the degree of infectivity to other species. For example, a strain of canarypox has been found that can infect chickens, quail (*Coturnix* sp.) and turkeys, but not House Sparrows (*Passer domesticus*) and Rock Doves (*Columba livia*); another canarypox strain infected chickens, Rock Doves, and House Sparrows (Karstad 1971). Irons (1934) found a strain of avian pox from the Rock Dove that produced lesions in the House Sparrow after a series of blind passages. Dobson (1937) described a poxvirus strain isolated from Ring-necked Pheasants (*Phasianus colchicus*) that was transmissible to chickens and Rock Doves. Many of the poxviruses of wild birds are not pathogenic for chickens (for example, Tripathy et al. 2000).

Avian poxvirus strains from one host can provide reciprocal immunity to other host species, and cross-immunity has been proven for several strains of avian pox. For example, chickens may be vaccinated with live pigeonpox strains because they stimulate immunity to typical strains of avian poxviruses without causing serious disease (Cunningham 1972). Dobson (1937) demonstrated that Rock Dove poxvirus immunized birds against a pheasant strain. DuBose (1965) reported reciprocal immunization between strains of poxvirus from the Sage Grouse *(Centrocercus urophasianus)* and a strain isolated from the Blue Grouse *(Dendragapus obscurus)*. It seems probable that immunity to avian pox exists in a spectrum of continuous adaptation to various avian host species.

PUBLIC HEALTH CONCERNS

It has not yet been demonstrated that avian poxviruses are transmissible to humans, as are some of the mammalian strains such as cow and sheep poxviruses (Robinson and Kerr 2001).

DOMESTIC ANIMAL HEALTH CONCERNS

Due to the host specificity demonstrated by most avian poxviruses (see the "Etiology" and "Immunity" sections in this chapter), wild birds are presently not considered a significant reservoir of the virus for domestic animals. Kirmse (1966) attempted to infect chickens with strains of poxvirus from the Northern Flicker, Dark-eyed Junco, Song Sparrow *(Melospiza melodia)*, and domestic canary. Only the Song Sparrow strain produced lesions in chickens. Conversely, three poultry strains were pathogenic for chickens but not for several species of wild birds, including the Red-winged Blackbird *(Agelaius phoeniceus)*, European Starling *(Sturnus vulgaris)*, Northern Oriole *(Icterus galbula)*, Gray Catbird *(Dumetella carolinensis)*, Song Sparrow, House Sparrow, White-throated Sparrow *(Zonotrichia albicollis)*, American Robin *(Turdus migratorius)*, Evening Grosbeak (*Coccothraustes vespertinus)*, Indigo Bunting *(Passerina cyanea)*, American Goldfinch *(Spinus tristis)*, Brown Thrasher *(Toxostoma rufum)*, Eastern Kingbird *(Tyrannus tyrannus)*, and Common Grackle *(Quiscalus quiscula)*. These results may be taken as evidence of host specificity and suggest that pox infections in migratory birds do not presently constitute a threat to the domestic poultry industry.

There is recent evidence that anthropogenic movement of birds can cause avian pox problems for wild as well as captive bird populations. Krone et al. (2004) demonstrated avian pox mortality in Peregrine Falcons that were pen-reared and released in northern Germany. In the Arabian Gulf region, Remple (1988) found that avian pox is common in many of the captive falcons that are used for falconry. In captive parrots, avian pox has become a concern around the world (Petrak 1982; Hitchner and Clubb 1980). In the United States, poxvirus infections are among the more significant health risks associated with releasing pen-reared or game-farm birds such as Wild Turkeys and Northern Bobwhites into the wild for hunting purposes (Davidson et al. 1982; Davidson and Wentworth 1992). Such releases should be discouraged or prohibited, but if they are allowed to occur, only healthy pen-reared birds should be used (Forrester and Spalding 2003).

WILDLIFE POPULATION IMPACTS

Little is known about mortality rates from poxvirus infection in naturally infected, free-flying wild birds. The majority of wild-bird avian pox infections have been reported as mild and self-limiting. In pheasants, quail, and Wild Turkeys, mortality rates are probably similar to chickens with regard to the severity and course of avian pox infections. Davidson et al. (1980) estimated that during an epornitic of avian pox in Northern Bobwhites, morbidity was approximately 2% and mortality varied between 0.6 and 1.2% in a 13,000-km^2 region of Georgia and Florida. During a survey from 1968 through 1984 of 1,052 Wild Turkeys in southern Florida, Forrester and Spalding (2003) reported 15 cases of avian pox. Dobson (1937) reported extensive losses in Ring-necked Pheasants affected by the diphtheritic form of avian pox. Karstad (1965) documented that eyelid lesions prevented feeding and were responsible for extensive losses among captive Impiyan Pheasants (now called Himalyan Monal [*Lophophorus impejanus*]). The outbreak occurred in the fall and subsided after frosts had reduced mosquito populations.

Extremely high mortality rates have been recorded in some epizootics. Gallagher (1916) reported 85% mortality in quail (of unstated species) imported from Mexico, where lesions were present on the unfeathered skin and in the mouth. In the Galapagos Mockingbird (*Nesomimus parvulus*), Vargus (1987) found 13 of 18 healthy fledglings after two months but failed to find any of the 14 young birds that previously had been observed with avian pox lesions. With avian pox now introduced into the Canary Islands (Medina et al. 2004), there exists the potential for transmission to native birds and future epizootics (for example, Smits et al. 2005).

Avian pox infections in Hawaii have been demonstrated to have negative effects on many populations of native birds (van Riper and Scott 2001). Warner (1968) demonstrated extensive poxlike lesions on Laysan Finches that he had brought from Laysan Island to the island of Oahu. Jenkins et al. (1989) reported that avian poxvirus had a negative impact on the few remaining Hawaiian Crows (*Corvus hawaiiensis*) that inhabit the island of Hawaii. In the Elepaio (*Chasiempis sandwichensis*) on Hawaii, VanderWerf (2001) demonstrated a population decline on Mauna Kea Volcano in the year following an epizootic of poxlike lesions. In a larger-scale study, van Riper et al. (2002) recorded high avian pox prevalences (up to 47%) in native birds that inhabit the mid-elevational forests of Mauna Loa, Hawaii. They demonstrated that where vectors and native birds (Hawaiian honeycreepers) had their greatest overlap, avian pox had the greatest negative influence on forest bird populations (Figure 6.9). In controlled laboratory experiments, the authors also demonstrated that avian poxvirus will kill some species of native birds (for example, Hawaii Amakihi), but is mild and self-limiting in the introduced bird species such as the House Finch. Atkinson et al. (2005) found a similar situation in the Hawaii Amakihi in other forests on Mauna Loa, Hawaii.

Avian pox in captive situations (especially canaries) may be associated with extensive losses (Bigland et. al. 1962). Transmission is facilitated by housing large numbers of birds in close quarters. In such situations, transmission may occur by direct and indirect contact, or by inhalation of virus-laden dust. Poxviruses are very resistant to inactivation by drying and, therefore, dust that contains contaminated particles of feathers, skin, or scabs may be highly infective. Under conditions of aerosol exposure, canaries may die with rather acute, apparently generalized systemic infections.

TREATMENT AND CONTROL

For outbreaks in which avian poxvirus is being transmitted by vectors, control should be targeted at reduction of those vector populations. For example, adult mosquitoes can be directly targeted for reduction or, as is most often the case, breeding areas can be manipulated either through direct reduction of larvae or via indirect reduction through biocontrol agents (Service 1976). Control can also be achieved by preventing vector access to birds (for example, by screening) in the case of captive birds. Where birds are being artificially concentrated, such as at home feeders or in aviaries, feeders and perches should be sterilized at least every two weeks (Bleitz 1958). Any strong antiseptic cleaning agent can be used, including bleach. In holding areas or aviaries, diseased birds should be kept in separate, isolated, screened cages.

On occasion, it may be useful to try vaccination where avian pox occurs in captive wild birds. Ideally, one should select for vaccination an avian poxvirus strain that causes a mild infection that would be limited to the skin at the site of vaccine application. Vaccination such as this may prove practical in certain situations, such as with endangered species (see Tripathy et al. 2000). For additional vaccination techniques and information, see Cunningham (1972). If avian pox infections are dust borne, as may occur in some aviaries and outdoor pens, control of dust will be an important factor.

For captive birds that do become infected, Arnall and Keymer (1975) have found success by applying flowers of sulfur directly to the lesion or giving it orally. Removal of the lesions and washing in bicarbonate soda may prove useful, but caution needs to be taken not to further spread the virus. Applying silver

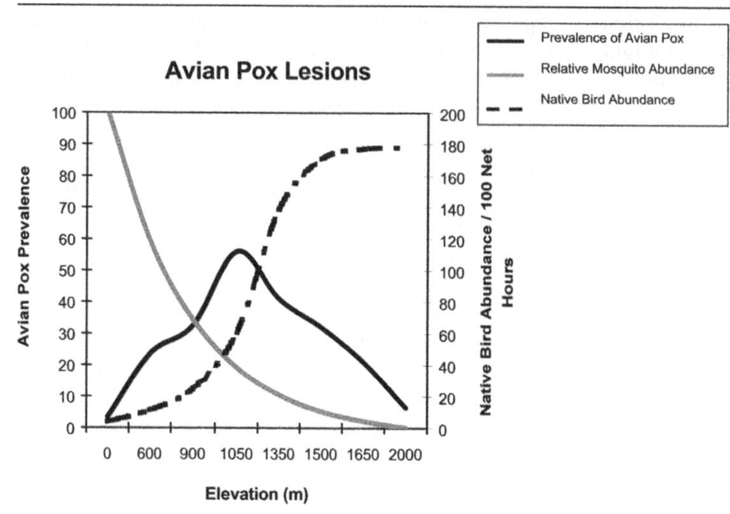

Figure 6.9. Avian pox prevalence compared to relative mosquito and native bird abundances on Mauna Loa Volcano, Hawaii. Values for the solid black line were derived from avian pox prevalence of 3,122 wild forest birds captured from 1977–1980 along a sea-level-to-tree-line elevational gradient on Mauna Loa Volcano, Hawaii. The gray line indicates relative mosquito abundance, whereas the broken line denotes native bird abundances along the elevational gradient.

nitrate, iodine, or 1–2% saline solution directly to the lesion has also shown some success in reducing the level of infection. All techniques are targeted at sterilizing around the lesion, and this is why bathing the infected area seems to help. In fact, broad-spectrum antibiotics are routinely given to birds with avian pox in an attempt to reduce the chance of secondary bacterial infection.

No matter what treatment is used, the disease will run its course. In most situations, prevention is the best treatment against avian pox infection. Keeping areas clean and disinfected is important. Any reduction in potential vector numbers will also help. In highly susceptible avian species, many individuals will probably succumb to infection (for example, Landolt and Kocan 1976). In the more resistant species, immunity quickly develops and the infection is usually gone within a short time period, with minimal damage to the bird.

MANAGEMENT IMPLICATIONS

For the majority of wild bird populations, avian pox appears to be a self-limiting disease. However, in localities where conditions are propitious for transmission (for example, an extremely heavy rainfall year), avian pox prevalences can reach high levels and negatively impact wild bird populations. For example, following an extremely wet year in southern Georgia and northern Florida, Davidson et al. (1980) reported a 12-fold avian pox increase in Northern Bobwhites. The authors estimated that this increase in avian pox infections resulted in an additional 12 to 24 deaths per 1,000 birds. This reduction in total population size had a negative impact on the allowed bag limits for that year. Forrester (1991) postulated that an abnormally early rainy season over a two-year period resulted in a widespread avian pox epizootic, which caused a significant decline in Wild Turkey populations in Florida throughout the 1960s. During these situations it might be wise to reduce the bag limits or shorten the hunting seasons on these game birds.

With the continued increase of bird feeding stations over the world, the concentrated numbers of birds utilizing those feeding stations predisposes them to enhanced transmission of poxviruses. This has been documented by a number of wild bird enthusiasts (for example, Bleitz 1958) and continues to be a problem.

The artificially increased host densities of wild birds at feeding stations is paralleled with what captive breeders are finding in regard to the transmission of avian pox. Donnelly and Crane (1984) described an epornitic of avian pox in a research aviary (Graham 1978; Petrak 1982). The situation becomes even more of a management concern when one is dealing with the captive breeding of endangered species such as Whooping Cranes (*Grus Americana*), Hawaiian honeycreepers, or Bali Mynas (*Leucospar rothschildi*).

Another situation in which land and wildlife managers must be concerned with the implications of avian pox infection is on the more remote islands of the world. For example, in Hawaii, where the native birds have had only a short history of co-evolution with the introduced avian poxvirus, the distribution and numbers of many native species are presently being negatively impacted by this disease (Warner 1968; van Riper et al. 2002; Atkinson et al. 2005). In the Galapagos Islands, Vargas (1987) demonstrated that in some years avian poxvirus greatly impacts the numbers of Galapagos Mockingbird young that survive to adulthood. The first detection of avian pox in the Canary Islands (Medina et al. 2004) should be followed closely by wildlife managers because the native birds on that island are probably very susceptible to *Avipoxvirus avium*. Although islands are indeed unique situations, on islands such as Trinidad that are closer to continents, Tikasingh et al. (1982) suggested that avian pox might not always greatly impact native birds.

In summary, wherever avian pox is a potential concern, monitoring of bird populations would assure early detection of infected birds. Programs such as MAPS (Monitoring Avian Productivity and Survivorship) developed by DeSante (1996) would provide wildlife managers with an early detection of any increase of avian pox lesions in wild bird populations. When infected birds are collected, some sort of standardized necropsy and reporting protocol should be developed, one like that developed by van Riper and van Riper (1980). Another example of a survey and reporting system that could be emulated is the "House Finch Disease Survey" (http://www.birds.cornell.edu/hofi/index.html) initiated by the Cornell Laboratory of Ornithology and described in Dhondt et al. (1998). This Web-based system documents the spread of conjunctivitis in the House Finch and could be easily modified to be used for a survey of avian pox. Following receipt of presence/absence information on lesions, more detailed laboratory analyses (see the "Diagnosis" section of this chapter) can be undertaken. It has been clearly shown that detecting disease in its early stages of spread is the preferred method of wildlife disease management (Friend 1987). After avianpox prevalence becomes high, this disease will "run its course" and has the potential to greatly impact certain wild bird populations.

Table 6.1. Orders, families, and representative species of birds throughout the world recorded with avian pox. Taxonomy of avian orders, families and species follows Clements (2000), as does common family and common species names. Representative literature citations are included for each country in which avian pox has been reported. For those avian orders and families where avian pox has not been reported, lines in the table are blank.

Order	Family	Common Family Name	Species	Common Species Name	Country Reported	References
Struthioniformes	Struthionidae	Ostrich	*Struthio camelus*	Ostrich	Israel	Perelman et al. 1988
			Struthio camelus	Ostrich	South Africa	Allwright et al. 1994
			Struthio camelus	Ostrich	Australia	Raidal et al. 1996
			Struthio camelus	Ostrich	Italy	Cerrone et al. 1999
	Rheidae	Rheas	*Rhea americana*	Greater Rhea	Spain	Vogelsang 1938
	Casuariidae	Cassowaries				
	Dromaiidae	Emu				
	Apterygidae	Kiwis				
Tinamiformes	Tinamidae	Tinamous				
Sphenisciformes	Spheniscidae	Penguins	*Spheniscus humboldti*	Humboldt Penguin	Poland	Landowska-Plazewska and Plazewski 1968
			Spheniscus demersus	Jackass Penguin	Cape Town, South Africa	Stannard et al. 1998
Gaviiformes	Gaviidae	Loons				
Podicipediformes	Podicipedidae	Grebes	*Podiceps cristatus*	Great Crested Grebe	Switzerland	Bouvier 1946
Procellariiformes	Diomedeidae	Albatrosses	*Phoebastria immutabilis*	Laysan Albatross	Midway Atoll, Pacific Ocean	Sileo et al. 1990
	Procellariidae	Shearwaters & Petrels	*Puffinus puffinus*	Manx Shearwater	Great Britain	Miles and Stocker, 1948; Nuttall et al. 1985
	Hydrobatidae	Storm-Petrels				
	Pelecanoididae	Diving-Petrels				
Pelecaniformes	Phaethontidae	Tropicbirds	*Phaethon lepturus*	White-tailed Tropicbird	Bermuda	Wingate et al. 1980
			Phaethon rubricauda	Red-tailed Tropicbird	Hawaii, U.S.A.	Locke et al. 1965
	Pelecanidae	Pelicans				

(*Continued*)

Table 6.1. (Continued)

Order	Family	Common Family Name	Species	Common Species Name	Country Reported	References
	Sulidae	Boobies & Gannets				
	Phalacrocoracidae	Cormorants	*Phalacrocorax bougainvillii*	Guanay Cormorant	Peru	Avila 1966
	Anhingidae	Anhinga & Darters				
	Fregatidae	Frigatebirds				
Ciconiiformes	Ardeidae	Herons, Egrets & Bitterns	*Ardea herodias*	Great Blue Heron	Florida, U.S.A.	Forrester and Spalding 2003
			Ardea alba	Great Egret	Florida, U.S.A.	Forrester and Spalding 2003
			Egretta rufescens	Reddish Egret	Florida, U.S.A.	Forrester and Spalding 2003
			Egretta thula	Snowy Egret	Florida, U.S.A.	Forrester and Spalding 2003
	Scopidae	Hamerkop				
	Ciconiidae	Storks	*Ciconia ciconia*	White Stork	Switzerland	Zangger and Muller 1990
			Ciconia nigra	Black Stork	Switzerland	Zangger and Muller 1990
	Balaenicipididae	Shoebill				
	Threskiornithidae	Ibis & Spoonbills	*Ajaia ajaja*	Roseate Spoonbill	Florida, U.S.A.	Spalding and Forrester 1991
Phoenicopteriformes	Phoenicopteridae	Flamingos	*Phoenicopterus chilensis*	Chilean Flamingo	—	Arai et al. 1991
Anseriformes	Anhimidae	Screamers				
	Anatidae	Ducks,	*Anser anser*	Greylag Goose	Germany	Ihlenburg 1972
		Geese & Swans	*Anser anser*	Greylag Goose	China	Zhang et al. 1996
			Anser cygnoides	Swan Goose	Germany	Ihlenburg 1972
			Anser cygnoides	Swan Goose	China	Zhang et al. 1996
			Anser fabalis	Bean Goose	Great Britain	Kear and Brown 1975
			Branta sandvincensis	Hawaiian Goose	Great Britain	Kear and Brown 1975
			Branta canadensis	Canada Goose	Canada	Cox 1980

			Cereopsis novaehollandiae	Cape Barren Goose	Australia	Wobeser 1981
			Anser indicus	Bar-headed Goose	China	Zhang et al. 1996
			Cygnus columbianus	Tundra Swan	Maryland, U.S.A.	Montgomery et al. 1980
			Cygnus olor	Mute Swan	New York, U.S.A.	Leibovitz 1969
			Chenopis atrata	Black Swan	Australia	Harrigan et al. 1975
			Anas sp.	Duck	India	Rao 1965
			Anas sp.	Duck	Canada	Kirmse 1967b
			Anas platyrhynchos	Mallard	China	Zhang et al. 1996
			Anas crecca	Green-winged Teal	Alaska, U.S.A.	Morton and Dietrich 1979
			Anas clypeata	Northen Shoveler	India	Mathur et al. 1972
			Anas penolope	European Wigeon	India	Mathur et al. 1972
			Cairina moschata	Muscovy Duck	Germany	Ihlenburg 1972
			Aix galericulata	Mandarin Duck	France	Megnin 1878
			Aix sponosa	Wood Duck	Florida, U.S.A.	Spalding and Forrester 2003
			Nettion crecca	Common Teal	India	Mathur et al. 1972
			Tadorna ferruginea	Ruddy Shelduck	China	Zhang et al. 1996
			Melanitta nigra	Black Scoter	Pennslyvania, U.S.A.	Ratcliff 1967
			Bucephala clangula	Common Goldeneye	Saskatchewan, Canada	Wobeser 1981
			Aythya affinia	Lesser Scaup	Alberta, Canada	Wobeser 1981
Falconiformes	Cathartidae	New World Vultures				
			Cathartes aura	Turkey Vulture	Florida, U.S.A.	Forrester and Spalding 2003
			Vultur gryphus	Andean Condor		Kim et al. 2003
	Pandionidae	Osprey				
	Accipitridae	Hawks, Eagles & Kites				
			Accipiter nisus	Eurasian Sparrowhawk	Iraq	Tantawi et al. 1981
			Accipiter gentilis	Northern Goshawk	Germany	Polowinkin 1901
			Accipiter gentilis	Northern Goshawk	France	Heusinger 1844

(*Continued*)

Table 6.1. (Continued)

Order	Family	Common Family Name	Species	Common Species Name	Country Reported	References
			Aquila chrysaetos	Golden Eagle	Germany	Gratzl 1953
			Aquila chrysaetos	Golden Eagle	Canada	Moffatt 1972
			Aquila chrysaetos	Golden Eagle	California, . U.S.A	Hill and Bogue 1977
			Aquila chrysaetos	Golden Eagle	Washington, U.S.A.	Garner 1989
			Aquila heliaca	Imperial Eagle	Spain	Hernadez et al. 2001
			Buteo platyptera	Broad-winged Hawk	Canada	Kuntze et al. 1968
			Buteo jamaicensis	Red-tailed Hawk	Missouri, U.S.A.	Halliwell 1972
			Buteo jamaicensis	Red-tailed Hawk	N. Dakota, U.S.A.	Pearson and Pass 1975
			Buteo jamaicensis	Red-tailed Hawk	Washington, U.S.A.	Fitzner et al. 1985
			Buteo jamaicensis	Red-tailed Hawk	California, U.S.A.	Wheeldon et al. 1985
			Buteo lagopus	Rough-legged Hawk	N. Dakota, U.S.A.	Pearson and Pass 1975
			Buteo lagopus	Rough-legged Hawk	California, U.S.A.	Wheeldon et al. 1985
			Buteo buteo	Eurasian Buzzard	Austria	Loupal et al. 1985
			Circus pygargus	Montagu's Harrier	Germany	Englemann 1928
			Circus cyaneus	Northern Harrier	N. Dakota, U.S.A.	Wheeldon et al. 1985
	Sagittariidae	Secretary-bird				
	Falconidae	Falcons & Caracaras	*Falco peregrinus*	Peregrine Falcon	Arabian Gulf	Cooper 1969
			Falco peregrinus	Peregrine Falcon	United Arab Emirates	Kiel 1985
			Falco peregrinus	Peregrine Falcon	Germany	Krone et al. 2004
			Falco rusticolus	Gyrfalcon	United Arab Emirates	Samour and Cooper 1993
			Falco cherrug	Saker Falcon	Arabian Gulf	Greenwood and Blakemore 1973
			Falco cherrug	Saker Falcon	Germany	Grimm and Jacobi 1977

			Falco cherrug	Saker Falcon	Afganistan	Winteroll et al. 1979
			Falco cherrug	Saker Falcon	United Arab Emirates	Kiel 1985
			Falco jugger	Laggar Falcon	Arabian Gulf	Greenwood and Blakemore 1973
			Falco tinnunculus	Eurasian Kestrel	Germany	Kitzing 1980
Galliformes	Megapodiidae	Megapodes				
	Cracidae	Guans, Chachalacas & Allies				
	Meleagridae	Turkeys	*Meleagris gallopavo*	Wild Turkey	France	Heusinger 1844
			Meleagris gallopavo	Wild Turkey	Germany	Bollinger 1877
			Meleagris gallopavo	Wild Turkey	India	Pandey and Mallick 1974
			Meleagris gallopavo	Wild Turkey	Florida, U.S.A.	Akey et al. 1981
			Meleagris gallopavo	Wild Turkey	Georgia, U.S.A.	Wheeldon et al. 1985
			Meleagris gallopavo	Wild Turkey	Malaysia	Ideris and Ibrahim 1986
			Meleagris gallopavo	Wild Turkey	Oregon, U.S.A.	Lutz and Crawford 1987
	Tetraonidae	Grouse	*Tetrastes bonasia*	Common Hazelhen	France	Cruasson 1946
			Dendragapus obscurus	Blue Grouse	Oregon, U.S.A.	Dickenson 1967
			Dendragapus obscurus	Blue Grouse	Canada	Syverton and McTaggert Cowan 1944
			Lagopus mutus	Rock Ptarmigan	Japan	Horiuchi et al. 1965
			Tetrao tetrix	Black Grouse	Denmark	Christiansen 1949
			Bonasa umbellus	Ruffed Grouse	U.S.A.	Bump et al. 1947
			Centrocercus urophasianus	Sage Grouse	Texas, U.S.A.	Dubose 1965
			Tympanuchus cupido	Greater Prairie-Chicken	Virginia, U.S.A.	Dubose 1965
	Odontophoridae	New World Quail	*Callipepla squamata*	Scaled Quail	Texas, U.S.A.	Wilson and Crawford 1988

(*Continued*)

Table 6.1. (Continued)

Order	Family	Common Family Name	Species	Common Species Name	Country Reported	References
			Callipepla gambelii	Gambel's Quail	Arizona, U.S.A.	Blankenship et al. 1966
			Callipepla californica	California Quail	Oregon, U.S.A.	Crawford et al. 1979
			Callipepla californica	California Quail	Hawaii, U.S.A.	Perkins 1903
			Colinus virginianus	Northern Bobwhite	Georgia & S. Carolina, U.S.A.	Stoddard 1931
			Colinus virginianus	Northern Bobwhite	Georgia & Florida, U.S.A.	Davidson et al. 1980
			Colinus virginianus	Northern Bobwhite	Malaysia	Reed and Schrader 1989
	Phasianidae	Pheasants & Partridge				
			Alectoris rufa	Red-legged Partridge	Spain	Buenestado et al. 2004
			Chrysolophus pictus	Golden Pheasant	Germany	Bollinger 1873
			Crossoptilon crossoptilon	White Eared-Pheasant	California, U.S.A.	Ensley et al. 1978
			Crossoptilon crossoptilon	White Eared-Pheasant	China	Hu Hongguan 1982
			Crossoptilon auritum	Blue Eared-Pheasant	California, U.S.A.	Ensley et al. 1978
			Phasianus colchicus	Ring-necked Pheasant	Oregon, U.S.A.	Crawford et al. 1979
			Phasianus colchicus	Ring-necked Pheasant	Hawaii, U.S.A.	Perkins 1903
			Phasianus colchicus	Ring-necked Pheasant	China	Hu Hongguan, 1982; Zhang et al. 1996
			Phasianus colchicus	Ring-necked Pheasant	Iraq	Al-Ani, 1986
			Phasianus colchicus	Ring-necked Pheasant	Texas, U.S.A.	Wilson and Crawford 1988
			Lophura diardi	Siamese Fireback	California, U.S.A.	Ensley et al. 1978

			Gallus gallus	Red Junglefowl	California, U.S.A.	Ensley et al. 1978
			Tragopan satyra	Satry Tragopan	France	Megnin 1878
			Tragopan temminckii	Temminck's Tragopan	China	Hu Hongguan 1982
			Perdix perdix	Gray Partridge	Germany	Stadie 1931
			Perdix perdix	Gray Partridge	Denmark	Christiansen 1949
			Perdix perdix	Gray Partridge	Great Britain	Pomeroy 1962
			Perdix perdix	Gray Partridge	Austria	Loupal et al. 1985
			Perdix perdix	Gray Partridge	Italy	Mani et al. 1990
			Coturnix coturnix	Common Quail	Mexico	Gallagher 1916
			Coturnix coturnix	Common Quail	Italy	Rinaldi et al. 1972
			Coturnix coturnix	Common Quail	China	Zhang et al. 1996
			Lophophorus impejanus	Himalayan Monal	Canada	Karstad 1965
			Lophophorus impejanus	Himalayan Monal	California, U.S.A.	Ensley et al. 1978
			Lophophorus impejanus	Himalayan Monal	Austria	Loupal et al. 1985
			Pavo cristatus	Indian Peafowl	Iraq	Alfalluji et al. 1979
			Pavo cristatus	Indian Peafowl	China	Hu Hongguan 1982
	Numididae	Guineafowl	*Numida meleagris*	Helmeted Guineafowl	Germany	Tietz 1932
Opisthocomiformes	Opisthocomidae	Hoatzin				
Gruiformes	Mesithornithidae	Mesites				
	Turnicidae	Buttonquail				
	Gruidae	Cranes	*Grus grus*	Common Crane	Germany	Zhang et al. 1996
			Grus japonensis	Red-crowned Crane	China	Zhang et al. 1996
			Grus canadensis	Sandhill Crane	Florida, U.S.A.	Simpson et al. 1975; Forrester and Spalding 2003
			Anthropoides virgo	Demoiselle Crane	China	Zhang et al. 1996
	Aramidae	Limpkin				
	Psophiidae	Trumpters				
	Rallidae	Rails, Gallinules & Coots	*Fulica atra*	Eurasian Coot	India	Mathur et al. 1972
	Helionorithidae	Finfoots				
	Rhynochetidae	Kagu				
	Eurypygidae	Sunbittern				
	Cariamidae	Seriemas				
	Otididae	Bustards	*Otis tarda*	Great Bustard	Rumania	Cociu et al. 1972
			Otis tarda	Great Bustard	Germany	Seidel 1972
			Chlamydoitis undulata	Houbara Bustard	United Arab Emirates; Middle East	Samour et al. 1996; Bailey et al. 2002

(Continued)

Table 6.1. (Continued)

Order	Family	Common Family Name	Species	Common Species Name	Country Reported	References
Charadriiformes	Jacanidae	Jacanas				
	Rostratulidae	Painted-Snipes				
	Dromadidae	Crab Plover				
	Haematopodidae	Oystercatchers	*Haematopus ostralegus*	Eurasian Oystercatcher	Great Britain	Green 1969
	Ibidorhynchidae	Ibisbill				
	Recurvirostridae	Avocets & Stilts				
	Burhinidae	Thick-knees				
	Glareolidae	Pratincoles & Coursers				
	Charadriidae	Plovers & Lapwing	*Vanellus vanellus*	Northern Lapwing	Denmark	Christiansen 1949
			Pluvialis apricaria	Eurasian Golden-Plover	Denmark	Christiansen 1949
	Pluvianellidae	Magellanic Plover				
	Scolopacidae	Sandpipers	*Pelidna alpina*	Dunlin	Great Britain	Green 1969
			Numenius arquata	Eurasian Curlew	Germany	Von Schauberg 1901
			Calidris alba	Sanderling	Florida, U.S.A.	Krueder et al. 1999
	Pedionomidae	Plains-wanderer				
	Thinocoridae	Seedsnipes				
	Chionididae	Sheathbills				
	Stercorariidae	Skuas & Jaegers				
	Laridae	Gulls	*Larus canus*	Mew Gull	Denmark	Christiansen 1949
			Larus argentatus	Herring Gull	Great Britain	Miles and Stocker 1948
	Sternidae	Terns	*Sterna masima*	Royal Tern	Florida, U.S.A.	Jacobson et al. 1980
			Sterna fuscata	Sooty Tern	Australia	Annuar et al. 1983
			Anous stolidus	Brown Noddy	Australia	Annuar et al. 1983
			Anous tenuirostris	Lesser Noddy	Australia	Annuar et al. 1983
	Rynchopidae	Skimmers				
	Alcidae	Auks, Murres & Puffins	*Uria aalge*	Common Murre	California, U.S.A.	Harris et al. 1978; Hill and Bogue 1978
Pterocliformes	Pteroclidae	Sandgrouse				

Columbiformes	Columbidae	Pigeons & Doves	*Columba sp.*	Pigeon	Germany	Hartig and Frese 1973
			Columba livia	Rock Dove or Feral Pigeon	The Netherlands	de Jong 1912
			Columba livia	Rock Dove or Feral Pigeon	Austria	Loupal et al. 1985
			Columba livia	Rock Dove or Feral Pigeon	Florida, U.S.A.	Forrester and Spalding 2003
			Columba junoniae	Laurel Pigeon	Canary Islands, Spain	Medina et al. 2004
			Columba palumbus	Common Wood-Pigeon	Great Britain	Jennings 1954
			Columba palumbus	Common Wood-Pigeon	Germany	Salhoff 1937
			Columba palumbus	Common Wood-Pigeon	Sweden	Hulphers 1943
			Columba palumbus	Common Wood-Pigeon	Norway	Holt and Krogsrud 1973; Weli et al. 2004
			Columba palumbus	Common Wood-Pigeon	New York, U.S.A.	Tangredi 1974
			Columba araucana	Chilean Pigeon	Chile	Cubillos et al. 1979
			Zenaida macroura	Mourning Dove	Illinois, U.S.A.	Kossack and Hanson 1954
			Zenaida macroura	Mourning Dove	Florida, U.S.A.	Forrester and Spalding 2003
			Streptopelia decaocto	Eurasian Collard-Dove	Iraq	Al-Ani 1986
Psittaciformes	Cacatuidae	Cockatoos & Allies	*Nyphicus hollandicus*	Cockatiel	Japan	Iwata et al. 1986
	Psittacidae	Parrots, Macaws & Allies	*Loriculus vernalis*	Vernal-Hanging Parrot	Germany	Pilaski et al. 1990
			Agapornis roseicollis	Rosy-faced Lovebird	Germany	Kraft and Teufel 1971
			Agapornis roseicollis	Rosy-faced Lovebird	Florida, U.S.A.	Hitchner and Clubb 1980
			Agapornis roseicollis	Rosy-faced Lovebird	Japan	Tsai et al. 1997

(*Continued*)

Table 6.1. (Continued)

Order	Family	Common Family Name	Species	Common Species Name	Country Reported	References
			Agapornis fischeri	Fischer's Love bird	Florida, U.S.A.	Hitchner and Clubb 1980
			Agapornis personatus	Yellow-collared Lovebird	Germany	Kraft and Teufel 1971
			Agapornis personatus	Yellow-collared Lovebird	California, U.S.A.	Emanuelson et al. 1978
			Agapornis personatus	Yellow-collared Lovebird	Florida, U.S.A.	Hitchner and Clubb 1980
			Agapornis personatus	Yellow-collared Lovebird	Japan	Iwata et al. 1986
			Amazona finschi	Lilac-crowned Parrot	Florida, U.S.A.	Hitchner and Clubb 1980
			Amazona finschi	Lilac-crowned Parrot	Indiana, U.S.A.	Boosinger et al. 1982
			Amazona autumnalis	Red-lored Parrot	Florida, U.S.A.	Hitchner and Clubb 1980
			Amazona albifrons	White-fronted Parrot	Mexico	Graham 1978
			Amazona albifrons	White-fronted Parrot	Florida, U.S.A.	Hitchner and Clubb 1980
			Amazona aestiva	Blue-fronted Parrot	Bolivia	Hitchner and Clubb 1980
			Amazona aestiva	Blue-fronted Parrot	California, U.S.A.	McDonald et al. 1981
			Amazona aestiva	Blue-fronted Parrot	Mexico	Olmos et al. 1986
			Amazona aestiva	Blue-fronted Parrot	Japan	Iwata et al. 1986
			Amazona aestiva	Blue-fronted Parrot	South Africa	Petrak 1982
			Amazona ochrocephala	Yellow-crowned Parrot	Florida, U.S.A.	Hitchner and Clubb 1980
			Amazona ochrocephala	Yellow-crowned Parrot	Indiana, U.S.A.	Boosinger et al. 1982
			Amazona orchrocephala	Yellow-crowned Parrot	U.S.A.	Minsky and Petrak 1982

Amazona farinosa	Mealy Parrot	Florida, U.S.A.	Hitchner and Clubb 1980
Deroptyus accipitrinus	Red-fan Parrot	Florida, U.S.A.	Hitchner and Clubb 1980
Pionus fuscus	Dusky Parrot	Florida, U.S.A.	Hitchner and Clubb 1980
Pionus senilis	White-crowned Parrot	Florida, U.S.A.	Hitchner and Clubb 1980
Pionus maximiliani	Scaly-headed Parrot	Florida, U.S.A.	Hitchner and Clubb 1980
Pionus menstruus	Blue-headed Parrot	Florida, U.S.A.	Hitchner and Clubb 1980
Pionus melano-cephalus	Black-headed Caique	Florida, U.S.A.	Hitchner and Clubb 1980
Ara rubrogenys	Red-fronted Macaw	Florida, U.S.A.	Hitchner and Clubb 1980
Ara ararauna	Blue-and-Yellow Macaw	U.S.A.	Minsky and Petrak 1982
Ara chloroptera	Red-and-green Macaw	South America	Kroesen 1977
Ara militaris	Military Macaw	Texas, U.S.A.	Clark et al. 1988
Anodorhynchus hyancinthinus	Hyacinth Macaw	South America	Kroesen 1977
Psittacara holochlora	Green Parakeet	Indiana, U.S.A.	Boosinger et al. 1982
Aratinga mitrata	Mitred Parakeet	Florida, U.S.A.	Hitchner and Clubb 1980
Aratinga solstitialis	Sun Parakeet	Mexico	Olmos et al. 1982
Aratinga canicularis	Orange-fronted Parakeet	Mexico	Olmos et al. 1982
Enicognathus leptorhynchus	Slender-billed Parakeet	Florida, U.S.A.	Hitchner and Clubb 1980
Aprosmictus erythropterus	Red-winged Parrot	Germany	Winteroll et al. 1979
Brotogeris pyrrhoptera	Grey-cheeked Parrot	Florida, U.S.A.	Hitchner and Clubb 1980

(*Continued*)

Table 6.1. (Continued)

Order	Family	Common Family Name	Species	Common Species Name	Country Reported	References
			Psephotus haemotonotus	Red-rumped Parrot	Florida, U.S.A.	Hitchner and Clubb 1980
			Platycercus eximius	Eastern Rosella	Florida, U.S.A.	Hitchner and Clubb 1980
			Melopsittacus undulatus	Budgerigar	Illinois, U.S.A.	Sharma et al. 1968
			Melopsittacus undulatus	Budgerigar	Philadelphia, U.S.A.	Petrak 1982
Cuculiformes	Musophagidae	Turacos				
	Cuculidae	Cuckoos	*Chrysococcyx caprius*	Dideric Cuckoo	South Africa	Markus 1974
Strigiformes	Tyonidae	Barn-Owls				
	Strigidae	Typical Owls				
			Otus asio	Eastern Screech-Owl	Florida, U.S.A.	Deem et al. 1997; Forrester and Spalding 2003
			Asio otus	Northern Long-eared Owl	Italy	Chiocco 1992
			Asio otus	Northern Long-eared Owl	Florida, U.S.A.	Forrester and Spalding 2003
			Bubo bubo	Eurasian Eagle-Owl	Italy	Maggiora and Valenti 1903
			Bubo virginianus	Great Horned Owl	Florida, U.S.A.	Forrester and Spalding 2003
			Strix varia	Barred Owl	Florida, U.S.A.	Deem et al. 1997; Forrester and Spalding 2003
Caprimulgiformes	Steatornithidae	Oilbird				
	Aegothelidae	Owlet-Nightjars				
	Podargidae	Frogmouths				
	Nyctibiidae	Potoo				
	Caprimuligidae	Nightjar & Allies				
Apodiformes	Apodidea	Swifts	*Chaetura pelagica*	Chimney Swift	Pennsylvania, U.S.A.	Worth 1956
	Hemiprocnidae	Treeswifts				
	Trochilidae	Humminbirds				

Coliiformes	Coliidae	Mousebirds				
Trogoniformes	Trogonidae	Trogon				
Coraciiformes	Alcedinidae	Kingfisher				
	Todidae	Todies				
	Momotidae	Motmot				
	Meropidae	Bee-eaters				
	Coraciidae	Typical Rollers				
	Brachypteraciidae	Ground-Roller				
	Leptosomidae	Cuckoo-Roller				
	Upupidae	Hoopoes	*Phoeniculus purpureus*	Red-billed Wood-Hoopoe	France	Megnin 1878
	Phoeniculidae	Woodhoopoes				
	Bucerotidae	Hornbills				
Piciformes	Galbulidae	Jacamars				
	Bucconidae	Puffbirds				
	Capitonidae	Barbets				
	Ramphastidae	Toucans				
	Indicatoridae	Honeyguides				
	Picidae	Woodpeckers & Allies	*Colaptes auratus*	Northern Flicker	Illinois, U.S.A.	Labisky and Mann 1961
			Colaptes auratus	Northern Flicker	Ontario, Canada	Kirmse, 1967c, 1969; Karstad 1971
			Colaptes auratus	Northern Flicker	Florida, U.S.A.	Forrester and Spalding 2003
Passeriformes	Eurylaimidae	Broadbills				
	Philepittidae	False-sunbirds (Asities)				
	Funariidae	Ovenbirds				
	Dendrocolapitidae	Woodcreepers				
	Thanmophilidae	Typical Antbirds				
	Formicariidae	Antthrushes & Antpittas				
	Conopophagidae	Anteaters				
	Rhinocryptidae	Tapaculos				
	Phytotomidae	Plantcutters				
	Cotingidae	Cotingas	*Cotinga maculata*	Banded Cotinga	Germany	Pilaski et al. 1990
	Pipridae	Manakins	*Manacus vitellinus*	Golden-collared Manakin	Panama	Kirmse and Loftin 1969

(*Continued*)

Table 6.1. (Continued)

Order	Family	Common Family Name	Species	Common Species Name	Country Reported	References
			Manacus manacus	White-bearded Manakin	Trinidad	Tikasingh et al. 1982
			Pipra erythrocephala	Golden-headed Manakin	Trinidad	Tikasingh et al. 1982
			Pipra mentalis	Red-capped Manakin	Panama	Kirmse and Loftin 1969
	Tyrannidae	Tyrant Flycathers	*Empidonax traillii*	Willow Flycatcher	Panama	Kirmse and Loftin 1969
			Empidonax traillii	Willow Flycatcher	Costa Rica, Arizona, U.S.A.	van Riper, pers. observation
	Oxyruncidae	Sharpbill				
	Pittidae	Pittas				
	Atrichornithidae	Scrub-birds				
	Menuridae	Lyrebirds				
	Acanthisittidae	New Zealand Wrens				
	Alaudidae	Larks	*Alauda arvensis*	Sky Lark	Denmark	Christiansen 1949
			Galerida cristata	Crested Lark	Spain	Groth 1963
			Calandrella rufescens	Lesser Short-toed Lark	Canary Islands, Spain	Smits et al. 2005
	Hirundinidae	Swallows				
	Motacillidae	Wagtails & Pipits	*Anthus novae-seelandiae*	Australasian Pipit	New Zealand	Westerkov 1953
			Anthus novae-seelandiae	Australasian Pipit	New Zealand	Quinn 1971
			Anthus berthelotti	Berthelot's Pipit	Canary Islands, Spain	Smits et al. 2005
	Campephagidae	Cuckoo-shrikes	*Coaracina novaehollandiae*	Black-faced Cuckoo-shrike	Australia	Sutton and Fillipich 1983
	Pycnonotidae	Bulbuls	*Pycnonotus jocosus*	Red-whiskered Bulbul		van Riper et al. 1979
	Regulidae	Kinglets				
	Chloropseidae	Leafbirds	*Chloropsis aurifrons*	Golden-fronted Leafbird	Germany	Hertig 1966

Aegithinidae	Ioras				
Ptilogonatidae	Silky-flycatchers				
Bombycillidae	Waxwings				
Hypocoliidae	Hypocolius				
Dulidae	Palmchat				
Cinclidae	Dipper				
Troglodytidae	Wrens	*Troglodytes troglodytes*	Wren	Denmark	Christiansen 1949
Mimidae	Mockingbirds & Thrashers	*Mimus polyglottus*	Northern Mockingbird	Spain	Oros et al. 1997
		Mimus polyglottus	Northern Mockingbird	Canada	Kirmse, 1966; Karstad 1971
		Mimus polyglottus	Northern Mockingbird	Florida, U.S.A.	Forrester and Spalding 2003
		Nesomimus parvulus	Galapagos Mockingbird	Galapagos Islands	Vargus 1987; Thiel et al. 2005
		Dumetella caroloinsis	Gray Catbird	New Jersey, U.S.A.	Kirmse et al. 1966
Prunellidae	Accentors	*Prunella collaris*	Apline Accentor	Austria	Loupal et al. 1985
		Prunella modularis	Dunnock	France	Mercier and Poisson 1923
		Prunella modularis	Dunnock	Great Britain	Edwards 1955
Turdidae	Thrushes & Allies	*Turdus migratorius*	American Robin	New Jersey, U.S.A.	Kirmse et al. 1966
		Turdus migratorius	American Robin	U.S.A.	Goodpasture and Anderson 1962
		Turdus migratorius	American Robin	Ontario Canada	Kirmse 1966
		Turdus migratorius	American Robin	California, U.S.A.	Hill and Bogue, 1977
		Turdus merula	Eurasian Blackbird	Italy	Maggiora and Valenti 1903
		Turdus philomelos	Song Thrush	Denmark	Christiansen 1949
		Turdus nudigenis	Bare-eyed Thrush	Trinidad	Tikasingh et al. 1982
		Turdus pilaris	Fieldfare	Italy	Maggiora and Valenti 1903
		Catharus minimus	Gray-cheeked Thrush	Ontario Canada	Kirmse 1966

(*Continued*)

Table 6.1. (Continued)

Order	Family	Common Family Name	Species	Common Species Name	Country Reported	References
			Catharus minimus	Grey-cheeked Thrush	Panama	Kirmse and Loftin 1969
			Catharus fuscescens	Veery	Panama	Kirmse and Loftin 1969
			Catharus ustulatus	Swainson's Thrush	Canada	Kirmse, 1966
			Hylocichla mustelina	Wood Thrush	U.S.A.	Goodpasture and Anderson 1962
			Hylocichla mustelina	Wood Thrush	Canada, Panama	Kirmse 1966; Kirmse and Loftin 1969
			Myadestes obscurus	Omao	Hawaii, U.S.A.	van Riper and van Riper 1985; van Riper et al. 2002
	Cistiocolidae	Cisticolas & Allies				
	Sylviidae	Old World Warblers	*Sylvia curruca*	Lesser Whitethroat	Denmark	Christiansen 1949
			Sylvia atricapilla	Blackcap	Czech Republic, Austria	Rajchard 2001
	Polioptilidae	Gnatcatchers				
	Muscicapidae	Old World Flycatchers	*Copsychus malabaricus*	White-rumped Shama	Germany	Hartig 1966
			Eumyias thalassina	Verditer Flycatcher	Germany	Hartig 1966
			Grandala coelicolor	Grandala	U.S.A.	Goodpasture and Anderson 1962
			Chasiempis sandwichensis	Elepaio	Hawaii, U.S.A.	Perkins 1903; van Riper and van Riper 1985; VanderWerf 2001; van Riper et al., 2002; Atkinson et al. 2005
	Platysteiridae	Wattle-eyes				
	Rhipiduridae	Fantails				
	Monarchidae	Monarch Flycatchers				
	Pteroicidae	Australasian Robins				

Pachycephalidae	Whistlers & Allies				
Picathartidae	Rockfowl				
Timaliidae	Babblers				
Pomatostomidae	Pseudo-babblers				
Paradoxornithidae	Parrotbills				
Orthonychidae	Logrunner & Chowchilla				
Cinclosomatidae	Whipbirds & Quail-thrushes				
Aegithalidae	Long-tailed Tits				
Maluridae	Fairywrens				
Acanthizidae	Thornbills & Allies				
Epthianuridae	Australian Chats				
Neosittidae	Sitellas				
Climacteridae	Australasian Treecreepers				
Paridae	Chickadees & Tits	*Baeolophus bicolor*	Tufted Titmouse	U.S.A.	Goodpasture and Anderson 1962
		Parus major	Great Tit	Germany	Polowinkin 1901
		Parus major	Great Tit	Norway	Holt and Krogsrud 1973
Sittidae	Nuthatches				
Tichidromidae	Wallcreeper				
Certhiidae	Creepers	*Certhia familiaris*	Tree-Creeper	Canada	Kirmse 1966
Rhabdornithidae	Phillippine Creepers				
Remizidae	Penduline Tits				
Nectarinidae	Sunbirds & Spiderhunters				
Melanocharitidae	Berrypeckers & Longbills				
Paramythiidae	Tit Berrypecker & Crested Berrypecker				
Dicaeidae	Flowerpeckers				
Pardalotidae	Pardalotes				
Zosteropidae	White-eyes	*Zosterops lateralis*	Silver-eye	New Zealand	Austin et al. 1973
		Zosterops lateralis	Silver-eye	Australia	Harrigan et al. 1975
		Zosterops lateralis	Silver-eye	Australia	Annuar et al. 1983

(Continued)

Table 6.1. (Continued)

Order	Family	Common Family Name	Species	Common Species Name	Country Reported	References
			Zosterops palpebrosus	Oriental White-eye	Japan	Kawashima 1962
			Zosterops japonicus	Japanese White-eye	Hawaii, U.S.A.	van Riper and van Riper 1985; van Riper et al. 2002
	Promeropidae	Sugarbirds				
	Meliphagidae	Honeyeaters				
	Oriolidae	Old World Orioles				
	Irenidae	Fairy-bluebirds				
	Laniidae	Shrikes	*Lanius sp.*	Shrike	Southern Africa	Abrey 1993
	Malaconotidae	Bushshrikes & Allies				
	Prionopidea	Helmetshrikes				
	Vangidae	Vangas				
	Dicruridae	Drongos				
	Callaeidae	Wattlebirds				
	Grallinidae	Mudnest-builders	*Grallina cyanoleuca*	Magpie-Lark	Australia	Harrigan et al. 1975; Annuar et al. 1983
	Corcoracidae	White-winged Chough & Apostlebird				
	Artimidae	Woodswallow				
	Pityriaseidae	Bristlehead				
	Cracticidae	Bellmagpies & Allies	*Gymnorhina tibicen*	Australian Magpie	Australia	Burnet and Stanley 1959; Harrigan et al. 1975; Chung and Spradbow 1977; Annuar et al. 1983
	Paradisaeidae	Birds-of-Paradise				
	Ptilonorhynchidae	Bowerbirds				
	Corvidae	Crows, Jays & Magpies	*Coleus monedula*	Jackdaw	The Netherlands	Jansen 1942
			Corvus frugilegus	Rook	Denmark	Christiansen 1949
			Corvus corax	Common Raven	Denmark	Christiansen 1949
			Corvus corone	Carrion Crow	Denmark	Christiansen 1949

		Corvus corone	Carrion Crow	Great Britain	Poulding 1960
		Corvus corone	Carrion Crow	Germany	Grzimek 1939
		Corvus hawaiiensis	Hawaiian Crow	Hawaii, U.S.A.	Jenkins et al. 1989; Tripathy et al. 2000
		Cyanocitta cristata	Blue Jay	Pennsylvania, U.S.A.	Worth 1956
		Pica pica	Black-billed Magpie	Denmark	Christiansen 1949
		Pica pica	Black-billed Magpie	Norway	Holt and Krogsrud 1973
		Cyanocitta cristata	Blue Jay	Florida, U.S.A.	Forrester and Spalding 2003
Sturnidae	Starlings	*Gracula religiosa*	Common Hill Myna	Malaysia	Karpinski and Clubb 1986
		Gracula religiosa	Common Hill Myna	Malaysia	Reed and Schrader 1989
		Leucopsar rothschildi	Bali Myna	Washington, U.S.A.	Landolt and Kochan 1976
		Sturnus vulgaris	European Starling	U.S.A.	Goodpasture and Anderson 1962
		Sturnus vulgaris	European Starling	Germany	Hartig 1966
		Sturnus vulgaris	European Starling	Germany	Luthgen 1983
		Sturnus vulgaris	European Starling	Austria	Loupal et al. 1985
		Cosmopsarus regius	Regal Starling	Germany	Pilaski et al. 1990
		Lamprotornis sp.	Glossy Starling	Germany	Luthgen 1983
Passeridae	Old World Sparrows	*Passer domesticus*	House Sparrow	Brazil	Reis and Nobrega 1937
		Passer domesticus	House Sparrow	U.S.A.	Coulston and Manwell 1941
		Passer domesticus	House Sparrow	Washington, U.S.A.	Giddens et al. 1971
		Passer domesticus	House Sparrow	Norway	Holt & Krogsrud 1973; Weli et al. 2004
		Passer domesticus	House Sparrow	California, U.S.A.	Hill and Bogue 1977
		Passer domesticus	House Sparrow	Germany	Herbst and Krauss 1989

(*Continued*)

Table 6.1. (Continued)

Order	Family	Common Family Name	Species	Common Species Name	Country Reported	References
			Passer domesticus	House Sparrow	Canada	Mikaelian and Martineau 1996
			Passer domesticus	House Sparrow	Hawaii, U.S.A.	van Riper and van Riper 1985
			Passer melanurus	Cape Sparrow	South Africa	Markus 1974
			Passer montanus	Tree Sparrow	Japan	Honma and Chiva 1976
	Ploceidae	Weavers & Allies	*Ploceus velatus*	African Masked-Weaver	South Africa	Markus 1974
			Quelea quelea	Red-headed Quelea	Africa	Barre 1975
	Estrildidae	Waxbills & Allies	*Padda oryzivora*	Java Sparrow	Germany	Kikuth and Gollub 1932
	Viduidae	Indigobirds				
	Vireonidae	Vireos & Allies				
	Fringillidae	Siskins, Crossbills & Allies	*Fringilla coelebs*	Chaffinch	Germany	Eberbeck and Kayser 1932
			Fringilla coelebs	Chaffinch	Great Britain	Keymer and Blackmore 1964
			Carduelis cucullata	Red Siskin	Germany	Kaleta and Marschall 1982
			Carduelis pinus	Pine Siskin	California, U.S.A.	Bigland et al. 1962
			Carduelis spinus	Eurasian Siskin	Germany	Hartwigk and Lange 1964
			Carduelis spinus	Eurasian Siskin	Austria	Loupal et al. 1985
			Carduelis carduelis	European Goldfinch	Germany	Polowinkin 1901
			Carduelis carduelis	European Goldfinch	Great Britain	Keymer and Blackmore 1964
			Carduelis carduelis	European Goldfinch	Germany	Kaleta and Ebert 1969

		Carduelis chloris	European Greenfinch	Great Britain	Keymore and Blackmore 1964
		Carduelis chloris	European Greenfinch	Germany	Kaleta and Ebert 1969
		Pyrrhula phrrhula	Common Bullfinch	Germany	Polwinkin 1901
		Pyrrhula phrrhula	Common Bullfinch	The Netherlands	De Jong 1912
				Germany	Stadie 1931
		Pyrrhula phrrhula	Common Bullfinch	Germany	Kaleta and Ebert 1969
		Pyrrhula phrrhula	Common Bullfinch	Austria	Loupal et al. 1985
		Linaria cannabina	Eurasian Linnet	Germany	Polowinkin 1901
		Linaria cannabina	Eurasian Linnet	Germany	Hartwigk and Lang 1964
		Serinus canaria	Island Canary	Germany	Hartig 1966; Kikuth and Gollub 1932; Michel and Lindner 1964
		Serinus canaria	Island Canary	Tunisia	Loir and Ducloux 1894
		Serinus canaria	Island Canary	Uruguay	Wolffhugel 1919
		Serinus canaria	Island Canary	Japan	Sato et al. 1962
		Serinus canaria	Island Canary	New York, U.S.A.	Donnely and Crane 1984
		Serinus canaria	Island Canary	Austria	Loupal et al. 1985
		Serinus canaria	Island Canary	Oklahoma, U.S.A.	Johnson and Castro 1986
		Carpodacus mexicanus	House Finch	California, U.S.A.	Power and Human 1976; Hill and Bogue 1977
		Carpodacus mexicanus	House Finch	Idaho, U.S.A.	Docherty and Long 1986
		Leucosticte tephrocotis	Gray-crowned Rosy-Finch	Alaska, U.S.A.	Bergstrom 1952
Drepanididae	Hawaiian Honeycreepers	*Paroreomyaz maculata*	Lanai Creeper	Hawaii, U.S.A.	Munro 1944
		Hemignathus obscurus	Akialoa	Hawaii, U.S.A.	Perkins 1903

(*Continued*)

Table 6.1. (Continued)

Order	Family	Common Family Name	Species	Common Species Name	Country Reported	References
			Himatione sanguinea	Apapane	Hawaii, U.S.A.	Perkins 1903; Amadon 1950; van Riper and van Riper 1985; Tripathy et al. 2000; van Riper et al. 2002; Atkinson et al. 2005
			Psittirostra psittacea	Ou	Hawaii, U.S.A.	Perkins 1903
			Rhodacanthus spp. (n=3)	Koa Finches	Hawaii, U.S.A.	Perkins 1903
			Telespiza cantans	Laysan Finch	Hawaii, U.S.A.	Warner 1968; van Riper and van Riper 1985; van Riper et al. 2002
			Loxops coccineus	Akepa	Hawaii, U.S.A.	Henshaw 1902
			Hemignathus virens	Hawaii Amakihi	Hawaii, U.S.A.	van Riper and van Riper 1985; van Riper et al. 2002; Atkinson et al. 2005
			Vestiaria coccinea	Iiwi	Hawaii, U.S.A.	Warner 1968; van Riper and van Riper 1985; van Riper et al. 2002
	Peucedramidae	Olive Warbler				
	Parulidae	New World Warblers	*Oporornis philadelphia*	Mourning Warbler	Panama	Kirmse and Loftin 1969
			Seiurus aurocapillus	Ovenbird	Panama	Kirmse and Loftin 1969
			Seiurus motacilla	Louisiana Waterthrush	Panama	Kirmse and Loftin 1969
			Dendroica tigrina	Cape May Warbler	New Jersey, U.S.A.	Kirmse et al. 1966
			Dendroica petechia	Yellow Warbler	Galapagos Islands	Thiel et al. 2005

		Icteria virens	Yellow-breasted Chat	New Jersey, U.S.A.	Kirmse et al. 1966
		Geothlypis trichas	Common Yellowthroat	New Jersey, U.S.A.	Kirmse et al. 1966
Coerebidae	Banaquit				
Thraupidae	Tanagers & Allies	*Thraupis episcopus*	Blue-grey Tanager	Panama	Kirmse and Loftin 1969
		Chlorospingus ophthalmicus	Common Bush-Tanager	Panama	Kirmse and Loftin 1969
		Piranga rubra	Summer-Tanager	Panama	Kirmse and Loftin 1969
		Euphonia violacea	Violaceous Euphonia	Trinidad	Tikasingh et al. 1982
		Tangra guttata	Speckled Tanager	Germany	Pilaski et al. 1990
Emberizidae	Buntings, Sparrows, Seedeaters & Allies	*Plectrophenax nivalis*	Snow Bunting	Maryland, U.S.A.	Irons 1934
		Spizella passerina	Chipping Sparrow	U.S.A.	Baldwin 1922
		Spizella passerina	Chipping Sparrow	Georgia, U.S.A.	Musselmann 1928
		Spizella passerina	Chipping Sparrow	Ontario Canada	Kirmse 1966
		Spizella passerina	Chipping Sparrow	Florida, U.S.A.	Stevenson and Anderson 1994
		Spizella arborea	American Tree Sparrow	U.S.A.	Bergstrom 1952
		Spizella pussilla	Field Sparrow	Tennessee & Mississippi, U.S.A.	Goodpasture and Anderson 1962
		Spizella pussilla	Field Sparrow	Ontario Canada	Kirmse 1966
		Passerculus sandwichensis	Savannah Sparrow	Canada	Karstad 1971
		Junco hyemalis	Dark-eyed Junco	New Jersey, U.S.A.	Worth 1956
		Junco hyemalis	Dark-eyed Junco	Tennessee & Mississippi, U.S.A.	Goodpasture and Anderson 1962
		Junco hyemalis	Dark-eyed Junco	U.S.A.	Beaver and Cheatham 1963
		Junco hyemalis	Dark-eyed Junco	Ontario Canada	Kirmse 1966
		Melospiza melodia	Song Sparrow	New York, U.S.A.	Coulston and Manwell 1941

(*Continued*)

Table 6.1. (Continued)

Order	Family	Common Family Name	Species	Common Species Name	Country Reported	References
			Melospiza melodia	Song Sparrow	Ontario Canada	Kirmse 1966
			Passurella iliaca	Fox Sparrow	New Jersey, U.S.A.	Worth 1956
			Pipilo erythrophtalmus	Eastern Towhee	Tennesseee & Mississippi, U.S.A.	Goodpasture and Anderson 1962
			Pipilo erythrophtalmus	Eastern Towhee	Canada	Kirmse 1966
			Pipilo chlorurus	Green-tailed Towhee	Canada	Kirmse 1966
			Zonotrichia atricapilla	Golden-crowned Sparrow	Washington, U.S.A.	Giddens et al. 1971
			Zonotrichia albicollis	White-throated Sparrow	New Jersey, U.S.A.	Worth 1956
			Zonotrichia albicollis	White-throated Sparrow	Canada	Kirmse 1966
			Zonotrichia leucophrys	White-crowned Sparrow	Washington, U.S.A.	Giddens et al. 1971
			Sporophila corvina	Variable Seedeater	Panama	Kirmse and Loftin 1969
			Sporophila sp.	Seedeater	Brazil	Reis and Nobrega 1937
			Sicalis flaveola	Saffron Finch	Brazil	Reis and Nobrega 1937
			Oryzoborus angolensis	Chestnut-bellied Seed-Finch	Brazil	Reis and Nobrega 1937; Kirmes and Loftin 1969
			Oryzoborus funereus	Thick-billed Seed Finch	Panama	Kirmse and Loftin 1969
			Aimophila cassinii	Cassin's Sparrows	Kansas, U.S.A.	Savage and Dick 1969
			Geospiza spp.	Ground Finches	Galapagos Islands	Thiel et al. 2005
	Cardinalidae	Caltators, Cardinals & Allies	*Cardinalis cardinalis*	Northern Cardinal	Tennessee & Mississippi, U.S.A.	Goodpasture and Anderson 1962
			Cardinalis cardinalis	Northern Cardinal	Austria	Loupal et al. 1985

		Cardinalis cardinalis	Northern Cardinal	Hawaii, U.S.A.	van Riper and van Riper 1985
		Cyanoloxia cyanea	Ultramarine Grosbeak	Brazil	Reis & Nobrega 1937
		Cyanocompsa cyanoides	Blue-black Grosbeak	Panama	Kirmse and Loftin 1969
Icteridae	Troupials & Allies	*Quiscalus sp.*	Grackle	Texas, U.S.A.	Docherty et al. 1991
		Quiscalus quiscula	Common Grackle	Florida, U.S.A.	Forrester and Spalding 2003
		Quiscalus quiscula	Common Grackle	Maryland, U.S.A.	Herman et al. 1962
		Quiscalus quiscula	Common Grackle	U.S.A.	Emmel 1930
		Molothrus ater	Brown-headed Cowbird	Pennsylvania, U.S.A.	Locke 1961
		Molothrus ater	Brown-headed Cowbird	Maryland, U.S.A.	Herman et al. 1962
		Molothrus ater	Brown-headed Cowbird	Alabama, U.S.A.	Stewart 1963
		Agelaius phoeniceus	Red-winged Blackbird	Florida, U.S.A.	Fisk 1972

ACKNOWLEDGEMENTS

Grateful acknowledgement is made of the groundwork for this chapter by Lars Karstad, who authored the "Avian Pox" chapter in the first edition of this book.

LITERATURE CITED

Abrey, A.N.S. 1993. Diseases of wild birds in southern Africa. In *Zoo and Wild Animal Medicine. Current Therapy 3,* M.E. Fowler (ed.). W.B. Saunders Co., Philadelphia, U.S.A., pp. 163–166.

Akey, B.L., J.K. Nayar, and D.J. Forrester. 1981. Avian pox in Florida wild turkeys: *Culex nigripalpus* and *Wyeomyia vanduzeei* as experimental vectors. *Journal of Wildlife Diseases* 17:597–599.

Al-Ani, M. O. A. 1986. An outbreak of pox among pheasants in Iraq. *Avian Pathology* 15:795–796.

Al Falluji, M.M., H.H. Tantawi, A. Al-Bana, and S. Sheikhly. 1979. Pox infections among captive peacocks. *Journal of Wildlife Diseases* 15:597–600.

Alicata, J.E. 1964. *Parasitic infections of man and animals in Hawaii.* Hawaii Agriculture Experiment Station Technical Bulletin No. 61. Honolulu, HI, U.S.A., 138 pp.

Allwright, D.M., W.P. Burger, A. Geyer, and J. Wessels. 1994. Avian pox in ostriches. *Journal of the South African Veterinary Association* 65:23–25.

Amadon, D. 1950. The Hawaiian Honeycreepers (Drepaniidae). *Bulletin of the American Museum of Natural History* 95:151–262.

Annuar, B.O., J.S Mackenzie, and P. A. Lalor. 1983. Isolation and characterization of avipoxvirus from wild birds in Western Australia. *Archives of Virology* 76:217–229.

Andrews, C.H.G. Pereira, and P. Wildy. 1978. *Viruses of Vertebrates,* 4th Ed. Bailliere Tindall, London, pp. 356–389.

Arai, S., C. Arai, M. Fujimaki, Y. Iwamoto, M. Kawarada, Y. Saito, Y. Nomura, and T. Suzuki. 1991. Cutaneous tumor-like lesions due to poxvirus infection in Chilean flamingos. *Journal of Comparative Pathology* 104:439–441.

Arhelger, R.B., R.W. Darlington, L.G. Gafford, and C.C. Randall. 1962. An electron microscopic study of fowlpox infection in chicken scalps. *Laboratory Investigation* 11:814–825.

Arhelger, R.B., and C.C. Randall. 1964. Electron microscopic observations on the development of fowlpox virus in chorioallantoic membrane. *Virology* 22:59–66.

Arnall, L, and I.F. Keymer. 1975. *Bird Diseases.* T. F.H. Publications, Neptune, NJ, U.S.A.

Atkinson, C.T., J.K. Lease, R.J. Dusek, and M.D. Samuel. 2005. Prevalence of pox-like lesions and malaria in forest bird communities on leeward Mauna Loa Volcano, Hawaii. *Condor*107:537–546.

Austin, F.J., P.C. Bull, and M.A. Chaudry. 1973. A poxvirus isolated from silvereyes (*Zosterops lateralis*) from Lower Hutt, New Zealand. *Journal of Wildlife Diseases* 9:111–114.

Avila, E. 1953. El Epteleioma contagiese en el guanay belet. Cientifico de la Cia. Admor. Guano (cited in Kirmse, 1967).

Baily, T.A., C. Silvanose, R. Manvell, R.E. Gough, J. Kinne, O. Combreau, and F. Launay. 2002. Medical dilemmas associated with rehabilitating confiscated houbara bustards (*Chlamydotis undulate macqueenii*) after avian pox and paramyxovirus type 1 infection. *Journal of Wildlife Diseases* 38:518–532.

Baldwin, S. P. 1922. Adventures in bird-banding in 1921. *Auk* 39:210–224.

Barre, N. 1975. Une infection variolque de Quelea quelea (L.) (Passeriformes, Ploceinae). *Revue d'Elevage et de Medicine Veterinarie des Pays Tropicaux* 28:105–113.

Beaver, D.L., and W.J. Cheatham. 1963. Electron microscopy of junco pox. *American Journal of Pathology* 42:23–39.

Bergstrom, E.A. 1952. Avian Pox in the Gray-crowned Rosy Finch in Alaska. *Auk* 39:210–224.

Bigland, C.H., G.R. Whenham, and F.E. Graesser. 1962. A pox-like infection of canaries: report of an outbreak. *Canadian Veterinary Journal* 3:347–351.

Blakenship, L.H., R.E. Reed, and H.D. Irby. 1966. Pox in mourning doves and Gambel's quail in southern Arizona. *Journal of Wildlife Management* 30:253–257.

Bleitz, D. 1958. Treatment of foot pox at a feeding and trapping station. *Auk* 75:474–475.

Bohart, R.M., and R.K. Washino. 1978. Mosquitoes of California. *Division of Agricultural Science Publication No. 4084,* Berkeley, California, U.S.A., 153 pp.

Bollinger, O. 1873. Ueber menschen- und thierpocken, ueber den ursprung der kuhpocken und ueber intrauterine vaccination. *Volkmann's sammlung klinischer vortraege* 116:1021–1060.

Bollinger, O. 1877. Ueber epithelioma contagiosum beim haushuhn und die sogenannten pocken des gefluegels. *Archiv für pathologiosche anatomie und physiologie und für klinische medizin* 58:349–361.

Bolte, A.L., J. Meurer, and E.F. Kaleta. 1999. Avian host spectrum of avipoxviruses. *Avian Pathology* 28:415–432.

Boosinger, T.R., W.R. Winterfield, D.S. Feldman, and A.S. Dhillon. 1982. Psittiacine pox virus: virus isolation and identification, transmission and cross-challenge studies in parrots and chickens. *Avian Diseases* 26:437–444.

Borrel, A. 1904. Sur les inclusions de l'epithelioma contagieux des oiseaux (*Molluscum contagiosum*). *Comparative Rend. Society of Biology* 2:642–643.

Bouvier, G. 1946. Observations sur les maladies du gibier, de quelques animaux sauvages et des poissones

(1942–1945). *Schweizerisches Archive Tierheilkunde* 88:268–274.

Buenestado, F., C. Gortazar, J. Millan, U. Hofle, and R. Villafurte. 2004. Descriptive study of an avian pox outbreak in wild red-legged partridges (*Alcetoris rufa*) in Spain. *Epidemiology and Infection* 132:369–374.

Bump, G., R.W. Darrow, F.C. Edminster, and W.F. Crissey. 1947. *The Ruffed Grouse: Life History, Propagation, Management.* New York Conservation Department, Albany, NY, U.S.A.

Burnet, F.M., and W.M. Stanle. 1959. Animal viruses. In *The Viruses. Biochemical, Biological and Biophysical Properties,* Vol. III. Academic Press, New York, 428 pp.

Bush, A.O., K.D. Lafferty, J.M. Lotz, and A.W. Shostak. 1997. Parasitology meets ecology on its own terms: Margolis et al. revisited. *Journal of Parasitology* 83:575–583.

Cerrone, A., M. Blasone, A. Piccirillo, F. Mariani, and L.F. Menna. 1999. Clinical findings observed in some ostrich-farms in Campania during the period 1997–1998. *XXXVII Convegno della Societa Italiana di Patologia Avirae,* Flori, Italy, *Selezione-Veterinaria* 1999, 8–9:653–661.

Cheevers, W.P., D.J. O'Callaghan, and C.C. Randall. 1968. Biosynthesis of host and viral deoxyribonucleic acid during hyperplastic fowlpox infection in vivo. *Journal of Virology* 2:421–429.

Cheville, N.F. 1966. Cytopathologic changes in fowlpox (turkey origin) inclusions body formation. *American Journal of Pathology* 49:723–737.

Chiocco, D. 1992. Owlpoxvirus isolation and cross-challenge studies in chickens. *Acta Medica Veterinaria* 38:261–266.

Chung, Y.S., and P.B. Spradbow. 1977. Studies on poxviruses isolated from a magpie in Queensland. *Australian Veterinary Journal* 53:334–336.

Clark, F.D., G.M. Hume, and E.S. Hayes. 1988. An isolated case of avian pox in a military macaw (*Ara militaris mexicana*). *Companion Animal Practice* 2:34–35.

Clements, J.F. 2000. *Birds of the World: A Checklist.* Ibis Publ. Co., Vista, California, U.S.A.

Cociu, M., G. Wagner, N. Micu, E. Tuschak, and G. Mihaescu. 1972. Gefluegelpocken bei einer trappe (Otis tarda). *Diseases of Zoo Animals, 14th International Symposium,* Wroclaw, Poland, pp. 81–83.

Conti, J.A., D.J. Forrester, and R.T. Paul. 1986. Parasites and diseases of Reddish Egrets (*Egretta rufescens*) from Texas and Florida. *Transactions of the American Microscopical Society* 105:79–82.

Cooper, J. E. 1978. *Veterinary Aspects of Captive Birds of Prey.* Standfast Press, Gloucester.

Cooper, J.E. 1969. Two cases of pox in recently imported peregrine falcons (*Falco peregrinus*). *Veterinary Record* 85:683–684.

Coulston, F., and R.D. Manwell. 1941. Successful chemotherapy of a virus disease of the canary. *American Journal of Veterinary Research* 2:101–107.

Coupar, B.E.H., T. Teo, and D.B. Boyle. 1990. Restriction endonuclease mapping of the fowlpox virus genome. *Virology* 179:159–167.

Cox, W.R. 1980. Avian pox infection in a Canada goose (*Branta canadensis*). *Journal of Wildlife Diseases* 16:623–626.

Crawford, J.A. 1986. Differential prevalence of avian pox in adult and immature California quail. *Journal of Wildlife Diseases* 22:564–566.

Crawford, J.A., R.M. Oates, and D.H. Helfer. 1979. Avian pox in California Quail from Oregon. *Journal of Wildlife Diseases* 15:447–449.

Cubillos, A., R. Schlatter, V. Cubillos. 1979. Diftero-vireula aviar en torcaza (*Columba araucana,* Lesson) del sur del Chile. *Journal of Veterinary Medicine B,* 26:430–432.

Curasson, G. 1946. Variole aviaire. In *Maladies Infectieuses des Animaux Domestique.* Vol 1. Paris, pp. 152–160.

Cunningham, C.H. 1966. *A Laboratory Guide in Virology,* 6th Ed. Burguss Publishing Company, Minneapolis, MN, U.S.A.

Cunningham, C.H. 1972. Avian Pox. In *Diseases of Poultry,* 6th Ed., M.S. Hofstad, B.W. Calnek, C.F. Helmboldt, W.M. Reid, and H.W. Yoder, Jr. (eds.). Iowa State University Press, Ames, Iowa, U.S.A., pp. 707–724.

Davidson, W.R., and E.J. Wentworth. 1992. Population influences: diseases and parasites. In *The Wild Turkey—Biology and Management,* J.G. Dickson (ed.). Stackpole Books, Harrisburg, PA, U.S.A., pp. 101–118.

Davidson, W.R., F.E. Kellogg, and G.L. Doster. 1980. An epornitic of avian pox in wild Bobwhite Quail. *Journal of Wildlife Diseases* 16:293–298.

Davidson, W.R., F.E. Kellogg, and G.L. Doster. 1982. An overview of diseases and parasitism in southeastern bobwhite quail. *Proceedings of the National Bobwhite Quail Symposium* 2:64–68.

Deem, S.L., D.J. Heard, and J.H. Fox. 1997. Avian pox in Eastern Screech Owls and Barred Owls from Florida. *Journal of Wildlife Diseases* 33:323–327.

De Jong, D.A. 1912. Epithelioma contagiosum bij *Pyrrula vulgaris. Tijdskrift Veartsenigk* 39:734–736.

DeSante, D.F. 1992. MAPS (Monitoring avian productivity and survivorship). General Instruction. Institute For Bird Populations, Box 1346, Point Reyes Station, CA, U.S.A.

Dobson, N. 1937. Pox in pheasants. *Journal of Comparative Pathology* 50:401–404.

Docherty, D.E., and R.I.R. Long. 1986. Isolation of a poxvirus from a house finch, *Carpodacus mexicanus* (Muller). *Journal of Wildlife Diseases* 22:420–422.

Docherty, D.E., R.I.R. Long, E.L. Flickinger, and L.N. Locke. 1991. Isolation of poxvirus from debiltating cutaneous lesions on four immature grackles (*Quiscalus* sp.). *Avian Diseases* 35:244–47.

Dhondt, A.A., D.L. Tessaglia, and R.L. Slothower. 1998. Epidemic mycoplasmal conjunctivitis in house finches from eastern North America. *Journal of Wildlife Diseases* 34:265–280.

Donnelly, T.M., and L.A. Crane. 1984. An epornitic of avian pox in a research aviary. *Avian Diseases* 28:517–25.

DuBose, R.T. 1965. Pox in the sage grouse. *Bulletin of the Wildlife Disease Association* 1:6.

Eberberk, E., and W. Kayser. 1932. Ueber das vorkommen von pockenerkrankunge n von kanarienvoegeln, buchfinken und sperlingen. *Archive Für Wissenschaftliche und Praktische Thierheilkunde* 65:307–310.

Edwards, G.R. 1955. Excrescenses about the eyes and on the legs and feet of dunocks. *British Birds* 48:186–187.

Emanuelson, S., J. Carney, and J. Saito. 1978. Avian pox in two black-masked conures. *Journal of the American Veterinary Association* 173: 1249–1250.

Emmel, M.W. 1930. Epidermoid cancers on the feet of wild birds. *Journal of the American Veterinary Association* 77:641–644.

Englemann, F. 1928. Die Raubvogel Europas. Radebeul: Neumann-Neudamm, pp 691.

Ensley, P.K., M.P. Anderson, M.L. Costello, H.C. Powell, and R. Cooper. 1978. Epornitic of avian pox in a zoo. *Journal of the American Veterinary Medical Association* 173: 1111–1114.

Fenner, F. 1968. *The Biology of Animal Viruses,* Vol. I. Academic Press, New York, NY, U.S.A.

Fisk, E.J. 1972. Injuries and disease observed at a south Florida banding station, 1971. *Eastern Bird Banding Association News* 35:62.

Fitzner, R.E., R.A. Miller, C.A. Pierce, and S. E. Rowe. 1985. Avian pox in a red-tailed hawk (*Buteo jamaicensis*). *Journal of Wildlife Diseases* 29:298–301.

Forrester, D.J. 1991. The ecology and epizootiology of avian pox and malaria in Wild Turkeys. *Bulletin of the Society for Vector Ecology* 16:127–148.

Forrester, D.J. 1992. A synopsis of disease conditions found in Wild turkeys (*Meleagris gallopavo* L.) from Florida, 1969–1990. *Florida Field Naturalist* 20:29–56.

Forrester, D.J., and M. G. Spalding. 2003. *Parasites and Diseases of Wild Birds in Florida.* University Press of Florida, Gainesville, FL, U.S.A., 1,132 pp.

Fowler, M.E. 1981. *Wildlife Diseases of the Pacific Basin and Other Countries.* Fruitridge Printing, Sacamento, CA, U.S.A., 262 pp.

Francki, R.B., C.M. Fauguet, D.L. Knudson, and F. Brown (eds.). 1991. Classification and nomenclature of viruses. Fifth Report on the International Committee on Taxonomy of Viruses. *Archives of Virology, Supplement* 2:94–95. Springer-Verlag Wien, New York, NY, U.S.A.

Friend, M. 1987. *Field Guide to Wildlife Diseases.* U.S. Dept. Interior, Fish and Wildlife Service Resource Publ. No. 167, Washington, D.C., 225 pp.

Gallagher, B. 1916. *Epithelioma contagiosum* of quail. *Journal of the American Veterinary Medical Association* 50:366–369.

Garner, M.M. 1989. Bumblefoot associated with poxvirus in a wild golden eagle (*Aquila chrysatos*). *Companion Animal Practice* 19:17–20.

Giddens, W.E., L.J. Swango, J.D. Henderson, R.A. Lewis, D. S. Farner, A. Carlos, and W. C. Dolowy. 1971. Canary pox in sparrows and canaries (Fringillidae) and in weavers (Ploceidae). *Veterinary Pathology* 8:260–280.

Goodpasture, E.W., and K. Anderson. 1962. Isolation of a wild avian pox virus inducing both cytoplasmic and nuclear inclusions. *American Journal of Pathology* 40:437–453.

Graham, C.L. 1978. Poxvirus infection in a spectacled Amazon parrot (*Amazona albifrons*). *Avian Diseases* 22:340–343.

Gratzl, E. 1953. Diphterie bei einem Steinalder. *Der Falkner* 3:2.

Green, G.H. 1969. Suspected pox virus infection of a dunlin. *British Birds* 62:26–27.

Greenwood, A.G., and W.F. Blakemore. 1973. Pox infection in falcons. *Veterinary Record* 93:468–469.

Grimm, F. and J. Jacobi. 1977. Krankheiten bei patienten der klinik des lehrstuhls und krankheiten des hausgfluegels, der zier-und wildvoegel Munchen, 1976. *Berliner und Muenchener Tieraerztliche Wochenschrift* 90:123–125.

Groth, W. 1963. Ein beitrag zur geschwulstbildung bei wildlebenden voegeln. *Berliner und Muenchener Tieraerztliche Wochenschrift* 76:192–194.

Grzimek, B.1939. Die pockendiptherie. In *Krankes Guefluegel,* Vol 2, Pfennigstorff, Berlin, pp. 56–63.

Halliwell, N.H. 1972. Avian pox in an immature Red-tailed Hawk. *Journal of Wildlife Diseases* 8:104–105.

Hansen, W.R. 1987. Avian pox. In *Field Guide to Wildlife Diseases: Fish and Wildlife Service Resource Publication* 167, M. Friend (ed.). Washington, D.C., U.S.A., pp. 135–141.

Harrigan, K.E., I.K Barker, and M.J. Studdert. 1975. Poxvirus infection in the white-backed magpie and pox-like conditions in other birds in Australia. *Journal of Wildlife Diseases* 11:343–346.

Harris, J.M., A.S. Williams and F. R. Dutra. 1978. Avian pox in a group of common (California) murres (*Uria aalgae*). *Veterinary Medicine Small Animal Clinic* 73:918–919.

Hartig, F. 1966. Verhuetung und bekaempfung der kanarienpocken. *Kanarienfreund* 19:215–217.

Hartig, F., and K. Frese. 1973. Tumor-forming pigeon and canary smallpox. *Zentralblatt Veterinarmedizin B* 20:153–160.

Hartwigk, H., and Lange, W. 1964. Vakzinierungsversuch und bei kanarienvoegeln gegen pocken. *Deutsche Tieraerzzliche Wochenschrift* 71:180–183.

Henshaw, H.W. 1902. Complete list of the birds of the Hawaiian possessions, with notes on their habits. *Thrum's Hawaiian Almanac and Annual* 1902:54–106.

Herbst, W., and H. Krauss. 1989. Isolation of a poxvirus from a sparrow (*Passer domesticus*). *Journal of Veterinary Medicine B,* 36:477–479.

Hernandez, M., C. Sanchez, M.E. Galka, L. Dominguez, J. Goyache, J. Oria, and M. Pizarro. 2001. Avian pox infection in Spanish Imperial eagles. (*Aquila adalberti*). *Avian Pathology* 30:91–97.

Herman, C.M., L.N. Locke, and G. M. Clark. 1962. Foot abnormalities in wild birds. *Bird-banding* 33:191–198.

Heusinger, C.F. 1844. *Recherches de Pathologie Comparee* 1:649. Cassel: Henri Hotop.

Hill, J.R., and G. Bogue. 1977. Epornitic of pox in a wild bird population. *Journal of the American Veterinary Medical Association* 171:993–994.

Hill, J.R., and G. Bogue. 1978. Natural pox infection in a common murre (*Uria aalge*). *Journal of Wildlife Diseases* 14:337–338.

Hitchner, S.B., and S.L. Clubb. 1980. Relationship between poxvirus of parrots and of other birds. In *Proceedings 29th* Western Poultry Disease Conference, Acapulco, Mexico, pp. 149–151.

Holt, G., and J. Krogsrud. 1973. Pox in wild birds. *Acta Veterinaria Scandinavica* 14:201–203.

Honma, Y., and A. Chiba. 1976. A case of avian pox in a tree sparrow *Passer montanu. Journal of the Yamashina Institute of Ornithology* 8:101–107.

Horiuchi, T., H. Kawamura, S. Shoya, and S. Umikawa. 1965. Avian pox of a Japanese ptarmigan (*Lagopus mutus japonicus*). *National Institute of Animal Health Quarterly* 5:125–129.

Hu Hongguan. 1982. Pox in phasianids. *Animal Science Veterinary Medicine, Najing* 14:236.

Hulphers, G. 1943. Meddelande, fraan Svenska jagerfoebundets viltundersoekning. *Svenska Jägareförbundet* 81:375–380.

Ideris, A., and A.L. Ibrahim. 1986. Poxvirus infection in turkeys. *Kajian Veterinar* 18:85–87.

Ihlenburg, H. 1972. Zur Pockeninfektion beim Wassergeflugel. *Diseases of Zoo Animals,* 14th International Symposium Wroclaw, Poland, pp. 77–80.

Irons, V. 1934. Cross-species transmission studies with different strains of bird pox. *American Journal of Hygiene* (*now American Journal of Epidemiology*) 20:329–357.

Iwata, Y., H. Fukushe, Y. Suzuki, and K Hirai. 1986. Poxvirus infection in Psittacine birds. *Research Bulletin of the Faculty of Agriculture,* Gifu University 51:201–205.

Jacoboson, E.R., B.L. Raphael, H.T. Nguyen, E.C. Greiner, and T. Gross. 1980. Avian pox infection, aspergillosis and renal trematodiasis in a royal tern. *Journal of Wildlife Diseases* 16:627–630.

Jansen, J. 1942. Pokken bij de kavw. *Tijdskrift vor Diergeneskunde* 69:128–131.

Jenkins, C.D., S.A. Temple, C. van Riper III, and W. R. Hansen. 1989. Disease-related aspects of conserving the endangered Hawaiian Crow. In *Disease and Management of Threatened Bird Populations,* J. E. Cooper (ed.). ICBP Technical Publication Series No. 10, Cambridge, England, pp 77–87.

Jennings, A. R. 1954. Diseases in wild birds. *Journal of Comparative Pathology* 64:128–131.

Johnson, B.J., and A.E. Castro. 1986. Canary pox causing a high mortality in an aviary. *Journal of the American Veterinary Medical Association* 189:1345–1347.

Kaleta, E.F., and U. Ebert. 1969. Zur prophylaxe und therapie der karnarienpocken. *Deutsche Tieraeziliche Wochenschrift* 76:690–691.

Kaleta, E.F., and H.J. Marschall. 1982. Pox in Red Siskins (*Cardulis cucullata*). *Zentralblatte Veterinarmedizin, B.* 29:776–781.

Karpinski, L.G., and S.L. Clubb. An outbreak of pox in imported mynahs. *Proceedings of the Annual Meeting of the Association of Avian Veterinarians,* Miami, FL, U.S.A., pp. 35–37.

Karstad, L. 1965. An outbreak of pox in Impiyan pheasants. *Bulletin of the Wildlife Disease Association* 1:3.

Karstad, L. 1971. Pox. In *Infectious and Parasitic Diseases of Wild Birds,* J. W. Davis, R. C. Anderson, L. Karstad, and D. O. Trainers (eds.). Iowa State University Press, Ames, Iowa, U.S.A., pp. 34–41.

Kawashima, H. 1962. Die forschung ueber die Gefluegelpocken. *Japanese Journal of Veterinary Sciences* 24:19–28, 53–64, 122–132, 225–235.

Kear, J., and M. Brown. 1976. A pox-like condition in the Hawaiian Goose. *International Zoo Yearbook* 16:133–134.

Keymer, I.F., and D.K. Blackmore. 1964. Disease of the skin and soft parts of wild birds. *British Birds* 57: 175–179.

Kiel, H. 1985. Pockeninfektion bei Jagdfalken In *Proceedings of the II DVG-Tagung uber Vogelkrankheiten,* Munchen, Germany, pp. 202–206.

Kikuth, W., and H. Gollub. 1932. Versuche mit einem filtrierbarem virus bei einer uebertragbaren kanarienbogelkrankheit. *Zentralblatt Bakteriologie* 125:313–320.

Kim, T.J., W.M. Schnitzlein, D. McAloose, A.P. Pessier, and D.N. Tripathy. 2003. Characterization of an avianpox virus isolated from an Andean condor (*Vulur gryphus*). *Veterinary Microbiology* 96:237–246.

Kirmse, P. 1966. New wild bird hosts for pox viruses. *Bulletin for the Wildlife Diseases Association* 2:30–33.

Kirmse, P. 1967a. Pox in wild birds: an annotated bibliography. *Wildlife Disease* 49:1–10.

Kirmse, P. 1967b. Experimental pox infection in waterfowl. *Avian Diseases* 11:209.

Kirmse, P. 1967c. Host specificity and long persistence of pox infection in the flicker (*Colaptes auratus*). *Bulletin of the Wildlife Disease Association* 3:14–20.

Kirmse, P. 1969. Host specificity and pathogenecity of pox virus from wild birds. *Bulletin of the Wildlife Disease Association* 5:376–386.

Kirmse, P., and H. Loftin. 1969. Avian pox in migrant and native birds in Panama. *Bulletin of the Wildlife Disease Association* 5:103–107.

Kirmse, P., L. Karstad, and M. Warburton. 1966. New bird pox cases from New Jersey. *Ontario Bird Banding* 2:15–18.

Kitzing, D. 1980. Neuere erkenntnisse ueber das falkenpockenvirus. *Der Praktische Tierazt* 61:952–956.

Kohn, F.G. 1927. Epitheliosa curtis beim rebhuhn in freier wildbahn. *Prager Archiv für Tiermedizin* 7:181–190.

Kossack, C.W., and H.C. Hanson. 1954. Fowlpox in the mourning dove. *American Journal of the Veterinary Medical Association* 124:199–201.

Kraft, V., and P. Teufel. 1971. Nachweis eines pockenvirus bei zwergpapageien (*Agapornis personata* und *Agapornis rosecollis*). *Berliner und Muenchener Tieraerzliche Wochenschrift* 84:83–87.

Krone, O., S. Essbauer, G. Wibbelt, G. Isa, M. Rudolph, and R.E. Gough. 2004. Avipoxvirus infection in peregrine falcons (*Falco peregrinus*) from a reintroduction programme in Germany. *Veterinary Record* 2004:110–113.

Kreuder, C., A.R. Irizarry-Rovira, E.B. Janovitz, P.J. Deitschel, and D.B. DeNicola. 1999. Avian pox in sanderlings from Florida. *Journal of Wildlife Diseases* 35:582–585.

Kuntz, A., H.D. Schroder, and R. Ippen. 1968. Geflugelpocken bei Breitschwingenbussarden (Buteo platypterus). *Diseases of Zoo Animals,* 10th International Symposium, Salzburg, Austria, pp. 161–163.

Labisky, R.F., and S.H. Mann. 1961. Observation of avian pox in a yellow-shafted flicker. *Auk* 78:642.

Landowska-Plazewska, E., and L. Plazewski. 1968. Ausbruch von vogelpocken bei Humboldttpinguinen im Warschauer Zoo. *Diseases of Zoo Animals,* 10th International Symposium, Salzburg, Austria, pp. 159–159.

Landolt, M., and R.M. Kocan. 1976. Transmission of avian pox from Starlings to Rothchild's Mynahs. *Journal of Wildlife Diseases* 12:353–356.

LaPointe, D.A. 2000. Avian malaria in Hawaii: the distribution, ecology and vector potential of forest-dwelling mosquitoes. Ph.D. dissertation, University of Hawaii, Honolulu, HI, U.S.A.

Leibovitz, L. 1969. Natural occurrence and experimental study of pox and Haemoproteus in a mute swan. *Bulletin of the Wildlife Disease Association* 5:130–136.

Locke, L.N., W.O. Wirtz II, and E.E. Brown. 1965. Pox infection and a secondary cutaneous mycosis in a red-tailed tropicbird (*Phaethon rubricauda*). *Bulletin of the Wildlife Disease Association* 1:60–61.

Loir, A., and E. Ducloux. 1894. Contribution a l'etude de la dipthterie aviaire in Tunisie. *Annales de l'Institute Pasteur* 8:599–607.

Loupal, G., M. Schonbauer, and J. Jahn. 1985. Pocken bei zoo- und wildvogeln. *Journal of Veterinary Medicine B,* 32:326–336.

Luthgen, W. 1983. Untersckhungen ueber die bildung praezipitieren-der antikoeper bei der pockenerkrankung der tauben. *Journal of Veterinary Medicine B,* 15:772–781.

Lutz, R.S, and J.A. Crawford. 1987. Prevalence of poxvirus in a population of Merriam's wild turkeys in Oregon. *Journal of Wildlife Diseases* 23:306–307.

Maggiora, A., and G.L. Valenti. 1903. Ueber eine infektioese krankheit beim genus Turdus. *Zentralblatt für Bakteriologie* 34:326–335.

Mani, P., O. Fabiani, S. Bellini, and M. Fontanellli. 1990. Caratteristiche di crescita, morfologico-struttural i ed antigeniche di uno stipite di avipoxvirus isolato dalla stama (*Perdix perdix*). *Zootecnica International* 28. Convegno Forli, 147–152.

Markus, M.B. 1974. Arthropod-borne disease as a possible factor limiting the distribution of birds. *International Journal for Parasitology* 4:609–612.

Mathur, B.B., K.C. Verma, K. Agarwal, and S. Kumar. 1972. Serological survey for the detection of certain common respiratory infections in migratory birds: a note. *Indian Journal of Animal Science* 42:144–145.

McClure, H.E. 1989. Epizootic lesions of House Finches in Ventura County, California. *Journal of Field Ornithology* 60:421–430.

McDonald, S.E., L.J. Lowenstine, and A.A. Ardans. 1981. Avian pox in blue-fronted Amazon parrots. *Journal of the American Veterinary Medical Association* 179:1218–1222.

McGaughey, C.A., and F.M. Burnet. 1945. Avian pox in wild sparrows. *Journal of Comparative Pathology and Therapeutics* 55:201–205.

Medina, F.M., G.A. Ramirez, and A. Hernandez. 2004. Avian pox in White-tailed Laurel-pigeons from the Canary Islands. *Journal of Wildlife Diseases* 40:351–355.

Megnin, M.P. 1878. Observations de pathologie ornithologique. *Recueil de Medicine Veterinaire* 6:1052–1063.

Mercier, L. and R. Poisson. 1923. Un cas d'epithelioma contagieux chez un oisseau sauvage. *Compte Rendu de Semanas de la Societe de Biologie* 89:1196–1198.

Michael, H., and K.E. Lendner. 1964. Ueber das auftreten von pockenerkrankungen bei kanarien im Raum Leipzig. *Monatshefte für die Veterinaermedizin* 19:902–904.

Mikaelian, I., and D. Martineau. 1996. Cutaneous avian pox in a house sparrow. *Canadian Veterinary Journal* 37:434.

Miles, J.A., and M.G. Stocker. 1948. Puffinois, a virus epizootic of the Manx Shearwater (Puffinus puffinus). *Nature* 161:1016–1017.

Minsky, L., and M.L. Petrak 1982. Diseases of the digestive system. In *Diseases of Cage and Aviary Birds,* M.L. Petrak (ed.). Lea & Febiger, Philadelphia, PA, U.S.A., pp 432–448.

Moffat, R.E. 1972. Natural pox infection in a golden eagle. *Journal of Wildlife Diseases* 8:161–162.

Montgomery, R. D., K. A. Chowdvry, and J. G. Reeses. 1980. Avian pox in a whistling swan. *Journal of the American Veterinary Medical Association* 177: 930–931.

Morton, J.K., and R.A. Dieterich. 1979. Avian pox in an American green-winged teal (*Anas crecca carolinensis*) in Alaska. *Journal of Wildlife Diseases* 15:451–453.

Munro, G.C. 1944. Birds of Hawaii. Bridgeway Press, Rutland, Vermont.

Murphy, F.A., E.P.J. Gibbs, M.C. Horzinek, and M.J. Studdert. 1999. *Veterinary Virology,* 3rd Ed. Academic Press, New York, NY, U.S.A., 629 pp.

Musselman, T.E. 1928. Foot disease of chipping sparrow (*Spizella passerina*). *Auk* 45:137–147.

Nuttall, P.A., M. De L Brooke, and C.M. Perrins. 1985. Poxvirus infection of the Manx Shearwater (*Puffinus puffinus*). *Journal of Wildlife Diseases* 21:120–124.

Olmos, P.R., B.L. Martinez, J.E. Lopez, and L.P. Martinez. 1986. Patogenicidad y antigenidad de un aislamiento sospechoso de viruela de los loror (*Amazona stivae*), en gallinas. *Veterinario Mexico* 17:104–109.

Oros, J., F. Rodriquez, C. Bravo, A. Fernandez. 1997. Debilitating cutaneous poxvirus infection of a Hodgson's grandala (*Grandala coelicolor*). *Avian Diseases* 41:481–483.

Pearson, G.L., D.A. Pass, and E.C. Beggs. 1975. Fatal Pox infection in a Rough-legged Hawk. *Journal of Wildlife Diseases* 11:224–228.

Perelmann, B., A. Gur-Lavie, and Y. Samberg. 1988. Pox in ostriches. *Avian Pathology* 17:735–739.

Perkins, R.C.L. 1903. Vertebrata (Aves). In *Fauna Hawaiiensis,* Vol. 1, Part 4, David Sharp (ed.). The University Press, Cambridge, England, pp. 368–465.

Petrak, M.L. 1982. *Diseases of Cage and Aviary Birds,* 2nd Ed. Lea and Febiger, Philadelphia, PA, U.S.A., 679 pp.

Pettingill, O.S., Jr. 1985. *Ornithology in Laboratory and Field,* 5th Ed. Academic Press, Orlando, FL, U.S.A., 403 pp.

Pilaski, J.L. Rotschuh, and W. Encke. 1990. Ein pockenausbruch in einem ziervogelbestand des Krefelder Zoologischen Gartens. *Verhandlungsberichete des 32 Internationalen Symposiums ueber die Erkrankungen der Zoo- und Wildtiere,* Eskilstuna, Sweden.

Polowinkin, P. 1901. Beitrag zur pathologischen Anatomie der Taubenpocke. *Archiv Tierheilkunde* 27:86–109.

Pomeroy, D.E. 1962. Birds with abnormal bills. *British Birds* 55:49–72.

Poulding, R.H. 1960. Fowlpox in a carrion crow. *British Birds* 53:174–175.

Power, D.M., and G. Human. 1976. A local occurrence of avian pox in the House Finch. *Condor* 78:262–263.

Quinn, P.J. 1971. Suspected case of bird pox in a small population of New Zealand pipits. *Nortornis* 18:217.

Raidal, S.R., J.H. Gill, and G.M. Cross. 1966. Pox in ostrich chicks. *Australian Veterinary Journal* 73:32–33.

Rajchard, J., and V. Rachc. 2001. Find of bird-pox (*Variola avium*) in blackcap (*Sylvia atricapilla*). *Veterinarni Medicina* 46:78–79.

Rao, C.G. 1965. Studies on pox in ducks in Andhra Pradesh. *Indian Veterinary Journal* 42:151–155.

Ralph, C.J., and C. van Riper III. 1985. Historical and current factors affecting Hawaiian native birds. In *Bird Conservation,* Vol. II, S. Temple (ed.). University of Wisconsin Press, Madison, WI, U.S.A., pp. 7–42.

Ratcliff, H.L. 1967. Report of the Penrose Research Laboratory of the Zoological Society. Philadelphia, PA, U.S.A., pp. 11–12.

Reed, W.M., and D.L. Schrader. 1989. Pathogenicity and immunogenicity of mynah pox virus in chicken and bobwhite quail. *Poultry Science* 68:631–638.

Reis, J., and P. Nobrega. 1937. Sobre um virus tripathogenico de bouba de carario. *Archivos do Instituto Biologico, Sao Paulo Brasilia* 8:211–214.

Remple, J.D. 1988. An overview of Arab falconry, its medical lore, and the introduction of avian medicine in the Arabian Gulf. In *Peregrine Falcon Populations: Their Management and Recovery,* T.J.K. Cade, J.H. Enderson, C.G. Thelander, and C.M. White (eds.).

The Peregrine Fund, Inc., Boise, Idaho, U.S.A., pp. 825–830.

Rinaldi, A.H. Mahnel, L. Nardelli, G.C. Andelli, G. Cervio, A. Valeri. 1972. Charakterisierung eines wachtelpockenvirus. *Journal of Veterinary Medicine B,* 19:199–212.

Robinson, A.J., and P.J. Kerr. 2001. Poxvirus infections. In *Infectious Diseases of Wild Mammals,* E.S. Williams and I.K. Barker (eds.). Iowa State University Press, Ames, Iowa, U.S.A., pp. 179–201.

Rosen, M.N. 1959. Killing them with kindness. *Outdoor California* 20:12–13.

Salhoff, S. 1937. Pockendiptherie biei wildtauben. *Tieaerzliche Wochenschrift* 53:349.

Sato, T., T. Sugimori, and S. Ishii. 1962. Etiologic study on an outbreak of canary pox in Japan 1958. *Japanese Journal of Experimental Medicine* 32: 247–261.

Savage, H., and J.A. Dick. 1969. Fowl pox in Cassin's sparrow, *Amophila cassinii. Condor* 71:71–72.

Samour, J.H., and J.E. Cooper. 1993. Avian pox in birds of prey (Order: Faliconiformes) in Bahrain. *Veterinary Record* 132:342–345.

Samour, J.H., O.R. Kaaden, U. Wernery, and T.A. Bailey. 1996. An epornitic of avian pox in houbara bustards (Chlamydotis undulata macqueenii). *Zentralbl Veterniarmed B* 43:287–92.

Schnitzlein, W.M., G. Ghildyal, and D.N. Tripathy. 1988. Genomic and antigenic characterization of avipoxviruses. *Virus Research* 10:65–76.

Scott, J.M., S. Mountainspring, F.L. Ramsey, and C.B. Kepler. 1986. Forest bird communities of the Hawaiian Islands: Their dynamics, ecology, and conservation. *Studies in Avian Biology* Number 9.

Seidel, B. 1972. Zu einigen erkrankungen der haut und ihrer anhangsorgan e bei zootieren. *Diseases of Zoo Animals, 14th International Symposium,* Wrocaw, Poland, pp. 171–181.

Senne, D.A. 1989. Virus propagation in embryonating eggs. In *A Laboratory Manual for the Isolation and Identification of Avian Pathogens,* 3rd Ed. American Association of Avian Pathologists, Kennett Square, PA, U.S.A., pp. 176–181.

Service, M.W. 1976. *Mosquito Ecology: Field Sampling Methods.* John Wiley and Sons, New York, NY, 583 pp.

Sevoian, M. 1960. A quick method for the diagnosis of avian pox and infectious laryngotracheitis. *Avian Diseases* 4:474–477.

Sharma, V.K., J. Simon, and L.E. Hanson. 1968. Histologic study of tissue reaction in canaries, chicken embryos infected with a pox agent. *Avian Diseases* 12:594–606.

Shirinov, F.B., A.I. Ibragimova, and Z.G. Misirov. 972. Spread of fowl pox virus by the mite *Dermanyssus gallinae. Veterinariya* 4:48–49.

Sileo, L., P.R. Sievert, and M.D. Samuel. 1990. Causes of mortality of Albatross chicks at Midway Atoll. *Journal of Wildlife Diseases* 26:329–338.

Simpson, C.F., D.J. Forrester, and S.A. Nesbitt. 1975. Avian pox in Florida Sandhill Cranes. *Journal of Wildlife Diseases* 11:112–115.

Smits, J.E., J.L. Tella, M. Carrete, D, Serrano, and G. Lopez. 2005. An epizootic of avian pox in endemic short-toed larks (*Calandrella rufescens*) and Berthelot's Pipits (*Anthus berthelotti*) in the Canary Islands, Spain. *Vet. Pathology* 42:59–65.

Spalding, M.G., and D.J. Forrester. 1991. Effects of parasitism and disease on the reproductive success of colonial wading birds (Ciconiiformes) in southern Florida. Final Report. Florida Game and Fresh Water Fish Commission, Tallahassee, 121 pp.

Stadie, R. 1931. Gefluegelpockenklrankheit bei Rebhuehnem. *Deutsches Weidwerk* 36:572.

Stannard, L.M., D. Marias, D. Kow, and K.R. Dumbell. 1998. Evidence for incomplete replication of a penguin poxvirus in cells of mammalian origin. Journal of General Virology 79:1637–1646.

Stevenson, H.M., and B.H. Anderson. 1994. *The Birdlife of Florida.* University Press of Florida, Gainsville, Florida, U.S.A., 892 pp.

Stewart, P.A. 1963. Abnormalities among brown-headed cowbirds trapped in Alabama. *Bird-banding* 34:199–202.

Stoddard, H.L. 1931. *The Bobwhite Quail: Its Habits, Preservation and Increase.* Charles Scribner's Sons, New York, NY, U.S.A., 559 pp.

Stroud, R. 1933. *Diseases of Canaries.* T.F.H. Publications, Inc., Neptune City, New Jersey, U.S.A., 239 pp.

Sutton, R.H., and L.J. Fillipich. 1983. Poxvirus infection in a black-faced cuckoo-shrike (*Coracina novaehollandiae*). *Australian Veterinary Journal* 60:673–675.

Syverton, J.T., and I. McTaggerty Cowan. 1944. Bird pox in the sooty grouse (*Dedragapus fuliginosus fuliginosus*)with recovery of the virus. *American Journal of Veterinary Research* 5:215–222.

Tajima, M., and T. Ushijima. 1966. Electron microscopy of avian pox viruses with special reference to the significance of inclusion bodies in viral replication. *Japanese Journal of Veterinary Science* 28:107–118.

Tangredi, B.P. 1974. Avian pox in a mourning dove. *Veterinary Medicine, Small Animal Clinician* 69:700–701.

Tantawai, H.H., S. Al Sheikhly and F.K. Hassan. 1981. Avian pox in buzzard (*Accipter nisus*) in Iraq. *Journal of Wildlife Diseases* 17:145–146.

Tantawai, H.H., M.M. Al Falluji, and M.O. Shony. 1979. Heat-selected mutants of pigeon poxvirus. *Acta Virologica* 23:249–252.

Thiel, T, Whiteman, N.K., Tirape, A., Baquero, M.I., Cedeno, V., Walsh, T., Uzcategui, G. J., Parke,

P.G. 2005. Characterization of canarypox-like viruses infecting endemic birds in the Galapagos Islands. *Journal of Wildlife Diseases* 41:342–53.

Tietz, G. 1932. Ueber die emfaenglichkeit verschiedener vogelarten für eine infektion mit originaerem huehner— und taubenpockenvirus. *Archiv für Wissenschaftliche und Praktische Thierheilkunde* 65:244–255.

Tikasingh, E.S., C.B. Worth, L. Spence, and T.H.G. Aitken. 1982. Avian pox in birds from Trinidad. *Journal of Wildlife Diseases* 18:133–139.

Trapp, J.L. 1980. Avian pox in the Gray-crowned Rosy Finch in Alaska. North American Bird Bander 5:146–147.

Tripathy, D.N. 1993. Avipox viruses. In *Virus Infections of Vertebrates—Virus Infections of Birds,* J. B. McFerran and M. S. McNulty (eds.). Elsevier Science Publishers B. V., Amsterdam, The Netherlands, pp. 5–15.

Tripathy, D.N. 2000. Molecular techniques for the diagnosis of fowlpox. 137th AVMA Convention Notes, pp. 655–656.

Tripathy, D.N., L.E. Hanson, and R.A. Crandall. 1981. Poxviruses of veterinary importance: Diagnosis of infections. *In Comparative Diagnosis of Viral Diseases,* E. Kurstak and C. Kurstak (eds.). Academic Press, New York, NY, U.S.A., pp. 267–346.

Tripathy, D.N., and W.M. Reed. 2003. Pox. In *Diseases of Poultry,* 11th Ed., Y.M. Saif, H.J. Barnes, J.R. Glisson, A.M. Fadly, and L.R. McDougald (eds.). Iowa State University Press, Ames, Iowa, U.S.A., pp. 253–269.

Tripathy, D.N., W.M. Schnitzlein, P.J. Morris, D.L. Janssen, J.K. Zuba, G. Massey, and C.T. Atkinson. 2000. Characterization of poxviruses from forest birds in Hawaii. *Journal of Wildlife Diseases* 36: 225–230.

Tsai, S.S., T.C. Chang, S.F. Yang, Y.C. Chi, R.S. Cher, M.S. Chien, and C. Itakura. 1997. Unusual lesions associated with avian poxvirus infection in rosy-faced lovebirds (*Agapornis roseicollis*). *Avian Pathology* 26:75–82.

VanderWerf, E. 2001. Distribution and potential impacts of avian poxlike lesions in ‘Elepaio at Hakalau Forest National Wildlife Refuge. In *Studies in Avian Biology,* Vol. 22, J.M. Scott, S. Conant, and C. van Riper III (eds.). Allen Press, Lawrence, Kansas, U.S.A., pp. 247–253.

van Riper, C., III, and J.M. Scott. 2001. Limiting factors affecting Hawaiian native birds. In *Studies in Avian Biology,* Vol. 22, J. M. Scott, S. Conant, and C. van Riper III (eds.). Allen Press, Lawrence, Kansas, U.S.A., pp. 221–233.

van Riper, C., III, and S.G. van Riper. 1980. A necropsy procedure for sampling disease in wild birds. *Condor* 82:85–98.

van Riper, C., III, S.G. van Riper, and A.J. Berger. 1979. The Red whiskered Bulbul in Hawaii. *Wilson Bulletin* 91:323–328.

van Riper, C. III, S.G. van Riper, and W. Hansen. 2002. The epizootiology and effect of avian pox on Hawaiian forest birds. *Auk* 119:929–942.

van Riper, S.G., and C. van Riper III. 1985. A summary of known parasites and diseases from the avifauna of the Hawaiian Islands. In *The Preservation and Management of Terrestrial Hawaiian Ecosystems,* C. Stone and J.M. Scott (eds.). University Press of Hawaii, Honolulu, Hawaii, U.S.A., pp. 298–374.

Van Tyne, J., and A.J. Berger. 1976. *Fundamentals of Ornithology,* 2nd Ed., John Wiley & Sons, New York, NY, U.S.A., 808 pp.

Vargas, H. 1987. Frequency and effect of pox-like lesions in Galapagos Mockingbirds. *Journal of Field Ornithology* 58:101–102.

Vogelsang, E.G. 1938. Viruela aviaria en el Ñandú (*Rhea americana*). *La Semana Médica* 45:556–557.

von Schauberg, R. 1901. Eine monstroese schnabelbidung. Ornithologische Monatsberichte 9:18–19.

Warner, R.E. 1961. Susceptibility of the endemic Hawaiian avifauna to mosquito-borne malaria and bird pox. *10th Pacific Science Congress Abstracts,* p.487.

Warner, R.E. 1968. The role of introduced diseases in the extinction of the endemic Hawaiian avifauna. *Condor* 70:101–120.

Weli, S.C., M.I. Okeke, M. Tryland, O. Nilssen, and T. Traavik. 2004. Characterization of avipoxviruses from wild birds in Norway. *Canadian Journal of Veterinary Research* 68:140–145.

Westerskov, K. 1953. Bird pox in a New Zealand Pipit (*Anthys novaeseelandiae*). *Notornis* 5:168–170.

Wheeldon, E.B., C.J. Sedgwick, and T.A. Schulz. 1985. Epornitic of avian pox in a raptor rehabilitation center. *Journal of the American Veterinary Medical Association* 187:1202–1204.

Wilson, M.H., and J.A. Crawford. 1988. Pox-virus in scaled quail and prevalences of poxvirus-like lesions in northern bobwhites and scaled quail in Texas. *Journal of Wildlife Diseases* 24:360–363.

Wilner, B.K. 1969. A classification of the major groups of human and other animal viruses, 4th Ed. Burgess Publishing Co., Minneapolis, MN, U.S.A.

Wingate, D.B., I.K. Barker, and N.W. King. 1980. Poxvirus infection of the white-tailed tropicbird (*Phaethon lepturus*) in Bermuda. *Journal of Wildlife Diseases* 16:619–622.

Winteroll, G.,S. Mousa, and M. Akrae. 1979. Pockenisolate aus psittaciden und falken – Naehere Charakterisierung. *DVG-Fachgruppe Gefluegel – Tagung Krankheiten der Voegel, Muenchen,* pp. 117–125.

Wobeser, G.A. 1981. *Diseases of wild waterfowl.* Plenum Press, New York, NY, U.S.A., 324 pp.

Woodruff, C.E., and E.W. Goodpasture. 1930. The relation of the virus of fowl-pox to the specific cellular inclusions of the disease. *American Journal of Pathology* 6:713–720.

Worth, C.B. 1956. A pox virus of the slate-colored junco. *Auk* 73:230–234.

Zahn, S.N., and S.I. Rothstein. 1999. Recent increase in male house finch plumage variation and its possible relationship to avian pox disease. *Auk* 116:35–44.

Zangger, N., and M. Muller. 1990. Endemic poxvirus infection in white storks (*Ciconia ciconia*) and black storks (*Ciconia nigra*) in Switzerland. *Schweizerisches Archiv Tierheilkunde* 132:135–138.

Zhang, -DeLing, Jia-Jun Yuan, Chen FuWand, Wie-WanRen, Zang-Chen Hu, Wu-LianHua. 1996. Serological investigation of 16 infectious diseases in rare birds in the Lhanzou area. *Chinese Journal of Veterinary Medicine* 22:22.

7
Orthoreoviruses

Tuula Hollmén and Douglas E. Docherty

INTRODUCTION

The genus Orthoreovirus is classified in the family Reoviridae and contains viruses isolated from mammals and birds (Robertson and Wilcox 1986). Avian orthoreoviruses have been associated with a variety of disease syndromes in domestic and captive wild birds, including arthritis/tenosynovitis, growth retardation, enteritis, bursal and thymic atrophy, and chronic respiratory disease in chickens (*Gallus domesticus*); tenosynovitis and sudden death in domestic turkeys (*Meleagris gallopavo*); respiratory disease in captive Northern Bobwhite (*Colinus virginianus*); necrotizing hepatitis in psittacines; and pericarditis, necrotizing hepatitis, and splenitis in Muscovy Ducks (*Cairina moschata*)(Robertson and Wilcox 1986; McNulty 1993). Reoviruses have been isolated both from healthy and clinically ill quarantined birds, including psittacines, and are implicated as a potential disease agent associated with translocation of birds (Rigby et al. 1981). Reoviruses also have been associated with mortality in free-ranging birds, including Common Eiders (*Somateria mollissima*) and American Woodcock (*Scolopax minor*) (Docherty et al. 1994; Hollmén et al. 2002).

Overall, reoviral diseases of domestic poultry have been well characterized in scientific literature, whereas significantly less information is available on reoviruses as pathogens of wild birds. This chapter provides an overview of orthoreoviruses and describes specific disease syndromes associated with reovirus infections in free-ranging birds and in wild species held in captivity.

HISTORY

An organism first named the Fahey-Crawley agent was isolated in 1954 from chickens with respiratory disease in North America, and classified in 1957 as an avian reovirus (van der Heide 2000). The causative agent of synovitis in broilers was later also identified as a reovirus, and these first isolations were followed by reports of tenosynovitis in chickens from several locations in the U.S. and elsewhere (van der Heide 2000). Although most of the subsequent research on avian reoviruses has focused on arthritis and tenosynovitis in domestic chickens and turkeys, viruses within this group have been associated with a wide variety of other diseases and avian species (Robertson and Wilcox 1986; McNulty 1993; Rosenberger and Olson 1997). Reoviruses have been identified in wild avian species held in captivity in importation quarantine facilities and, more recently, have been associated with mortality events in wild avian populations (Rigby et al. 1981; Docherty et al. 1994; Hollmén et al. 2002).

DISTRIBUTION

Reoviruses have been reported in birds from several continents including the Americas, Australia, and Eurasia, and are probably ubiquitous.

HOST RANGE

Reoviruses have been isolated from species in several orders of birds, including Anseriformes, Charadriiformes, Columbiformes, Falconiformes, Galliformes, Gruiformes, Passeriformes, Piciformes, and Psittaciformes (Jones and Guneratne 1984; Robertson and Wilcox 1986; Gough et al. 1988; Takehara et al. 1989). In addition, serologic evidence of reovirus infections has been reported from Sphenisciformes (Karesh et al. 1999). The host range of reoviruses is likely even wider than that reported to date, due to a limited number of studies conducted on reoviruses in free-ranging birds.

ETIOLOGY

Orthoreovirus particles are non-enveloped with an icosahedral double-shelled capsid and measure approximately 60–80 nm in diameter. The genome consists of 10 segments of linear double-stranded RNA. Orthoreoviruses are resistant to heat, low pH, and most disinfectants, but may be inactivated by 70% ethanol, 0.5% organic iodine, and 5% hydrogen peroxide (McFerran and McNulty 1993; McNulty 1993; Rosenberger and Olson 1997).

At least 11 avian serotypes or antigenic subtypes have been described, with considerable cross-neutralization among heterologous types (Robertson and Wilcox 1986; McNulty 1993). The heterogeneity of avian reoviruses has also been demonstrated at the genetic level. Analysis of migration patterns of viral RNA by electrophoresis has produced evidence of genetic polymorphism among strains (Gouvea and Schnitzer 1982), and amino acid and nucleotide sequences obtained from avian reovirus strains originating from different species and continents have shown relatively low homology (Liu and Giambrone 1997; Le Gall-Reculé et al. 1999).

EPIZOOTIOLOGY

Determining whether an orthoreovirus is the etiologic agent or simply an opportunistic or coincidental finding in a wildlife mortality event poses challenges. Clinical signs, prevalence, and incidence of the disease in specific populations are rarely available. Experimental reproduction of the disease may be difficult because many of the wild species cannot be properly maintained in captivity, and experimental conditions usually differ from those encountered in the wild. The heterogeneity of avian orthoreoviruses and concurrent or secondary pathogens often associated with infections further complicate investigations of etiology.

It is possible that several of the avian reoviruses are species specific, although at least some are capable of cross-infections among species. Some isolates from turkeys, ducks, and a Wedge-tailed Eagle (*Aquila audax*) have been shown to be infectious to chickens, and an isolate from Common Eiders was found to be infectious to Mallards (*Anas platyrhyncos*) (Jones and Guneratne 1984; Nersessian et al. 1986; Hollmén et al. 2002). Little is known about virus persistence in wild birds, but asymptomatic carriers have been implicated as sources of infection in domestic birds. Persistently infected birds may shed viruses even when circulating antibodies are present. Both horizontal and vertical transmission have been documented for reoviruses, with fecal-oral transmission being considered the most likely route of natural infections (Rosenberger and Olson 1997). The incubation period in wild birds is unknown.

Little is known about the epizootiology of reoviruses in wild avian populations, and only few reports of reovirus associated mortality events in wild birds have been published. Some epizootiologic data have been gathered on reovirus prevalence in declining Common Eider populations in the Baltic Sea and American Woodcock in the eastern U.S.A.

In an effort to determine the prevalence of the woodcock reovirus, 421 American Woodcock were sampled from the eastern and central U.S.A. populations (Docherty et al. 1994). The woodcock reovirus was not isolated from any of these apparently healthy birds, and to date it has been isolated only from dead birds.

In the Baltic Sea, reoviruses were isolated in association with a mortality event of Common Eider ducklings in 1996, when it was estimated that up to 99% of 7,500 ducklings that hatched in a breeding area in the Finnish archipelago died before fledging (Hollmén et al. 2002). During the following three years (1997–1999), reovirus seroprevalences were monitored in nesting females in three breeding areas in the Baltic Sea. Reovirus antibody prevalence in nesting females ranged from 0 to 86%, and the highest seroprevalences coincided with high (98%) duckling mortality at one of the locations in 1999 (Hollmén et al. 2002). Serologic evidence of reovirus exposure was also found in Common Eider colonies in eastern (Maine) and northern (Alaska) U.S.A. (Hollmén, unpublished data).

CLINICAL SIGNS AND PATHOLOGY

Clinical signs and pathologic lesions associated with orthoreoviruses vary greatly due to viral heterogeneity, and variation in virulence among strains may result in different disease manifestations even within the same host species (Robertson and Wilcox 1986; McNulty 1993; Rosenberger and Olson 1997). Many reoviruses are asymptomatic in their natural hosts. Predisposing factors, such as translocation of birds, and secondary or concurrent infections may play an important role in reoviral diseases by altering host susceptibility (McNulty 1993). The pathogenesis of most avian reovirus infections, especially those involving free-ranging birds, has not been fully characterized.

Psittacines

It has been suggested that Old World psittacines are more susceptible to reovirus infections than those from the New World (Clubb et al. 1985). Clinical signs of psittacine reovirus infection include anorexia, lethargy, weight loss, dyspnea, and nasal discharge. Anemia and leucocytosis followed by leucopenia are common findings. Serum biochemistry changes include decreased albumin and increased globulin concentrations, and elevated aspartate aminotransferase and lactate dehydrogenase activities during late stages of disease, consistent with hepatic disease (Clubb et al. 1985). Macroscopic postmortem findings include hepatomegaly and splenomegaly, and microscopic lesions include acute multifocal or diffuse coagulative necrosis of the liver, with or without mononuclear inflammatory cell infiltrations. Intravascular thrombi or microthrombi are common. Co-infections with bacteria and fungi may complicate the interpretation of pathologic findings (Clubb et al. 1985). However, reoviruses have been shown to act as primary pathogens in African Gray Parrots (*Psittacus erithacus*) under experimental conditions without concurrent bacterial or fungal infections (Graham 1987).

Northern Bobwhite

In captive young Northern Bobwhites, reoviruses have been associated with respiratory distress, lethargy, and high mortality (up to 95%) in two- to 24-day-old chicks (Magee et al. 1993). Necrotizing hepatitis was the primary pathologic lesion described, and survivors were unthrifty.

Pigeons

Diarrhea and hepatitis have been associated with reovirus infections in pigeons (*Columba spp.*) (McFerran et al. 1976; Vindevogel et al. 1982). However, attempts to reproduce the lesions experimentally have failed, suggesting that other factors may be involved with the naturally occurring disease (Vindevogel et al. 1982).

American Woodcock

Reoviruses were isolated from American Woodcock involved in a mortality event at Cape Charles, Virginia, during the winters 1989–1990 (Docherty et al. 1994) and 1993–1994 (1994 case files, National Wildlife Health Center). No clinical signs were observed. Emaciation was the only abnormality noted. The infection appeared to be systemic because virus isolates were obtained from a variety of tissues including intestines, brains, hearts, lungs, and swabs from the cloaca.

Common Eiders

Reoviruses were isolated from Common Eider ducklings during a die-off in the northern Baltic Sea in 1996 (Hollmén et al. 2002). Clinical signs were nonspecific, and up to 99% of the 7,500 ducklings that hatched died at one to three weeks of age. Concurrent infections with intestinal helminths, renal coccidia, and pulmonary staphylococci were common. Reoviruses were isolated from the bursa of Fabricius of affected birds and the birds had lymphoid necrosis, suggesting an immunosuppressive effect. Multifocal hepatic necrosis was also found in reovirus-positive ducklings. The Common Eider reovirus was infectious to Mallard ducklings under experimental conditions. Elevations of serum creatine kinase, aspartate aminotransferase, and lactate dehydrogenase, suggestive of muscle and liver damage, were seen in the infected ducklings. No mortality was observed, but infected ducklings had focal hemorrhages in thymus, liver, spleen, myocardium, and/or bursa of Fabricius (Hollmén et al. 2002).

Muscovy Ducks

A disease of young Muscovy Ducks caused by an orthoreovirus has been described in South Africa, France, and Israel. The disease usually affects ducklings between two and four weeks of age, and clinical signs include general malaise, diarrhea, and stunted growth (Malkinson et al. 1981; Heffels-Redmann et al. 1992). The disease may cause up to 50% mortality. Postmortem lesions include hepatomegaly and splenomegaly with multifocal coagulative necrosis, pericarditis, coagulative necrosis of pancreas, synovitis, and lymphoid depletion in the bursa of Fabricius and the thymus. When the pathogenicity of two reovirus strains isolated from Muscovy Ducks was evaluated by experimental infections, it was seen that one produced lesions characteristic of natural infections, whereas the other was avirulent (Malkinson et al. 1981; Heffels-Redmann et al. 1992).

DIAGNOSIS

Differential diagnoses include a wide variety of infectious and noninfectious diseases because pathological findings associated with reoviruses may vary from emaciation to specific organ lesions. Diagnosis of a reovirus infection is best achieved by virus isolation and identification (McNulty 1993). Reoviruses are relatively stable, and samples intended for virus isolation can be stored at 4°C in transport medium for several days, or at −20°C or −70°C for longer periods. Several avian cell lines can be used for virus isolation, including chicken embryo liver and kidney cells, chicken embryo fibroblasts, and Muscovy Duck embryo fibroblasts, but their susceptibility to different virus strains may vary. Mammalian cell lines, especially Vero cells, also support the growth of some avian reoviruses. Reoviruses produce syncytial-type cytopathic effects in cultured cells. Embryonated eggs can also be used for virus isolation, and the inoculation of chorioallantoic membrane has been reported to be more successful than the allantoic cavity for virus propagation. Identification is based on size and morphology of virus particles determined by electron microscopy, stability of virus in low pH, and electropherotype of virus determined by electrophoresis of viral RNA segments. Orthoreovirus group-specific antigen may be demonstrated with the agar gel precipitin (AGP), fluorescent antibody (FA), and complement fixation (CF) tests. Orthoreoviruses can be further classified antigenically using serotype-specific antisera, and differences among strains also have been compared using genome sequence information (McNulty 1993; Rosenberger and Olson 1997).

Several techniques, including serum neutralization assays, enzyme-linked immunosorbent assay (ELISA), indirect fluorescent antibody (IFA) assay, AGP test, and Western blotting, have been used to detect reovirus antibodies in serum samples (McNulty 1993). Commercially available antibody tests generally use reagents derived from reoviruses of poultry origin, and assays specific to reoviruses originating from wild avian species have been developed and used for research projects. When serologic methods are used to monitor antibody levels or to determine whether birds have been exposed to reoviruses, the interpretation of results must be considered carefully due to antigenic cross-reactions among serotypes, the ubiquitous nature of reoviruses, and the possibility of subclinical and asymptomatic infections. Because reoviruses are frequently recovered from asymptomatic birds, further characterization of viral pathogenicity (that is, by experimental infectivity studies) is usually required to assess the significance of new isolates.

IMMUNITY

Both group-specific and serotype-specific antigens are present in avian reoviruses. Neutralizing and precipitating antibodies may be detected in serum after seven to 10 days post-infection, and neutralizing antibodies persist longer in circulation. The role of antibodies in resistance to re-infection is not well understood, but maternal antibodies may provide at least some immunity against natural and experimental infections in young birds. Survival and recovery from infection probably also requires T-cell-mediated immunity (Rosenberger and Olson 1997).

PUBLIC HEALTH CONCERNS

Avian orthoreoviruses present no known danger to human health.

DOMESTIC ANIMAL HEALTH CONCERNS

Viral arthritis/tenosynovitis is economically the most important reoviral disease in domestic poultry. Too little is known of the occurrence of arthritis/tenosynovitis virus in wild birds to evaluate their role as a source of poultry infections. Although experimental studies have shown that reoviruses isolated from wild birds can be infective to domestic poultry (Jones and Guneratne 1984), nothing is known about their significance as a poultry pathogen.

TREATMENT AND CONTROL

Until the epizootiology of reovirus infections in wild birds is elucidated, only general disease control methods can be recommended. Removal of carcasses during a die-off reduces the possibility of virus transmission and contamination of the environment. Control of reoviruses may be important in imported and quarantined wild birds, such as psittacines. Treatment is limited to supportive care and control of secondary bacterial infections that are typically associated with reoviruses. Reoviruses are difficult to eliminate from the environment because of their resistance to chemical and physical disinfectants, but clorhexidine has been used successfully to control contamination (Clubb et al. 1985). Commercially available poultry vaccines have not been found to provide protection against reovirus infections in other species of birds, but autogenous vaccines were considered effective in reducing morbidity and mortality in a psittacine study (Clubb et al. 1985).

MANAGEMENT IMPLICATIONS

Although little is known about reoviruses in wild birds, evidence is emerging indicating that these viruses contribute to disease and mortality in free-ranging populations. Investigations of mortality events in wild birds should consider previously unrecognized viruses, such as reoviruses. Because there is evidence of concurrent infections in association with reoviruses, complex interactions of infectious and parasitic agents should be considered. In captive situations, monitoring birds for signs of illness, serological testing, and disinfection of cages may help prevent the spread of disease to wild birds.

LITERATURE CITED

Clubb, S.L., J. Gaskin, and E.R. Jacobson. 1985. Psittacine reovirus: an update including a clinical description and vaccination. In *Proceedings of the Association of Avian Veterinarians,* pp. 85–90.

Docherty, D.E., K.A. Converse, W.R. Hansen, and G.W. Norman. 1994. American woodcock (*Scolopax minor*) mortality associated with a reovirus. *Avian Diseases* 38:899–904.

Gough, R.E., D.J. Alexander, M.S. Collins, S.A. Lister, and W. J. Cox. 1988. Routine virus isolation or detection in the diagnosis of diseases in birds. *Avian Pathology* 17:893–907.

Gouvea, V.S., and T.J. Schnitzer. 1982. Polymorphism of the migration of double-stranded RNA genome segments of avian reoviruses. *Journal of Virology* 43: 465–471.

Graham, D.L. 1987. Characterization of a reo-like virus and its isolation from and pathogenicity for parrots. *Avian Diseases* 31:411–419.

Heffels-Redmann, U., H. Müller, and E.F. Kaleta. 1992. Structural and biological characteristics of reoviruses isolated from Muscovy Ducks (*Cairina moschata*). *Avian Pathology* 21:481–491.

Hollmén, T., J.C. Franson, M. Kilpi, D.E. Docherty, W.R. Hansen, and M. Hario. 2002. Isolation and characterization of a reovirus from common eiders (*Somateria mollissima*) from Finland. *Avian Diseases* 46:478–484.

Jones, R.C., and J.R.M. Guneratne. 1984. The pathogenicity of some avian reoviruses with particular reference to tenosynovitis. *Avian Pathology* 13:173–189.

Karesh, W.B., M.M. Uhart, P. Gandini, W.E. Braselton, H. Puche, and R. A. Cook. 1999. Health evaluation of free-ranging rockhopper penguins (*Eudyptes chrysocomes*) in Argentina. *Journal of Zoo and Wildlife Medicine* 30:25–31.

Le Gall-Reculé, G., M. Cherbonnel, C. Arnauld, P. Blanchard, A. Jestin, and V. Jestin. 1999. Molecular characterization and expression of the S3 gene of muscovy duck reovirus strain 89026. *Journal of General Virology* 80:195–203.

Liu, H.G., and J.J. Giambrone. 1997. Amplification, cloning, and sequencing of the sigma C-encoded gene of avian reovirus. *Journal of Virological Methods* 63: 203–208.

Magee, D.L., R.D. Montgomery, W.R. Maslin, C. Wu, and S. W. Jack. 1993. Reovirus associated with excessive mortality in young bobwhite quail. *Avian Diseases* 37:1130–1135.

Malkinson, M., K. Perk, and Y. Weisman. 1981. Reovirus infection of young muscovy ducks (*Cairina moschata*). *Avian Pathology* 10:433–440.

McFerran, J.B., T.J. Connor, and R.M. McCracken. 1976. Isolation of adenoviruses and reoviruses from avian species other than domestic fowl. *Avian Diseases* 20:519–524.

McFerran, J.B., and M.S. McNulty. 1993. Reoviridae. In *Virus Infections of Birds,* J.B. McFerran and M.S. McNulty (eds.). Elsevier Science Publishers, Amsterdam, the Netherlands, pp. 177–179.

McNulty, M.S. 1993. Reovirus. In *Virus Infections of Birds,* J. B. McFerran and M. S. McNulty, (eds.). Elsevier Science Publishers, Amsterdam, the Netherlands, pp. 181–193.

Nersessian, B., M.A. Goodwin, R.K. Page, S.H. Kieven, and J. Brown. 1986. Studies on orthoreoviruses isolated from young turkeys. III. Pathogenic effects in chicken embryos, chicks, poults, and suckling mice. *Avian Diseases* 30:585–592.

Rigby, C.E., J.R. Pettit, G. Papp-Vid, J.L. Spencer, and N.G. Willis. 1981. The isolation of Salmonellae, Newcastle disease virus and other infectious agents from quarantined imported birds in Canada. *Canadian Journal of Comparative Medicine* 45:366–370.

Robertson, M.D., and G.E. Wilcox. 1986. Avian reovirus. *Veterinary Bulletin* 56:155–174.

Rosenberger, J.K., and N.O. Olson. 1997. Viral arthritis. In *Diseases of Poultry,* 10th Ed., B.W. Calnek, H.J. Barnes, C.W. Beard, L.R. McDonald, and Y.M. Saif (eds.). Iowa State University Press, Ames, Iowa, U.S.A., pp. 711–719.

Takehara, K., C. Kawai, A. Seki, N. Hashimoto, and M. Yoshimura. 1989. Identification and characterization of an avian reovirus isolated from black-tailed gull (*Larus crassirostris*). *Kitasato Archives of Experimental Medicine* 62:187–198.

Van der Heide, L. 2000. The history of avian reovirus. *Avian Diseases* 44:638–641.

Vindevogel, H., G. Meulemans, P. Pastoret, A. Schwers, and C. Calberg-Bacq. 1982. Reovirus infection in the pigeon. *Annales de Recherches Veterinaires* 13: 149–152.

8
Avian Adenoviruses

Scott D. Fitzgerald

INTRODUCTION

Adenoviruses are ubiquitous in domestic and wild birds throughout the world. Although adenoviral infections are a significant cause of economic loss to the commercial poultry industry, less is known about adenoviral infections in wild bird populations. Much of what is known about avian adenoviruses comes from extensive study in domestic and captive birds, with data extrapolated and supplemented by anecdotal reports in low numbers of wild birds. Some adenoviral infections can cause disease and mortality on their own, whereas other adenoviruses cause disease only in combination with other immunosuppressive infectious agents. In general, adenoviral infections in wild birds are subclinical or cause only sporadic disease in local bird populations over a limited geographic area. Many descriptions of adenoviral-induced disease in wild bird species are limited to birds held in captivity.

Adenoviruses are divided into several genera: those infecting mammals or Mastadenoviridae, and those infecting birds that are members of the *Aviadenoviridae,* the *Siadenoviridae,* or the *Atadenoviridae. Aviadenoviruses* are composed of five species of fowl adenovirus (fowl adenovirus A though E) divided into 12 serotypes, as well as tentative species of duck, pigeon, and turkey adenoviruses. Important diseases in the *Aviadenovirus* genus include inclusion body hepatitis, quail bronchitis, and hydropericardium syndrome. The *Siadenvirus* genus consists of viruses that are typically capable of producing disease without any immunosuppressive factors, and include the viruses producing hemorrhagic enteritis of turkeys, marble spleen disease of pheasants, and splenomegaly of chickens. The *Atadenovirus* genus is limited to a single entity, the egg drop syndrome virus affecting chickens but originating from ducks. There are additional recently described adenoviruses from various wild bird species that do not appear to match characteristics with any of the three avian adenovirus genera and remain unclassified at this time.

HISTORY

The first *aviadenovirus* recognized and serving as the type virus for the genus was chicken embryo lethal orphan (CELO) virus. CELO virus was inadvertently isolated from embryonated chicken eggs in 1957, and although it caused death in embryos (chicken embryo lethal), it produced no disease or lesions when inoculated into chickens (orphan) (McFerran 2003). The first avian adenovirus associated with clinical disease was isolated from Northern Bobwhite (*Colinus virginianus*) in West Virginia suffering from respiratory lesions in 1949 (Reed and Jack 2003). It has been subsequently shown that the CELO virus and the quail bronchitis virus (QBV) are both fowl adenovirus A, serotype 1, and indistinguishable by conventional methods. The vast majority of published reports of *aviadenovirus* infections have come from captive birds, including domestic chickens, turkeys, and ducks, as well as captive-reared Northern Bobwhite. However, one study conducted in 1976 demonstrated the presence of *aviadenovirus* in the ceca and livers of free-living Northern Bobwhite. Subsequent surveillance showed that 23% of the local Northern Bobwhite population exhibited titers against QBV, indicating previous exposure (King et al. 1981). Additional *aviadenovirus* reports from wild bird species have included inclusion body hepatitis in captive-reared Gambel's Quail (*Callipela gambelii*) chicks exhibiting significant mortality (Bradley et al. 1994), and inclusion body hepatitis from captive reared pigeons in Europe, Japan, Australia, and North America (Vindevogel et al. 1981; Takase et al. 1990; Ketterer et al, 1992). In 1978 an outbreak of hemorrhagic enteritis and inclusion body hepatitis occurred in a captive colony of American Kestrels (*Falco sparverius*) at the Patuxent Wildlife Research Center, Maryland, which was associated with adenoviral particles consistent with *aviadenovirus* (Sileo et al. 1983).

The second genus of avian adenoviruses is the *Siadenovirus.* Hemorrhagic enteritis (HE) virus of turkeys was the first of the three siadenoviruses identified; it was initially reported from domestic turkeys in Minnesota in 1937 (Pierson and Fitzgerald 2003). HE is now an important worldwide disease of captive turkeys; however, limited serologic surveys have failed to identify serologic titers in wild turkeys (*Meleagris gallopavo*). Marble spleen disease (MSD) of pheasants was first recognized in captive Ring-necked Pheasants (*Phasianus colchicus*) in Italy in 1958 (Fitzgerald and Reed 1989). Since then, MSD has become an important cause of mortality in captive pheasants on at least three continents; again, there is no evidence of its spread into wild pheasants in spite of frequent release of captive birds to the wild. Splenomegaly virus of chickens was the most recently recognized member of the *siadenovirus* genus. It was initially reported in 1979 that broiler chickens in the southeastern U.S.A. had splenomegaly due to an avian adenovirus similar to HE and MSD viruses. Generally, splenomegaly in chickens is a subclinical disease, although there is at least one report of low mortality associated with pulmonary edema (Pierson and Fitzgerald 2003).

The avian adenovirus in the genus *atadenovirus* is one of the more recently recognized. The initial outbreak of egg drop syndrome (EDS) occurred in domestic laying hens from the Netherlands in 1976 (McFerran and Adair 2003b). Egg drop syndrome is characterized by a marked decrease in rate of lay, accompanied by poor egg quality including decreased shell pigment, thin or soft-shelled eggs, and even shell-less eggs. This disease affects laying hens with reductions in egg production of up to 40%, so it has serious economic consequences. Since the initial report, EDS virus and/or antibodies against this virus have been found repeatedly in various domesticated ducks and geese, as well as serologic evidence in a variety of wild waterfowl species, throughout the world (Scholer 1979; Gulka et al. 1984; Hlinak et al. 1998). Although infected ducks develop no disease themselves, they may shed the virus to domestic poultry through their droppings, leading to sporadic outbreaks. It is now believed that EDS virus originated in ducks, and it is classified as a duck adenovirus, serotype 1 (McFerran and Adair 2003b).

DISTRIBUTION

Aviadenoviruses are present worldwide in domestic chickens, captive-reared quail, and pigeons. The aviadenoviruses are sporadically reported in captive ducks and geese, ostriches, turkeys, and captive psittacine birds. The few free-living wild bird reports (kestrels, Gambel's Quail) are generally limited to one or two reports, with the exception of more widespread occurrences of QBV (Sileo et al. 1983; Bradley et al. 1994). Siadenoviruses are represented by HE virus of captive turkeys worldwide; by MSD virus in captive-reared pheasants in North America, Europe, and Australia; and by splenomegaly of chickens restricted to the U.S.A. The atadenovirus, EDS virus, occurs worldwide in domestic fowl, ducks, and geese, as well as serologic evidence in wild waterfowl (see Table 8.1).

HOST RANGE

Aviadenoviruses have been identified and sometimes isolated from chickens, ducks, turkeys, Guinea fowl, kestrels, Northern Bobwhite, Gambel's quail, pigeons, ostriches, and assorted psittacine birds, including Budgerigars (*Melopsittacus undulatus*), lovebirds, Cockatiels (*Nymphicus hollandicus*), cockatoos, conures, macaws, parrots, and parakeets (Table 8.1). Siadenoviruses have been isolated from turkeys, captive pheasants, and chickens. *Atadenovirus,* specifically the virus causing EDS, has been isolated from chickens and from captive ducks and geese, and serologic evidence has been detected in many wild waterfowl including Ruddy Ducks (*Oyxura jamaicensis*), Ring-necked Ducks (*Aythya collaris*), Wood Ducks (*Aix sponsa*), Buffleheads (*Bucephala albeola*), Muscovy Ducks (*Cairina moschata*), Mallards (*Anas platyrhynchos*), mergansers (*Mergus spp.*), Lesser Scaups (*Aythya affinis*), Gadwalls (*Anas strepera*), Northern Shovelers (*Anas clypeata*), American Coots (*Fulica americana*), grebes (*Podiceps & Podilymbus spp.*), Canada Geese (*Branta canadensis*), Bean Geese (Anser fabalis) and White-fronted Geese (*Anser albifrons*)(Gulka et al. 1984; Hlinak et al. 1998). Several unclassified avian adenoviruses have been reported in Common Eiders (*Somateria mollisima*), Long-tailed Ducks (Clangula hyemalis), Common Murres (*Uria aalge*), and Herring Hulls (*Larus argentatus*) (Lowenstine and Fry 1985; Leighton 1984; Hollmen et al. 2003a; Hollmen et al. 2003b).

ETIOLOGY

As previously stated, avian adenoviruses are divided into three genera. The *aviadenovirus* genus is further divided into five species (A–E) based on restriction enzyme fragmentation patterns and genome sequencing data. These species are further differentiated into 12 serotypes based on cross neutralization assays. The *siadenovirus* genus includes three diseases associated with serotype 3 of a turkey adenovirus. The *atadenovirus* genus consists of a single species of duck adenovirus serotype 1, which produces EDS in chickens (Benko et al. 2000; McFerran 2003) (Table 8.1).

All avian adenoviruses have non-enveloped, icosahedral, 70 to 90 nm diameter virions. Their virions are composed of 252 capsomeres, with capsomeres arranged in triangular faces with six capsomeres on each edge, accounting for 240 capsomeres. The final

Table 8.1. Summary of avian adenoviruses including classification, bird species affected, and geographic distribution.

Genus	Old Classification	Disease	Adenovirus Species & Serotype[a]	- Host Species Common	Host Species-Scientific	First report (Year & Location)	Current Distribution[b]	Free or Captive	Disease Assoc.	VI or Serology[c]
Aviadenovirus	Group I avian adenovirus	Inclusion Body Hepatitis	FAdVA-E-1-10,12	Chickens	*Gallus gallus*	unknown	Worldwide	Captive	Yes	VI
			unknown	Kestrels	*Falco sparverius*	1983–U.S.A.	First report	Captive	Yes	No
			unknown	Gambel's Quail	*Callipepla gambelli*	1994–Arizona	First report	Captive	Yes	VI
		Quail Bronchitis Virus	FAdVA-1	Bobwhite Quail	*Colinus virginianus*	1949–W. Virginia	Worldwide	Captive & Free	Yes	VI
		Hydropericardium Syndrome	FAdVC-4	Chickens	*Gallus gallus*	1987–Pakistan	Asia, Central& South America	Captive	Yes	VI
		Duck Adenovirus	DAdV-2	Ducks & Geese	Multiple	1984–Canada	Canada	Captive	Yes	VI
		Turkey Adenovirus	TAdV-1,2	Turkeys	*Meleagris gallapavo*	1977–U.S.A.	U.S.A.	Captive	Yes	VI
		Pigeon Adenovirus	PIAdV	Pigeons	*Columba livia*	1992–Australia	Worldwide	Captive	Yes	VI
		Ostrich Adenovirus	unknown	Ostriches	*Struthio camelus*	1993–U.S.A.	North America, England	Captive	Yes	VI
		Psittacine Adenovirus	unknown	Psittacines	Multiple	unknown	Worldwide	Captive	Yes	VI
Siadenovirus	Group II avian Adenovirus	Hemorrhagic Enteritis	TAdV-3	Turkeys	*Meleagris gallopavo*	1937–Minnesota	Worldwide	Captive	Yes	VI
		Marble Spleen Disease		Pheasants	*Phasinius colchicus*	1965–Italy	North America, Europe, Australia	Captive	Yes	VI

		Splenomegaly		Chickens	*Gallus gallus*	1979– U.S.A.	U.S.A.	Captive	No	VI
Atadeno-virus	Group III avian adenovirus	Egg Drop Syndrome	DAdV-1	Chickens	*Gallus gallus*	1976– Netherlands	Worldwide	Captive	Yes	VI
				Ducks & geese	Multiple	unknown	Worldwide	Captive Free	No No	VI Serology
Unclassi fied		Duck Mortality	unknown	Long-tailed ducks	*Clangula hyemalis*	2003– Alaska	First report	Free	Yes	VI
		Eider Impaction	unknown	Common Eiders	*Somateria mollissima*	2003– Finland	First report	Free	Yes	VI
		Gull bursal adenovirus	unknown	Herring gulls	*Laurus argentatus*	1984– Newfoundland	First report	Free	No	No
		Murre renal adenovirus	unknown	Common Murre	*Urie alge*	1985– California	First report	Captive	No	No

[a] Current adenoviral classification includes FAdV (Fowl adenoviruses, 5 species (A–E), 12 serotypes), DAdV (Duck adenoviruses, 2 serotypes), TAdV (Turkey adenoviruses, 3 serotypes), PiAdV (Pigeon adenoviruses).

[b] Current distribution indicates known regions with infection of this virus; first report indicates no additional spread of the virus since its first report.

[c] VI indicates virus isolated from tissue, whereas serology indicates presence of antibodies only. "No" indicates neither virus isolation nor antibody detection; description based on microscopic and electron-microscopic morphology.

12 capsomeres form the vertex capsomeres, and each has one or more fiber projections (two fibers in aviadenoviruses, one fiber in the siadenovirus). The density of the virions varies between 1.32 and 1.37 gm/ml in cesium chloride. The genome is not segmented and composed of a single molecule of double-stranded DNA. DNA composes between 11.3 to 13.5 percent of the total virion, with the remainder consisting of proteins (McFerran and Adair 2003a).

Fowl adenovirus serotype 1 (FAdV-1) is the prototype of aviadenoviruses. The guanine-cytosine (G-C) component of its DNA is 54%. Between 11 and 14 structural polypeptides have been described for FAdV-1; these include several capsid proteins, two fiber proteins, and several core proteins (McFerran and Adair 2003a). In addition, nonstructural polypeptides include a DNA polymerase and a replicase enzyme. The complete genome of CELO virus, an FAdV-1, was sequenced in 1996, consisting of 43,804 base pairs in length (Chiocca et al. 1996).

HE virus, of the *siadenovirus* genus, was completely sequenced in 1998 (Pitcovski et al. 1998). Its genome measures 26,263 base pairs in length. The G-C component of 34.9% is significantly less than that of aviadenoviruses. The virus contains 11 structural polypeptides. EDS virus, of the *atadenovirus* genus, has the smallest genome of the avian adenoviruses, and has a very high A-T content, and contains 13 structural polypeptides (McFerran and Adair 2003b).

All three genera of avian adenoviruses are resistant to lipid solvents and are stable over a pH range from 3 to 9. All avian adenoviruses show greater heat stability than mammalian adenoviruses, but heating HE virus at 70°C for one hour, or heating EDS virus at 60°C for 30 minutes, will inactivate them. Infectivity of these viruses is destroyed after treatment with 0.5% formaldehyde, or treatment with a variety of disinfectants (0.0086% sodium hypochlorite, 1.0% sodium lauryl sulfate, 0.4% Chlorocide, 0.4% Phenocide, 0.4% Wescodyne, or 1.0% Lysol) (McFerran and Adair 2003a; Pierson and Fitzgerald 2003).

EPIZOOTIOLOGY

Aviadenoviruses are typically spread by horizontal transmission, through fecal shedding, urates, or nasal secretions. The viruses are usually shed in the feces at peak levels between four and six weeks post-infection, but have been detected up to 14 weeks (McFerran and Adair 2003a). Because these viruses are moderately resistant to heat, they may be spread by fomites and persist in the environment for a number of days. Vertical transmission through the egg also occurs. Incubation periods for these viruses are short (one to two days). Several of the fowl aviadenoviruses, such as QBV of Northern Bobwhite and the virus producing hydropericardium syndrome in commercial chickens, are highly pathogenic. In general, these viruses are most pathogenic in juvenile birds; QBV is most pathogenic in quail under six weeks of age, and hydropericardium mortality peaks in chickens from four to five weeks of age (McFerran and Adair 2003a; Reed and Jack 2003). Many of the other aviadenoviruses are considerably less pathogenic. The fowl adenoviruses associated with inclusion body hepatitis in chickens may cause disease and mortality, frequently in association with immunosuppressive viruses such as infectious bursal disease virus or chicken infectious anemia virus. Aviadenoviruses isolated from turkeys, pigeons, ducks, and geese have been isolated from birds with no clinical illness. In turkeys, efforts to reproduce disease through experimental infections have been unsuccessful (McFerran and Adair 2003a).

Siadenoviruses are transmitted only horizontally, through fecal shedding, infected carcasses, and contaminated litter. Both HE virus and MSD virus are primary pathogens, although they produce significantly more mortality in juvenile birds (turkeys are most affected between four and 11 weeks of age; pheasants are most affected between three and eight months of age)(Pierson and Fitzgerald 2003). The early post-hatch periods when birds are refractory to infection are likely due to the presence of maternal antibodies. Both HE and MSD viruses have been shown to cause immunosuppression in birds post-infection (McFerran and Fitzgerald 2003). The adenovirus of splenomegaly in chickens usually produces subclinical infection. These siadenoviruses likely persist in the environment for days due to their heat resistance. Interestingly, neither HE nor MSD viruses have been reported as causing clinical disease in wild bird populations, suggesting that captive rearing of birds at high density may be a necessary condition for virus transmission (Pierson and Fitzgerald 2003).

EDS *atadenovirus* can spread horizontally through feces and oviductal secretions, or vertically through the embryonated egg. Therefore, several different disease outbreak manifestations may be encountered. Vertically infected birds may reactivate the virus during egg production, leading to decreased egg quality and production as well as virus shedding. The virus may spread by slow horizontal transmission through an endemically infected flock, causing prolonged decreased egg production. Or a layer flock may be infected as a sudden sporadic episode due to drinking water contaminated by ducks or geese. The onset of EDS following exposure tends to be longer than for other avian adenoviruses, varying from seven to 17 days post-infection. This virus is also somewhat resistant to heat and may persist for days in the environment, especially in fecal-contaminated water (McFerran and Adair 2003b).

CLINICAL SIGNS

Aviadenoviruses have been associated with variable clinical manifestations ranging from subclinical infection to syndromes with high mortality. QBV produces a rapid disease course (one to three weeks) in young birds and is characterized by rales, coughing, sneezing, depression, and mortality rates from 10 to 100% (Reed and Jack 2003). A similar range of upper respiratory signs has been reported in turkeys infected by an aviadenovirus producing inclusion body tracheitis; however, species and strain characterization were not performed (Crespo et al. 1998). The other commonly manifested syndrome associated with aviadenoviruses is hepatitis, referred to as inclusion body hepatitis. Adenoviral hepatitis has been reported in Northern Bobwhite, Gambel's Quail, pigeons, and domestic chickens. Inclusion body hepatitis is characterized by a rapid disease course (one to three weeks), diarrhea, decreased appetite, lethargy, and low to moderate mortality rates (less than 10% to 30%) (McFerran and Adair 2003a). In Northern Bobwhite, bronchitis and inclusion body hepatitis have been seen simultaneously in both natural and experimental infections (Reed and Jack, 2003). Hemorrhagic enteritis associated with inclusion body hepatitis has been described in captive American Kestrels, with both juvenile and adults affected (Sileo et al. 1983). Signs were limited to cloacal hemorrhage and sudden death. This was initially attributed to a group II adenovirus (*siadenovirus*) based on the hemorrhagic enteritis. However, it is now presumed to be an *aviadenovirus,* although definitive virus isolation and classification studies have not been reported. A recently recognized syndrome associated with an *aviadenovirus* infection is hydropericardium syndrome in chickens, which is identical to inclusion body hepatitis but is associated with higher mortality rates and the presence of marked pericardial effusion for which the syndrome is named (McFerran and Smyth 2000). A wide variety of pet psittacine birds have had adenoviral inclusions found microscopically or the causative virus isolated. Reported signs range from depression, anorexia, central nervous system signs, diarrhea, and death, to totally asymptomatic birds (Ritchie 1995a).

Siadenovirus produces marble spleen disease in young (two to eight months old) pheasants, which usually results in sudden death without premonitory signs, although there is occasional respiratory distress or nasal discharge in some birds (Fitzgerald and Reed 1989). Hemorrhagic enteritis in turkeys is characterized by bloody diarrhea, lethargy, and low to moderate mortality rates in young (one to three months old) poults (Pierson and Fitzgerald 2003). Splenomegaly virus infection of chickens is usually subclinical, although one report describes pulmonary distress and low mortality.

The *atadenovirus* that produces egg drop syndrome appears to be a clinical problem only in domestic laying hens. Signs include production of smaller-than-normal eggs, soft-shelled, thin-shelled, or shell-less eggs, and either a rapid or extended loss in egg production of up to 40%. Clinical signs are generally limited to poor egg quality and production losses (McFerran and Adair 2003b).

PATHOGENESIS

Quail bronchitis/hepatitis virus is one of the best studied of the fowl adenoviruses affecting wild bird species (Jack and Reed 1990; Jack et al. 1994b). Younger birds are most susceptible to infection, with highest morbidity and mortality in birds three weeks of age or less. Intratracheally inoculated birds exhibit viremia within 8 hours of inoculation, with virus being present in the lungs, liver, spleen, bursa of Fabricius, and cecal tonsils at that time. Highest levels of virus titers are present at four to six days post-infection, which corresponds with the most severe tracheal lesions.

There has been extensive investigation into the pathogenesis of both HE and MSD viruses, with MSD virus being perhaps the more important of the two for wild bird species. The disease course is rapid, with mortality occurring three to six days post-infection and the outbreak usually lasting one to two weeks. Young birds up to three months of age exhibit highest mortality rates. The viruses replicate in the spleen because they have affinity for B lymphocytes and histiocytes. Viremia occurs, and pheasants generally die of pulmonary edema, whereas turkeys develop severe hemorrhagic enteritis. The reason for the difference between the two viral-induced syndromes is not completely known; it may be the result of species variation in the host birds, although some researchers believe that mast cells mediate the enteric response in turkeys with HE (Pierson and Fitzgerald 2003). The pulmonary edema seen in MSD may be related to unknown environmental factors or secondary infections, because this lesion is not generally reproduced in experimental infections (Fitzgerald and Reed 1989). Both viruses result in significant post-infection immunosuppression (Pierson and Fitzgerald 2003).

The *atadenovirus* of EDS undergoes viremia and viral replication in lymphoid tissues and the infundibulum by three to four days post-infection. Between seven and 20 days post-infection, there is massive viral replication in the shell gland and other portions of the oviduct with an associated inflammatory reaction, which corresponds with production of abnormal eggs (McFerran and Adair 2003b).

PATHOLOGY

Infection with fowl adenovirus A, serotype 1 (FAdVA-1) produces the disease quail bronchitis, resulting in catarrhal, fibrinous, or necrotizing tracheitis and bronchitis, and disseminated pale 1 to 3 mm diameter foci throughout the liver (Reed and Jack 2003). Microscopically, large basophilic intranuclear inclusions are found within epithelial cells in the upper airways and sometimes in hepatocytes, as well as occasionally in the lungs and bursa of Fabricius. The respiratory epithelium may vary from hyperplastic to necrotic, with a predominantly lymphocytic infiltrate. The hepatic lesions consist of multifocal necrosis with a mixed lymphocytic and heterophilic infiltrate. Other organs exhibiting histologic lesion include: spleens with lymphoid depletion, histiocytic hyperplasia, and fibrinoid necrosis; and lymphoid depletion and necrosis in the bursa of Fabricius (Jack et al. 1994). Turkeys with tracheitis due to *aviadenovirus* exhibit deciliation, mucosal necrosis, and lymphoplasmacytic infiltrates in the airway epithelium, as well as intranuclear inclusions similar to those found in quail (Crespo et al. 1998).

Inclusion body hepatitis associated with fowl adenoviruses in chickens has also been described in captive Gambel's Quail chicks (Bradley et al. 1994). The livers had disseminated pale foci of hepatocellular necrosis, with mixed lymphocytic and heterophilic infiltrates. Hepatocytes contained both small eosinophilic and larger basophilic intranuclear inclusions (Figure. 8.1). Numerous cases of adenoviral hepatitis in racing and show pigeons have been reported (Vindevogel et al. 1981; Takase et al. 1990; Ketterer et al. 1992). In chickens, it has been demonstrated several times that co-infection with immunosuppressive viruses such infectious bursal disease virus or chicken infectious anemia virus predispose to inclusion body hepatitis and increase both lesion severity and mortalities (McFerran and Adair 2003a). The situation in other avian hosts is less well studied, but there are reports of co-infection with papovavirus and aviadenoviruses being seen and possibly exacerbating the resulting clinical disease and lesions in Budgerigars (Tsai et al. 1994). Circovirus infections are reported in juvenile pigeons, which appear to have immunosuppressive effects as in chickens, and could lead to similar severe co-infections with pigeon adenovirus (Ritchie 1995b). Gross and microscopic lesions of inclusion body hepatitis in these other avian hosts are similar to those described in quail.

All siadenoviral infections are characterized by macroscopic splenic enlargement with diffuse mottling (Figure. 8.2). Other gross lesions are pulmonary edema in pheasants infected with MSD, and congestion, hemorrhages and necrosis of the intestinal mucosa in turkeys with HE. Microscopically, spleens exhibit marked reticuloendothelial cell hyperplasia, lymphoid depletion and necrosis, and characteristic intranuclear inclusions in lymphoid cells (Fitzgerald and Reed 1989). These inclusions cause marked nuclear enlargement with margination of chromatin, and vary from palely eosinophilic to basophilic (Figure. 8.3). The intestines of turkeys with HE have congestion, hemorrhages, and necrotic villous tips. The intestinal lamina propria contains mixed inflammatory infiltrates and variable numbers of typical

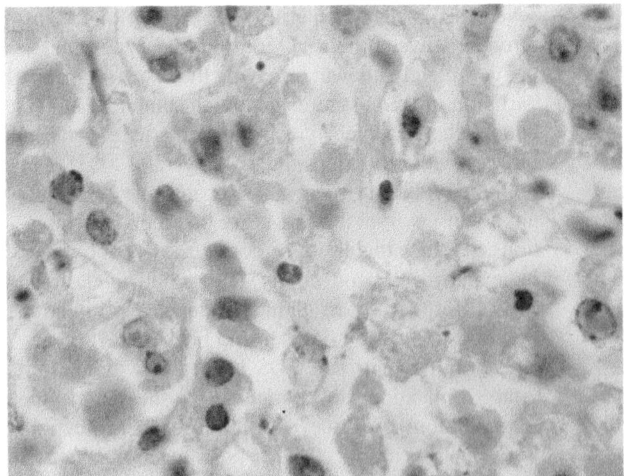

Figure 8.1. Photomicrograph of the liver from a chicken with inclusion body hepatitis. There is widespread necrosis, and multiple hepatocyte nuclei contain intranuclear inclusions. H&E. 100X

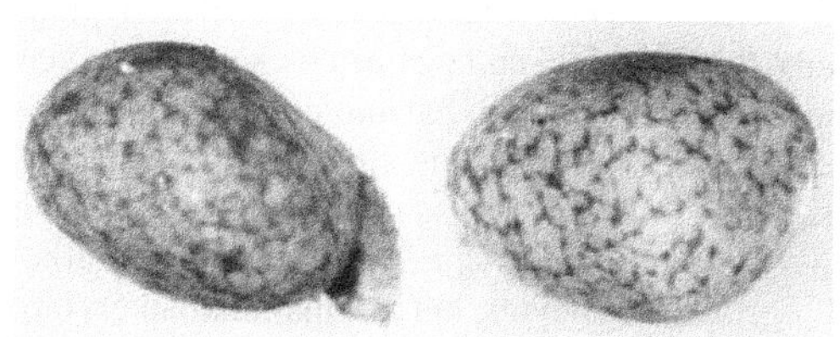

Figure 8.2. Two spleens removed from pheasants inoculated with MSD virus five days earlier. The spleens are markedly enlarged and show classic marbling.

intranuclear inclusions within mononuclear leukocytes (Pierson and Fitzgerald 2003).

EDS virus in both natural and experimental outbreaks creates minimal gross lesions, principally oviduct edema in acute stages, and atrophied oviducts in more chronic stages. Microscopically, mucosal epithelial cells contain typical intranuclear adenoviral inclusions, and a moderate to severe mixed inflammatory infiltrate composed of lymphocytes, plasma cells, macrophages, and heterophils is present (McFerran and Adair 2003b).

There have been several case reports of adenoviruses identified in wild birds, but the viruses were either not isolated, or, if isolated, the viruses have not been fully classified to date. Juvenile Herring Gulls that had been captured and captive-housed for a crude oil toxicity study exhibited large basophilic intranuclear inclusions within lymphocytes in the medullary portion of their bursas associated with heterophilic infiltration. Electron microscopy revealed non-enveloped virions similar to other avian adenoviruses; however, virus isolation was not performed (Leighton 1984). Another report described a Common Murre captured after an oil spill, which was euthanatized in captivity. Its kidneys had prominent intranuclear inclusions within epithelial cells lining multiple collecting ducts. Electron microscopy again revealed typical adenoviral virions; however, virus isolation was not performed (Lowenstine and Fry 1985). Both reports involved subclinical adenoviral infections in wild birds, with no further classification or experimental pathogenesis studies available. More recently, wild Long-tailed Ducks off the north coast of Alaska in the Beaufort Sea exhibited a die-off, with lesions of hemorrhagic enteritis. An adenovirus isolated failed a neutralization assay with antiserum against all three of the known avian adenovirus genera (Hollmén et al. 2003a). Finally, a die-off of Common Eiders occurred in the Baltic Sea. These birds demonstrated intestinal impaction and mucosal necrosis, but the adenovirus isolated again was not neutralized by antisera against any of the three adenovirus genera (Hollmén et al. 2003b). These cases suggest that subclinical adenoviral infections may be widespread in a variety of wild bird species with various organs involved, and in some cases may result in epizootic mortalities in specific host species over a limited geographic area.

DIAGNOSIS

Avian adenoviral infections may be suspected based upon a combination of clinical signs, gross lesions, and

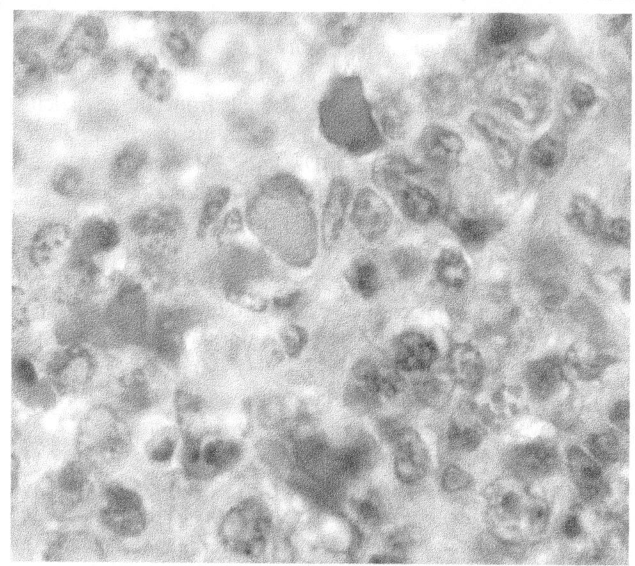

Figure 8.3. Photomicrograph of the spleen from a turkey infected with HE virus. Multiple macrophages contain enlarged nuclei with typical intranuclear inclusion bodies. H&E. 100X

typical intranuclear inclusions as described previously. Techniques for definitive confirmation of the etiologic agent and classification to genus, species, and serotype may include immunohistochemistry, electron microscopy, serology, virus isolation, and various molecular techniques. An immunohistochemical staining technique that cross-reacts with the viral antigen of all members of the siadenoviruses has been described for use on formalin-fixed paraffin-embedded tissues; however, its sensitivity is not significantly greater than routine histopathology (Fitzgerald et al. 1992). Typical viral particles can be detected from feces, liver, spleen, kidney, or other affected tissues using standard transmission electron microscopic techniques. Of the various serologic methods, enzyme-linked immunosorbent assay (ELISA) has been used for detection of all three genera and exhibits the highest sensitivity (McFerran and Adair 2003a). An agar gel precipitin (AGP) assay, also known as double immunodiffusion, has been frequently utilized for aviadenovirus detection and is the standard method of diagnosis employed for siadenoviruses. Hemagglutination-inhibition (HI) has been used only for *atadenovirus* because this is the only avian adenovirus that uniformly agglutinates avian erythrocytes (McFerran 1998; McFerran and Adair 2003b). Virus isolation and identification accompanied by molecular techniques including PCR and sequencing are the current gold standards for diagnosis. Aviadenoviral-infected tissues are made into a suspension and inoculated onto chicken embryo liver or kidney cell lines. QBV may be isolated by chorioallantoic inoculation of nine- to 11-day embryonated chicken eggs. After several passages, cells may be stained with a fluorescent-labeled antibody and virus neutralization performed with reference antisera to determine the serotype (McFerran 1998). PCR has become a rapid and reliable method of confirmation. Restriction enzyme fragmentation patterns and sequencing were initially used to classify aviadenoviruses into five genotypes (designated A–E). Currently, primer sequences based on the virus hexon gene are used to segregate the five *aviadenovirus* species into 12 serotypes in some laboratories, whereas other laboratories continue to utilize cross neutralization tests using reference antibodies (Benko et al. 2000; Hess 2000).

Siadenoviruses are extremely difficult to isolate in cell culture, requiring either a lymphoblastoid B cell line (MTDC RP-19) or peripheral blood leukocytes (Pierson et al. 1998). These closely related viruses are indistinguishable by AGP and ELISA methods; however, isolates can be differentiated by restriction endonuclease fingerprinting or monoclonal antibody affinity testing (Pierson and Fitzgerald 2003).

Atadenovirus is best propagated by inoculation into either embryonated duck or goose eggs, or onto duck or goose embryo cell lines, because it will grow more readily than on chicken eggs or chicken embryo cell lines (McFerran 1998). Allantoic fluid from these inoculated eggs needs to be checked following each passage for HA activity against avian erythrocytes. EDS virus agglutinates chicken, duck, goose, turkey, and pigeon erythrocytes, but not mammalian erythrocytes (McFerran and Adair 2003b). The sensitivities of various serologic assays, including AGP, ELISA, HI, and serum neutralization, are similar for detecting antibodies to EDS virus. HI testing is the most commonly employed method for serologic detection of EDS. Although PCR and genetic sequencing have been utilized to detect EDS virus and to identify three different genotypes, these techniques are not routinely employed because only a single serotype is recognized (McFerran and Adair 2003b).

IMMUNITY

Fowl aviadenoviruses share a common group antigen across the five species and 12 serotypes; however, there are differences between the different serotypes in reactivity to this antigen (McFerran and Adair 2003a). This suggests that some cross protection is provided following exposure to other serotypes, but likely only partial protection. Rapidly developing antibodies occur one to three weeks after infection and correlate with an end of virus shedding; however, humoral immunity appears relatively short lived because reinfection is possible within approximately eight weeks after the initial infection (McFerran and Adair 2003a). Maternal antibody protects against infection by natural routes, but infection following intra-abdominal inoculation, which avoids local immunity, can still occur. Less is known about immunity in other aviadenoviruses such as those found in ducks, turkeys, and pigeons.

Siadenoviruses also possess a shared common group antigen that is distinct from the aviadenoviruses. In fact, HE has been used to immunize pheasants against MSD, and MSD has been used similarly in turkeys to produce immunity against HE. Passive immunity can be utilized by injection of convalescent serum into naïve birds. A number of studies have shown that both HE and MSD viruses are immunosuppressive, causing reduced humoral and cellular immunity post-infection for several weeks (Pierson and Fitzgerald 2003). Maternal antibodies can be detected for these viruses up to three to six weeks post-hatching using ELISA techniques.

EDS *atadenovirus* produces antibodies as early as five days post-infection, with peak levels reached in approximately four to five weeks post-infection. These antibodies prevent clinical drops in egg production, but infected layers will continue to shed viruses in spite of high antibody titers (McFerran and Adair 2003b). Maternal antibody is transferred to the embryo through the yolk sac, and these antibodies are generally undetectable by four to five weeks post-hatch.

PUBLIC HEALTH CONCERNS

There is no evidence that avian adenoviruses are infectious to humans.

DOMESTIC ANIMAL HEALTH CONCERNS

Aviadenoviruses are ubiquitous and likely cycle between domestic poultry, other captive birds, and wild bird species. However, with the exceptions of QBV and hydropericardium syndrome, most of these viruses are not highly pathogenic. Siadenoviruses have been isolated from or had serologic titers demonstrated only in domestic birds, so wild birds apparently do not serve as a reservoir for these viruses. Atadenovirus has been shown to be widespread serologically in many species of wild waterfowl, and it is likely that some outbreaks of EDS in domestic chickens are due to contamination by the feces of free-ranging infected birds. Stringent biosecurity measures, including not using potentially contaminated surface waters, will help to avoid outbreaks in domestic birds (McFerran and Adair 2003b).

WILDLIFE POPULATION IMPACTS

To date, with the exceptions of QBV and EDS virus, most birds suffering from either clinical disease or exhibiting antibodies against avian adenoviruses have been captive. It appears, at least for the aviadenoviruses and siadenoviruses, that high bird densities are needed for the transmission of these diseases. Therefore, the direct impact on wild bird populations has been minimal. Of course, large numbers of captive-reared gamebirds (pheasants, Northern Bobwhite, turkeys) are released annually into the wild. In addition, pigeons are held in captivity but allowed to fly freely over long distances for racing and exhibition purposes. Furthermore, modern poultry biosecurity practices are designed to protect domestic poultry from introduction of outside disease agents, not to prevent the release of infectious agents and their exposure to free-ranging birds. Practices such as raising turkeys on range, open-air pen-rearing of game birds, outdoor composting of poultry carcasses, and transport of poultry to farms, slaughter houses, or rendering facilities in open trucks all allow for the potential spill-over of infectious agents including adenoviruses to free-ranging birds.

Antibodies against the EDS *atadenovirus* have been documented in many waterfowl species, at significant prevalence rates, and over a wide geographic area (Gulka et al. 1984; Hlinak et al. 1998; Schloer 1979). Because this virus predominantly results in decreased egg quality, it is not likely to create clinical disease and mortality in wild birds. However, it could potentially impact the reproductive efficiency of wild waterfowl species and might play a role in the declining populations of some waterfowl species currently occurring in North America.

TREATMENT AND CONTROL

Most aviadenoviruses are not considered primary pathogens, and because they are ubiquitous and transmitted both vertically and horizontally, control is difficult. QBV is an important primary pathogen; however, attempts at using the Indiana C (chicken-origin adenovirus isolate) as a vaccine are of questionable value because research indicates that it produces identical lesions and mortality to those produced by QBV. The use of Indiana C virus as a vaccine against QBV was done prior to recognizing that both these viruses were closely related FAdV-1 strains (Jack and Reed 1994a).

Another important aviadenovirus-induced disease is hydropericardium syndrome. Inactivated homogenates from livers of infected chickens have been used extensively in Pakistan and provided protection against the disease in boilers (McFerran and Adair 2003a; McFerran and Smyth 2000). In general, autogenous vaccines have not been widely used because there are 12 different aviadenovirus serotypes, and they share only partial reactivity against the group antigen. In field situations, birds with aviadenoviruses are frequently shedding multiple different serotypes simultaneously, further complicating vaccination strategies (McFerran and Adair 2003a).

Siadenoviruses share a group-specific antigen, so HE virus has been used as a vaccine against MSD in pheasants, and MSD virus used as an HE vaccine in turkeys. These viruses are spread only by the horizontal route, so live-virus vaccines administered through the water, cell-culture-propagated vaccines, and genetically engineered subunit vaccines have all been used successfully to control the diseases. Virus remains virulent in carcasses for some time, so removal of dead birds helps aid control during an outbreak. These siadenoviruses are also immunosuppressive, so post-outbreak prophylactic antibacterials in the feed or water may help to control secondary bacterial infections and associated mortality (Pierson and Fitzgerald 2003).

Atadenovirus is transmitted both vertically and horizontally, so control is difficult. Waterfowl shed the virus into surface water, so use of chlorinated or well water for captive waterfowl and poultry is recommended. An oil-adjuvant inactivated vaccine is available and efficacious in domestic fowl; however, it remains unproven in waterfowl species (McFerran and Adair 2003b).

MANAGEMENT IMPLICATIONS

Because all three genera of avian adenovirus are present worldwide, and because both domesticated and wild birds are susceptible to these pathogens, there are several management recommendations. First, all the aviadenovirus- and siadenovirus-associated clinical disease outbreaks have been reported only in captive birds, with the exception of QBV. This suggests that either the high bird density found in captivity, or stresses associated with captive rearing, play a major role in promoting adenoviral disease outbreaks. Decreasing bird densities, rearing birds on wire to decrease fecal-oral contamination, and rapid removal of sick and dead birds that are sources of virus will all help decrease mortality rates. The practice of routinely reintroducing captive wild bird species back into the wild, through the release of captive-reared game bird species, allows for the potential introduction of avian adenoviruses into wild bird populations. Game bird managers and pigeon fanciers have a responsibility to limit release of clinically sick or recently recovered birds that may be shedding adenoviruses into the wild. Because the EDS atadenovirus is widespread in wild waterfowl, there is a need for high biosecurity of captive poultry and waterfowl to prevent their exposure to this disease. Finally, monitoring of wild bird species for the presence of aviadenoviruses or serologic evidence of previous exposure to these viruses should be continued and expanded. To date, predominantly aquatic bird species have been shown to have either subclinical or localized mortalities related to as yet unclassified avian adenoviruses. These viruses may turn out to be new species, or opportunistic infections of established viruses that are signaling the stresses associated with environmental degradation and contamination on wild bird populations.

LITERATURE CITED

Benko, M., B. Harrah, and W.C. Russel. 2000. Family Adenoviridae, Virus Taxonomy. In *Seventh Report of the International Committee on Taxonomy of Viruses,* M.H.V. van Regenmortel, C.M. Fauguet, D.H.L. Bishop, E.B. Carsten, M.K. Estes, S.M. Lemon, J. Maniloff, M.A. Mayo, D.J. McGeoch, C.R. Pringle, and R.B. Wickner (eds.). Academic Press, New York and San Diego, U.S.A., pp. 227–238.

Bradley, G.A., M.R. Shupe, C. Reggiardo, T.H. Noon, F. Lozano-Alarcon, and E.J. Bicknell. 1994. Inclusion body hepatitis in Gambel's quail (*Callipepla gambelii*). *Journal of Wildlife Diseases* 30:281–284.

Chiocca, S., R. Kurzbauer, G. Schaffner, A. Baker, V. Mautner, and M. Cotton. 1996. The complete DNA sequence and genomic organization of the avian adenovirus CELO. *Journal of Virology* 70:2939–2949.

Crespo, R., H.L. Shivaprasad, R. Droual, R.P. Chin, P.R. Woolcock, and T.E. Carpenter. 1998. Inclusion body tracheitis associated with avian adenovirus in turkeys. *Avian Diseases* 42:589–596.

Fitzgerald, S.D., and W.M. Reed. 1989. A review of marble spleen disease of ring-necked pheasants. *Journal of Wildlife Diseases* 25:455–461.

Fitzgerald, S.D., W.M. Reed, and T. Burnstein. 1992. Detection of type II adenoviral antigen in tissues sections using immunohistochemical staining. *Avian Diseases* 36:341–347.

Gulka, C.M., T.H. Piela, V.J. Yates, and C. Bagshaw. 1984. Evidence of exposure of waterfowl and other aquatic birds to the hemagglutinating duck adenovirus identical to EDS-76 virus. *Journal of Wildlife Diseases* 20:1–5.

Hess, M. 2000. Detection and differentiation of avian adenoviruses: a review. *Avian Pathology* 29:195–206.

Hlinak, A., T. Muller, M. Kramer, R.U. Muhle, H. Liebherr, and K. Ziedler. 1998. Serologic survey of viral pathogens in bean and white-fronted geese from Germany. *Journal of Wildlife Diseases* 34:479–486.

Hollmen, T.E., J.C. Franson, P.L. Flint, J.B. Grand, R.B. Lanctot, D.E. Docherty, and H.M. Wilson. 2003a. An adenovirus linked to mortality and disease in long-tailed ducks (*Clangula hyemalis*) in Alaska. *Avian Diseases* 47:1434–1440.

Hollmen, T.E., J.C. Franson, M. Kilpi, D.E. Docherty, and V. Myllys. 2003b. An adenovirus associated with intestinal impaction and mortality of male common eiders (*Somateria mollissima*) in the Baltic Sea. *Journal of Wildlife Diseases* 39:114–120.

Jack, S.W., and W.M. Reed. 1990. Pathology of experimentally induced quail bronchitis. *Avian Diseases* 34:44–51.

Jack, S.W., and W.M. Reed. 1994a. Experimental infection of bobwhite quail with Indiana C adenovirus. *Avian Diseases* 38:325–328.

Jack, S.W., W.M. Reed, and T. Burnstein. 1994b. The pathogenesis of quail bronchitis. *Avian Diseases* 38:548–556.

Ketterer, P.J., B.J. Timmins, H.C. Prior, and J.G. Dingle. 1992. Inclusion body hepatitis associated with an adenovirus in racing pigeons in Australia. *Australian Veterinary Journal* 69:90–91.

King, D.J., S.R. Pursglove, and W.R. Davidson. 1981. Adenovirus isolation and serology from wild bobwhite quail (*Colinus virginianus*). *Avian Diseases* 25:678–682.

Leighton, F.A. 1984. Adenovirus-like agent in the bursa of Fabricius of herring gulls (*Larus argentatus pontoppidan*) from Newfoundland, Canada. *Journal of Wildlife Diseases* 20:226–230.

Lowenstine, L.J., and D.M. Fry. 1985. Adenovirus-like particles associated with intranuclear inclusion bodies in the kidney of a common murre (*Uria aalge*). *Avian Diseases* 29:208–213.

McFerran, J.B. 1998. Adenoviruses. In *A Laboratory Manual for the Isolation and Identification of Avian Pathogens,* 4th Ed., D.E. Swayne, J.R. Glisson, M.W. Jackwood, J.E. Pearson, and W.M. Reed (eds.). American Association of Avian Pathologists, Kennett Square, Pennsylvania U.S.A., pp. 100–105.

McFerran, J.B. 2003. Adenovirus infections: introduction. In *Diseases of Poultry,* 11th ed., Y.M. Saif, H.J. Barnes, J.R. Glisson, A.M. Fadly, L.R. McDougald, and D.E. Swayne (eds.). Iowa State Press, Ames, Iowa, U.S.A., pp. 213–214.

McFerran, J.B., and B.M. Adair. 2003a. Group I adenovirus infections. In *Diseases of Poultry,* 11th Ed., Y.M. Saif, H.J. Barnes, J.R. Glisson, A.M. Fadly, L.R. McDougald, and D.E. Swayne (eds.). Iowa State Press, Ames, Iowa, U.S.A., pp. 214–227.

McFerran, J.B., and B.M. Adair. 2003b. Egg drop syndrome. In *Diseases of Poultry,* 11th Ed., Y.M. Saif, H.J. Barnes, J.R. Glisson, A.M. Fadly, L.R. McDougald, and D.E. Swayne (eds.). Iowa State Press, Ames, Iowa, U.S.A., pp. 227–237.

McFerran, J.B., and J.A. Smyth. 2000. Avian adenoviruses. *Reviews of Science and Technology* 19:589–601.

Pierson, F.W., and S. D. Fitzgerald. 2003. Hemorrhagic enteritis and related infections. In *Diseases of Poultry,* 11th Ed., Y.M. Saif, H.J. Barnes, J.R. Glisson, A.M. Fadly, L.R. McDougald, and D.E. Swayne (eds.). Iowa State Press, Ames, Iowa, U.S.A., pp. 237–247.

Pierson, F.W., C.H. Domermuth, and W.B. Gross. 1998. Hemorrhagic enteritis of turkeys and marble spleen disease of pheasants. In *A Laboratory Manual for the Isolation and Identification of Avian Pathogens,* 4th Ed., D.E. Swayne, J.R. Glisson, M.W. Jackwood, J.E. Pearson, and W.M. Reed (eds.). American Association of Avian pathologists, Kennett Square, PA, U.S.A., pp. 106–110.

Pitcovski, J., M. Mualem, Z. Rei-Koren, S. Krispel, E. Shmueli, Y. Peretz, B. Gutter, G.E. Gallili, A. Michael, and D. Goldberg. 1998. The complete DNA sequence and genome organization of the avian adenovirus, hemorrhagic enteritis virus. *Virology* 249:307–315.

Reed, W.M., and S.W. Jack. 2003. Quail bronchitis. In *Diseases of Poultry,* 11th Ed., Y.M. Saif, H.J. Barnes, J.R. Glisson, A.M. Fadly, L.R. McDougald, and D.E. Swayne (eds.). Iowa State Press, Ames, Iowa, U.S.A., pp. 248–251.

Ritchie, B.W. 1995a. Adenoviridae. In *Avian Viruses Function and Control.* Winger's Publishing, Inc., Lake Worth, Florida, pp. 313–322.

Ritchie, B.W. 1995b. Circoviridae. In *Avian Viruses Function and Control.* Winger's Publishing, Inc., Lake Worth, Florida, pp. 223–252.

Schloer, G.M. 1979. Frequency of antibody to adenovirus 127 in domestic ducks and wild waterfowl. *Avian Diseases* 24:91–98.

Sileo, L., J.C. Franson, D.L. Graham, C.H. Domermuth, B.A. Rattner, and O.H. Pattee. 1983. Hemorrhagic enteritis in captive American kestrels (*Falco sparverius*). *Journal of Wildlife Diseases* 19:244–247.

Takase, K., N. Yoshinaga, T. Egashira, T. Uchimura, and M. Yamamoto. 1990. Avian adenovirus isolated from pigeons affected with inclusion body hepatitis. *Nippon Juigaku Zasshi* 52:207–215.

Tsai, S.S., J.H. Park, B.M. Iqbal, K. Ochiai, K. Hirai, and C. itakura. 1994. Histopathological study on dual infections of adenovirus and papovavirus in budgerigars (*Melopsittacus undulatus*). *Avian Pathology* 23:481–487.

Vindevogel, H.U., L. Dagenais, B. Lansival, and P.P. Pastoret. 1981. Incidence of rotavirus, adenovirus and herpesviruses infection in pigeons. *Veterinary Record* 109:285–286.

Zsak, L., and J. Kisary. 1984. Grouping of fowl adenoviruses based upon the restriction patterns of DNA generated by BAM HI and HIND III. *Intervirology* 22:110–114.

9
Circovirus

Jean A. Paré and Nadia Robert

INTRODUCTION

The Circoviridae is a family of very small, non-enveloped viruses that contain a covalently closed, circular single-stranded DNA (ssDNA) genome and infect mammals and birds (Todd 2000). Because several newly described viruses possessing circular ssDNA await official classification, this family is currently in some taxonomical flux. As a rule, avian circovirus infections are either clinically silent or are characterized by a combination of feather abnormalities and/or secondary infections subsequent to viral-induced immune compromise (Todd 2000). Chicks and juvenile birds seem particularly affected, and damage to the bursa of Fabricius is often conspicuous. Large intracytoplasmic, basophilic, botryoid (in the shape of a cluster of grapes) inclusion bodies in the bursa of Fabricius or other lymphoid tissue and/or in growing feathers and feather follicles are pathognomonic for avian circovirus infection but are not always present.

This chapter addresses infections with psittacine beak and feather disease virus, pigeon circovirus, Laughing (Senegal) Dove (*Streptopelia senegalensis*) circovirus, gull circovirus, goose circovirus, duck circovirus, ostrich circovirus, canary circovirus, and finch circovirus. Of these viruses, the first four are known to affect wild birds. Psittacine beak and feather disease is a serious threat to conservation efforts for endangered wild psittacines. The impact of PiCV, Senegal dove CV, and gull circovirus infection for feral and wild birds is currently undetermined.

ETIOLOGY

The type genus Circovirus is well established and consists of the type species Porcine Circoviruses 1 and 2 (PCV1 and PCV2), as well as the Psittacine beak and feather disease virus (PBFDV). Inclusion in this genus of pigeon circovirus (PiCV) and goose circovirus (GoCV) is pending (Todd 2004). Recent cloning and sequencing of the genomes of a canary circovirus (CaCV) and a duck circovirus (DuCV) suggest that they also are novel species within the genus (Phenix et al. 2001; Todd et al. 2001a; Hattermann et al. 2003). Because of molecular and organizational (negative sense) genomic differences, chicken anemia virus (CAV), the former type species for the genus Circovirus, has recently been transferred to Gyrovirus, a novel genus within the Circoviridae for which it is the type species and sole representative (Pringle 1999). TorqueTenovirus (TTV) and TorqueTenoVirus-like Mini Virus (TLMV) are recently discovered human viruses that were tentatively assigned to the Circoviridae (Bendinelli et al. 2001; Biagini 2004), but their taxonomy is unsettled. Some authors argue that the genomes of these two viruses present sufficient molecular and biophysical differences from circoviruses to justify their reassignment in a novel family for which the name Circinoviridae has been proposed (Mushahwar et al. 1999). Other authors argued that TTV, TLMV, and SEN virus (SENV, another human circular ssDNA genome virus) were more similar to Gyrovirus than to Circovirus, yet were different enough to warrant inclusion in a novel genus, Anellovirus (Hino 2002). Circular ssDNA genome plant viruses such as banana bunchy top virus and subterranean clover stunt virus were formerly classified as circoviruses but have recently been accommodated in the novel genus Nanovirus outside the Circoviridae (Randles et al. 2000).

The family Circoviridae currently consists of animal viruses belonging to two genera, Circovirus and Gyrovirus. Chicken anemia virus (CAV), in the genus Gyrovirus, causes chicken infectious anemia but is not specifically discussed in this text because it has yet to be documented in a species other than the domestic chicken (*Gallus domesticus*). Chicken infectious anemia has been reviewed by Schat (2003).

Porcine and avian circoviruses are non-enveloped, 15–26 nm icosahedral viruses with 1.7 to 2.3 kb, ambisense (negative and positive), circular ssDNA genomes (Todd 2004). Pathogenicity has not been established for PCV1, but PCV2 has been implicated as the cause of post-weaning multisystemic wasting syndrome (PMWS) in pigs. Although one report exists of a bovine circovirus in cattle with respiratory disease and abortions in Canada (Nayar et al. 1999), PCV1 and PCV2 are the only two officially recognized circoviruses known from mammalian hosts. In contrast to the porcine circoviruses, avian circoviruses have yet to be grown in cell culture systems, and circoviruses and circovirus-like viruses have been identified in a spectrum of avian species encompassing psittacines, columbids, passerines (estrildids, fringillids), larids, anatids, phasianids, haematopodids, and struthionids. Many have only very recently been discovered, and others are likely to be described in the future. CaCV and PiCV are more closely related to PBFDV than to GoCV (Todd et al. 2001a; Todd et al. 2001b; Phenix et al. 2001), based on nucleotide sequence analysis, and DuCV is closely related to GoCV (Hattermann et al. 2003).

EPIZOOTIOLOGY

The ecology and epidemiology of circoviruses in captive and free-ranging birds remain largely unknown. Infection with circoviruses is often subclinical or latent, and disease is often insidious so that viral infection is unsuspected or is easily overlooked. For example, the detection and description of TTV (Miyata et al. 1999) in a single human patient in 1998 preceded serologic surveys that, using PCR technology, demonstrated that TTV infection in humans is common and occurs worldwide, and may well have been overlooked in the past (Handa et al. 2000; Bendinelli et al. 2001; Biagini 2004). Similarly, psittacine beak and feather disease and chicken infectious anemia were well-defined disease entities long before their respective causative agents were identified as circoviruses (Ritchie et al. 1989; Gelderblom et al. 1989). Inclusion bodies characteristic of circovirus were retrospectively demonstrated in archived histological sections from Rock Pigeons dating as far back as 1986, four years prior to the first description of PiCV disease and seven years before the virus was identified (Woods at al. 1994). The emergence of circoviruses may therefore reflect increased awareness among the scientific community and refinement in viral diagnostic and investigative tools rather than the emergence of newly evolved viruses.

Infected birds readily shed viruses in feces, crop secretions, and in feathers and, based on studies of PCV and CAV, virions are highly stable and are very resistant to chemical inactivation and environmental degradation (Todd 2000).

Circumstances surrounding the identification of circoviruses in aviary finches and canaries, commercial domestic geese (*Anser sp.*), and farmed Mulard ducks, ostriches, and Ring-necked Pheasants (*Phasianus colchicus*) are also described in this chapter because their host range remains undetermined and the status of wild passerine, waterfowl, or pheasant populations with regard to circovirus is unknown. Even if these viruses were to be detected only in domestic and farmed birds, several factors suggest that the threat of spread to wild species should not be downplayed, because prevalence of circovirus may be very high in aviary and farmed species, as has been demonstrated in pigeons and in geese. Furthermore, the insidious nature of circoviral disease in birds, the stability of the virus outside the host, and efficacious viral shedding and dissemination via feces and feather dander are all factors that favor contagion. It therefore seems prudent to promote awareness among wildlife scientists of these farmed and aviary bird viruses until serological surveys of wild waterfowl, estrildid finches, or ostriches provide us with data to confirm or dismiss their susceptibility to infection.

Psittacine Beak and Feather Disease

SYNONYMS

PBFD, psittacine circovirus infection, psittacine circovirus disease, French moult.

HISTORY

Psittacine beak and feather disease (PBFD) has been recognized in free-ranging birds for more than a hundred years. Feather abnormalities observed in wild Red-rumped Parrots (*Psephotus haematonotus*) as early as 1887 were possibly the first account of PBFD, long before the name was coined for a syndrome characterized by plumage and beak abnormalities in various species of cockatoos in Australia (Perry 1981). Psittacine beak and feather disease is currently the most common infectious disease of wild psittacines in Australia (Raidal et al. 1993) and has become a disease of major importance in pet and captive psittacines around the world. Detailed reviews of PBFD are available in the literature (Latimer et al. 1991; Ritchie 1995).

DISTRIBUTION

Psittacine beak and feather disease is thought to have originated in and around the Australian continent but has now been identified in captive psittacines in Asia, Europe, Africa, and North America (Ritchie 1995), probably as a result of the trade in pet birds occurring on a worldwide scale. Disease in wild psittacines is documented in Australia and New Zealand (Julian and McKenzie 1985; Raidal et al. 1993) and is reported in wild Cape Parrots (*Poicephalus robustus*) and Black-cheeked Lovebirds (*Agapornis nigrigenis*) in Africa (Kock et al. 1993; Perrin 1999; Warburton and Perrin 2002; Heath et al. 2004; Warburton, personal communication).

HOST RANGE

All Psittaciformes are considered susceptible to this virus. There are few surveys on prevalence of PBFDV in wild birds. The disease is endemic in wild populations of Sulphur-crested Cockatoos (*Cacatua galerita*) in Victoria and New South Wales, Australia, in Galahs (*Eolophus roseicapillus*), Little Corellas (*Cacatua sanguinea*), and Long-billed Corellas (*C. tenuirostris*) in New South Wales (Raidal et al. 1993) as well as in populations of wild Budgerigars (*Melopsittacus undulatus*) (Ritchie 1995). Psittacine beak and feather disease has also been diagnosed in wild Major Mitchell's Cockatoos (*C. leadbeateri*) and Gang-gang Cockatoos (*Callocephalon fimbriatum*) in Australia, and may be endemic in other Cacatua populations across the Australian continent (Raidal et al. 1993). Orange-bellied Parrots (*Neophemachrysogaster*), Swift Parrots (*Lathamus discolor*), and Crimson Rosellas (*Platycercus elegans*) have also been diagnosed with PBFD (Raidal et al. 1993). Antibodies to PBFDV were demonstrated in wild Mallee Ringneck Parrots (*Barnardius barnardi*) and Rainbow Lories (Trichoglossus haematodus). Feather abnormalities consistent with PBFD were observed in wild Eastern Rosellas (*P. eximius*) in New Zealand (Julian and McKenzie 1985). In Africa, PBFD was identified in captive Black-cheeked Lovebirds (*Agapornis nigrigenis*) (Kock et al. 1993), prior to its being diagnosed in wild, free-ranging birds (Warburton and Perrin 2002; Warburton, personal communication). Infection with PBFDV has also been observed in captive and free-ranging Cape Parrots, an endangered South African species (Perrin 1999; Warburton, personal communication).

ETIOLOGY

PBFDV is a 14 to 16 nm, non-enveloped virion with circular ssDNA (Ritchie 1995). Evidence exists to suggest some genetic diversity among and between Australian, European, and South African PBFDV isolates (Bassami et al. 2001; Raue et al. 2004; Heath et al. 2004). There is evidence to suggest a link between PBFDV genotype and host, based on studies of isolates from pet cockatoos and lorikeets in New Zealand (Ritchie et al. 2003). C1 gene fragment analysis of PBFDV isolates from various parrots in Germany revealed that isolates from lories clustered together as one lineage (Raue et al. 2004). Nucleic acid primers currently used for PBFDV failed to detect circoviral DNA in lories (Loriinae) with feather dystrophy (Ritchie et al. 2000), further suggesting that a distinct genotype occurs in the Loriinae. In a PBFD outbreak in captive lovebirds in Zimbabwe, 100% of Black-cheeked and Nyasa Lovebirds (*Agapornis lilianae*) died, whereas most of Peach-faced (A. roseicollis) and all Fischer's Lovebirds (*A. fischeri*) housed in close contact were unaffected (Kock et al. 1993), suggesting some PBFDV strain or genotype host specificity.

EPIZOOTIOLOGY AND TRANSMISSION

In populations of wild psittacines in which PBFD is endemic, seroprevalence of antibodies was as high as 94% and disease prevalence reached 20% (Ritchie 1995). Transmission of disease from sick birds can occur both horizontally and vertically (Ritchie 1995). Vertical transmission was demonstrated in the Little Corella, when eggs from a PBFD-positive hen were artificially incubated and the hatchlings, raised independently from the hen, developed PBFD (Latimer et al. 1991). Inhalation of aerosolized viral particles and ingestion of contaminated material are believed to constitute the major routes of horizontal transmission (Ritchie 1995). Viral shedding in feces, crop secretions, and feather dander of infected birds has been demonstrated. Nestlings and fledglings may become infected when food is regurgitated during feeding by infected parents. Shedding of virus particles in feather dander and in feces of infected individuals can result in heavy contamination of the environment, especially in captive situations. Clinical PBFD has been experimentally produced in baby Budgerigars, Galahs, African Gray Parrot (*Psittacus erithacus erithacus*), and White Cockatoo (*Cacatua alba*) by oral, intracloacal, and intranasal routes of virus inoculation (Ritchie et al. 1991).

CLINICAL SIGNS

Clinical signs depend on how rapidly the disease progresses. Bilateral and symmetrical feather loss, progressing from contour feathers to remiges and rectrices, is the typical clinical picture observed in infected wild birds with the chronic form of PBFD. Affected birds may become completely bald. The incubation period may range from three weeks to a year (Ritchie 1995). Necrosis of the beak and claws may or may not follow plumage abnormalities (Figures. 9.1, 9.2). PBFDV is immunosuppressive, and additional clinical signs often reflect secondary infections that may be fatal. A peracute form of the disease, in which neonatal birds are found dead without premonitory signs, does sometimes occur (Ritchie 1995) and is likely under-reported in the wild. An

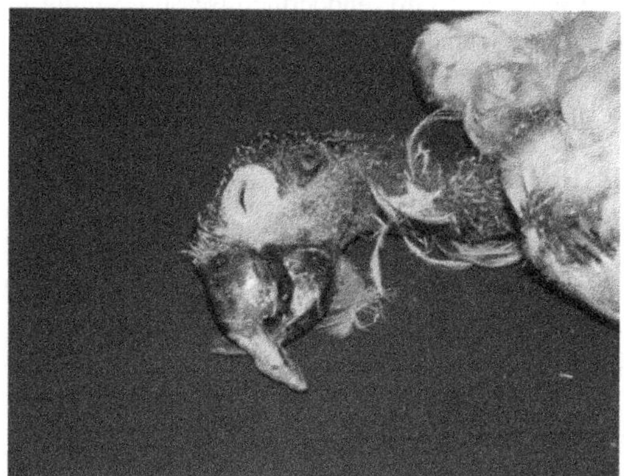

Figure 9.1. Sulphur-crested Cockatoo (*Cacatua galerita*) with Psittacine Beak and Feather Disease (PBFD) showing extensive feather loss and necrosis and deformity of the beak.

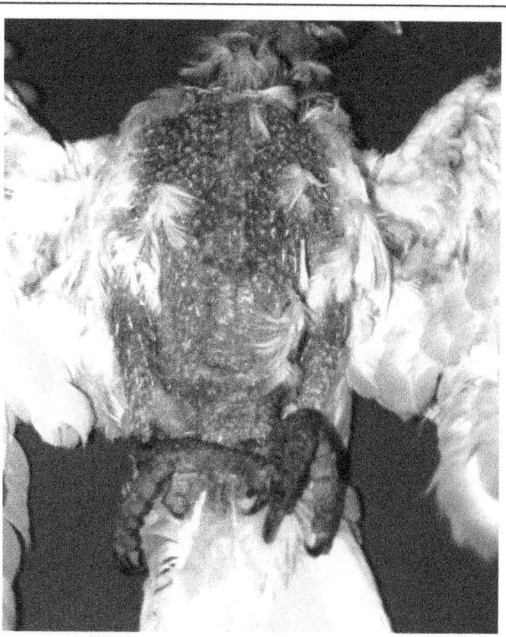

Figure 9.2. Sulphur-crested Cockatoo (same birds as in Figure 9.1) with PBFD showing the extensive feather dystrophy over much of the body.

acute form of PBFD also occurs in nestlings and fledglings and is characterized by depression, followed by changes in growing feathers such as dystrophy, necrosis, or hemorrhage. These feather changes may be subtle and may be eclipsed by more overt systemic signs such as diarrhea, weakness, and depression. Death typically ensues within one or two weeks (Ritchie 1995). In many birds, PBFDV triggers a vigorous immune response, especially in healthy adults, with subsequent clearing of the virus and no evidence of clinical disease.

PATHOGENESIS

PBFDV exhibits epitheliotropism and lymphotropism (Latimer et al. 1991). Following infection in a susceptible bird, there is hematogenous dissemination of the virus to the cutaneous follicular epithelium resulting in plumage abnormalities, and to the bursa of Fabricius and thymus where the virus causes immune dysfunction. Many birds succumb to infection, but others may recover and some become asymptomatic carriers (Latimer et al. 1991). Recovery from clinical PBFD has been documented in macaws (*Ara spp.*) and pionus parrots (*Pionus spp.*) as well as in the Loriinae (Ritchie 1995).

PATHOLOGY

Hematology and serum chemistries are often of little value in trying to establish a diagnosis of PBFD (Ritchie 1995), although severe leucopenia, anemia, and liver necrosis were consistent findings in one outbreak of PBFD in African Gray Parrots in Germany (Schoemaker et al. 2000). Typically, however, when blood abnormalities are noted, they are not specific and more likely reflect secondary infections. In acute and chronic cases, plumage abnormalities predominate and are highly suggestive of PBFD. Dystrophic or necrotic feathers, pulp hemorrhage within feather shafts, constriction and distortion of the shaft of emerging feathers, sheath retention, and clubbing or curling of feathers is highly suggestive of PBFD (Figure 9.3). Necrosis of the beak and nails, when it occurs, is usually seen late in protracted cases, but may rarely occur in presence of minimal feathering abnormalities. Plumage abnormality may sometimes be minor or very subtle. In the peracute form of the disease, gross necropsy findings may be more consistent with acute septicemia.

The large, basophilic, botryoid, intracytoplasmic inclusion bodies in both feather and follicular epithelial cells and in macrophages are characteristic of circovirus (Ritchie 1995). Intranuclear basophilic inclusions are typically less numerous. Inclusion bodies are often associated with necrosis and inflammation. Inclusion bodies may also be found in the bursa of Fabricius, thymus, and other lymphoid tissue, with varying degrees of inflammation and necrosis. Ultrastructurally, inclusions consist of tightly packed paracrystalline arrays, circles, or semicircles of small, 14–16 nm viral particles.

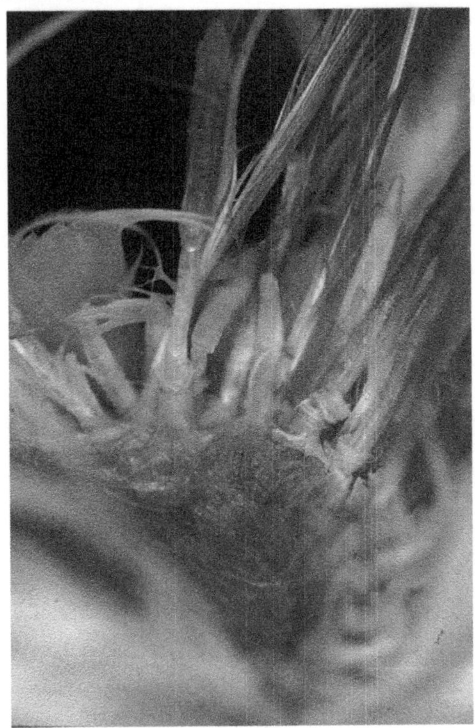

Figure 9.3. Crest feathers of a Salmon-crested Cockatoo (*Cacatua moluccensis*) with PBFD. Note the distortion and pinching of the feathers and their failure to erupt from the feather sheathes. Photo courtesy of Dr. Bruce Hunter, with permission.

DIAGNOSIS

Although signs and lesions in sick birds are highly suggestive of PBFD, the diagnosis should be confirmed through demonstration of virus, viral antigen, or viral nucleic acid within lesions. This can be done using viral-specific DNA probes to detect PBFDV nucleic acid in plucked feathers or whole or heparinized blood (Ritchie 1995). Alternatively, HA assays may be used (Riddoch et al. 1996). Serologic assays to assess immune response in individuals or antibody prevalence in parrot population are also available (Ritchie 1995; Riddoch et al. 1996). Diagnostic methods performed on histological sections include PCR with DNA dot-blot hybridization, and immunoperoxidase staining (Latimer et al. 1991).

Differential Diagnoses

The clinical picture of PBFD in a population of wild birds is rather unequivocal, but polyomavirus infection needs to be ruled out, especially in Budgerigars. Dual infection with PBFDV and polyomavirus is possible. In the individual bird, endocrine disease resulting in symmetrical feather loss may be considered, as well as bacterial, fungal, parasitic, or even psychogenic dermatoses.

IMMUNITY

Individual immune response to PBFDV exposure depends on several host and environmental factors. Birds naturally exposed to PBFDV may remain clinically normal and mount a protective immune response. Immune hens may transfer antibodies in the egg, imparting transient protection to the progeny. Less than adequate or timely humoral response may result in a peracute, acute, or protracted clinical course (Ritchie 1995).

CONTROL AND TREATMENT

Control of PBFD in the field meets with practically insurmountable logistic difficulties. Control in a captive environment resides in prevention. Proper quarantine and testing of any new psittacine being added to an existing collection is critical. Tests to detect both antigen and antibody should be used. A commercial vaccine is available in some countries (Australia) and may be useful in a captive setting. Hygiene and good husbandry practices are essential. Based on information gathered from studies on disinfectants and their effect on CAV and PCV, PBFDV should be regarded as stable and persistent in the environment. Iodine, 10% sodium hypochlorite, 0.4% beta-propriolactone, 1% glutaraldehyde, and 80°C heating for one hour were shown to inactivate CAV and may be considered as options for disinfection (Ritchie 1995). Various glutaraldehyde, formaldehyde, and formic acid–based disinfectants also inactivated PCV2, but only after prolonged contact (Yilmaz and Kaleta 2004).

Treatment of affected individuals is supportive, although the use of interferon has been documented in an African Gray Parrot (Stanford 2004).

PUBLIC HEALTH CONCERNS

There is no current evidence to indicate that PBFD virus is pathogenic for people.

DOMESTIC ANIMAL HEALTH CONCERNS

There is no current evidence to implicate PBFD virus in causing disease in commercial poultry. PBFD is, however, a significant and economically important disease in the pet bird industry and a significant concern for psittacine aviaries, breeding establishments, and captive collections.

MANAGEMENT IMPLICATIONS

The implications of this disease for wild parrots, and especially for threatened and endangered species, are serious. Wild parrot populations do not easily lend themselves to disease management, with the possible exception of localized sedentary populations of flightless species such as the Kakapo (*Strigops habroptilus*). Management of captive propagation programs and *in situ* conservation efforts involving psittacine species, as well as reintroduction protocols, should include provisions for careful PBFDV testing and screening. The Australia Department of the Environment and Heritage has drafted a Threat Abatement Plan for Psittacine Circoviral (Beak and Feather) Disease Affecting Endangered Psittacine Species (Department of Environment and Heritage 2004) in which priorities and guidelines for control of PBFD in wild parrots are addressed; these could be used as a blueprint for other countries. Although the disease has been found in wild parrots in Australia, New Zealand, and southern Africa, escaped pet psittacines have become established in many other subtropical and tropical locales, including the U.S.A., and represent a constant threat for dissemination of the virus to native species.

Pigeon Circovirus Infection

HISTORY

Circovirus infection was identified in Rock Pigeons (*Columba livia*) in 1993 (Woods et al. 1993). Retrospective studies demonstrated that pigeon circovirus (PiCV) infection had been overlooked in histological sections for years (Woods et al. 1994).

DISTRIBUTION AND HOST RANGE

Pigeons are the only known host for PiCV (Woods and Latimer 2000). Infection has been documented in various areas of North America, Europe, and Australia (Woods and Latimer 2000) and is probably more widespread than reports indicate. Investigations showed infection prevalence of up to 89% among birds tested in Ireland, Germany, and the U.S.A. (Smyth et al. 2001; Soike et al. 2001; Roy et al. 2003).

ETIOLOGY

Pigeon circovirus (PiCV) appears to be a typical circovirus and measures 14–17 nm in diameter. Although PiCV is distinct from PBFDV, the two share homologous DNA sequences (Woods et al. 1994). The relationship of PiCV to Senegal dove circovirus has not been investigated. Columbid circovirus (CoCV) is used synonymously with PiCV but may lead to confusion with the circovirus of Senegal dove and the circovirus-like inclusions observed in wood pigeons (see later), and until the relationship between these viruses is established, the term PiCV should be used.

EPIZOOTIOLOGY, TRANSMISSION AND CLINICAL SIGNS

Documented cases of PiCV infection have occurred in racing, meat, and other breeds of domestic pigeons, but rarely in truly feral pigeons. This probably stems from a sampling bias, because birds from commercial lofts are more likely to be presented for necropsy. Pigeon circovirus infection may be clinically silent in a loft and therefore go unnoticed (Paré et al. 1999), or it may present as mortality outbreaks of varying magnitude in unweaned squabs (Woods and Latimer 2000). Disease is rare in adult birds, but morbidity ranges from 0–100% in young birds (Woods and Latimer 2000). Ill thrift, poor performance, and diarrhea are often reported but respiratory and upper gastrointestinal signs are also possible.

Circoviral damage to lymphoid tissue results in infected squabs becoming more susceptible to viral, bacterial, and fungal pathogens. Severity and type of clinical signs, mortality, and lesions may depend more on the virulence of secondary pathogens in sick birds, as well as on the quality of husbandry and hygiene within the loft (Paré et al. 1999; Woods and Latimer 2000). A single documented case in which the clinical presentation consisted of feathering abnormalities in PiCV-infected pigeons is the exception rather than the rule (Woods et al. 2000). Horizontal transmission via the fecal oral route or via crop milk is likely (Woods et al. 2000), and there is circumstantial evidence to suggest that vertical transmission also occurs (Paré et al. 1999). Racing events and intermingling of commercial pigeons with feral birds may well promote dissemination of the virus to naïve lofts or feral pigeon populations.

PATHOGENESIS AND PATHOLOGY

PiCV appears to exhibit primary bursotropism, with subsequent systemic spread to non-bursal lymphoid organs (Abadie et al. 2001). The hallmark of pigeon circovirus infection is the presence of typical botryoid, basophilic intracytoplasmic circoviral inclusions in lymphoid tissue (Figure 9.4), and especially the bursa of Fabricius (Woods et al. 1994), but inclusions within bursal epithelial cells may be intranuclear. Ultrastructurally, PiCV inclusions are indistinguishable from those of PBFDV and consist of nonmembrane-bound, paracrystalline, semicircular, or layered arrays of tightly packed icosahedral, non-enveloped, 14 to 21 nm virions. Inclusions are usually accompanied by varying degree of necrosis and histiocytosis, but may be observed in the absence of noticeable histopathological changes in the bursa (Paré et al. 1999). Other microscopic lesions are almost always attributable to secondary pathogens, as are most macroscopic lesions.

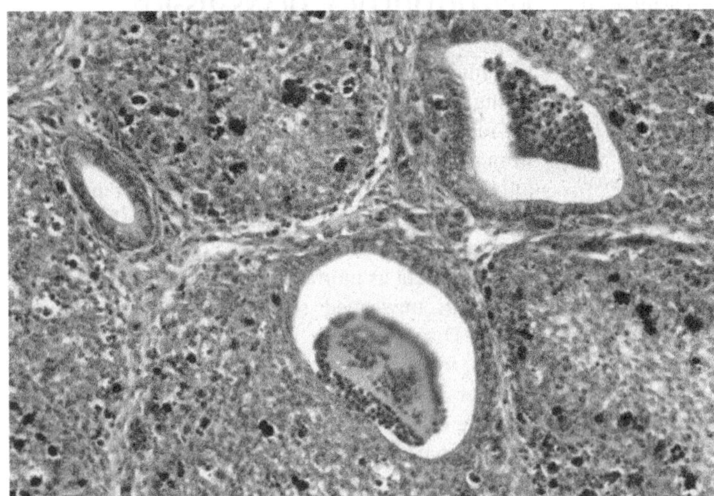

Figure 9.4. Histological section of the bursa of Fabricius from a young Rock Dove (*Columba livia*) with pigeon circovirus infection. Note the marked depletion of lymphocytes in both cortical and medullary areas and the numerous dark, botryoid inclusions typical of circovirus. H&E × 400. Photo courtesy of Dr. Bruce Hunter, with permission.

Circovirus-induced bursal and lymphoid damage in infected squabs is likely to result in immunosuppression, with the aforementioned consequences. Hematology did not correlate with histopathologic changes in PiCV-infected squabs (Paré et al. 1999).

DIAGNOSIS

Diagnosis of PiCV infection has relied mostly on demonstration of typical inclusion bodies in histopathologic sections, usually in the bursa. However, *in situ* hybridization using specific PiCV DNA probe on bursal tissue sections has shown to be more sensitive for detection of infection (Smyth et al. 2001). A nested PCR test performed on dried blood samples has shown promise for diagnosis of PiCV infection in live birds (Hattermann et al. 2002) and may become useful in assessing infection status of lofts. Because secondary infections are responsible for the clinical signs observed, the list of differential diagnoses is long. However, underlying PiCV infection should be suspected in any disease outbreaks affecting young pigeons.

IMMUNITY

There is some evidence to suggest that, at least in some instances, PiCV-infected squabs will recover, even if moderate to severe bursal damage has occurred (Paré et al. 1999). However, the role of humoral and cell-mediated immune response has yet to be investigated.

CONTROL AND TREATMENT

Prevention and control of PiCV infection may be impossible to achieve, but in a captive setting, sound husbandry and good hygiene may reduce morbidity (Paré et al. 1999).

Laughing (Senegal) Dove Circovirus

HISTORY

In 1994, a syndrome consisting of feathering abnormalities and resembling PBFD was described in Laughing (Senegal) Doves in Australia (Pass et al. 1994). Hemagglutination and hemagglutination inhibition studies further demonstrated that Senegal Dove circovirus was serologically distinct from PBFDV (Raidal and Riddoch 1997). The disease has been observed in Senegal Dove in Western Australia and Spotted Doves (*Streptopelia chinensis*) in the Sydney metropolitan area (Raidal and Riddoch 1997). Both are introduced species to Australia.

The agent has not been fully characterized but appears to be a circovirus antigenically distinct from PBFDV (Raidal and Riddoch 1997). Round, negatively stained viral particles, averaging 16 nm in diameter, were identified in impression smears of feathers (Pass et al. 1994).

The modalities of transmission have not been determined, and the epidemiology is unclear. Horizontal transmission, similar to that of PBFDV appears plausible. Clinical signs are limited to feathering abnormalities, mimicking PBFD (Pass et al. 1994). Macroscopic and microscopic lesions are practically identical to those of PBFD but are limited to feathers. Botryoid, basophilic intracytoplasmic inclusions are seen in macrophages within affected feathers (Pass et al. 1994; Raidal and Riddoch 1997).

Diagnosis is based on clinical signs and pathological features. The presence of classic circovirus inclusion bodies in feathers is highly suggestive, but a definitive diagnosis relies on identification of typical viral particles on electron microscopy. In the individual bird, the list of differential diagnoses includes dermatoses of other origin or even feather trauma from a cat attack (Raidal and Riddoch 1997).

Gull Circovirus

Circovirus-like infection was identified in a single juvenile southern Kelp Gull (*Larus dominicanus*) in New Zealand (Twentyman et al. 1999). Subsequently, similar inclusions were identified in juvenile Ring-billed Gulls (*L.* delawarensis) in Ontario and Saskatchewan, Canada, and electron microscopy demonstrated typical circovirus-like virions (Campbell 1999). Furthermore, retrospective examination of archived histological sections indicated that circovirus infection in gulls might have been present as early as 1983 (Campbell 1999; Velarde, unpublished data).

The Kelp Gull, which has a holantarctic distribution, may be a definitive host for the virus or may represent an accidental host. Infection also occurs in gulls (*Larus sp.*) in North America (Campbell 1999; Velarde, unpublished data) and characteristic bursal inclusions were observed in a Black-headed Gull (*L. ridibundus*) in the Netherlands (Kuiken et al. 2002).

Based on typical inclusions in the bursa and on ultrastructural morphology, the virus is believed to be a circovirus (Twentyman et al. 1999; Campbell 1999; Velarde, unpublished data).

Little is known of the epizootiology and transmission modalities of this putative gull circovirus. Juvenile birds are affected. Dead birds were all from die-offs, but the exact role of the virus in those epornitics was unclear. Bursal damage and emaciation with or without secondary aspergillosis were recurrent findings and are consistent with the general circoviral clinicopathological picture. Sick birds in the Ontario die-off were weak or paralyzed, became recumbent, and died, and all birds tested had detectable antibodies to paramyxovirus 1 (Campbell 1999).

In the Kelp Gull, large intracytoplasmic, basophilic botryoid inclusion bodies in macrophages and in lymphoid cells of bursal follicles were observed. Bursal and splenic lymphoid depletion were noted histologically (Twentyman et al. 1999). Macroscopic and microscopic lesions referable to aspergillosis predominated and were the likely cause of death.

Diagnosis relies on demonstration of typical inclusion bodies in histological sections of the bursa. Underlying circoviral infection should be considered in die-offs of gulls, especially when juvenile gulls are predominantly affected.

Goose Circovirus

Goose circovirus (GoCV) was first identified when stunting and increased mortality were observed in a large flock of domestic Czech hybrid geese (*Anser sp.*) in Germany (Soike et al. 1999). Circovirus-like basophilic globular intracytoplasmic inclusion bodies were identified in the bursa only and were associated with lymphoid depletion of follicles. When present, gross lesions were consistent with those caused by secondary infections, chiefly aspergillosis or bacterial infections such as *Riemerella anatipestifer.* Since then, GoCV infection has been diagnosed in Hungary (Ball et al. 2004) and in Taiwan (Chen et al. 2003; Chen et al. 2004a). Genome sequence determination confirmed that GoCV belonged to the genus *Circovirus* but was more distantly related to PBFDV than was PiCV (Todd et al. 2001b). Nucleotide sequencing of 11 GoCV isolates from Taiwan identified two groups that differed from each other and from a German isolate by 7.0 to 7.7% (Chen et al. 2003). GoCV DNA was identified in more than 50% of sick and dead geese from commercial flocks in Hungary (Ball et al. 2004), and in 33% and 94.5% of geese sampled at slaughterhouses in Taiwan in 2002 and 2003 (Chen et al. 2004a). The risk for wild waterfowl populations is unknown, but the high prevalence of GoCV in farmed geese in Europe and Asia appears to justify investigating antibody seroprevalence in free-ranging waterfowl.

Duck Circovirus

A novel circovirus was identified in Muscovy Ducks(*Cairina moschata*) in Taiwan (Chen et al. 2004b) and in mulard ducks from a farm in Germany (Soike et al. 2004). Mulards are Muscovy × Pekin Duck hybrids that are intensively raised for the meat industry in Taiwan. The Mulard ducks in Germany had been purchased from a French breeder and exhibited poor growth and marked feather dystrophy, which was especially noticeable over the dorsum. Hemorrhage was noted in the shaft of feathers. Inclusion bodies were absent, but necrosis and histiocytosis along with lymphoid depletion was observed in the bursa of Fabricius, and secondary infection with *Riemerella anatipestifer* suggested some degree of immunosuppression (Soike et al. 2004). Duck circovirus (DuCV) was identified in Taiwan by detection of circoviral DNA in the bursa of Fabricius of Muscovy Ducks using PCR (Chen et al. 2004b). Analysis of a German DuCV isolate from a Mulard duck by genome sequencing revealed sequences unique to DuCV and also provided evidence that DuCV is closely related to GoCV (Hatterman et al. 2003).

Canary Circovirus

Circovirus-like infection was suspected in an aviary experiencing 90% mortality in neonate Common Canaries (*Serinus canaria*) in the United States (Goldsmith 1995). Macroscopic abnormalities included abdominal enlargement and congestion of the gall bladder that was readily seen through the translucent skin of nestlings, which led to the condition being dubbed "black spot disease" by aviculturists. A similar condition had been reported by canary breeders in Europe. In these nestlings, necrosis was observed in the bursa of Fabricius, the epithelium of the epidermal collar in the developing feather, and the oral epithelium and small 18 nm viral particles were identified in homogenates of tissues from sick neonates using electron microscopy (Goldsmith 1995). More recently, a condition characterized by dullness, anorexia, lethargy, and feather disorder was identified in canaries from an aviary in Italy. Ten to 15% of the birds in the aviary were affected, of which 50% died (Todd et al. 2001b). Pinpoint hemorrhages in the muscles were the only macroscopic finding. Electron microscopy on organ homogenates detected large numbers of virions that were morphologically consistent with circovirus. PCR techniques using specific circovirus primers confirmed the suspicion, and the virus was tentatively named canary circovirus (CaCV). Initial nucleotide and amino acid sequence analysis suggested that it was more closely related to PiCV than to PBFDV. Subsequent cloning and complete sequencing of CaCV corroborated these findings, confirmed that the virus belonged in the genus *Circovirus,* and further determined that CaCV was more similar to PiCV than to GoCV.

Finch Circovirus

Circovirus infection was suspected in fledgling Zebra Finches (*Poephilagustata*) with feather loss and lethargy. These birds had hepatic necrosis, and inclusion bodies in the spleen were suggestive of circovirus (Mysore et al. 1995). Circovirus infection has since been documented in a fledgling Gouldian Finch (*Chloebia gouldiae*) (Shivaprasad et al. 2004), an estrildid species closely related to the Zebra Finch. The fledgling was from an aviary experiencing respiratory disease and mortality. Characteristic inclusion bodies and lymphoid depletion were noted in the bursa of Fabricius. Virus particles measuring 15–18 nm were identified within the inclusions by electron microscopy and circovirus DNA was demonstrated by *in situ* hybridization using a circovirus-specific DNA probe. Coexisting bacterial and adenoviral infections were present in this bird (Shivaprasad et al. 2004). The role of the virus in regard to disease in the aviary was not ascertained.

Ostrich Circovirus

Circovirus-like particles were identified in the gut content of a captive Ostrich (*Struthio camelus*) (Els and Josling 1998), but the possibility that they were ingested plant nanovirus particles existed. More convincing was the identification using PCR, Southern Blot, and *in situ* hybridization, of circovirus DNA in tissues of dead-in-shell Ostrich embryos and chicks from a farm in the Netherlands experiencing a disease known locally as Fading Chick Syndrome (FCS). In FCS, chicks die after exhibiting nonspecific signs such as depression, weight loss, anorexia, and diarrhea (Eisenberg et al. 2003). PBFDV primers and specifically designed Ostrich primers were used for PCR, and the comparison of nucleotide sequences suggested that the Ostrich circovirus was closely related to PBFDV. Inclusion bodies were not seen but it is unclear whether cloacal bursae were actually examined histologically. Ostrich circovirus infection was tentatively linked with FCS (Eisenberg et al. 2003).

Other Avian Circoviruses

Circovirus-like particles were identified serendipitously on electron microscopy in kidney and intestine tissue homogenates from farmed Ring-necked Pheasants (*Phasianus colchicus*) in Italy (Terregino et al. 2001). Weakness, delayed growth, diarrhea, and mortality observed in 10- to 30-day-old chicks were attributed to co-infection with reovirus, but disease may have been compounded by circovirus infection and immunosuppression (Terregino et al. 2001). Bursal depletion was noted histologically but inclusion bodies were not seen. Interestingly, these pheasants were raised for repopulation and release purposes. Circovirus-like inclusion bodies were also found in histological sections of Wood Pigeons (*Columba palumba*) and Common Oystercatchers (*Haematopus ostralegus*) in the Netherlands (Kuiken et al. 2002) and await further characterization. Prevalence of circovirus in oystercatchers and other shorebirds would be interesting in the light of a recent study that provides evidence to suggest that oysters and mussels may be involved in the epidemiology of circoviruses, at least in regard to TTV and TLMV in humans (Myrmel et al. 2004).

MANAGEMENT IMPLICATIONS FOR CIRCOVIRAL DISEASES

Wildlife pathologists must be aware of the possibility of circovirus infection when investigating the causes of epornitics in wild populations of birds. Mortality events implicating various infectious agents and affecting primarily fledglings and juveniles in the presence of bursal depletion should especially raise suspicion. Evidence suggesting circoviral involvement should be explored through the use of electron microscopy and/or nucleic acid probes, because the mere absence of typical inclusion bodies in the bursa of Fabricius or feather epithelium does not rule out circovirus infection. Finally, there is a lack of data pertaining to the immune status of wild birds to circovirus. Serological surveys of wild birds are few and rarely include circovirus among the panel of infectious agents for which birds are tested. Such data could prove very helpful in developing species management plans and in monitoring reintroduction efforts.

UNPUBLISHED DATA

Rose Velarde. 2002. Investigation of viral infections of Ring-billed Gulls (*Larus delawarensis*) in southern Ontario, Canada. DVSc Thesis dissertation.

L. Warburton, Cape Parrot Working Group, School of Botany and Zoology, University of Natal, Scottsville, South Africa.

LITERATURE CITED

Abadie, J., F. Nguyen, C. Groizeleau, N. Amenna, B. Fernandez, C. Guereaud, L. Guigand, P. Robart, B. Lefebvre, and M. Wyers. 2001. Pigeon circovirus infection: pathological observations and suggested pathogenesis. *Avian Pathology* 30:149–158.

Ball, N.W., J.A. Smyth, J.H. Weston, B.J. Borghmans, V. Palya, R. Glávits, É. Ivanics, A. Dán, and D. Todd. 2004. Diagnosis of goose circovirus infection in Hungarian geese samples using polymerase chain reaction and dot blot hybridization tests. *Avian Pathology* 33:51–58.

Bassami, M.R., I. Ypelaar, D. Berryman, G.E. Wilcox, and S.R. Raidal. 2001. Genetic diversity of beak and feather disease virus detected in psittacine species in Australia. *Virology* 279:392–400.

Bendinelli, M., M. Pistello, F. Maggi, C. Fornai, G. Freer, and M.L. Vatteroni. 2001. Molecular properties, biology, and clinical implications of TT virus, a recently identified widespread infectious agent of humans. *Clinical Microbiology Reviews* 14:98–113.

Biagini, P. 2004. Human circoviruses. *Veterinary Microbiology* 98:95–101.

Campbell, D. 1999. Gull mortality—Kitchener. *Canadian Cooperative In Wildlife Health Center Newsletter,* Vol 6, No 2.

Chen, C.L., P.C. Chang, M.S. Lee, J.H. Shien, S.J. Ou, and H.K. Shieh. 2003. Nucleotide sequences of goose circovirus isolated in Taiwan. *Avian Pathology* 32:165–171.

Chen, C.L., P.C. Chang, J.H. Shien, S.R. Gong, M.S. Lee, C.H. Chen, and H.K. Shieh. 2004a. Molecular epidemiology and virus quantification of goose circovirus in Taiwan. *Taiwan Veterinary Journal* 30:156–162.

Chen C.-L., P.-C. Chang, H.K. Shieh, M.-S. Lee, S.-J. Ou, C.-H. Chen, and J.-H. Shien. 2004b. Detection of goose circovirus in waterfowls by polymerase chain reaction. *Taiwan Veterinary Journal* 30:84–90.

Department of Environment and Heritage, Commonwealth of Australia. 2004. Threat Abatement Plan for Psittacine Circoviral (Beak and Feather) Disease Affecting Endangered Psittacine Species. Threatened Species and Threat Abatement Section, Canberra Act 2601. [Online.] Retrieved from the World Wide Web: www.deh.gov.au/biodiversity/threatened/tap/index.tml.

Eisenberg, S.W.F., A.J.A.M. van Asten, A.M. vanEderen, and G.M. Dorrestein. 2003. Detection of circovirus with a polymerase chain reaction in the ostrich (*Struthio camelus*) on a farm in the Netherlands. *Veterinary Microbiology* 95:27–38.

Els, H.J., and D. Josling. 1998. Viruses and virus-like particles identified in ostrich gut contents. *Journal of the South African Veterinary Association* 69:74–80.

Gelderblom, H.S. King, R. Lurz, I. Tischer, and V. von Bülow. 1989. Morphological characterization of chicken anaemia agent (CAA). *Archives of Virology* 109:115–120.

Goldsmith, T.L. 1995. Documentation of passerine circovral infection. *Proceedings of the Annual Conference of the Association of Avian Veterinarians,* Philadelphia, PA, U.S.A., pp. 349–350.

Handa, A., B. Dickstein, N.S. Young, and K.E. Brown. 2000. Prevalence of the newly described human circovirus, TTV, in United States blood donors. *Transfusion* 40:245–251.

Hattermann, K., D. Soike, C. Gund, and A. Mankertz. 2002. A method to diagnose pigeon circovirus infection *in vivo*. *Journal of Virological Methods* 104:55–58.

Hatterman, K., C. Schmitt, D. Soike, and A. Mankertz. 2003. Cloning and sequencing of Duck circovirus (DuCV). *Archives of Virology* 148:2471–2480.

Heath L., D.P. Martin, L. Warburton, M. Perrin, W. Horsfield, C. Kingsley, E.P. Rybicki, and A.L. Williamson. 2004. Evidence of unique genotype of beak and feather disease virus in Southern Africa. *Journal of Virology* 78:9277–9284.

Hino, S. 2002. TTV, a new human virus with single stranded circular DNA genome. *Reviews in Medical Virology* 12:151–158.

Julian, A.F., and P. McKenzie. 1985. Feather disease in eastern rosellas. *Ornithological Society of New Zealand News* 36:1.

Kock, N.D., P.U. Hangartner, and V. Lucke. 1993. Variation in clinical disease and species susceptibility to psittacine beak and feather disease in Zimbabwean lovebirds. *Onderstepoort Journal of Veterinary Research* 60:159–161.

Kuiken, T., R. Fouchier, and A. Osterhaus. 2002. Circovirus in wild birds in the Netherlands. *Supplement to the Journal of Wildlife Diseases,* January issue.

Latimer, K.S., P.M. Rakich, F.D. Niagro, B. W. Ritchie, W.L. Steffens III, R.P. Campagnoli, D.A. Pesti, and P.D. Luckert. 1991. An updated review of psittacine beak and feather disease. *Journal of the Association of Avian Veterinarians* 5:211–220.

Miyata, H., H. Tsunoda, A. Kazi, A. Yamada, M.A. Khan, J. Murakami, T. Kamahora, K. Shiraki, and S. Hino. 1999. Identification of a novel GC-rich 113-nucleotide region to complete the circular, single-stranded DNA genome of TT virus, the first human circovirus. *Journal of Virology* 73:3582–3586.

Mushahwar, I.K., J.C. Erker, A.S. Muerhoff, T.P. Leary, J.N. Simons, L.G. Birkenmeyer, M.L. Chalmers, T.J. Pilot-Matias, S.M. Dexai. 1999. Molecular and biophysical characterization of TT virus: evidence for a new virus family infecting humans. *Proceedings National Academy of Science,* USA 96:3177–3182.

Myrmel, M., E. M.M. Berg, E. Rimstad, and B. Grinde. 2004. Detection of enteric viruses in shellfish from the Norwegian Coast. *Applied and Environmental Microbiology* 70:2678–2684.

Mysore, J., D. Read, and B. Draft. 1995. Circovirus-like particles in finches (abstract). In *Proceedings of the Annual Meeting of the American Association of Veterinary Laboratory Diagnosticians,* Histopathology Section, Reno, Nevada, U.S.A., p. 2.

Nayar, G.P., A.L. Hamel, L. Lin, C. Sachvie, E. Grudeski, and G. Spearman. 1999. Evidence for circovirus in cattle with respiratory disease and from aborted bovine fetuses. *Canadian Veterinary Journal* 40:277–278.

Paré, J.A., M.L. Brash, D.B. Hunter, and R.J. Hampson. 1999. Observations on pigeon circovirus infection in Ontario. *Canadian Veterinary Journal* 40:659–662.

Pass, D.A., S.L. Plant, and N. Sexton. 1994. Natural infection of wild doves (*Streptopelia senegalensis*) with the virus of psittacine beak and feather disease. *Australian Veterinary Journal* 71:307–308.

Perrin, M., C. Downs, and C. Symes. 1999. Final blows for the Cape parrot? *PsittaScene* 11:12.

Perry, R.A. 1981. A psittacine combined beak and feather syndrome. In *Proceedings 55 of Courses for Veterinarians, Cage and Aviary Birds,* T. G. Hungerford (ed.). Sidney, Australia, The Post Graduate Committee Veterinary Science 55:73, 81–108.

Phenix, K.V., J.H. Weston, I. Ypelaar, A. Lavazza, J.A. Smyth, D. Todd, G.E. Wilcox, and S.E. Raidal. 2001. Nucleotide sequence analysis of a novel circovirus of canaries and its relationship to other members of the genus Circovirus of the family Circoviridae. *Journal of General Virology* 82:2805–2809.

Pringle, C.R. 1999. Virus taxonomy at the XIth *International Congress of Virology,* Sidney, Australia, 1999. *Archives of Virology* 144:2065–2070.

Raidal, S. R., C. L. McElnea, and G. M. Cross. 1993. Seroprevalence of psittacine beak and feather disease in wild psittacine birds in New South Wales. *Australian Veterinary Journal* 70:137–139.

Raidal, S.R., and P.A. Riddoch. 1997. A feather disease in Senegal doves (*Streptopelia senegalensis*) morphologically similar to psittacine beak and feather disease. *Avian Pathology* 26:829–836.

Randles, J.W., P.W.G. Chu, J.L. Dale, R. Harding, J. Hu, L. Katul, M. Kojima, K.M. Makkouk, Y. Sano, J.E. Thomas, and H.J. Vetten. 2000. Genus Nanovirus. In *Virus Taxonomy—Classification and Nomenclature of Viruses,* M.H.V. van Regenmortel, C.M. Fauquet, D.H.L. Bishop, E.B. Carstens, M.K. Estes, S.M. Lemon, J. Maniloff, M.A. Mayo, D.J. McGeoch, C.R. Pringle, and R.B. Wickner (eds.). R.B. Academic Press, San Diego, CA, U.S.A., pp. 303–309.

Raue, R., J. Reimar, L. Crosta, M. Bürkle, H. Gerlach, and H. Müller. 2004. Nucleotide sequence analysis of a C1 gene fragment of psittacine beak and feather disease virus amplified by real-time polymerase chain reaction indicates a possible existence of genotypes. *Avian Pathology* 33:41–50.

Riddoch, P.A., S.R. Raidal, and G.M. Cross. 1996. Psittacine circovirus antibody detection and an update on the methods for diagnosis of psittacine beak and feather disease. *Australian Veterinary Practitioner* 26:34–139.

Ritchie, B.W. 1995. Circoviridae. In *Avian Viruses, Function and Control,* B.W. Ritchie (ed.). Wingers Publishing, Inc., Lake Worth, Florida, pp. 223–252.

Ritchie, B.W., F.D. Niagro, P.D. Luckert, W.L. Steffens, and K.S. Latimer. 1989. Characterization of a new virus from cockatoos with psittacine beak and feather disease. *Virology* 171:38–88.

Ritchie, B.W., F.D. Niagro, K.S. Latimer, W.L. Steffens, D. Pesti, J. Ancona, and P.D. Lukert. 1991. Routes and prevalence of shedding of psittacine beak and feather disease virus. *American Journal of Veterinary Research* 52:1804–1809.

Ritchie, B.W., C.R. Gregory, K.S. Latimer, R.P. Campagnoli, D. Pesti, P. Ciembor, M. Rae, H.H. Reed, B.L. Speer, B.G. Loudis, H.L. Shivrapasad, and M.M. Garner. 2000. Documentation of a PBFD virus variant in lories. *Proceedings of the Annual Conference of the Association of Avian Veterinarians,* Portland, Oregon, pp. 263–268.

Ritchie, P.A., I.L. Anderson, and D.M.Lambert. 2003. Evidence of specificity of psittacine beak and feather disease viruses among avian hosts. *Virology* 306:109–115.

Roy, P., A.S. Dhillon, L. Lauerman, and H.L. Shivaprasad. 2003. Detection of pigeon circovirus by polymerase chain reaction. *Avian Diseases* 47:218–222.

Schat, K.A. 2003. Chicken infectious anemia. In *Diseases of Poultry,* 11th Ed., Y.M. Saif, H.J. Barnes, J.R. Glisson, A.M. Fadly, L.R. McDougald, and D.E. Swayne (eds.). Iowa State Press, Ames, Iowa, U.S.A., pp. 182–201.

Schoemaker. N.J., G.M. Dorrestein, K.S. Latimer, J.T. Lumeij, M.J.L. Kik, M.H. van der Hage, and R.P. Campagnoli. 2000. Severe leucopenia and liver necrosis in young African grey parrots (*Psittacus erithacus erithacus*) infected with psittascine circovirus. *Avian Diseases* 44:470–478.

Smyth, J.A., J. Weston, D.A. Moffett, and D. Todd. 2001. Detection of circovirus infection in pigeons by in situ hybridization using cloned DNA probes. *Journal of Veterinary Diagnostic Investigation* 13:475–482.

Soike, D., B. Köhler, and K.Albrecht. 1999. A circovirus-like infection in geese related to a runting syndrome. *Avian Pathology* 28:199–202.

Soike, D., K. Hattermann, K. Albrecht, J. Segalés, M. Domingo, C. Schmiit, and A. Mankertz. 2001. A diagnostic study on columbid circovirus infection. *Avian Pathology* 30:605–611.

Soike, D., K. Albrecht, K. Hattermann, C. Schmitt, and A. Mankertz. 2004. Novel circovirus in mulard ducks with developmental and feathering disorders. *The Veterinary Record* 154:792–793.

Stanford, M. 2004. Interferon treatment of circovirus infection in grey parrots (*Psittacus e. erithacus*). *Veterinary Record* 154:435–436.

Terregino, C., F. Montesi, F. Mutinelli, I. Capua, and A. Pandolfo. 2001. Detection of a circovirus-like agent from farmed pheasants in Italy. *Veterinary Record* 149:340.

Todd, D. 2000. Circoviruses: immunosuppressive threats to avian species: a review. *Avian Pathology* 29:373–394.

Todd, D. 2004. Avian circovirus diseases: lessons for the study of PMWS. *Veterinary Microbiology* 98:169–174.

Todd, D., J.H. Weston, D. Soike, and J.A. Smyth. 2001a. Genome sequence determinations and analyses of novel circoviruses from goose and pigeon. *Virology* 286:354–362.

Todd, D., J. Weston, N.W. Ball, B.J. Borghmans, J.A. Smyth, L. Gelmini, and A. Lavazza. 2001b. Nuceotide sequence-based identification of a novel circovirus of canaries. *Avian Pathology* 30:321–325.

Twentyman, C.M., M.R. Alley, J. Meers, M.M. Cooke, and P. J. Duignan. 1999. Circovirus-like infection in a southern black-backed gull (*Larus dominicanus*). *Avian Pathology* 28:513–516.

Warburton, L.S., and M.R. Perrin. 2002. Evidence of psittacine beak and feather disease in wild black-cheeked lovebirds in Zambia. *Papageien* 5:166–169.

Woods, L.W., K.S. Latimer, B.C. Barr, F.D. Niagro, R.P. Campagnoli, R.W. Nordhausen, and A.E. Castro. 1993. Circovirus-like infection in a pigeon. *Journal of Veterinary Diagnostic Investigation* 5:609–612.

Woods, L.W., K.S. Latimer, F.D. Niagro, C. Riddell, A.M. Crowley, M.L. Anderson, B.M. Daft, J.D. Moore, R. P. Campgnoli, and R. H. Nordhausen. 1994. A retrospective study of circovirus infection in pigeons: nine cases (1986–1993). *Journal of Veterinary Diagnostic Investigation* 6:156–164.

Woods, L.W., and K.S. Latimer. 2000. Circovirus infection of nonpsittacine birds. *Journal of Avian Medicine and Surgery* 14:154–163.

Yilmaz, A., and E.F. Kaleta. 2004. Disinfectant tests at 20 and 10 degrees C to determine the virucidal activity against circoviruses. *Deutsch Tierarztl Wochenschr* 111: 248–251.

10 Papillomaviruses and Polyomaviruses

David N. Phalen

INTRODUCTION

Historically, the papillomaviruses and polyomaviruses were considered to be two genera within a single family, the papovaviruses. Characterization of the genomes of these viruses, however, show that they are fundamentally different and therefore are now placed in their own families, the *Papillomavirnidae* and *Polyomaviridae* (Howley and Lowy 2001). There are two known avian papillomaviruses (Terai et al. 2002: the *Fringilla coelebs* papillomavirus (FPV) and the *Psittacus erithacus timneh* papillomavirus (PePV). There are also two known avian polyomaviruses: the avian polyomavirus (APV) and the goose hemorrhagic polyomavirus (GHPV) (Guerin et al. 2000).

Papillomaviruses

HISTORY

Papillomatous lesions consistent with those caused by FPV were first reported in the 1960s and early 1970s on the feet of wild Common Chaffinches (*Fringilla coelebs*) and Brambling (*Fringilla montifringilla*) in Great Britain and Europe by Blackmore and Keymer 1969; Groth and Abs 1967; Lima et al. 1973; Keymer and Blackmore 1974. Virus from the lesions on a Common Chaffinch was purified and shown to have the characteristics of a papillomavirus in 1977 (Osterhaus et al. 1977). The virus was subsequently cloned and sequenced in its entirety, proving that it was a papillomavirus (Terai et al. 2002). The first report of a papillomavirus in parrots was published in 1983 (Jacobson et al. 1983). This bird, an African Gray Parrot (*Psittacus erithacus timneh*), had extensive papillomatous lesions of the face that contained virions of appropriate size and morphology to be a papillomavirus, and they stained with a papillomavirus-specific antibody. The virus has subsequently been cloned, partially (O'Banion et al. 1992) and then completely sequenced (Terai et al. 2002), proving that it is also a papillomavirus.

HOST RANGE

FPV has been reported to cause papillomas in wild Common Chaffinch, Brambling, and Eurasian Bullfinch (*Pyrrhuyla pyrrhula*) (Blackmore and Keymer 1969; Groth and Abs 1967; Lima et al. 1973; Keymer and Blackmore 1974; Osterhaus et al. 1977). Virions consistent with papillomaviruses have also been identified in cutaneous lesions of captive European Greenfinches (*Carduelis chloris*) (Sironi and Gallazzi 1992) and Common Canaries (*Serenus canaria*) (Dom et al. 1993). Cutaneous papillomas have been described in captive Yellow-crowned Parrots (*Amazona ochrocephala*) and African Gray Parrots (*Psittacus erithacus*), Budgerigars (*Melopsittacus undulatus*), a Quaker Parrot (*Mylopsitta monachus*), and a Cockatiel (*Nymphicus hollandicus*) (reviewed by Phalen 1997). Cutaneous papillomas of confirmed papillomavirus etiology in parrots have been documented only in an African Gray Parrot (Jacobson et al. 1983). Cutaneous papillomas have also been described in macaws (*Ara* spp.) and cockatoos (*Cacatua* spp.). However, these lesions appear to contain herpesviruses (Lowenstine et al. 1983).

ETIOLOGY

Papillomaviruses are epitheliotrophic, non-enveloped, double-stranded, icosahedral DNA viruses that are approximately 52–55 nm in diameter. These viruses replicate in differentiated epithelial cells. Except in complex systems, these viruses cannot be grown *in vitro* (Reviewed in Howley and Lowy 2001). FPV and PePV have been completely sequenced. Their genomes range in size from 7,304 bp (FPV) to 7,729 bp (PePV). The genomes of these viruses are similarly organized and contain six open reading frames corresponding to two early proteins (E1 and E2) and two late proteins (L1 and L2) found in all other papillomaviruses. Two unique open reading frames, designated E7 and X-ORF, are also present. Phylogenic analysis shows the avian papillomaviruses to be most closely related to each other and in a separate grouping from other known papillomaviruses (Terai et al. 2002).

EPIZOOTIOLOGY

Virtually nothing is known about the epizootiology of these viruses. It can only be assumed that the viruses require direct contact between birds for spread. Moderate numbers of affected Common Chaffinches and Eurasian Bullfinches are reported to be caught each year by bird banders in Europe (Pennycott 2003), so it appears that this infection has a continuous presence in the populations of these birds. There are only two cases of cutaneous papillomas reported in African Gray Parrots (Jacobson et al. 1983). Both were wild-caught birds, suggesting that this disease may occur in nature, but both had been imported into the U.S.A., and the possibility that the papillomavirus infections may have originated from contact with another bird species cannot be ruled out.

CLINICAL SIGNS

Papillomas in finches occur predominantly on the skin of the toes and the distal tarsometatarsus. Lesions of the face are rare (Moreno-Lopez et al. 1984). Grossly, the lesions are hyperplastic, locally extensive, and papilliferous. They have some resemblance to other skin lesions, including those caused by poxviruses and knemidocoptes mites. The two affected African Gray Parrots had papilliferous plaques on the commissures of the beak, the eyelids, and the face. The original case was followed for a year after presentation, during which time the lesions became more extensive (Jacobson et al. 1983).

PATHOGENESIS

The pathogenesis of these viruses has not been studied. It is assumed that virus transmission occurs as the result of direct contact from an infected bird to a non-infected bird, as do papillomavirus infections in mammals. It is also assumed that the papillomas seen in birds result from alterations in cell proliferation rates caused by viral proteins, as are papillomas of other species (Reviewed by Howley and Lowy 2001).

PATHOLOGY

Microscopically, the lesions in finches were characterized by a thick layer of keratinized epidermis with widespread vacuolization of the keratinocytes (Lima et al. 1973). Histologically, the African Gray Parrot papillomas consisted of finger-like projections of hyperplastic epidermis that contained a thin fibrovascular core. Nuclei persisted into the stratum corneum and some appeared to contain pan-nuclear eosinophilic inclusions (Jacobson et al. 1983).

DIAGNOSIS

A diagnosis strongly suggestive of FPV is made by microscopic examination of a cutaneous biopsy or cutaneous sections taken at necropsy. Hyperplastic skin diseases, other cutaneous tumors, and poxvirus lesions can look like cutaneous papillomas grossly but can be differentiated histologically. Histological findings of cutaneous papillomas of the African Gray parrot are also highly suggestive of this disease. However, a local periocular papilloma, believed to be caused by Psittacid Herpesviruses 2 (PsHV-2), has also been reported (Styles et al. 2005), and therefore a herpesviruses infection must be considered as an alternative diagnosis for the cause of facial cutaneous papillomas in this species. The presence of FPV and PePV can be confirmed by immunohistochemistry using papillomavirus-specific antibodies or detection of virions with electron microscopy (Jacobson et al. 1983). Primers capable of amplifying both FPV and PePV DNA have been developed, and PCR could be used to confirm the presence of this virus in suspect lesions. PsHV-2 can also be detected with the appropriate primers and PCR (Styles et al. 2005).

IMMUNITY

Nothing is known about the immune system and its relationship to these diseases.

PUBLIC HEALTH CONCERNS

There is no evidence of transmission of these viruses to humans.

DOMESTIC ANIMAL HEALTH CONCERNS

There is no evidence of transmission of these viruses to domestic animals.

WILDLIFE POPULATION IMPACTS

The most detailed report of papillomas in wild birds was made by Lina et al. (1973). The vast majority of birds with lesions were Chaffinches, and a prevalence rate of approximately 1.8% was observed. Papillomas were estimated to weigh up to 5% of the birds' body weight, yet they were not associated with poor conditioning in the affected birds. Therefore, there is no evidence that these lesions significantly impact wild populations of these species.

Papillomas in wild African Gray Parrots have not been reported.

TREATMENT AND CONTROL

There are no reports of treatment of cutaneous papillomas in finches. If a high prevalence of infection is noted in wild populations of finches, it might be prudent to reduce finch concentrations by encouraging the public to discontinue feeding them.

MANAGEMENT IMPLICATIONS

Avian papilloma viruses do not appear to have management-related implications. However, if susceptible species were to be bred in captivity, efforts should be made to isolate birds with clinical signs.

Polyomaviruses

SYNONYMS

Papovavirus, Budgerigar Fledgling Disease Virus.

HISTORY

APV was first isolated from nestling Budgerigars obtained from aviaries in the United States and Canada in the early 1980s experiencing a high rate of nestling mortality (Bernier et al. 1981; Davis et al. 1981). APV was subsequently shown to cause disease in parent-raised lovebirds (*Agapornis* spp.) and several species of hand-raised nestling parrots (Jacobson et al. 1993; Graham et al. 1987). A similar and possibly the same virus has been detected in several species of passerines (reviewed by Phalen 1997). It was assumed that this virus was originally present in wild birds, but conclusive evidence of wild bird infection was not shown until 1998 when antibodies to APV were detected in the serum of wild-caught Sulphur-crested Cockatoos (*Cacatua gallerita*) in Australia (Raidal et al. 1998). APV has subsequently been isolated from a small sampling of diurnal raptors in Europe (Johne and Müller 1998).

A second avian polyomavirus, named the goose hemorrhagic polyomavirus (GHP), has recently been isolated and characterized from farm-raised geese (species not provided) in France (Guerin et al. 2000). Sequence analysis of the amino acids of the GHP-encoded proteins shows that this virus is most closely related to APV, and it has been suggested that both viruses be included in a new subgenus *Avipolyomavirus*.

DISTRIBUTION

Avian polyomavirus has a worldwide distribution and has been reported in domestically raised parrots in Japan, Australia, Great Britain, Europe, Canada, South Africa, and the United States of America (reviewed by Phalen 1997). GHP has been described only in Europe (Lacroux et al. 2004; Payla et al. 2004).

HOST RANGE

The only confirmed natural host for APV is the sulphur-crested cockatoo. It is likely, however, that many more wild birds will be found to be naturally infected with this virus. Infection in captive-raised birds is widespread. It is likely that all psittacine birds and many other species of birds are susceptible to infection. A serologic survey of birds, in an aviary where a Green Aracari (*Pteroglossus viridis*) died with APV, found neutralizing antibody in Zebra Finches (*Poephila guttata*), a Ross's Turaco (*Musophaga rossae*), and even a Kookaburra (*Dacelo novaeguineae*) (Lafferty et al. 1998). Although unapparent infection is common in adult and nestling birds, disease is generally limited to parent-fed Budgerigar and lovebird nestlings and hand-fed nestling non-Budgerigar parrots, particularly macaws, conures (*Aratinga* and *Pyrhurra* spp.), Ring-necked Parakeets (*Psittacula krameri*), caiques (*Pionites* spp.), and Eclectus Parrots (*Eclectus roratus*). Mortality is occasionally seen in other nestling parrots, such as Amazon parrots (*Amazona* spp.) and cockatoos, but much less commonly (reviewed by Phalen 1997).

A survey of wild Dusky-headed Conures (*Aratinga weddellii*) reported low levels of neutralizing activity to APV virus neutralizing antibody (Gilardi et al. 1995). Subsequent investigations, however, have shown that this neutralizing activity was nonspecific and not caused by antibody (Phalen 1997).

Avian polyomavirus has been isolated from wild Buzzards (*Buteo buteo*) and a Eurasian Kestrel (*Falco tinnunculus*) in Europe. The cause of death in these birds is not known, so it is not known whether these birds represent a natural host species or not (Johne and Müller 1998). An APV-like disease is reported in captive-bred finches, particularly Gouldian finches (*Chloebia gouldiae*) (reviewed in Phalen 1997). It is not known what the relationship is of this virus to APV, nor is it known whether they are the natural hosts for the virus. To date, the GHPV has been isolated only from domestic geese.

ETIOLOGY

APV is a naked, approximately 40–50 nm iscosahedral virus that has a 4984 bp circular double-stranded DNA genome. The genome of this virus is organized in a similar manner to other polyomaviruses. It contains two early proteins, the large T and small t antigens, which interact with cellular proteins and regulate virus replication. There are four structural proteins, the VP 1, 2, and 3 and the agno protein. VP1 is the major capsid protein and the other structural proteins are involved in packaging the viral DNA. Between the open-reading frame for the T antigens and the agno protein is the presumed origin of replication and adjacent regulatory domains (Rott et al. 1988). A small degree of genetic variation has been found in the open reading frames of all but one of the APVs sequenced to date (Johne and Müller 2003; Lafferty et al. 1998; Phalen et al. 1999). Partial duplications of some of the regulatory elements have been documented in viruses that have been grown *in vitro* (Phalen et al. 1999). However, a duplication has also been identified in virus DNA amplified directly from tissue, so these duplications may also occur *in vivo* to a lesser extent (Phalen et al. 2001). In general, there is little evidence to suggest that these genetic variants have mutations that impart host specificity to the virus (Johne and Müller 1998; Phalen et al. 1999). One exception, however, is the variant found in cockatoos with pneumonitis. Although these viruses are still capable of causing disease in other parrots, there appears to be very specific point mutations that allow this virus to cause pneumonitis in cockatoos (Phalen et al. 2001).

EPIZOOTIOLOGY

Avian polyomavirus is maintained in captive populations of parrots though a number of mechanisms. Infections in susceptible non-Budgerigar species that are of the appropriate age result in a rapidly fatal disease, but slightly older nestlings survive and shed virus in feces and possibly through feather dander for up to 16 weeks. These birds are important sources for infections in other birds. APV infection is widespread in budgies and lovebirds. In Budgerigars, virus shedding is believed to continue for up to six months. Concurrent APV and Psittacine Beak and Feather Disease virus (PBFDV) infection, particularly in lovebirds, may permit persistent shedding of APV. The common practice of taking birds to bird shows and sales where birds from multiple aviaries are present and stocking pet stores with birds from multiple sources perpetuates infections (Phalen 1998).

Infection trials and the rapid rate of dissemination of this virus suggest that infection occurs through the respiratory tract. Egg transmission was suggested in a study with Budgerigars, however, these nestlings could have also contracted the infection at hatch if the eggs were contaminated (Bernier et al. 1984). Actual deaths in the egg caused by APV have recently been documented, but the aviculturalist was feeding baby birds that were shedding virus and then handling the eggs. It is likely that virus infection of the eggs was the result of the owner contaminating the eggs as opposed to vertical transmission (Pesaro et al. 1995).

Although APV infection has been documented in wild Sulphur-crested Cockatoos in Australia, it is not known how this virus is maintained in these birds. Given that the prevalence of PBFDV is high in this species, it may be that birds with concurrent infections continuously shed virus. The virus is also believed to be environmentally stable and might survive from one year to the next in nest cavities. How the virus infected European birds of prey is not known. GHPV has caused sporadic outbreaks in domestic geese in Europe since 1977, but the epizootiology of this virus is not known.

CLINICAL SIGNS

The common presenting sign in Budgerigar aviaries is a sudden onset of mortality in chicks that are 10–20 days old. Live nestlings are typically stunted, have distended abdomens, and may have feather dystrophy. Intention tremors are seen in some outbreaks but not in all. A variable percentage of nestlings survive the outbreaks with only a feather dystrophy. These birds appear healthy except that they have no remiges and retrices or the remiges and rectrices develop partially and fail to unsheath. Hemorrhage within the feather shaft is common. Because the psittacine PBFDV is a common co-infection in this species, feather dystrophy may also be a manifestation of concurrent infection with this virus (Reviewed in Phalen 1997).

In hand-fed nestling parrots, most affected birds die suddenly with little or no prodromal period. Clinical signs, when they occur, last for less than 24 hours and include weakness, pallor, subcutaneous hemorrhage, prolonged bleeding times, anorexia, dehydration, inappetence, and crop stasis (Graham et al. 1987; Phalen et al. 1997). Because of the associated liver necrosis, the plasma concentrations of the alanine aminotransferase will be expected to be elevated.

There are two atypical presentations of APV. The first occurs in chicks that survive the acute form of the disease. These birds develop a generalized edema and ascites. It is thought that these lesions develop as a result of hypoproteinemia that is secondary to liver necrosis and/or is the result of progressive glomerular damage. A second atypical presentation occurs when nestling cockatoos are infected with a genetic variant of APV. These birds develop slowly, fail to gain weight and become severely dyspneic before they die. The dyspnea is the result of a severe diffuse interstitial pneumonia and pulmonary edema (Phalen et al. 2001).

APV infection or an APV-like infection has been reported in several non-psittacine species. A Green Aracari infected with APV died following a short course of a nonspecific disease. This bird had a leukocytosis, heterophilia, anemia, and a marked elevation in the amino asparate transferase. In this study, in contact birds including Zebra Finches, a Kookaburra and a Ross's Turaco became seropositive but did not develop disease (Lafferty et al.1998). Several species of finches have been reported to have an APV-like disease, but the virus causing these lesions has not been characterized (reviewed by Phalen 1997). Finches with APV disease generally die without signs that are recognized by the owner. Gouldian Finches that have been in aviaries where APV infections have been documented occasionally develop an abnormal elongate, conical beak.

Signs of GHPV infection are nonspecific. Disease typically occurs in geese that are three to 16 weeks old but birds as young as four days of age and as old as 20 weeks have been diagnosed with disease. Signs were not observed in most birds. Signs when they occurred included tremors and ataxia, bloody diarrhea, and subcutaneous hemorrhages. Morbidity and mortality ranged from 4 to 67% (Lacroux et al. 2004; Payla et al. 2004).

PATHOGENESIS

The incubation period for APV is approximately 10–14 days. Initial virus replication may occur in the respiratory tract but this is still to be proved. Birds rapidly develop a viremia (Phalen et al. 2000). Virus replication occurs in many organ systems in Budgerigars and lovebirds. The majority of virus replication is confined to phagocytic cells of the immune system in non-Budgerigar psittacine birds (Graham et al. 1987). The characteristic hemorrhagic lesions seen in these birds may be the result of an immune-complex glomerulopathy (Phalen et al. 1996). Liver necrosis may be the result of cytokine-induced apoptosis and not necessarily direct viral infection of hepatocytes (Pesaro et al. 2005).

PATHOLOGY

APV causes a subacute, generally fatal, disease of nestling captive Budgerigars. At necropsy, birds are typically stunted, have abnormal feather development, skin discoloration, abdominal distension, ascites, hepatomegaly with localized areas of necrosis, and scattered areas of hemorrhage. Histologically, virus inclusion bodies are found in cells of multiple organ systems, including the liver, spleen, kidney, feather follicles (Figure 10.1), skin, esophagus, brain, and heart. Inclusion bodies are pan-nuclear, clear to lightly basophilic or amphophilic, and are associated with a pronounced karyomegaly (Bernier et al. 1981; Davis et al. 1981). They are fairly specific, but in some cases may be difficult to distinguish from inclusion bodies caused by adenoviruses or herpesviruses.

Non-Budgerigar parrot nestlings with APV disease die suddenly. Necropsy findings include generalized pallor, with subcutaneous and subserosal hemorrhage and enlargement of the spleen and liver (Figure 10.2). Less commonly, ascites and pericardial effusion may be present. Hallmark histological findings include massive hepatic necrosis that may spare only the periportal regions (Figure 10.3) and the presence of characteristic inclusion bodies in the spleen (Figure 10.4), mesangial cells of the kidney, and Kupffer cells of the liver. Necrosis of splenic cells is often massive. Less commonly, virus inclusions are found in other organ systems including the feather follicles (Graham et al. 1987). An immune complex glomerulopathy occurs in a significant percentage of the birds with this disease (Figure 10.5) (Phalen et al. 1996). Birds surviving the acute form of the disease may subsequently develop a glomerulosclerosis, ascites and anasarca (Phalen et al. 2001). Uncommonly, a chronic debilitating disease

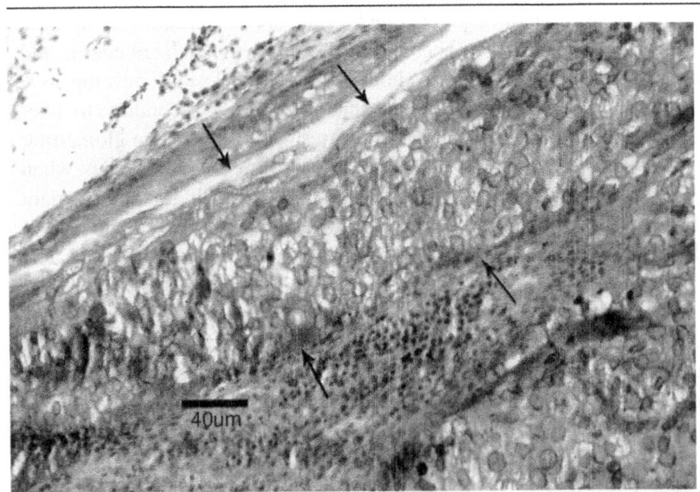

Figure 10.1. Avian polyomavirus inclusions (see arrows) in the feather follicle epithelium of a feather from a nestling Budgerigar. Bar = 40 μm

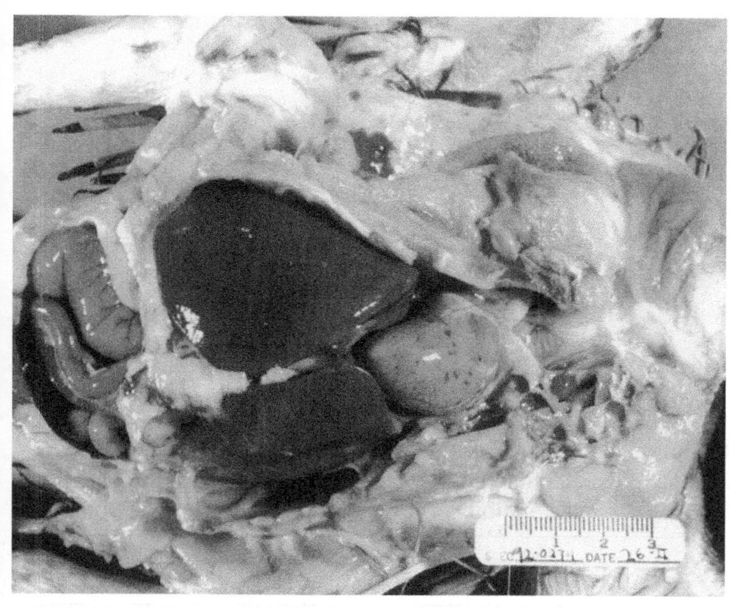

Figure 10.2. Six-week-old Scarlet Macaw *(Ara macao)* with avian polyomavirus disease. There is generalized pallor of all muscles, subcutaneous, intra-abdominal, and subserosal hemorrhage. There is also a marked hepatomegaly.

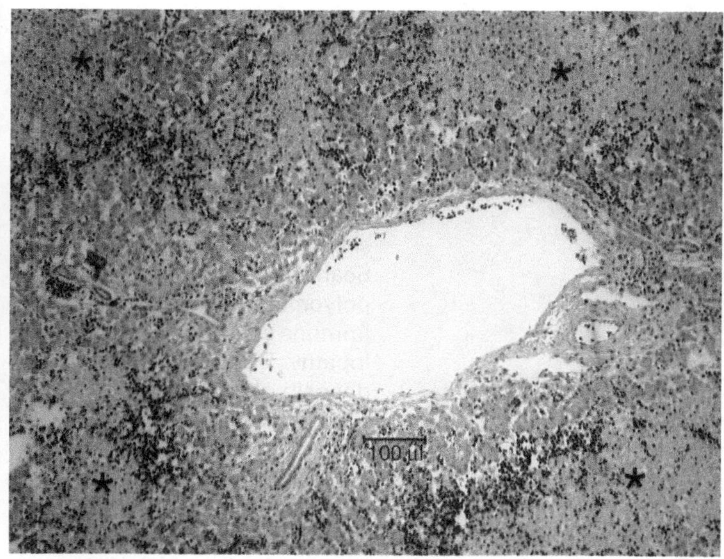

Figure 10.3. H&E stained section of liver from the macaw in Figure 10.2. Massive necrosis (*), sparing only the hepatocytes surrounding the portal vein. Bar = 100 μm

occurs in nestling cockatoos. Histologically, the cockatoos have a severe diffuse pneumonitis with abundant inclusion bodies (Schmidt 2003).

Lesions found in geese with GHPV included edema and acites, subcutaneous hemorrhage, hydropericardium, hemorrhage into the lumen of the intestine, and red discoloration and edema of the kidney. Histologically, there was proximal tubular necrosis with varying degrees of urate nephrosis, hepatitis, and hemorrhagic enteritis with necrosis of cells lining the intestinal crypts. Importantly, inclusion bodies were not found, nor were virus particles detected with electron microscopy (Lacroux et al. 2004; Payla et al. 2004).

DIAGNOSIS

The diagnosis of avian polyomavirus infection in parrots is readily made by characteristic gross and microscopic findings. Confirmation can be made by PCR, using virus-specific primers (Phalen et al. 1991), by immunohistochemistry, using anti-APV

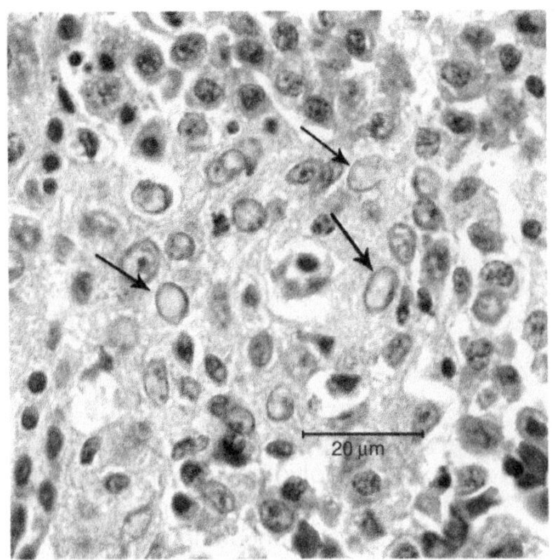

Figure 10.4. H&E-stained section of spleen from an Eclectus Parrot. Many, possibly most of the splenic cells exhibit karyomegaly (arrows). Bar = 20 µm

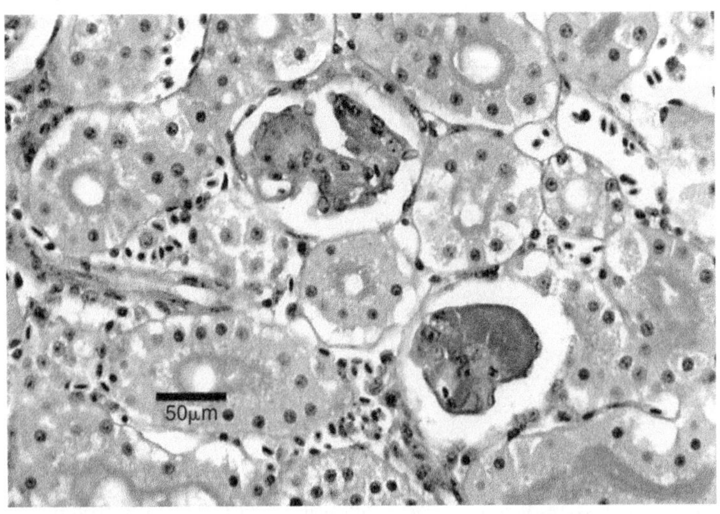

Figure 10.5. PAS-stained section of a kidney from a Scarlet Macaw with avian polyomavirus-associated immune complex glomerulopathy. The darkly staining deposits are immune complexes. Bar = 50 µm

antibodies (Graham et al. 1987), and *in situ* hybridization using APV-specific probes (Garcia et al. 1994). Polyomaviruses are non-enveloped, 42 to 48 nm and icosahedral. Transmission electron microscopy of fixed tissues or partially purified homogenates of fresh tissues will often demonstrate virions. APV has been isolated in chicken embryo fibroblasts. APV can be purified with isopyknic ultracentrifugation and has a buoyant density of 1.34 gm/ml (Rott et al. 1988).

GHPV should be suspected in young geese with edema, diffuse hemorrhage, proximal tubule necrosis, and a hemorrhagic enteritis. PCR with virus specific primers is currently the only definitive diagnostic assay (Lacroux et al. 2004; Payla et al. 2004).

IMMUNITY

Birds that survive APV infections develop circulating antibody, and antibody can be detected for five years or more after infection. All evidence suggests that infection results in a life-long immunity. It is possible that immunization results in protective circulating antibodies, but the ability of the current APV vaccine to prevent infection remains controversial (Phalen et al. 2000). After a bird is infected, it appears that cell-mediated immunity is necessary for elimination of infection, because antibody positive birds may remain viremic for several weeks (Phalen et al. 2000). The age of the bird and presumably the maturation stage of the immune system appears to play a key role in the outcome of an APV infection in birds that are susceptible to disease. Disease is typically confined to nestlings of susceptible species that are in a very specific stage of development (Graham et al. 1987).

PUBLIC HEALTH CONCERNS

There are no indications that avian polyomaviruses causes disease in humans.

DOMESTIC ANIMAL HEALTH CONCERNS

APV has been isolated from the feces and drinking water of a flock of chickens experiencing an outbreak of infectious bursal disease (Stoll et al. 1993). Additionally, virus inclusion bodies and virions characteristic of those of APV were found in the cecal epithelium of a chicken. Results of *in situ* hybridization with probes derived from the sequence of APV suggested that this virus was genetically similar, but not identical, to the APV (Goodwin et al. 1996). There have not been subsequent reports of APV-like infections in poultry.

The GHPV has only been identified in domestic geese. Sporadic outbreaks of this disease have been seen in Europe since 1979. Outbreaks of GHPV have resulted in up to 100% mortality (Lacroux et al. 2004; Payla et al. 2004).

WILDLIFE POPULATION IMPACTS

There is strong evidence that APV occurs in wild birds on multiple continents. A high prevalence of anti-APV antibody was found in free-ranging greater Sulphur-crested Cockatoos in Australia (Raidal et al. 1998). APV disease has not been reported to occur in wild Australian birds, but a disease with characteristic APV lesions was induced in a cockatoo infected with a preparation of PBFDV derived from the feathers of a wild bird, suggesting that APV was present in these tissues and was co-purified with the psittacine beak and feather disease virus (Raidal et al. 1995). Recently APVs were identified in five buzzards and a kestrel in Europe. Genetically, the sequence of the falcon virus was nearly identical to other APV variants of psittacine origin and the virus in the buzzard amplified with PCR primers derived from the sequence of the original APV isolated from a Budgerigar. Although virus concentrations were high and in the range typically found in birds with APV-disease, the carcasses of the buzzards were severely autolyzed and histological evaluation of the tissues was not possible. The falcon was reported to have a chronic illness, but the nature of the illness and whether this bird was a wild bird or was kept in a collection was not reported (Johne and Müller 1998).

Lesions characteristic of APV infection were reported in Red-faced Lovebirds (*Agapornis pullaria*) recently captured in Mozambique and held in quarantine for three weeks (Enders et al. 1997). The sequence of this virus was again very similar to those seen in other psittacine birds (Johne and Müller, 1998). The timing of this infection, three weeks after the onset of quarantine suggested that the birds may have acquired the infection while in quarantine from other birds. However, details on the possibility of exposure to other birds were not provided.

Preliminary evidence that APV may occur in wild birds in North America also exists. A House Sparrow (*Passer domesticus*) was found to have a glomerulopathy with characteristic APV-like inclusions within mesangial cells and PAS positive deposits within the mesangium and glomerular capillaries (Phalen 1997).

The significance of the GHPV to wildlife remains unclear, but the lesions seen in these geese are unlike any seen in other polyomavirus infections previously described, and karyomegaly was not reported, suggesting that this virus could be easily overlooked (Guerin et al. 2000). Contact between wild and domestic geese could be a possible means of dissemination of this virus.

Perhaps the greatest concern for APV or any virus found in domestically raised parrots is its introduction into a wild naive population of parrots. Re-introduction of captive-raised parrots is an increasingly popular idea. If birds come from sources where avian polyomavirus has been present, their release creates a potential scenario where wild populations of birds could be infected with APV.

TREATMENT AND CONTROL

There is no known treatment for polyomavirus infection. Control in captive populations of birds is done through management and testing. Breeding facilities can prevent the introduction of this disease by keeping a closed nursery, the prudent use of quarantine, and the prudent use of testing. Most birds shed virus for only 16 weeks or less, so birds would not be expected to be shedding virus after 16 weeks in quarantine. However, birds concurrently infected with the PBFDV may continuously shed APV. Therefore, birds that are high risk for PBFDV infection should be tested for both viruses before being allowed to leave quarantine. Budgerigars and lovebirds should not be kept in the same facilities as other parrots unless they are all tested (Phalen 1998).

Virus shedding begins within two weeks of infection and unapparently infected birds shed virus for up to 16 weeks. Viremia and virus shedding can be detected with polymerase chain reaction assays (PCR) of blood and combined oral and cloacal swabs. Antibody titers persist for years and possibly for life in some birds even though virus shedding is transient (Phalen et al. 2000). Therefore, serology is of little use in predicting virus shedding.

MANAGEMENT IMPLICATIONS

There is considerable interest in re-introducing captive-raised parrots back into the wild. Given the uncertain status of APV infection in most wild populations of parrots, any released bird should be negative for APV by PCR assays or by serology.

LITERATURE CITED

Bernier, G., M, Morin, and G. Marsolais. 1981. A generalized inclusion body disease in the budgerigar (*Melopsittacus undulatus*) caused by a papovavirus-like agent. *Avian Diseases* 25:1083–1092.

Bernier, G., M, Morin, and G. Marsolais. 1984. Papovirus induced feather abnormalities and skin lesions in the budgerigar: clinical and pathological findings. *Canadian Veterinary Journal* 25:307–310.

Blackmore, D.K., and I.F. Keymer. 1969. Cutaneous diseases of wild birds in Britain. *British Birds* 62:316–331.

Dom, P., R.Ducatelle, G. Charlier, and P. De Herdt. 1993. Papilloma-like virus infection in canaries (*Serinus canaria*). *Proceedings The 1993 European Conference on Avian Medicine and Surgery.* Utrecht, Netherlands, pp. 224–231.

Davis, R.B., L.H, Bozeman, D. Gaudry, O.J. Fletcher, P.D. Lukert, and M.J. Dykstra. 1981. A viral disease of fledgling budgerigars. *Avian Diseases* 25:179–183.

Enders, F., M. Gravendyck, H. Gerlach, and E.F. Kaleta. 1997. Fatal avian polyomavirus infection during quarantine in adult wild-caught red-faced lovebirds (*Agapornis pullaria*). *Avian Diseases* 41:496–498.

Howley, P.M., and D.R. Lowy. 2001. Papillomaviruses and their replication. In *Field's Virology,* D.M. Knipe, P.M. Howley, D.E. Griffen, R.A. Lamb, M.A. Martin, B. Roizman, and S.E. Straus (eds.). Lippincott Williams and Wilkins, Philadelphia, PA, U.S.A., pp. 2197–2229.

Graham, D.L., and B.W. Calnek. 1987. Papovavirus infection in hand-fed parrots: virus isolation and pathology. *Avian Diseases* 31:398–410.

Goodwin, M.A., K.S. Latimer, E.C. Player, F.D. Niagro, and P.R. Campagnoli. 1996. Polyomavirus inclusion bodies in chicken caecal epithelium. *Avian Pathology* 25:619–625.

Guerin, J.L., J. Gelfi, L. Dubois, A. Vuillaune, C. Boucraut-Barolon, and J.L. Pingret. 2000. A novel polyomavirus (goose hemorrhage polyomavirus) is the agent of hemorrhagic nephritis enteritis of geese. *Journal of Virology* 74:4523–4529.

Garcia, A., K.S. Latimer, F.D. Niagro, B.W. Ritchie, and R.P. Campagnoli. 1994. Diagnosis of polyomavirus-induced hepatic necrosis in psittacine birds using DNA probes. *Journal of Veterinary Diagnostic Investigation* 6:308–314.

Gilardi, K.V., L.J. Lowenstine, J.D. Gilardi, and C.A. Munn. 1995. A survey for selected viral, chlamydial, and parasitic diseases in wild dusky-headed parakeets (*Aratinga weddellii*) and tui parakeets (*Brotogeris sanctithomae*) in Peru. *Journal of Wildlife Diseases* 31:523–528.

Groth, W., and M. Abs. 1967. Papillomatosis in chaffinches. *Deutsche Tierarztliche Wochenschrift* 74:146–150.

Jacobson, E.R., C.R. Mladinich, S. Clubb, J. Sundberg, and W.D. Lancaster. 1983. Papilloma-like virus infection in an African gray parrot. *Journal of the American Veterinary Medical Association* 183:1307–1308.

Johne, R., and H. Müller. 1998. Avian polyomavirus in wild birds: genome analysis of isolates from *Falconiformes* and *Psittaciformes. Archives of Virology* 143:1501–1512.

Johne, R., and H. Müller. 2003. The genome of goose hemorrhagic polyomavirus, a new member of the proposed subgenus *Avipolyomavirus. Virology* 308:291–302.

Keymer, I.F., and D.K. Blackmore. 1974. Disease of the skin and soft parts of wild birds. *British Birds* 57:175–179.

Lafferty, S., A. Fudge, R. Schmidt, and D.N. Phalen. 1998. Avian polyomavirus infection in a green aracaris. *Avian Diseases* 43:577–585.

Lacroux, C., O. Andreoletti, B. Payre, J.L. Pingret, A. Disssais, and J.L. Guerin. 2004. Pathology of spontaneous and experimental infections by goose haemorrhagic polyomavirus. *Avian Pathology* 33:351–358.

Lima, P.H. C., M.J. Van Noord, and G.G. De Groot. 1973. Detection of virus in squamous papillomas of the wild bird species *Fringilla coelebs. Journal of the National Cancer Institute* 50:567–571.

Lowenstine, L.J., M.E. Fowler, and K. Flammer. 1983. Viral papillomas on the feet of cockatoos. In *Proceedings of the American Association of Zoo Veterinarians and International Symposium of Zoo and Wild Animal Medicine,* Vienna, Austria, pp. 85–87.

Moreno-Lopez, J., H. Ahola, A. Stenlund, A. Osterhaus, and U. Pettersson. 1984. Genome of an avian papillomavirus. *Journal of Virology* 51:872–875.

Osterhaus, A.D.M.E., D.J. Ellens, and M.C. Horzinek. 1977. Identification and characterization of a papillomavirus from birds (Fringillidae). *Intervirology* 8:351–359.

O'Banion, M.K., E.R. Jacobson, and J.P. Sundberg. 1992. Molecular cloning and partial characterization of a parrot papillomavirus. *Intervirology* 33:91–96.

Palya, V., É. Ivanics, R. Glávits, Á. Dán, T. Maltó, and P. Zarka. 2004. Epizootic occurrence of haemorrhagic nephritis enteritis virus infection of geese. *Avian Pathology* 33:244–250.

Pennycott, T.T. 2003. Scaly leg, papillomas and pox in wild birds. *Veterinary Record* 152:444.

Pesaro, S., R. Ceccherelli, C. Tarantino, S. Scoccianti, E. Bert, and G. Rossi. 1995. The first Italian outbreak of polyomavirus infection in macaws. In *Proceedings of the 7th* European Association of Avian Veterinarians and 6th Scientific Meeting of the European College of Avian Medicine and Surgery, Arles, France, pp. 321–326.

Phalen, D.N., V.G. Wilson, and D.L. Graham. 1991. Polymerase chain reaction assay for avian polyomavirus. *Journal Clinical Microbiology* 29:1030–1037.

Phalen D.N., V.G. Wilson, D.L. Graham. 1996. Characterization of the avian polyomavirus-associated immune complex glomerulopathy. *Avian Diseases* 40:140–149.

Phalen, D.N. 1997. Viruses. In *Avian Medicine and Surgery,* R.B. Altman, S.L. Clubb, G.M. Dorrestein, and K. Quesenberry, (eds.). W.B. Saunders Company, Philadelphia, PA, U.S.A., pp. 281–322.

Phalen, D.N. 1998. Avian polyomavirus: my thoughts. *American Federation of Aviculture Watchbird* 25:28–29.

Phalen, D.N., B. Dahlhausen, and S. Radabaugh. 1998. Avian polyomavirus: More pieces to the puzzle. In *Proceedings of the Association of Avian Veterinarians,* St. Paul, MN, U.S.A., pp. 151–158.

Phalen, D.N., V.G. Wilson, J.M. Gaskin, J.N. Derr, and D.L. Graham. 1999. Genetic diversity in 20 variants of the avian polyomavirus. *Avian Disease* 43:207–218.

Phalen, D.N. 2000. Avian viral diagnostics. In *Laboratory Medicine Avian and Exotic Pets,* A. Fudge (ed.). W.B. Saunders Company, Philadelphia, PA, U.S.A., pp. 111–123.

Phalen, D.N., C.S. Radabaugh R.D. Dahlhausen, and D.K. Styles. 2000. Antibody response and duration of viremia and cloacal virus in psittacine birds naturally infected with avian polyomavirus. *Journal of the American Veterinary Medical Association* 217:32–36.

Phalen, D.N., E. Tomaszewski, K. Boatwright, and S.L. Lafferty. 2001. Genetic diversity in avian polyomaviruses, clinical implications. In *Proceedings of the Association of Avian Veterinarians,* Orlando, FL, U.S.A., pp. 171–174.

Raidal, S.R., and G.M. Cross. 1995. Acute necrotizing hepatitis caused by experimental infection with psittacine beak and feather disease virus. *Journal of Avian Medicine and Surgery* 9:36–40.

Raidal, S.R., G.M. Cross, E. Tomaszewski, D.L. Graham, and D. N. Phalen. 1998. A serologic survey for avian polyomavirus and Pacheco's disease virus in Australian cockatoos. *Avian Pathology* 27:263–268.

Rott, O., M.Kroger, H.L. Müller, and G.Hobom. 1988. The genome of budgerigar fledgling disease virus, an avian polyomavirus. *Virology* 165:74–86.

Schmidt, R.,D. Reavell, and D.N. Phalen. 2003. *Pathology of Exotic Birds.* Iowa State University Press, Ames, IA, U.S.A.

Sironi, G., and D.Gallazzi. 1992. Papillomavirus infection in green finches (*Carduelis chloris*). *Journal of Veterinary Medicine* 39:454–458.

Styles, D.K., E.K. Tomaszewski, and D.N. Phalen. 2005. A novel psittacid herpesviruses in African gray parrots (*Psittacus erithacus erithacus*) *Avian Pathology* 34:150–15.

Terai, M., R.DeSalle, and R.D. Burk. 2002. Lack of canonical E6 and E7 open reading frames in birds papillomaviruses: *Fringilla coelebs* papillomavirus and *Psittacus erithacus timneh* papillomavirus. *Journal of Virology* 76:10020–10023.

11
Retroviral Infections

Mark L. Drew

INTRODUCTION

Avian retroviruses include a group of RNA viruses capable of inducing a variety of neoplastic diseases in birds, usually involving tissues of mesodermal origin.

The retroviruses are generally divided into two groups: the leukosis/sarcoma (L/S) viruses and the reticuloendotheliosis (RE) viruses. The L/S viruses are members of the genus *Alpharetrovirus* of the family Retroviridae (Regenmortel et al. 2000). These closely related viruses cause a variety of neoplastic conditions affecting mainly cells of the hematopoeitic system such as lymphoid, myeloid, or erythroid cell lines or tumors of mesenchymal origin such as sarcomas, endotheliomas, or fibromas. The RE group of retroviruses are unrelated to the L/S viruses and cause chronic lymphomas and an immunosuppressive runting disease syndrome described in commercial chickens and ducks. Both groups of retroviruses are well documented in commercial poultry and cause significant mortality and/or economic loss to the poultry industry worldwide. L/S viruses can infect a wide range of avian species under experimental and possibly natural conditions, but clinical disease in species other than chickens is uncommon. RE viruses also infect a wide range of species including chickens, turkeys, ducks, geese, pheasants, and quail, but naturally occurring clinical disease in species other than commercial chickens and turkeys occurs infrequently.

In wild birds, neoplasia is uncommon (Jennings 1968; Siegfried 1983), leading to an incomplete understanding of the prevalence and impact of these viral pathogens. Lymphoid, erythroid, and myeloid cell line tumors and some sarcomas occur sporadically in individual wild birds but the link between these neoplastic conditions and L/S retroviruses as seen in poultry is unclear.

Neoplasia associated with RE viruses has been reported in free-ranging Wild Turkey (*Meleagris gallopavo*), Attwater's (*Tympanuchus cupido attwateri*), and Greater Prairie Chicken (*T. cupido*) reared in a captive propagation project. This has raised concerns that release of these birds to the wild could have adverse health effects on endangered or threatened wild populations (Drew et al. 1998).

This chapter will provide an overview of some neoplastic diseases in wild and captive birds that are or may be associated with retroviruses. The neoplastic disease conditions associated with retroviruses in domestic poultry are well documented (Fadly and Payne 2003; Witter and Fadly 2003; Witter and Schat 2003) and will be only highlighted here. Comparison of the salient features of Marek's disease, lymphoid leukosis, and reticuloendotheliosis in domestic poultry are summarized in Witter and Schat (2003) and lymphoid neoplasia in pet birds is summarized in Coleman (1995).

Leukosis/Sarcoma Group

SYNONYMS

A variety of names have been given to neoplastic conditions associated with L/S viruses in poultry. These names are based on the tissue or cell type transformed by the viral infection. In captive and wild birds, these terms should be used with caution unless an association with a leukosis/sarcoma virus is known.

Hematopoietic Tumors

LYMPHOID TUMORS

Avian leukosis, visceral lymphoma, lymphomatosis, big liver disease, lymphatic leukosis, lymphocytoma, lymphoid leukosis.

ERYTHROID TUMORS

Intravascular lymphoid leukosis, erythroblastosis, erythroid leukosis.

MYELOID TUMORS

Leukemic myeloid leukosis, myeloblastosis, myelomatosis, myelocytoma.

Connective Tissue Tumors

Fibroma, fibrosarcoma, myoma, myxosarcoma, histiocytic sarcoma, chondroma.

Epithelial Tumors

Nephroma, nephroblastoma.

Endothelial Tumors

Hemangioma, angiosarcoma, endothelioma, mesothelioma.

Bone Tumors

Osteopetrosis, marble bone, thick leg disease.

CNS Tumors

Fowl glioma, meningioma.

HISTORY

Diseases caused by the Leukosis/Sarcoma group of retroviruses are common in domestic poultry, especially chickens, and include a wide variety of transmissible neoplasms. Leukosis in poultry has been recognized for more than 100 years, with the first report of lymphoid neoplasia in chickens appearing in 1868 (Roloff 1868, cited in Fadly and Payne 2003). Various presentations of leukosis and the pathology of lymphoid, myeloid, and erythroid neoplasia in the fowl was described in some detail as early as 1921 by Ellerman. Due to the spectrum of pathological presentations, many of these conditions were thought to be due to different pathogens (Payne and Purchase 1991; Iwata et al. 2002). Proof of a viral etiology for lymphoid leucosis was provided by Burmester (1947). The history of this virus complex in domestic poultry has been reviewed by Doughtery (1987) and Payne (1992).

Lymphoid and myeloid neoplastic conditions similar to those caused by L/S retroviruses have been recognized sporadically in wild birds in captivity and occasionally in free-ranging birds, but rarely has the causative agent been proven to be retroviruses. The use of molecular techniques to identify evidence of retroviral genome in tumor cells will undoubtedly help to better define the presence of retroviruses in these lesions.

DISTRIBUTION AND HOST RANGE

Neoplastic diseases caused by L/S retroviruses are found worldwide in domestic chickens (*Gallus gallus*), and exposure rates are very high (Fadly and Payne 2003). Lymphoid leukosis virus has been isolated from several captive species of pheasants (Fujita et al. 1974; Hanafusa et al. 1976), Gray Partridge (*Perdix perdix*) (Hanafusa et al. 1976), and Gambel's Quail (*Callipepla gambellii*) (Troesch and Vogt 1985). Experimental infections have been established in a variety of avian species including Helmeted Guineafowl (*Numida meleagris*), Pekin duck (*Anas platyrhynchos domesticus*), Rock Pigeon (*Columba livia*), turkey (*Meleagris* spp.) and Gray Partridge, but only with a limited number of virus subgroups (Fadly and Payne 2003). There have been no comprehensive surveys of captive or wild birds for antibodies to lymphoid leukosis. Antibodies have been found in captive pheasants and quail (Chen and Vogt 1977) and captive Ostrich (*Struthio camelus*) in Zimbabwe (Cadman et al. 1994). Antibodies to L/S virus subgroups A and B have been found in free-range chickens and feral Red Junglefowl (*Gallus gallus*) in Kenya and Malaysia (Morgan 1973).

A wide variety of lymphoreticular neoplastic conditions have been documented in individual captive and wild birds (Keymer 1972; Effron et al. 1977; Griner 1983) (Table 11.1), some of which may be associated with L/S retroviruses. The connection between neoplasia and the presence of L/S viruses in most captive or wild birds has not been demonstrated. However, there is some evidence for a causal relationship between L/S retroviruses and renal tumors in the Budgerigar (*Melopsittacus undulatus*) (Gardner et al. 1981; Neumann and Kummerfeld 1983; Gould et al. 1993), lymphoid neoplasia in pheasants (Dren et al. 1983), and possibly others.

ETIOLOGY

Viruses in the leukosis/sarcoma group are RNA viruses (Mathews 1982; Darcel 1996) recently placed in the genus *Alpharetrovirus* of the family Retroviridae (Regenmortel et al. 2000). These viruses are small, about 90 nm, with knobbed projections on the surface (Nowinski et al. 1973; Temin 1974), and are distinct from those that produce RE. Viruses in the L/S retroviruses are found in two forms, nondefective and defective, which affect the ability of the virus to replicate and express tumors in the bird. Defective viruses have incomplete genomes and many of these require the presence of a helper leukosis virus to enable them to replicate (Fadly and Payne 2003).

The L/S retroviruses affecting chickens have been divided into six subgroups (A, B, C, D, E, and J) based on the structure of their viral envelope glycoproteins (Payne et al. 1992; Sung et al. 2002; Fadly and Payne 2003). Subgroups F, G, H, and I represent endogenous retroviruses identified in captive gallinaceous species other than chickens, including pheasants, Gray

Table 11.1. Neoplastic diseases in captive or wild birds that are similar to tumors in domestic chickens or turkeys caused avian retroviruses. In most of these reports there was no attempt by the investigators to isolate or identify an avian retrovirus. In many of the reports the authors suggest that there could be a link with avian retroviruses

Species	Organ System	Lesion	Virus Isolation[a]	Serology[a]	Reference
Galliformes					
Peafowl (*Pavo* spp.)		Lymphomatosis	No	No	Sah et al. 1973
Common Peafowl (*Pavo* spp.)	Periocular tissue	Lymphosarcoma	REV	No	Miller et al. 1998
Common Peafowl (*Pavo cristatus*)	Liver, kidney, spleen	Lymphoblastic leukosis	No	No	Kaliner and Miringa 1972
Common Peafowl	Multiple organs	Lymphoid leucosis	No	No	Rao and Acharjyo 1984
Japanese Quail (*Coturnix japonica*)	Digestive tract, other visceral organs	Anaplastic mononuclear tumors	REV	No	Carlson et al. 1974
Wild Turkey (*Meleagris gallopavo*)	Spleen, esophagus	Lymphoreticular masses	REV	No	Hayes et al. 1992
Wild Turkey	Liver, spleen esophagus	Lymphoproliferative masses	REV	No	Ley et al. 1989
Turkey (*Meleagris* spp.)		Avian myeloblastosis	NA	NA	Mladenov et al. 1977
Attwater's Prairie Chicken (*Tympanuchus cupido attwateri*)	Skin, multiple organs	Lymphoreticular masses	REV	REV	Drew et al. 1998
Greater Prairie Chicken (*T. pinnatus*)	Skin, multiple organs	Lymphoreticular masses	REV	REV	Drew et al. 1998
Rock Partridge (*Alectoris graeca*)	Liver, spleen	Lymphoma	No	No	Ozgencil and Metin 1972

Gray Partridge (*Perdix perdix*)	Liver, crop, esophagus	Lymphoma	REV	No	Trampel et al. 2002
Chinese Bamboo-Partridge (*Bambusicola thoraciia*)		Lymphoma	NA	NA	Mladenov et al. 1977
Crested Wood Partridge (*Rollulus rouroul*)	Liver	Cholangiocellular adenocarcinoma	No	No	Mladenov et al. 1977
Crested Wood Partridge		Lymphoma	No	No	Mladenov et al. 1977
Ruffed Grouse (*Bonasa umbellus*)	Foot	Chondrosarcoma	No	No	Siegfried 1983
Golden Pheasant (*Chrysolophus pictus*)	Wing	Hemangiosarcoma	Negative		Suedmeyer et al. 2001
Ring-necked Pheasant (*Phasianus colchicus*)	Head, oral cavity, multiple organs	Pleomorphic lymphoblasts	REV	REV	Dren et al. 1983
Ring-necked Pheasant		Myeloid leukosis	No	No	Loupal 1984
Ring-necked Pheasant	Multiple organs	Lymphomatosis	No	No	Rosen and Mathey 1955
Ring-necked Pheasant	Lung	Angiosarcoma	No	No	Carter et al. 1983
Copper Pheasant (*Syrmaticus soemmerringii*)	Liver, spleen, kidney, thyroid	Lymphoblastic leukosis	No	No	Wadsworth et al. 1981
Gray Peacock Pheasant (*Polyplectron bicalcaratum*)		Lymphoid leukosis	No	No	Loupal 1984
Psittaciformes					
Amazon Parrot (*Amazona* spp.)	Periorbital tissue	Lymphoid leukosis	No	No	Campbell 1984

(*Continued*)

Table 11.1. (Continued)

Species	Organ System	Lesion	Virus Isolation[a]	Serology[a]	Reference
Orange-winged Parrot (*Amazona amazonia*)	Liver	Malignant lymphoma	No	No	de Wit et al. 2003
Blue-fronted Parrot (*Amazona aestria*)	Liver, spleen, kidney, duodenum	Malignant lymphoma	No	No	de Wit et al. 2003
Blue-and-yellow Macaw (*Ara ararauna*)	Skin of face	Pseudolymphoma	No	No	Kollias et al. 1992
Scarlet Macaw (*Ara macao*)	Periorbital tissue	Plasmycytoid lymphosarcoma	Negative	No	Ramos-Vara et al. 1997
African Gray Parrot	Periorbital tissue, liver, spleen	Lymphoreticular neoplasia	No	No	Paul-Murphy et al. 1985
African Gray Parrot	Liver, spleen	Lymphoblastic leukosis	No	No	Palmer and Stauber 1981
African Gray Parrot		Lymphoid leukosis	No	No	Loupal 1984
African Gray Parrot (*Psittacus erithacus*)	Beak, bones, syrinx, liver	Fibrosarcoma	No	No	Riddel and Cribb 1983
Budgerigar (*Melopsittacus undulatus*)	Kidney, liver	Nephroblastoma, lymphoma, adenocarcinoma	Negative	LL	Neumann and Kummerfeld 1983
Budgerigar		Lymphoid leukosis	No	No	Loupal 1984
Budgerigar		Myeloid leukosis	No	No	Loupal 1984
Budgerigar		Lymphoid leukosis	No	No	Bauck 1986
Budgerigar		Avian myeloblastosis	No	No	Mladenov et al. 1977
Cockatiel (*Nymphicus hollandicus*)		Lymphoid leukosis	No	No	Bauck 1986
Eastern Rosella (*Platycerus eximius*)		Lymphoid leukosis	No	No	Loupal 1984
Pale-headed Rosella (*Platycercus*	Liver, spleen	Malignant lymphoma	No	No	Griner 1983

adscitus)					
Fischer's Lovebird (*Agapornis fischeri*)		Myeloid leukosis	No	No	Loupal 1984
Cockatoo (*Cacatua* spp.)		Lymphosarcoma			Messonier 1992
Salmon-crested Cockatoo (*Cacatua moluccensis*)		Lymphoid leukosis	No	No	Bauck 1986
Salmon-crested Cockatoo	Muscle, skin	Lymphosarcoma	No	No	France and Gilson 1993
Sulfur-crested Cockatoo (*Cacatua galerita*)	Liver, spleen	Malignant lymphoma	No	No	Griner 1983
Superb Parrot (*Polytelis swainsonii*)	Lung, kidney	Malignant lymphoma	No	No	Griner 1983
Princes Parrot (*Polytelis alexandrae*)	Liver, spleen, mesentery	Lymphoblastic leukosis	No	No	Wadsworth et al. 1981
Turquoise Parrot (*Neophema pulchella*)		Myeloid leukosis	No	No	Loupal 1984
Pacific (*Forpus coelestis*)	Liver, kidney, bone marrow	Myeloblastic leukemia	No	No	Griner 1983
Passeriformes					
European Starling (*Sturnis vulgaris*)	Multiple organs	Multicentric lymphoma	RV	No	Wade et al. 1999
Hill Mynah (*Gracula religiosa*)	Liver	Lymphosarcoma	No	No	Hill et al. 1986
Hill Mynah	Liver	Lymphosarcoma	No	No	Griner 1983
Asian Pied Starling (Pied Mynah) (*Sturnuscontra*)		Lymphomatosis	No	No	Sah et al. 1973

(*Continued*)

Table 11.1. (Continued)

Species	Organ System	Lesion	Virus Isolation[a]	Serology[a]	Reference
Green-and-gold Tanager (*Tangara schrankii*)	Liver, spleen kidney	Lymphoblastic leukosis	No	No	Wadsworth et al. 1981
White-throated Laughingthrush (*Garrulax albogularis*)	Liver, spleen	Lymphoblastic leukosis	No	No	Wadsworth et al. 1981
Common Canary (*Serinus canaria*)	Intestine	Lymphoid leucosis	No	No	Blackmore 1966
Common Canary		Lymphoid leukosis	No	No	Bauck 1986
Common Canary		Stem cell leukosis	No	No	Loupal 1984
Red-cheeked Cordon-bleu Finch (*Uraeginthus bengalus*)		Lymphoid leukosis	No	No	Loupal 1984
American Goldfinch (*Carduelistristis*)	Duodenum	Neoplastic lymphocytic infiltrate	No	No	Middleton and Julian 1983
Blue-gray Tanager (*Thraupis episcopus*)	NA	Lymphosarcoma	No	No	Griner 1983
Red-cowled Cardinal (*Paroaria dominicana*)	NA	Lymphosarcoma	No	No	Griner 1983
Falconiformes					
Merlin (*Falco columbarius*)	Liver	Lymphoblastic lymphosarcoma	No	No	Higgins and Hannam 1985
Peregrine Falcon (*Falco peregrinus*)	Spleen	Lymphoblastic leukemia, malignant lymphoma	No	No	Rosskopf et al. 1987

Struthioniformes					
Ostrich (*Struthio camelus*)	Liver, heart, thoracic inlet	Multicentric lymphoma	No	No	Van der Heyden et al. 1992
Ostrich	Multiple organs	Immature lymphoid cells	No	No	Garcia-Fernandez et al. 2000
Casuariiformes					
Emu (*Dromaius novaehollandiae*)	Liver, spleen, kidney	Lymphocytic leukocytosis, disseminated lymphoma	No	No	Gregory et al. 1996
Columbiformes					
Rock Pigeon (*Columba livia*)	Periocular tissues, spleen	Lymphoblastic lymphoma	No	No	Rambow et al. 1981
Rock Pigeon		Lymphoma	No	No	Loupal 1984
Rock Pigeon	Eye, crop, liver, spleen, kidney	Multicentric lymphoblastic lymphoma	No	No	Chalmers 1986
Speckled Pigeon (*Columba guinea*)	Liver, spleen	Lymphoblastic leukosis	No	No	Wadsworth et al. 1981
European Turtle-Dove (*Streptopelia turtur*)	Liver, ascites	Lymphoblastic leukosis	No	No	Wadsworth et al. 1981
Eurasian Collared-Dove (*Streptopelia decaocto*)		Lymphoid leukosis	No	No	Loupal 1984
BlueCrowned Pigeon (*Goura cristata*)	Spleen, liver, kidney, lung	Leukemia, visceral lymphosarcoma	No	No	Griner 1983
Anseriformes					
Mallard (*Anas platyrhynchos*)	Lung, esophagus	Lymphoblastic lymphosarcoma	No	No	Siegfried 1983

(*Continued*)

Table 11.1. (Continued)

Species	Organ System	Lesion	Virus Isolation[a]	Serology[a]	Reference
Pekin Duck (*Anas platyrhynchos domesticus*)		Lymphocytic leukemia, malignant lymphoma	No	No	Newell et al. 1991
Muscovy Duck (*Cairina moschata*)	Small intestine	Lymphoproliferative disease	Negative	REV	Paul et al. 1978
Chestnut Teal (*Anas castanea*)		Lymphosarcoma	No	No	Griner 1983
Black Swan (*Cygnus atratus*)		Lymphosarcoma	No	No	Griner 1983
Brant Goose (*Branta bernicia*)		Lymphosarcoma	No	No	Griner 1983
Canada Goose (*Branta canadensis*)	Muscle, multiple organs	Spindle cell sarcoma	No	No	Gates et al. 1992
Canada Goose	Muscle	Multicentric liposarcoma	No	No	Doster et al. 1987
Canada Goose	Muscle	Multicentric lipomatosis/ fibromatosis	No	No	Daoust et al. 1991
Canada Goose	Muscle	Multicentric fibrosarcoma	No	No	Siegfried 1983.
Canada Goose	Leg, abdominal wall	Hemangiosarcoma	No	No	Siegfried 1983
Canada Goose	Muscle	Multicentric neurofibrosarcoma	No	No	Locke 1963
White-fronted Goose (*Anser albifrons*)	Muscle	Multicentric lipomatosis/ fibromatosis	No	No	Daoust et al. 1991
Eider (*Somateria* spp.)	Multiple organs	Lymphoma	NA	NA	Sigurdson et al. 1996

Gruiformes					
Common Crane (*Grus grus*)		Reticulosarcoma	NA	NA	Mladenov et al. 1977
Gough Island Moorhen (*Porphyriornis comeri*)		Lymphocytic leukemia	No	No	Montali 1978
Ciconiiformes					
Great Egret (*Ardea alba*)	Liver, spleen, kidney	Lymphoblastic leukosis	No	No	Nobel 1972
Sphenisciformes					
King Penguin (*Aptenodytes patagonica*)		Lymphoid leukosis	No	No	Loupal 1984

[a] No indicates that no attempt was made to identify virus; negative indicates that virus was looked for but not found; RV indicates that evidence of a retrovirus was identified, REV indicates reticuloendotheliosis virus was identified; LL indicates Lymphoid leucosis virus was identified; NA indicates information not available.

Partridge, and Gambel's Quail (Payne 1992). For example, L/S subgroup F viruses have been found in Ring-necked (*Phasianus colchicus*) and Green Pheasant (*Phasianus versicolor*) and subgroup G virus in Ghinghi, Silver (*Lophura nycthemera*), and Golden (*Chrysolophus pictus*) Pheasants. Subgroup H has been isolated from Gray Partridge and subgroup I from Gambel's Quail (Chen and Vogt 1977).

Avian leukosis viruses that are transmitted as infectious virus particles are termed exogenous viruses. There are several families of avian retrovirus elements that are part of the normal chicken genome and these are termed endogenous viruses and are transmitted genetically (Fadly and Payne 2003). A number of endogenous retrovirus-like viruses have been found in members of the Pheasanidae (Hanafusa et al. 1976; Chen and Vogt 1977), domestic chickens (Boyce-Jacino et al. 1989; Resnick et al. 1990), and Ostrich (Peach 1997).

Endogenous leukosis virus of subgroup E is found in most normal chickens (Payne and Purchase 1991). It has little or no oncogenicity and may even benefit the bird by providing protection against infection with certain exogenous L/S retroviruses.

Recent work demonstrated avian leukosis and sarcoma virus *gag* genes in 26 species of galliform birds from North America, Central America, eastern Europe, Asia, and Africa, including birds in the family Tetraoninidae (grouse and ptarmigan) (Dimcheff et al. 2000). Nineteen of the 26 host species from whom L/SVs were sequenced were not previously known to contain L/SVs. A new retrovirus, tetraonine endogenous retrovirus (TERV), has been isolated from Ruffed Grouse (*Bonasa umbellus*) (Dimcheff et al. 2001). These data suggest that retroviruses are present and transmitted genetically and possibly horizontally among some wild bird species and may be separate from those found in domestic chickens.

EPIZOOTIOLOGY

Source/Reservoir

Chickens are the natural host and reservoir for the leukosis/sarcoma group of viruses. Captive populations of pheasants and quail may also be infected, but the distribution and extent of disease in these species is unknown. Although surveys of free-ranging birds have not been done, it is likely that some wild birds that have contact with domestic chickens have been exposed to the virus.

Transmission

In chickens, the exogenous leukosis/sarcoma group viruses are capable of being transmitted vertically through the egg (Cottral et al. 1954) or horizontally by both direct and indirect contact (Rubin et al. 1961, 1962; Fadly and Payne 2003). The primary means of transmission is direct contact with infected birds in close proximity. Vertical transmission is important in maintaining the virus between generations (Rubin et al. 1961) and because congenitally infected birds are much more likely to develop clinical disease.

Endogenous L/S retroviruses are transmitted genetically in germ cells of both sexes. These rarely result in disease in the chicks and in some instances may impart some protection against infection with exogenous virus.

CLINICAL SIGNS

The clinical signs exhibited by chickens infected with leukosis/sarcoma virus are variable and depend on the tissues and organ systems involved. For example, chickens with osteopetrosis may be lame and have visible deformities of long bones. Chickens with hemangiomas of the skin may have raised skin lesions resembling blood blisters that are easily traumatized and hemorrhage. Chickens with fibromas or even myelocytomatosis may have lumps or skeletal abnormalities that are visible grossly. The clinical signs vary with the subgroup of virus as well as the immune status of the affected bird (Fadly and Payne 2003), but clinical signs for internal tumors such as lymphoid leukosis are generally nonspecific and include general malaise, depression, diarrhea, and dehydration. Clinical signs are seen after birds reach 14 weeks of age.

In captive and wild birds, clinical signs are generally nonspecific. Clinical evaluation of live birds may indicate some level of ill-thrift or specific organ dysfunction associated with the location of the tumors.

PATHOGENESIS AND PATHOLOGY

During viral infection, the transformation of normal cells to neoplastic cells is mediated by the formation of a DNA provirus (Weiss et al. 1982). Virally encoded reverse transcriptase mediates the conversion of the viral RNA genome into a DNA intermediate, enabling the integration into the host genome. The proviral genes are transcribed into viral RNA, which is used to produce new viral particles that escape from the host cell. The exception to this process is lymphoid leukosis virus, which lacks an oncogene, resulting in a prolonged time period for tumor development (Payne and Purchase 1991).

Clinical Pathology

No definitive clinical pathological changes are present in chickens infected with leukosis/sarcoma viruses. Affected birds may be anemic and there may be an increase in the number of immature forms of specific white or red blood cells in the peripheral blood. Peripheral leukocyte changes have been observed in some captive and wild birds reported to have lesions similar to that of lymphoid leukosis in poultry (Campbell 1984; Bauck 1986; Van Der Heyden 1992; Gregory et al. 1996; Ramos-Vara et al. 1997; Wade et al. 1999; Garcia-Fernandez et al. 2000; Suedmeyer et al. 2001; de Wit et al. 2003).

Cytology is rarely done in domestic poultry, but in valuable captive birds the technique may be useful to determine the cell types within the tumor.

Pathology

Macroscopic lesions of L/S retroviral infections depend on the strain of virus, the infectious dose, and immune status of the host. The gross pathological lesions associated with the various types of neoplasia in chickens are well described in Fadly and Payne (2003). In wild birds, lymphoid leukosis-like lesions are the most frequent tumor reported (Table 11.1). These are generally described as soft, smooth, white nodular-to-diffuse tumors affecting a variety of parenchymal organs, most commonly liver, spleen, kidney, and mesentery and often involving multiple organs.

Detailed descriptions of microscopic lesions associated with the various L/S virus–related tumors in poultry are found in Fadly and Payne (2003). In captive and wild birds, tumor classification depends on the cell lines affected, with lymphoblastic lymphoma being the most common neoplasm reported (Table 11.1). Most reports describe these as consisting of solid or infiltrating masses of quite uniform, immature lymphoblastic cells that infiltrate an organ and physically compress and alter the adjacent tissue architecture.

DIAGNOSIS

A tentative diagnosis of leukosis/sarcoma virus infection can be made based on the presence of neoplastic lesions either pre- or post-mortem. In valuable individual birds, clinical evaluation, hematology and biopsy/cytology may be useful in establishing a diagnosis.

Specific identification of the causative agent requires virus culture, detection of virus antigen or viral nucleic acid associated with the lesions, or serological evidence of infection. This level of diagnostic investigation has rarely been done in wild birds and hence there is incomplete evidence in most cases linking retroviruses to individual neoplastic conditions. Molecular analysis of the multiple strains of leukosis/sarcoma virus will result in development and use of new specific diagnostic tests for these agents in many avian species (Sacco et al. 2001). Not all tumor types produce sufficient virus within the tumor itself for viral isolation. Virus isolation is generally done in cell culture, but care must be taken to use permissive cell lines that are free of exogenous virus (Payne and Purchase 1991).

Antigen capture ELISA may be used to identify L/S viral antigens, provided that there is sufficient virus load in the tumor tissue. Detection of retroviral DNA provirus has been done using polymerase chain reaction (PCR) (Benkel et al. 1996; Garcia et al. 2003). RT-PCR can also be used to detect viral RNA.

Serologic tests have been developed that are capable of detecting the presence of antibodies to most leukosis/sarcoma viruses (Purchase and Fadley 1980). Serology can be used to test for antibodies using complement fixation or ELISA (Fadly et al. 1981). These serologic tests are generally not available through commercial laboratories and contact with a specialized avian pathology laboratory is required. The standard protocols and testing reagents used for poultry may not react with antibodies produced by other species. The development of species-specific test reagents will allow serological surveys to be done with more accurate results (Cadman et al. 1994; Ziedler et al. 1995).

In captive or free-ranging birds, the diagnosis of leukosis/sarcoma virus is usually based on the presence of tumors and the cell types within the tumors. Virus has been successfully isolated from pheasants, but not in other species of birds with lymphoreticular tumors thought to be similar to lymphoid leukosis (Table 11.1). Serology has been used to detect lymphoid leukosis antibodies in Japanese Quail (*Coturnix japonicus*) (Chambers et al. 1986), feral and wild Junglefowl (Morgan 1973; Sacco et al. 2001), and farmed Ostrich (Cadman et al. 1994).

Differential diagnoses that should be considered in birds suspected of having lesions due to leukosis/-sarcoma virus include Marek's disease, reticuloendotheliosis, lymphoproliferative disease, and other immunosuppressive conditions.

IMMUNITY

There is a fair amount known about immunity to L/S retroviruses in commercial chickens because control and eradication of these diseases in commercial breeder flocks has been a goal for many years. Immunity against L/S viruses in chickens is reviewed in Fadly and Payne (2003). Chickens of all ages that are exposed to these viruses tend to develop transient viremia with the development of antibodies that persist for the life of the bird (Rubin et al. 1962). Young birds may have passive immunity dependent on antibody titer of the hen (Witter et al. 1966). Infection and tumor development are dependent on age, sex, genetics, and exposure dose (Rubin et al. 1961, 1962; Fadly and Payne 2003). Young chicks are more prone to infection and tumor development than adults (Payne and Purchase 1991). Intact males are less susceptible to tumor development than intact females or castrated males (Burmester and Nelson 1945). Genetic resistance to both infection and tumor induction is well documented in chickens (Fadly and Payne 2003). Immune-tolerant infections with persistent viremia and no antibody production can develop in congenitally infected chicks (Payne and Purchase 1991). There has been almost no research on immunity to L/S viruses in wild bird species.

PUBLIC HEALTH CONCERNS

There is no known public health concern associated with L/S retroviruses.

DOMESTIC ANIMAL CONCERNS

Avian leukosis/sarcoma virus infections are common in commercial poultry throughout the world and uncommon or rare in wild birds. There is no evidence that wild birds infected with L/S viruses are a significant risk for commercial poultry flocks, and in fact where disease has been reported in captive gallinaceous species other than chickens, the source of infection has likely been commercial chickens. Disease from avian L/S viruses has not been documented in naturally infected mammals. Neoplasia, especially lymphoblastic lymphoma, has been reported in many species of captive birds. The link between neoplasia and infection with avian leukosis/sarcoma virus is still unclear.

WILDLIFE POPULATION IMPACTS

Neoplastic diseases with a similar pathological picture to lymphoid leukosis in poultry have been reported in wild birds. However, there is almost no information on the prevalence of infection in wild avian species. Free-ranging wild birds that develop slow growing and chronically debilitating tumors would be difficult to locate and most would be removed from the population through predation. The impact of infection and tumor development on individuals and wildlife populations is unknown, but the fact that there are individual cases reported is evidence that neoplasia possibly linked to avian retroviruses does occur in wild populations. With the recent detection of L/S virus *gag* genes in 26 species of galliform birds around the globe and the identification of TERV in Ruffed Grouse (Dimcheff et al. 2001), further work to identify retroviruses in wild bird species is certainly warranted. The sporadic development of neoplasia in captive and wild birds is unlikely to have negative effects on population levels.

TREATMENT AND CONTROL

Treatment of birds affected by leukosis/sarcoma virus is generally not attempted. In valuable birds with limited lesions, temporary relief may be obtained by surgical excision of lesions or radiation (Newell et al. 1991; Paul-Murphy et al. 1985; France and Gilson 1993). Development of a vaccine for poultry against leukosis viruses has not been successful (Okazaki et al. 1982).

Reticuloendotheliosis Group

SYNONYMS

Reticuloendotheliosis, RE, chronic lymphoid neoplasia, acute reticulum cell neoplasia, runting disease syndrome.

HISTORY, DISTRIBUTION, AND HOST RANGE

Reticuloendotheliosis (RE) was initially identified in domestic turkeys in 1958 (Robinson and Twiehaus 1974). RE occurs naturally in turkeys in many areas of the world, although it is not common (Witter 1991). It is also uncommon in chickens, although REV has been shown to induce lymphoma in chickens vaccinated with vaccines contaminated with the virus (Jackson et al. 1977; Fadly et al. 1996).

Natural infections with REV and tumor development have been described in a number of avian species other than domestic chickens and turkeys (Table 11.1) including domestic Pekin Duck, Ring-necked Pheasant, geese, and Japanese Quail (Chen et al. 1987; Witter 1991). Recently, captive Attwater's (*Tympanuchus cupido attwateri*) and Greater Prairie Chicken (*T. cupido*) were infected with REV (Drew et al. 1998). Experimental infections have been documented in Ring-necked Pheasants and Guinea Fowl (Dren et al. 1983; Witter 1991).

Serologic evidence of antibodies to REV have been found using agar gel immunodiffusion (AGID) tests in Pekin Duck and Ring-necked Pheasant in Japan (Sasaki et al. 1993), Rock Pigeon in Germany (Neumann et al. 1981), and Ostrich in Zimbabwe (Cadman et al. 1994). Only a few surveys of wild gallinaceous bird populations have been undertaken, but those that have been done in the U.S.A. show a very low prevalence of exposure to REV. These include surveys of Wild Turkey in Connecticut and Texas (Sasseville et al. 1988) and Attwater's Prairie Chicken and Lesser Prairie Chicken (*T. pallidicinctus*) in Texas (Peterson et al. 1998, 2002a,b; Wiedenfeld et al. 2002).

Neoplasia associated with REV has been documented in free-ranging Wild Turkey (Ley et al. 1989; Hayes et al. 1992), captive Attwater's and Greater Prairie Chickens (Drew et al. 1998) and captive Gray Partridge (Trampel et al. 2002). The low number of individuals and species of nondomestic gallinaceous birds in which the disease has been identified is likely due to minimal surveillance. The use of molecular techniques for surveillance will likely confirm the presence of RE in other wild bird species in the future.

ETIOLOGY

Viruses in the reticuloendotheliosis group are RNA viruses and they have been placed in the genus *Mammalian C-type* within the family Retroviridae. Based on host immunological responses, morphology, ultrastructure, and nucleic acid sequences, the REV are distinct from leukosis/sarcoma viruses (Coffin 1996). REV particles are about 100 nm with surface projections that are typical of retroviruses (Zeigel et al. 1966; Kang et al. 1975). Numerous strains of REV have been identified (Purchase and Witter 1975; Witter and Fadly 2003), but it is often difficult to distinguish one from another antigenically (Witter 1991), making definitive diagnosis of a specific disease syndrome problematic in some situations. Some of the viruses within this group include the Twiehaus-type strain of RE (Strain T), duck infectious anemia virus, spleen necrosis virus, and chicken syncytial virus (Gerlach 1994).

Within the REV group are two distinct virus types, nondefective and defective. Nondefective REV strains replicate in a similar fashion to L/S retroviruses. Defective REV strains require a nondefective RE helper virus for replication (Witter 1991).

EPIZOOTIOLOGY

Source, Reservoir

No definitive reservoir of REV has been identified. Although the virus is found most commonly in domestic turkeys, it is not widespread. Contamination of avian vaccines with REV has been documented (Jackson et al. 1977; Fadly et al. 1996) and may be a source of infection for domestic poultry. Extensive serologic surveys for the presence of REV in free-ranging avian species have not been done. The source of virus for infections in captive prairie chickens was never identified (Drew et al. 1998).

Transmission

REV can be transmitted from infected birds to susceptible birds by both vertical and horizontal routes. The primary means of transmission of the virus in commercial turkey or chicken flocks is unclear (Witter 1991), but direct contact with infective virus in feces, ocular and nasal secretions, and contaminated litter are likely the most common means of transmission (Peterson and Levine 1971; Paul et al. 1978; Bagust et al. 1981; Witter and Johnson 1985). However, direct contact between naive birds and infected birds or REV contaminated material rarely results in clinical disease (Peterson and Levine 1971; Witter and Johnson 1985).

Insects may play a role in the transmission of REV as the viruses have been transmitted mechanically to chickens via mosquitoes (Motha et al. 1984) and both mosquitoes and houseflies have been shown capable of harboring REV (Davidson and Braverman 2005). Infection rates of turkeys and chickens in the southern U.S.A. vary seasonally and the highest prevalence of infection occurs in the summer months (Motha et al. 1984; Witter and Johnson 1985), indirectly supporting the possibility of insect transmission. More research is needed to confirm the role of insects in spreading this disease. Mechanical transmission of REV by mosquitoes may explain the onset and seasonal occurrence of RE in captive prairie chickens (Drew et al. 1998).

Vertical transmission of REV has been shown to occur in domestic poultry (McDougall et al. 1980; Bagust et al. 1981; Motha and Egerton 1987; Witter 1991); however, its importance in maintaining the viruses is not clear.

CLINICAL SIGNS

Clinical signs of RE in birds are dependent on the species, age, and immune status of individuals. In domestic turkeys and chickens infected with REV, several distinct syndromes are recognized including acute reticular cell neoplasia, runting syndrome, and chronic lymphoma (Witter and Fadly 2003).

Acute reticular cell neoplasia occurs in newly hatched chickens or turkeys, but the birds show few clinical signs and mortality rates can be very high.

Runting syndrome in chickens is seen with a variety of non-neoplastic lesions associated with REV (Witter 1991). These birds are likely immunosuppressed, markedly stunted with pale extremities and mucus membranes. Chickens with runting syndrome may develop localized feather vane lesions characterized by a lack of development of feather barbules (termed Nakanuke) (Tajima et al. 1977). Runting syndrome has not been identified in wild birds.

Birds with chronic lymphoma due to infection with REV generally present with nonspecific clinical signs ranging from few or no signs in birds with lymphomas affecting internal organs to general malaise, wasting, and dehydration. External cutaneous lesions, generally on the head, have been described in turkeys (Hanson and Howell 1979), Ring-necked Pheasants (Dren et al.

1983), and Prairie Chickens (Drew et al. 1998). These lesions may affect vision and the ability of the bird to eat leading to clinical signs of ill-thrift.

PATHOLOGY

Of the three presentations of REV infection in birds (acute reticular cell neoplasia, chronic lymphoma, and runting disease syndrome), only lymphomas have been documented in captive and wild species other than domestic chickens and turkeys. Only changes associated with lymphomas are described here.

Clinical Pathology

No definitive clinical pathology changes have been described for wild birds infected with REV. Changes in hematology or clinical biochemistry may occur but are likely related to the effects of neoplasia on specific affected organs or alterations in normal body functions associated with chronic disease.

Macroscopic and Micropsopic Pathology

There are no pathognomonic lesions for RE in birds. Lesions of RE are similar to those caused by L/S viruses and Marek's disease virus and are reviewed in detail in Witter and Fadly (2003).

The gross lesions of RE are dependent on the location of the lymphoma. The majority of tumors develop in parenchymal organs or along peripheral nerves. Lesions generally vary from smooth enlargements of the spleen, liver, heart, thymus, or bursa to nodular lymphomas in visceral organs with or without necrosis (Witter and Fadly 2003). Lesions in ducks have included enlarged livers and spleens, lesions in intestine and lymphoid infiltrates in skeletal muscle, kidneys and heart (Li et al. 1983; Motha 1984). In addition to visceral lesions, cutaneous lymphomas on the face, eyelids, and feet have been reported in turkeys, Ring-necked Pheasants, and Prairie Chickens (Hanson and Howell 1979; Dren et al. 1983; Drew et al. 1998). These lesions may interfere with the ability of the bird to see or eat, and they may ulcerate and become encrusted with exudates and environmental debris.

Lymphomas from birds infected with REV are composed of uniform, usually blastic lymphoreticular cells (Li et al. 1983; Witter 1991; Drew et al. 1998). Inflammatory cells may be present depending on the size and location of the tumor. The specific cell type of the tumor associated with RE in wild or captive birds is usually not known.

DIAGNOSIS

A tentative diagnosis of RE in wild or captive species is based on the gross and microscopic lesions and confirmation of REV infection requires viral culture, detection of REV antigens, or REV nucleic acid associated with the lesions or the presence of RE viral antibodies in affected birds. Virus isolation can be done from tissue samples or whole blood using appropriate cell lines. PCR has been used to detect REV proviral-DNA, and RT-PCR may be useful to detect viral RNA (Aly et al. 1993). Viral antigen in tissues and cell cultures can be detected using monoclonal antibodies (Cui et al. 1986) or neutralization tests and monoclonal antibodies (Chen et al. 1987).

Serology can be used to screen birds for antibodies to REV using an ELISA (Cui et al. 1986, 1988) or virus neutralization tests (Witter 1989). These and other serologic tests are generally not available through commercial laboratories and contact with an avian pathology laboratory may be needed for assistance. In addition, the standard testing protocol and testing reagents used for poultry may not react with antibodies produced by other species.

Differential diagnoses that should be considered in birds suspected of having lesions of RE include Marek's disease, lymphoid leukosis, lymphoproliferative disease, and other immunosuppressive conditions. The variety of retroviral diseases that are known in domestic poultry and the difficulty in differentiating these viruses make it difficult to make a definitive diagnosis.

IMMUNITY

Immunity in chickens and turkeys to REV is described in Witter and Fadly (2003). Virtually nothing is known about immunity to REV in other avian species. Birds exposed via the embryo tend to develop tolerant infections with persistent viremias and the absence of antibodies. Adult birds exposed to the virus tend to have a transient viremia with the development of antibodies that appear to be protective. Maternal antibodies passed through the egg may provide some protection against infection in young chicks. Chronic lymphoid neoplasia develops in birds that do not develop antibodies and become persistently infected with REV. Some strains of nondefective REV cause immunosuppression, and both humoral and cellular immune responses may be depressed. No evidence of genetic resistance to RE has been documented in poultry (Witter 1991).

PUBLIC HEALTH CONCERNS

No public health concerns have been reported with REV.

DOMESTIC ANIMAL CONCERNS

There are no documented reports indicating that wild birds have been the source of virus for commercial poultry. Domestic poultry are likely the reservoir of REV for wild birds.

WILDLIFE POPULATION IMPACTS

The impact of RE on wild birds is unknown due to minimal surveys for the disease. Serologic surveys of Wild Turkey (Sasseville et al. 1988; Peterson et al. 2002a), Attwater's Prairie Chicken (Peterson et al. 1998), Greater Prairie Chicken (Wiedenfeld et al. 2002), and Lesser Prairie Chicken (Peterson et al. 2002b; Wiedenfeld et al. 2002) have found no evidence of widespread exposure to REV in these species in the U.S.A. To date, there are reports of only two Wild Turkeys that have died due to RE (Ley et al. 1989; Hayes et al. 1992) and only two individual birds serologically positive for REV (Peterson et al. 2002a). In free-ranging Greater and Lesser Prairie Chicken, only two birds have been found to be serologically positive for REV (Wiedenfeld et al. 2002).

TREATMENT AND CONTROL

Treatment of RE in domestic turkeys is generally not attempted. In valuable individual birds with limited lesions, temporary relief may be obtained by surgical excision of lesions, but these birds would remain potential sources of virus for other birds.

There are no vaccines for immunizing against REV in birds. REV contamination of commercial poultry vaccines (particularly avian fowl pox vaccines) has been documented (Diallo et al. 1998) and although a rare event, the possibility should be considered when developing vaccination protocols for rare or endangered species or for vaccinating birds in captive propagation and release programs.

Control of RE in poultry flocks is difficult due to the sporadic nature of the disease. Control of RE was attempted in a captive flock of Prairie Chickens by isolating birds with antibodies to and lesions suggestive of REV, preventing mosquito access to birds, and selective euthanasia (Drew et al. 1998). The effectiveness of these measures in reducing the prevalence of disease and the development of tumors is unclear, but to date, RE has not been found in any of the captive birds released into the wild.

MANAGEMENT IMPLICATIONS

The management implications of RE in wild populations of gallinaceous birds is of considerable importance for captive breeding of rare or endangered species and for translocation of birds (Peterson 2004). Because there are currently very few surveys for RE in wild birds, the potential risk of inadvertent introduction of RE into free-ranging populations through management actions is undefined. Many state wildlife management agencies in the U.S.A. conduct extensive translocation efforts of Wild Turkey and may spread RE or other infectious agents to naïve populations. The presence of RE in Attwater's and Greater Prairie Chickens raised in captive propagation facilities for release and reintroduction of birds into the wild is problematic from a biological, disease management, and genetic perspective (Drew et al. 1998; Peterson 2004). Serologic testing of Prairie Chicken, Wild Turkey, and other gallinaceous birds is needed to determine the presence, prevalence, and host range of REV in free-ranging populations.

LITERATURE CITED

Aly, M.M., E.J. Smith, and A.M. Fadly. 1993. Detection of reticuloendotheliosis virus infection using the polymerase chain reaction. *Avian Pathology* 22:543–554.

Bagust, T.J., T.M. Grimes, and N. Ratnamohan. 1981. Experimental infection of chickens with an Australian strain of reticuloendotheliosis virus. 3. Persistent infection and transmission by the adult hen. *Avian Pathology* 10:375–385.

Bauck, L. 1986. Lymphosarcoma/avian leukosis in pet birds:Case reports. In *Proceedings of the Association of Avian Veterinarians*, pp. 241–245.

Benkel, B.F., A.A. Grunder, D. Burke, and F.A. Ponce de Leon. 1996. A polymerase chain reaction based diagnostic test for the endogenous retroviral element ev-Ble of chickens. *Animal Genetics* 27:436–437.

Blackmore, D.K. 1966. The clinical approach to tumours in cage birds. I. The pathology and incidence of neoplasia in cage birds. *Journal of Small Animal Practice* 7:217–223.

Boyce-Jacino, M.T., R. Resnick, and A.J. Faras. 1989. Structural and functional characterization of the unusually short long terminal repeats and their adjacent regions of a novel endogenous avian retrovirus. *Virology* 173:157–166.

Burmester, B.R. and N.M. Nelson. 1945. The effect of castration and sex hormones upon the incidence of lymphomatosis in chickens. *Poultry Science* 24: 509–515.

Burmetser, B.R. 1947. Studies on the transmission of avian visceral lymphomatosis. II. Propagation of lymphomatosis with cellular and cell-free preparations. *Cancer Research* 7:786–797.

Cadman, H.F., P.J. Kelly, R. Zhou. 1994. A serosurvey using enzyme linked immunosorbent assay for antibodies against poultry pathogens in ostriches (*Struthio camelus*) from Zimbabwe. *Avian Diseases* 38:621–625.

Campbell, T.W. 1984. Lymphoid leukosis in an Amazon parrot—A case report. In *Proceedings of the Association of Avian Veterinarians*, pp. 229–234.

Carlson, H.C., G.L. Seawright, and J.R. Petit. 1974. Reticuloendotheliosis virus in Japanese quail. *Avian Pathology* 3:169–175.

Carter, J.K., S.J. Proctor, and R.E. Smith. 1983. Induction of angiosarcomas by ring-necked pheasant virus. *Infection and Immunity* 40:310–319.

Chalmers, G.A.1986. Neoplasms in two racing pigeons. *Avian Diseases* 30:241–244.

Chambers, J.A., A. Cywinski, P.J. Chen1986. Characterization of Rous sarcoma virus-related sequences in the Japanese quail. *Journal of Virology* 59:354–362.

Chen, P.Y., Z.Z. Cui, L.F. Lee, and R.L. Witter. 1987. Serologic differences among nondefective reticuloendotheliosis viruses. *Archives of Virology* 93:233–246.

Chen, Y.C. and P.K. Vogt. 1977. Endogenous leukosis viruses in the avian family Phasianidae. *Virology* 76:740–750.

Chubb, L.G., and R.F. Gordon. The avian leukosis complex—a review. Veterinary Review Annotated 32:97–120.

Coffin, J.M. 1996. Retroviridae:the viruses and their replication. In *Virology,* B.N. Fields, D.M. Knipe, and P.M. Howley (eds.). Lippincott-Raven Publishers, Philadelphia, PA, U.S.A., pp. 1767–1846.

Coleman, C.W. 1995. Lymphoid neoplasia in pet birds:A review. *Journal of Avian Medicine and Surgery* 9:3–7.

Cottral, G.E., B.R. Burmester, and N.F.Waters. 1954. Egg transmission of avian lymphomatosis. *Poultry Science* 33:1174–1184.

Cui, Z.Z, L.F. Lee, R.F. Silva, and R.L. Witter. 1986. Monoclonal antibodies against avian reticuloendotheliosis virus:Identification of strain-specific and strain-common epitopes. *Journal of Immunology* 136: 4237–4242.

Cui, Z.Z, L.F. Lee, R.F. Silva, R.L. Witter and T.S. Chang. 1988. Monoclonal-antibody-mediated enzyme -linked immunosorbant assay for detection of reticuloendothelial viruses. *Avian Diseases* 32:32–40.

Daoust, P.Y., G. Wobeser, D.J. Rainnie, and F.A. Leighton. 1991. Multicentric intramuscular lipomatosis/fibromatosis in free-flying white-fronted and Canada geese. *Journal of Wildlife Disease* 27: 135–139.

Darcel, C. 1996. Lymphoid leukosis viruses, their recognition as 'persistent' viruses and comparisons with certain other retroviruses of veterinary importance. *Veterinary Research Communications* 20:83–108.

Davidson, I. and Y. Braverman. 2005. Insect contribution to horizontal transmission of Reticuloendotheliosis virus. *Journal of Medical Entomology* 42:128–133.

de Wit, M., N.J. Schoemaker, M.J. Kik, and I. Westerhof. 2003. Hypercalcemia in two Amazon parrots with malignant lymphoma. *Avian Diseases* 47:223–228.

Diallo, I.S., M.A. MacKenzie, P. B.Spradbrow, and W.F. Robinson. 1998. Field isolates of fowlpox virus contaminated with reticuloendotheliosis virus. *Avian Pathology* 27:60–66.

Dimcheff, D.E., S.V. Drovetski, M. Krishnan, and D.P. Mindell. 2000. Cospeciation and horizontal transmission of avian sarcoma and leukosis virus *gag* genes in galliform birds. *Journal of Virology* 74:3984–3995.

Dimcheff, D.E., M. Krishnan, and D.P. Mindell. 2001. Evolution and characterization of Tetraonine endogenous retrovirus: a new virus related to avian sarcoma and leukosis viruses. *Journal of Virology* 75: 2002–2009.

Doster, A.R., J.L. Johnson, G.E. Duhamel, T. W. Bargar, and G. Nason. 1987. Liposarcoma in a Canada goose (*Branta canadensis*). *Avian Diseases* 31:918–920.

Doughtery, R.M. 1987. A historical review of avian retrovirus research. In *Avian Leukosis.* G.F. deBoer (ed.). Matrinus Nijhoff International, Boston, MA, U.S.A., pp. 1–27.

Dren, C.N., E. Saghy, R. Glavits, F. Ratz, J. Ping, and V. Sztojkov. 1983. Lymphoreticular tumour in pen-raised pheasants associated with a reticuloendotheliosis-like virus infection. *Avian Pathology* 12:55–71.

Drew, M.L., W.L. Wigle, D.L. Graham, C.P. Griffin, N.J. Silvy, A.M. Fadly, and R.L. Witter. 1998. Reticuloendotheliosis in captive greater and Attwater's prairie chickens. *Journal of Wildlife Disease* 34: 783–791.

Effron, M., L. Griner, and K. Benirschke. 1977. Nature and rate of neoplasia found in captive wild mammals, birds, and reptiles at necropsy. *Journal of the National Cancer Institute* 59:185–198.

Ellerman, V. 1921. *The leucosis of fowls and leucemia problems.* Gyldendal, London, UK.

Fadly, A.M., W. Okazaki, E.J. Smith, L.B. Cri, and J. Henden. 1981. Relative efficiency of test procedures to detect lymphoid leukosis virus infection. *Poultry Science* 60:2037–2044.

Fadly, A.M., and L.N. Payne. 2003. Leukosis/sarcoma group. In *Diseases of Poultry,* 11th Ed., Y.M. Saif, H.G. Barnes, J.R. Glisson, A.M. Fadly, L.R. McDougald, and D.E. Swayne (eds.). Iowa State University Press. Ames, IA, U.S.A., pp. 465–516.

Fadly, A.M.R.L. Witter, E.J. Smith, R.F. Silva, W.M. Reed, F.J. Hoerr, and M.R. Putman. 1996. An outbreak of lymphomas in commercial broiler breeder chickens vaccinated with a fowlpox vaccine contaminated with reticuloendotheliosis virus. *Avian Pathology* 25:35–47.

France, M., and S. Gilson. 1993. Chemotherapy treatment of lymphosarcoma in a Moluccan cockatoo. In *Proceedings of the Association of Avian Veterinarians,* pp. 15–19.

Fujita, D.J., Y.C. Chen, R.R. Friis, and P.K. Vogt. 1974. RNA tumor viruses of pheasants:Characteristics of avian leukosis subgroups F and G. *Virology* 60:558–571.

Garcia-Fernandez, R.A., C. Perez-Martinez, J. Espinosa-Alvarez, A. Escudero-Diez, J.F. Garcia-Marin, A. Nunez, and M.J. Garcia-Iglesias. 2000. Lymphoid leukosis in an ostrich (*Struthio camelus*). *Veterinary Record* 146:676–677.

Garcia, M., J. el Attrache, S.M. Riblet, V.R. Lunge, A.S. Fonsea, P. Villegas and N. Ikuta. 2003. Development and application of a reverse transcriptase nested polymerase chain reaction test for detection of exogenous avian leukosis virus. *Avian Diseases* 47:41–53.

Gardner, M.B., R.W. Rongey, P. Sarma, and P. Arnstein. 1981. Electron microscope search for retrovirus particles in spontaneous tumors of the parakeet. *Veterinary Pathology* 18:700–703.

Gates, R.J., A. Woolf, D.F. Caithamer, and W. E. Moritz. 1992. Prevalence of spindle cell sarcomas among wild Canada geese from southern Illinois. *Journal of Wildlife Disease* 28:666–668.

Gerlach, H. 1994. Viruses. *In Avian Medicine:Principles and Application.* B.W. Ritchie, G.J. Harrison, and L.R.Harrison. Wingers Publishing, Inc., Lake Worth, FL, U.S.A., pp. 862–948.

Gould, W.J., P.H. O'Connell, H.L. Shivaprasad, A.E. Yeager, K.A. Schat. 1993. Detection of retrovirus sequences in budgerigars with tumors. *Avian Pathology* 22:33–45.

Gregory, C.R., K.S. Latimer, E.A. Mahaffey, and T. Doker. 1996. Lymphoma and leukemic blood picture in an emu (*Dromaius novaehollandiae*). *Veterinary Clinical Pathology* 25:136–139.

Griner, L.A. 1983. *Pathology of Zoo Animals.* Zoological Society of San Diego, San Diego, CA, U.S.A., 608 pp.

Hanafusa, T., H. Hanafusa, C.E. Metrioka, W.S. Hayward, C.W. Rettemier, R.C. Sawyer, R.M. Doughtery, and H.S. DiStefano. 1976. Pheasant virus:New class of ribodeoxyvirus. In *Proceedings of the National Academy of Science USA* 73:1333–1337.

Hanson, J., and J. Howell. 1979. Suspected reticuloendotheliosis in turkeys with cutaneous lesions reminiscent of fowl pox. *Canadian Veterinary Journal* 20: 61–164.

Hayes, L.E., K.A. Langheinrich, and R.L. Witter. 1992. Reticuloendotheliosis in a wild turkey (*Meleagris gallopavo*) from coastal Georgia. *Journal of Wildlife Disease* 28:154–158.

Higgins, R.J. and D.A.R. Hannam. 1985. Lymphoid leukosis in a captive merlin (*Falco columbarius*). *Avian Pathology* 14:445–447.

Hill, J.E., D.L. Burke, and G.N. Rowland. 1986. Hepatopathy and lymphosarcoma in a mynah bird with excessive iron storage. *Avian Diseases* 30: 634–636.

Iwata, N., K. Ochiai, K. Hayashi, K. Ohashi, and T. Umemura. 2002. Avian retrovirus infection causes naturally occurring glioma:isolation and transmission of a virus from so-called fowl glioma. *Avian Pathology* 31:193–199.

Jackson, C.A.W., S.E. Dunn, D.I. Smith, P.T. Gilchrist, and P.A. MacQueen. 1977. Proventriculitis, "Nakanuke", and reticuloendotheliosis in chickens following vaccination with Herpesviruses of turkeys (HVT). *Australian Veterinary Journal* 53:457–458.

Jennings, A.R. 1968. Tumors of free-living wild mammals and birds in Great Britain. *Symposium of the Zoological Society of London* 24:273–287.

Kaliner, G., and E.N. Miringa. 1972. Malignant lymphoid neoplasia in a peahen (*Pavo cristatus*). *Avian Diseases* 16:1115–1117.

Kang, C.Y., T.C. Wong and K.V. Holmes. 1975. Comparative ultrastructure study of four reticuloendotheliosis viruses. *Journal of Virology* 16: 1027–1038.

Keymer, I.F. 1972. Diseases of birds of prey. *Veterinary Record* 90:579–594.

Kollias, G.V., B. Homer, and J.P. Thompson. 1992. Cutaneous pseudolymphoma in a juvenile blue and gold macaw (*Ara ararauna*). *Journal of Zoo and Wildlife Medicine* 23:235–240.

Ley, D.H., M.D. Fisker, D.T. Cobb and R.L. Witter. 1989. Histomoniasis and reticuloendotheliosis in a wild turkey (*Meleagris gallopavo*) in North Carolina. *Journal of Wildlife Disease* 25:262–265.

Li, J., B.W. Calnek, K.A. Schat, and D.L. Graham. 1983. Pathogenesis of reticuloendotheliosis infection in ducks. *Avian Diseases* 27:1090–1105.

Locke, L.N. 1963. Multicentric neurofibrosarcoma in a Canada goose, *Branta canadensis. Avian Diseases* 7:196–202.

Loupal, G. 1984. Leukosis among zoo and free-living birds. *Avian Pathology* 13:703–714.

Mathews, R.E.F. 1982. Fourth report of the international committee on taxonomy of viruses. Classification and nomenclature of viruses. *Intervirology* 17:1–199.

McDougall, J.S., R.W. Shilleto, and P. M. Biggs. 1980. Experimental infection and vertical transmission of reticuloendotheliosis virus in the turkey. *Avian Pathology* 9:445–454.

Messonier, S.P. 1992. Lymphosarcoma in a young cockatoo. *Journal of the Association of Avian Veterinarians* 6:207.

Middleton, A.L.A. and R.J. Julian. 1983. Lymphoproliferative disease in the American goldfinch, *Carduelis tristis. Journal of Wildlife Disease* 19:280–285.

Miller, P. E., J. Paul-Murphy, R. Sullivan, A.J. Cooley, R.P. Dubielzig, C.J. Murphy, and A.M. Fadly. 1998. Orbital lymphosarcoma associated with reticuloendotheliosis virus in a peafowl. *Journal of the American Veterinary Medical Association* 213:377–380.

Mladenov, Z., R. Ippen, and A. Konstantinov. 1977. Cases of leucosis and tumours in wild birds. *Obshch I Sravnitelna Patologiya* 3:83–93.

Montali, R.J. 1980. An overview of tumors in zoo animals. In *The Comparative Pathology of Zoo Animals,* R.J. Montali and G. Migaki (eds.). Smithsonian Institution Press, Washington, D.C., U.S.A., pp. 531–542.

Morgan, H.R. 1973. Avian leukosis-sarcoma virus antibodies in wildfowl, domestic chickens, and man in Kenya. In *Proceedings of the Society for Experimental Biology and Medicine* 144:1–4.

Motha, M.S.J. 1984. Distribution of virus and tumor formation in ducks experimentally infected with reticuloendotheliosis virus. *Avian Pathology* 13: 303–320.

Motha, M.X.J., J.R. Egerton, and A.W. Sweeney. 1984. Some evidence of mechanical transmission of reticuloendotheliosis virus by mosquitoes. *Avian Diseases* 28:858–867.

Motha, M.X.J. and J.R. Egerton. 1987. Vertical transmission of reticuloendotheliosis virus in chickens. *Avian Pathology* 16:141–147.

Neumann, U. and N. Kummerfeld. 1983. Neoplasms in budgerigars (*Melopsittacus undulatus*):Clinical, pathomorphological, and serological findings with special consideration of kidney tumours. *Avian Pathology* 12:353–362.

Neumann, U., T. Mikami, E.F. Kaleta, H.J. Busche, and U. Heffels. 1981. Serological survey on reticuloendotheliosis virus infection in poultry in northern Germany. *Deutsche Tierarztliche Wochenschrift* 88: 104–107.

Newell, S.M., M.C. McMillan, and F.M. Moore. 1991. Diagnosis and treatment of lymphocytic leukemia and malignant lymphoma in a Pekin duck (*Anas platyrhynchos domesticus*). *Journal of the Association of Avian Veterinarians* 5:83–86.

Nobel, T.A. 1972. Avian leucosis (lymphoid) in an egret (*Egretta alba*). *Avian Pathology* 1:75–76.

Nowinski, R.C., E. Fleissner, and N.H. Sarkar. 1973. Structural and serological aspects of the oncornaviruses. *Perspectives in Virology* 8:31–60.

Okazaki, W., H.G. Purchase, and L.B. Crittenden. 1982. Pathogenicity of avian leukosis viruses. *Avian Diseases* 26:553–559.

Ozgencil, B, and N. Metin. 1972. Malignant lymphoma in a partridge (*Alectoris graeca*). *Turkish Veterinarian* 42:22–25.

Palmer, G.H. and E. Stauber. 1981. Visceral lymphoblastic leukosis in an African Grey Parrot. *Veterinary Medicine/Small Animal Clinician* 76:1355.

Paul, P.S., K.H. Johnson, K.A. Pomeroy, B.S. Pomeroy, and P.S. Sarma. 1977. Experimental transmission of reticuloendotheliosis in turkeys with the cell-culture-propagated reticuloendotheliosis viruses of turkey origin. *Journal of the National Cancer Institute* 58:1819–1824.

Paul, P.S., R.E. Werdin, and B.S. Pomeroy. 1978. Spontaneously occurring lymphoproliferative disease in ducks. *Avian Diseases* 22:191–195.

Paul-Murphy, J., L. Lowenstine, J.M. Turrel, C.J. Murphy, and M.E. Fowler. 1985. Malignant lymphoreticular neoplasm in an African gray parrot. *Journal of the American Veterinary Medical Association* 187: 1216–1217.

Payne, L.N. 1992. Biology of avian retroviruses. In *The Retroviridae,* Vol. 1, J. Levy (Ed.), Plenum Press, New York, NY, U.S.A., pp. 299–404.

Payne, L.N., K. Howes, A.M. Gillespie, and L.M. Smith. 1992. Host range of Rous sarcoma virus pseudotype RSV (HPRS-103) in 12 avian species:support for a new avian retrovirus envelope subgroup, designated J. *Journal of General Virology* 73:2995–2997.

Peach, P. 1997. Detection of retroviral infections and their application to the detection of a novel retrovirus isolated in ostriches diagnosed with Ostrich Fading Syndrome. In *Proceedings of Association of Avian Veterinarians Australian Committee Annual Conference,* Perth, Western Australia, pp. 143–149.

Peterson, D.A., and A.S. Levine. 1971. Avian reticuloendotheliosis virus (strain T). IV. Infectivity in day-old cockerels. *Avian Diseases* 14:874–883.

Peterson, M.J. 2004. Parasites and infectious diseases of prairie grouse:should managers be concerned? *Wildlife Society Bulletin* 32:35–55.

Peterson, M.J., J.R. Purvis, J.R. Lichtenfels, T.M. Craig, N.O. Dronen, Jr., and N.J. Silvy. 1998. Serologic and parasitologic survey of the endangered Attwater's prairie chicken. *Journal of Wildlife Disease* 34:137–144.

Peterson, M.J., R. Aguirre, P.J. Ferro, D.A. Jones, T.A. Lawyer, M.N. Peterson, and N.J. Silvy. 2002a. Infectious disease survey of Rio Grande wild turkeys in the Edwards Plateau of Texas. *Journal of Wildlife Disease* 38:826–833.

Peterson, M.J., P.J. Ferro, M.N. Peterson, R.M. Sullivan, B.E. Toole, and N.J. Silvy. 2002b. Infectious disease survey of lesser prairie chickens in north Texas. *Journal of Wildlife Disease* 38:834–839.

Purchase, H.G. and A.M. Fadley. 1980. Leukosis and sarcomas. In *Isolation and Identification of Avian Pathogens.* S.B. Hitchner, C.H. Domermuth, H.G. Purchase, and J.E. Williams (eds.). American Association of Avian Pathologists, Kennett Square, PA, U.S.A., pp. 54–58.

Purchase, H.G. and R.L. Witter. 1975. The reticuloendotheliosis viruses. *Current Topics in Microbiology and Immunology* 71:103–124.

Rambow, V.J., J.C. Murphy, and J.G. Fox. 1981. Malignant lymphoma in a pigeon. *Journal of the American Veterinary Medical Association* 179:1266–1268.

Ramos-Vara, J.A., E.J. Smith, and G.L. Watson. 1997. Lymphosarcoma with plasmacytoid differentiation in a scarlet macaw (*Ara macao*). *Avian Diseases* 41: 499–504.

Regenmortel, M.H.V., C.M. Fauquet, D.H.L. Bishop, E.B. Carstens, M.K. Estes, S.M. Lemon, J. Maniloff, M.A. Mayo, D.J. McGeoch, C.R. Pringle, and R.B. Wickner (eds). 2000. *Virus Taxonomy Classification and Nomenclature of Viruses.* Academic Press, New York, NY, U.S.A., pp. 1162.

Rao, A.T. and L.N. Acharjyo. 1984. Causes of mortality in pea-fowls (*Pavo cristatus*) at Nandankanan Zoo. *Indian Veterinary Journal* 61:259–260.

Resnick, R.M., M.T. Boyce-Jacino, Q. Fu, and A.J. Faras. 1990. Phylogenetic distribution of the novel avian endogenous provirus family EAV-0. *Journal of Virology* 64:4640–4653.

Riddell, C., and P.H. Cribb. 1983. Fibrosarcoma in an African grey parrot (*Psittacus erithacus*). *Avian Diseases* 27:549–555.

Robinson, F.R. and M.J. Twiehaus. 1974. Isolation of the avian reticuloendothelial virus (strain T). *Avian Diseases* 18:278–288.

Rosen, M.N. and W.J. Mathey, Jr. 1955. Some new pheasant diseases in California. *Transactions of the North American Wildlife Conference* 20:220–228.

Rosskopf, W.J., R.W. Woerpel, J. LaBonde, D. Van de Water, and S. Martin. 1987. Malignant lymphoma in a peregrine falcon—a case report. In *Proceedings of the First International Conference on Zoological and Avian Medicine,* Oahu, Hawaii, U.S.A., pp. 325–331.

Rubin, H., A. Cornelius, and L. Fanshier. 1961. The pattern of congential transmission of an avian leukosis virus. In *Proceedings of the National Academy of Science USA* 47:1058–1060.

Rubin, H., L. Fanshier, A. Cornelius, and W.F. Hughes. 1962. Tolerance and immunity in chickens after congenital and contact infection with an avian leukosis virus. *Virology* 17:143–156.

Sacco, M.A., K. Howes, and K. Venugopal. 2001. Intact EAV-HP endogenous retrovirus in Sonnerat's jungle fowl. *Journal of Virology* 75:2029–2032.

Sah, R.L., L.N. Acharjyo, and G.C. Mohanty. 1973. Lymphomatosis in a peahen and a pied mynah. *Poultry Science* 52:1210–1212.

Sasaki, T., S. Sasaki, and H. Koyama. 1993. A survey of an antibody to REV virus in chickens and other avian species in Japan. *Journal of Veterinary Medical Science* 55:885–888.

Sasseville, V.G., B. Miller, and S.W. Nielsen. 1988. A pathological survey of wild turkeys in Connecticut. *Cornell Veterinarian* 78:353–364.

Siegfried, L.M. 1983. Neoplasms identified in free-flying birds. *Avian Disease* 27:86–99.

Suedmeyer, W.K., R.L. Witter, and A. Bermudez. 2001. Hemangiosarcoma in a golden pheasant (*Chrysolophus pictus*). *Journal of Avian Medicine and Surgery* 15:126–130.

Sung, H.W., J.H. Kim, S. Reddy, and A. Fadly. 2002. Isolation of subgroup J avian leukosis virus in Korea. *Veterinary Science* 3:71–74.

Tajima, M., T. Nunoya, and Y. Otaki. 1977. Pathogenesis of abnormal feathers in chickens inoculated with reticuloendotheliosis virus. *Avian Diseases* 21:77–89.

Temin, H.M. 1974. The cellular and molecular biology of RNA tumor viruses, especially avian leukosis-sarcoma virus and their relatives. *Advances in Cancer Research* 19:47–104.

Trampel, D.W., T.M. Pepper, and R.L. Witter. 2002. Reticuloendotheliosis in Hungarian partridge. *Journal of Wildlife Diseases* 38:438–442.

Troesch, C.D. and P.K. Vogt. 1985. An endogenous virus from Lophortyx quail is the prototype for envelope subgroup I of avian retroviruses. *Virology* 143: 595–602.

Van der Heyden, N, R.M. Fulton, D.B. DeNicola, and K. Hicks. 1992. Lymphoma in an ostrich (*Struthio camelus*). In *Proceedings of the Association of Avian Veterinarians,* pp. 310–312.

Wade, L.L., E.W. Polack, P.H. O'Connell, G.S. Starrak, N. Abou-Madi, and K.A. Schat. 1999. Multicentric lymphoma in a European starling. *Journal of Avian Medicine and Surgery* 13:108–115.

Wadsworth, P.F., D.M. Jones, and S.L. Pugsley. 1981. Some cases of lymphoid leukosis in captive wild birds. *Avian Pathology* 10:499–504.

Wiedenfeld, D.A., D.H. Wolfe, J.E. Toepfer, L.M. Mechlin, R.D. Applegate, and S.K. Sherrod. 2002. Survey for reticuloendotheliosis viruses in wild populations of Greater and Lesser Prairie-Chickens. *Wilson Bulletin* 114:142–144.

Weiss, R.A., N. Teich, H. Varmus, and J. Coffin. 1982. *RNA tumor viruses.* Cold Spring Harbor Laboratory, Cold Spring Harbor, NY, U.S.A.

Witter, R.L. 1989. Reticuloendotheliosis. A Laboratory Manual for the Isolation and Identification of Avian Pathogens. H.G. Purchase, L.H. Arp, C.H. Domermuth, and J.E. Pearson (eds.). American Association of Avian Pathologists, Kennett Square, PA, U.S.A., pp.143–148.

Witter, R.L. 1991. Reticuloendotheliosis. In *Diseases of Poultry,* 9th Ed. B.W. Calnek, H.J. Burns, C.W. Beard, W.M. Reid, and H.W. Yoder, Jr. (eds.). Iowa State University Press. Ames, IA, U.S.A., pp. 406–417.

Witter, R.L., B.W. Calnek, and P.P. Levine. 1966. Influence of naturally occurring parental antibody on visceral lymphomatosis virus infection in chickens. *Avian Diseases* 10:43–56.

Witter, R.L., and A.M. Fadly. 2003. Reticuloendotheliosis.In *Diseases of Poultry,* 11th Ed., Y.M. Saif, H.G. Barnes, J.R. Glisson, A.M. Fadly, L.R. McDougald, and D.E. Swayne(eds.). Iowa State University Press, Ames, IA, U.S.A., pp. 517–535.

Witter, R.L. and D.C. Johnson. 1985. Epidemiology of reticuloendotheliosis virus in broiler breeder flocks. *Avian Diseases* 29:1140–1154.

Witter, R.L., and K.A. Schat. 2003. Marek's disease. In *Diseases of Poultry, 11th Ed.,* Y.M. Saif, H.G. Barnes, J.R. Glisson, A.M. Fadly, L.R. McDougald, and D.E. Swayne (eds.). Iowa State University Press, Ames, IA, U.S.A., pp. 407–464.

Ziedler, K., A. Hlinak, G. Raetz, O. Werner, and D. Ebnere. 1995. Investigations on antibody titers in wild and zoo birds against pathogens of farm poultry. *Journal of Veterinary Medicine (Series B)* 42: 321–330.

Zeigel, R.F., G.H. Theilen, and M.J. Twiehaus. 1966. Electron microscope observations on reticuloendotheliosis virus (Strain T) that induces reticuloendotheliosis in turkeys, chickens and Japanese quail. *Journal of the National Cancer Institute* 37:7–9.

Section 2:
Bacterial and Fungal Diseases

12
Avian Cholera

Michael D. Samuel, Richard G. Botzler, Gary A. Wobeser

INTRODUCTION

Avian cholera is an infectious disease caused by *Pasteurella multocida,* an encapsulated Gram-negative bacterium whose shape may vary from a rod to a coccobacillus (Rimler and Glisson 1977). *Pasteurella multocida* is a heterogeneous species where pathogenicity of individual strains is highly variable and susceptibility to these bacterial strains varies considerably among avian species (Christensen and Bisgaard 2000). Epizootics of avian cholera typically occur in wetlands with abundant waterfowl populations or at breeding colonies with high densities of birds. Mortality often involves multiple species of birds.

The bacterium has a worldwide distribution and produces septicemic and respiratory disease in a wide variety of domestic and wild birds. Acute illness is common; infection can result in mortality within six to 12 hr after exposure, although one to two days is more typical (Friend 1999). Among wild birds, mortality from *P. multocida* is primarily reported from waterbirds, especially waterfowl of North America, but natural infection has occurred in more than 180 species representing at least 47 different families of birds. Most bird species can be infected under appropriate circumstances. Disease transmission among wild birds is believed to occur from bird-to-bird contact and by ingestion of bacteria or aerosol transmission within a contaminated environment. Discharge of pasteurellae from dead or diseased birds is considered an important source of wetland contamination and transmission to susceptible birds.

Despite its occurrence in domestic fowl on most continents, avian cholera seems best described as having a limited distribution and significance for most wild bird populations around the world (Botzler 1991). North American waterfowl are an exception in which the frequency and distribution of avian cholera mortality events increased greatly since the disease was first reported in 1943–1944. During recent decades, large epizootics killing more than 50,000 birds have taken place in Texas (U.S.A) and on several occasions in California (U.S.A), Nebraska (U.S.A), and the Chesapeake Bay of Maryland (U.S.A). The disease now occurs throughout most of North America and is a significant problem for wild populations (Friend 1999). As waterfowl have become increasingly concentrated on substantially diminished wetland habitats, transmission of this infectious disease has become a greater problem for wildlife managers. Although avian botulism (caused by a toxin) may affect more birds, avian cholera is the most important infectious disease and causes significant annual mortality of waterfowl in North America.

SYNONYMS

Fowl cholera, avian pasteurellosis, avian hemorrhagic septicemia, chicken cholera.

HISTORY

Avian cholera has been recognized as a distinct disease associated with domestic fowl for more than 200 years. An avian cholera-like disease was reported in domestic birds in Italy as early as 1600. However, avian (fowl) cholera was first described among domestic birds by veterinarians in France in the late 1700s (Gray 1913), and the infectious nature of the disease was not recognized until the 1850s (Hutyra et al. 1949). Epizootics occurred through the 1800s in domestic birds across several European countries, including France, Bohemia, Austria, Russia, Italy, and Hungary, as well as the East Indies (Gray 1913). Gray (1913) believed the disease was introduced to Germany between 1897 and 1899 when geese and other domestic fowl were imported from Russia, Poland, Silesia, and Italy. However, this theory conflicts with other accounts in which avian cholera was reported earlier among ducks, including domestic ducks and various hybrids, swans, and geese in Germany (Willach 1895). Interestingly,

Willach (1895) also noted that sparrows and other species were not affected during these early epizootics. The causative agent, "*Pasteurella,*" was named in honor of Louis Pasteur (Trevisan 1887, in Rosen 1971) who attenuated the bacterium and produced the first vaccine in the late 1800s (Rimler and Glisson 1997).

Avian cholera was noted among wild pheasants (presumably *Phasianus colchicus*) associated with domesticated pheasants in Germany (Sticker 1888). The disease had a high prevalence in Great Britain in 1900, and Gray (1913) speculated that it had been present there for about 40 years. Avian cholera declined in importance in northern, western, and central Europe in the early 1900s to the point of having little significance; however, it still was considered important in eastern and southern Europe. Avian cholera was present in South Africa and probably Australia and New Zealand in the early 1900s (Gray 1913). During this early period, the source of the disease was believed to be carrier animals; in some cases, free-living European Starlings *(Sturnus vulgaris)* were believed to spread the disease by ingesting contaminated food at infected farms and transmitting the disease to birds on other farms through contaminated feces (Hutyra et al. 1949).

Avian cholera was reported among domestic birds in the United States between 1880 and 1882 (Gray 1913). Cases also were recorded in the United States in 1898 and in Canada in 1899. In North America, the disease had its greatest impact in the winter months (Hutyra et al. 1949), whereas in Europe, most epizootics among domestic birds occurred from August to October. Among wild birds in North America, Green and Shillinger (1936) noted the occurrence of avian cholera epizootics in Ruffed Grouse (*Bonasa umbellus*), presumably in Minnesota (U.S.A). Later, avian cholera was reported in wild Ruffed Grouse and geese, ducks, turkeys, pheasants, pigeons, quail, and a large number of other wild birds in the United States were found to be susceptible (Shillinger and Morley 1942). It was not clear from their description which wild species besides Ruffed Grouse were naturally infected; however, the disease was rare among wild birds.

The first known epizootics in wild North American waterfowl occurred in 1943–1944 among ducks in Texas (Quortrup et al. 1946) as well as ducks, American Coots (*Fulica americana*), Tundra Swans (*Cygnus columbianus*), gulls, shorebirds, and other species in northern California (Rosen and Bischoff 1949). The epizootics in both Texas (Gordus 1993a) and California (Rosen and Bischoff 1949, 1950) were associated with nearby mortality in domestic fowl and suspected disposal of dead birds into the environment (Friend 1981).

The first report of avian cholera among wildfowl (wild birds) outside North America occurred during the same time period with the mortality of about 40 wild Egyptian (*Alopochen aegyptiacus*) and Spur-winged Geese (*Plectropterus gambensis*) on Lake Nakuru, Kenya, in 1940 (Hudson 1959). In 1941, avian cholera was reported among marine ducks, pelicans (probably *Pelecanus occidentalis*), and gulls in Chile (Suarez and Ilazabal 1941). In September 1945, avian cholera was found in Holland among migrating Mallards (*Anas platyrhynchos*) and Green-winged Teal (*Anas crecca*), as well as gulls; the epizootic occurred shortly before avian cholera was reported among domestic poultry in the same regions (Van den Hurk 1946). Subsequently, avian cholera was reported among Kelp Gulls (*Larus dominicanus*), Jackass Penguins (*Spheniscus demersus*), Cape Cormorants (*Phalacrocorax capensis*), and Sacred Ibis (*Threskiornis aethiopicus*) in South Africa (Kaschula and Truter 1951; Crawford et al. 1992). Avian cholera was occasionally reported among European waterfowl (Bezzel 1979; Mullié et al. 1979, 1980), but most reports among European wildlife involved doves, crows, and sparrows (Wetzel and Rieck 1972). The disease has also been reported in Great Skuas (*Catharacta skua*) from Antarctica (Parmelee et al. 1979) and Rockhopper Penguins (*Eudyptes crestatus*) from New Zealand (De Lisle et al. 1990).

It is not clear whether the rapid sequence of reports of avian cholera among the world's wildfowl resulted from increased awareness of the disease or from rapid human introduction of avian cholera to wild species. However, it seems likely that earlier large epizootics of avian cholera among wildfowl would have been documented because the disease was well known among domestic birds (Botzler 1991). In North America, the disease was present in domestic fowl at least 75 years before it was recognized in wild waterfowl (Heddleston and Rhoades 1978) and there is evidence that the disease was absent from waterfowl prior to 1944 (Phillips and Lincoln 1930; Friend 1981). The subsequent onset of reports coincided with proximity of wild birds to domestic poultry, significant changes in wildfowl habitat and land use practices, including large-scale use of pesticides, application of more intense agricultural methods, significant losses of wetland habitats (Botzler 1991), and increased concentrations of birds.

DISTRIBUTION

In domestic birds, avian cholera probably occurs worldwide (Rimler and Glisson 1997). Historical and recent reports of avian cholera in wild birds are considerably more limited in global distribution. Since about 1980, most reports of substantial epizootics in wild birds have occurred in North America, where significant epizootics occur almost annually. In other parts of the world, recurrent epizootics have been more limited. In the late 1970s, high mortality of Common Eiders (*Somateria mollissima*) occurred in the Netherlands in overcrowded winter areas such as blowholes in the ice (Mullié et al. 1979, 1980). Further epizootics were reported from breeding colonies in 1984 (Swennen and Smit 1991). In 1996, epizootics occurred on both wintering and breeding areas for Common Eiders in Denmark (Christensen 1996; Christensen et al. 1997). Substantial mortality recurred on breeding areas during 2001 (Pedersen et al. 2003). During these later epizootics, Great Cormorants (*Phalacrocorax carbo*), Eurasian Oystercatchers (*Haematopus ostralegus*), Herring Gulls (*Larus argentatus*), and Greater Black-backed Gulls (*Larus marinus*) were also affected (Christensen et al. 1998; Pedersen et al. 2003). Although avian cholera in domestic birds has been reported from many parts of eastern Asia and from wild species in zoological collections or farms in Japan (Fujihara et al. 1986; Sawada et al. 1999), it was not reported in wild birds until 2000, when an epizootic killed > 10,000 Baikal Teal (*Anas formosa*) in Korea (Kwon and Kang 2003).

In North America, the first reports of avian cholera in wild waterfowl occurred during the 1940s in Texas and California (Rosen 1971). During the next two to three decades, major epizootics were confined primarily to these two states, but small mortality events also occurred in the Atlantic and Mississippi Flyways (Friend 1981). The emergence of avian cholera as a widespread, significant disease of wild waterfowl in North America began with the increasing geographic distribution and frequency of disease epizootics during the 1970s (Friend 1981). By the end of the 1970s and early 1980s, large mortality events had spread to the Rainwater Basin in Nebraska, the Chesapeake Bay in Maryland, and near Hudson Bay in the Northwest Territories, Canada. The disease has now been reported in most areas of the United States and in many portions of Canada. Avian cholera is suspected to occur on waterfowl wintering areas in Mexico, but surveillance and diagnostic efforts have been limited. Since epizootics in 1998–1999, there has been a notable and unexplained decline in reported avian cholera mortality events throughout North America (National Wildlife Health Center, unpublished data).[1]

Within the United States there are several major enzootic areas for avian cholera: the California Central Valley; the Tule Lake and Klamath Basins in northern California and southern Oregon; the Playa Lakes and Gulf Coast regions in Texas; the Rainwater Basin in Nebraska; the Lower Missouri River Basin in Iowa and Missouri; and the Chesapeake Bay in Maryland (Figure 12.1). Mortality occurs almost annually in most of these regions except the Chesapeake Bay, where events are less frequent. Limited mortality also occurs in western Canada each spring among migrating Lesser Snow (*Chen c. caerulescens*) and Ross's (*Chen rossii*) Geese, and mortality of unknown extent occurs in many years on the Arctic breeding grounds of these species (Canadian Cooperative Wildlife Health Centre, unpublished data).[2]

Historically, avian cholera was considered a disease associated with wintering waterfowl. However, epizootics have occurred in all four North American waterfowl flyways, during both spring and fall migration in Canada (Wobeser 1997), during the nesting season for Common Eiders on the east coast of the United States and Canada (Gershman et al. 1964; Reed 1975; Korschgen et al. 1978; Jorde et al. 1989) and Lesser Snow Geese in the Arctic (Brand 1984; Wobeser et al. 1982; Samuel et al. 1999a), and during summer molt of Redheads (*Aythya americana*) in Saskatchewan (Canada) (Wobeser and Leighton 1988). Seasonal and geographic patterns of mortality closely follow the migration patterns of waterfowl, and the disease now occurs throughout the annual life cycle and in many waterfowl areas of North America (Figure 12.1). Within some of the major enzootic areas, mortality from avian cholera may occur over a prolonged period (for example, 2–4 mo), but in other areas mortality events may be brief (< 1 wk). In the Central Valley of California, avian cholera mortality may begin during fall and continue until the following spring. In contrast, avian cholera epizootics occur almost every year in conjunction with spring migration through Nebraska's Rainwater Basin, but epizootics are much less frequent in this area during the fall migration.

HOST RANGE

Pasteurella multocida has been reported from a wide variety of birds and mammals (Blackburn et al. 1975; Brogden and Rhoades 1983; Botzler 1991). More than 190 species of birds, from at least 44 families, have been reported as naturally infected with *P. multocida* (Table 12.1). Bird groups most frequently affected by avian cholera are waterfowl and coots, followed by scavengers (gulls, raptors, and crows), and to a lesser extent other water birds (waders, shorebirds, and cranes) and upland species. The first known reports of *P. multocida* isolations are presented in Table 12.1, along with new serotypes for the same host species in later studies; however, serotypes were not determined in reports prior to 1972 and only in some reports after that. Fourteen of the 16 known serotypes have been reported in avian species, with at least 31 different serotype combinations represented. It seems likely that most or all bird species are susceptible to avian cholera under appropriate circumstances.

The reports cited in Table 12.1 represent the first records for which it is reasonably certain that

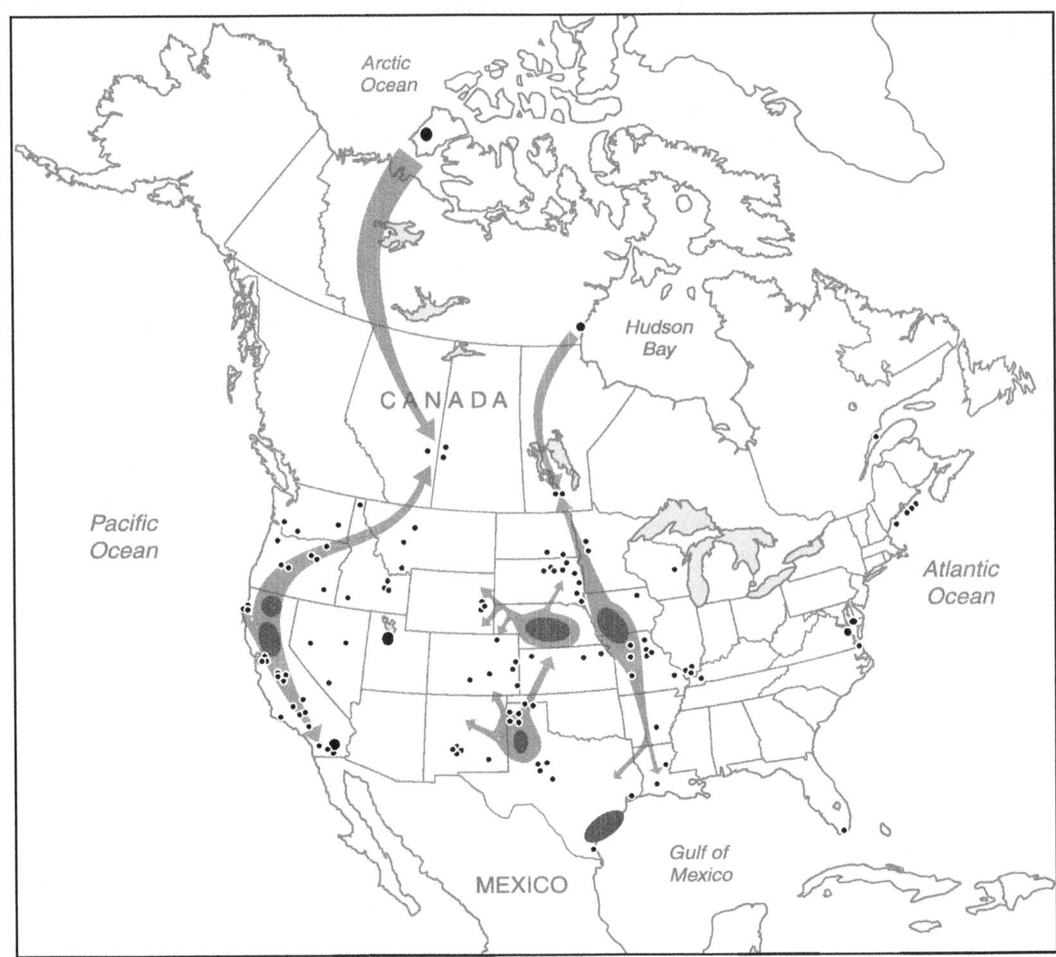

Figure 12.1. Avian cholera epizootic sites and bird migration routes associated with disease epizootics in North American waterfowl, 1944–2001. The occurrence of avian cholera is closely related to bird movements, especially west of the Great Lakes. Black dots represent epizootic sites; dark-gray zones are major enzootic areas; light-gray arrows portray major migratory pathways. (Figure follows that of Friend 1999: Figure 7.11).

P. multocida was isolated from each species. In addition, there have been claims of *P. multocida* infections in birds for which the documentation is uncertain. For example, septicemic pasteurellosis was reported as the cause of death for a captive King Vulture *(Sarcoramphus papa)* and acute pasteurellosis was reported in a Merlin *(Falco columbarius),* but no bacterial isolation or identification was provided for these diagnoses (Hill 1953; Cooper 1978). Ambiguous claims for pasteurellosis in Common (Atlantic) Puffins *(Fratercula arctica)* and other, unidentified species are also described in Botzler (1991).

The first known diagnoses of pasteurellosis in some species were for captive birds in zoos or private collections. In most of these situations the source of pasteurellosis can be difficult to assess because it often is not clear how long the wild birds had been in captivity before *P. multocida* was isolated. Thus in many cases these diagnoses represent potential species susceptibility, but not necessarily natural infection. For some species, *P. multocida* was first reported in captive birds and later observed in free-living birds of the same species.

The role of predators as the source of infection is confusing in a number of reported cases. In some situations, pasteurellosis clearly was associated with predator bites rather than natural infection, but in other cases, adequate information was not provided. For example, Korbel (1990) listed 22 wild bird species from which *P. multocida* was isolated. For three

Table 12.1. The natural occurrence of *Pasteurella multocida* among free-living and captive birds, where definitive information is available for host species and bacterial identification.

Scientific Name	Common Name	Serotypes Reported	Citations
Ostriches (Struthionidae)			
Struthio camelus	Ostrich	NR[a]	Okoh 1980
Penguins (Spheniscidae)			
Eudyptes crestatus	Rockhopper Penguin	NR	De Lisle et al. 1990
Spheniscus demersus	Jackass Penguins	NR	Crawford et al. 1992
Waterfowl—Geese and Swans (Anserinae)			
Anser albifrons	Greater White-fronted Goose	NR	Rosen 1969
Chen caerulescens	Snow Goose	1	Brogden and Rhoades 1983
		11	Wilson et al. 1995b
Chen rossii	Ross's Goose	NR	Rosen and Morse 1959
		1	Heddleston et al. 1972
Branta bernicia	Brant Goose	NR	Rosen 1971
Branta canadensis	Canada Goose	1	Brogden and Rhoades 1983
		1	USGS-NWHC[b]
		NR	Petrides and Bryant 1951
Alopochen aegyptiacus	Egyptian Goose	1; 3	Heddleston et al. 1972
Plectropterus gambensis	Spur-winged Goose	3,4	Montgomery et al. 1979
Cygnus olor	Mute Swan	NR	Hudson 1959[c]
Cygnus buccinator	Trumpeter Swan	NR	Hudson 1959[c]
		NR	Korbel 1990
Cygnus columbianus	Tundra Swan	NR	Gritman and Jensen 1965
		1	Wilson et al. 1995b
		NR	Rosen and Bischoff 1949
		1; 3	Brogden and Rhoades 1983
		3,4	Montgomery et al. 1979
Waterfowl—Ducks (Anatinae)			
Cairina moschata	Muscovy Duck	3,4	Montgomery et al. 1979
		1	USGS-NWHC
Aix sponsa	Wood Duck	NR	Rosen 1971
Anas strepera	Gadwall	NR	Vaught et al. 1967
		1	Brogden and Rhoades 1983
Anas americana	American Wigeon	NR	Rosen and Bischoff 1949
		1	Brogden and Rhoades 1983
Anas rubripes	American Black Duck	NR	Vaught et al. 1967
		1	Wilson et al. 1995b
Anas platyrhynchos	Mallard	NR	Quortrup et al. 1946
		1	Brogden and Rhoades 1983
		1,15; 1,13,15; 1,13,16	Windingstad et al. 1988
Anas fulvigula	Mottled Duck	1	USGS-NWHC
Anas wyvilliana	Hawaiian Duck	3	USGS-NWHC
Anas discors	Blue-winged Teal	NR	Klukas and Locke 1970
		1	Brogden and Rhoades 1983
Anas cyanoptera	Cinnamon Teal	NR	Rosen 1969
		1	Wilson et al. 1995b
Anas clypeata	Northern Shoveler	NR	Rosen and Bischoff 1949
		1	Brogden and Rhoades 1983

(Continued)

Table 12.1. (Continued)

Scientific Name	Common Name	Serotypes Reported	Citations
Anas acuta	Northern Pintail	NR	Quortrup et al. 1946
		1; 3	Brogden and Rhoades 1983
		3,4	Wilson et al. 1995b
Anas crecca	Green-winged Teal	NR	Petrides and Bryant 1951
		1; 3	Brogden and Rhoades 1983
Anas formosa	Baikal Teal	1,12,13	Kwon and Kang 2003
Netta peposaca	Rosy-billed Pochard	3	Fujihara et al. 1986
Aythya valisineria	Canvasback	NR	Rosen and Bischoff 1949
		1	Brogden and Rhoades 1983
Aythya americana	Redhead	NR	Wobeser et al. 1979
		1	Brogden and Rhoades 1983
Aythya collaris	Ring-necked Duck	1	Brogden and Rhoades 1983
Aythya fuligula	Tufted Duck	NR	Keymer 1958
Aythya marila	Greater Scaup	NR	Rosen 1971
Aythya affinis	Lesser Scaup	NR	Petrides and Bryant 1951
		1	Brogden and Rhoades 1983
Somateria mollissima	Common Eider	NR	Gerschman et al. 1964
		1	USGS-NWHC
		3; 3,4; 3,12; 4; 4,7; 4,12	Brogden and Rhoades 1983
Melanitta perspicillata	Surf Scoter	NR	Locke et al. 1970
		3,4	USGS-NWHC
Melanitta fusca	White-winged Scoter	NR	Locke et al. 1970
		1	Brogden and Rhoades 1983
		3	Heddleston et al. 1972
		3,4	Montgomery et al. 1979
Melanitta nigra	Black Scoter	NR	Montgomery et al. 1979
Clangula hyemalis	Long-tailed Duck	3; 3,4	Montgomery et al. 1979
		1	Brogden and Rhoades 1983
Bucephala albeola	Bufflehead	3,4	Montgomery et al. 1979
		1	Wilson et al. 1995b
Bucephala clangula	Common Goldeneye	NR	Locke et al. 1970
		1	USGS-NWHC
		3,4	Montgomery et al. 1979
Mergus merganser	Common Merganser	1	Brogden and Rhoades 1983
Mergus serrator	Red-breasted Merganser	NR	Montgomery et al. 1979
		3,4	USGS-NWHC
Oxyura jamaicensis	Ruddy Duck	NR	Petrides and Bryant 1951
		1; 6	Brogden and Rhoades 1983
Partridges, grouse, and		NR	Jennings 1954
turkeys (Phasianidae)		3,4	Miguel et al. 1998
Perdix perdix	Gray Partridge	NR	Rosen and Morse 1959
Coturnix coturnix	Common Quail	3	Heddleston et al. 1972
Phasianus colchicus	Ring-necked Pheasant	3,4; 3,12; 4,12; 7,12	Brogden and Rhoades 1983
Phasianus vesicolor	Green Pheasant	3	Sawada et al. 1999
Syrmaticus soemmerringii	Copper Pheasant	3	Sawada et al. 1999
Bonasa umbellus	Ruffed Grouse	NR	Green and Shillinger 1936
Lagopus lagopus	Willow Ptarmigan	NR	Jennings 1955
Tympanuchus sp.	Prairie Chicken	NR	USGS-NWHC
Meleagris gallopavo	Wild Turkey	3; 5	Brogden and Rhoades 1983
		1; 1,15; 1,13,15	Windingstad et al. 1988

Table 12.1. (Continued)

Scientific Name	Common Name	Serotypes Reported	Citations
Quail (Odontophoridae)			
Callipepla californica	California Quail	NR	Hinshaw and Emlen 1943
Loons (Gaviidae)			
Gavia immer	Common Loon	NR	Montgomery et al. 1979
Grebes (Podicipedidae)			
Podilymbus podiceps	Pied-billed Grebe	NR	Klukas and Locke 1970
		1	Wilson et al. 1995b
Podiceps auritus	Horned Grebe	3,4	Montgomery et al. 1979
Podiceps nigricollis	Eared Grebe	NR	Rosen 1971
		1	Wilson et al. 1995b
		3,4	Montgomery et al. 1979
Aechmophorus occidentalis	Western Grebe	1	Brogden and Rhoades 1983
Petrels and shearwaters (Procellariidae)			
Macronectes giganteus	Southern Giant Petrel	1	Leotta et al. 2003
Puffinus pacificus	Wedge-tailed Shearwater	1	USGS-NWHC
Gannets and boobies (Sulidae)			
Sula sula	Red-footed Booby	3; 3,4	USGS-NWHC
Pelicans (Pelecanidae)			
Pelecanus erythrorhynchus	American White Pelican	1	Wilson et al. 1995b
Pelecanus occidentalis	Brown Pelican	NR	Suarez and Ilazabal 1941[d]
Cormorants (Phalacrocoracidae)			
Phalacrocorax auritus	Double-crested Cormorant	NR	Montgomery et al. 1979
Phalacorcorax carbo	Great Cormorant	3	Christensen 1996
Phalacrocorax capensis	Cape Cormorant	NR	Crawford et al. 1992
Herons, egrets and bitterns (Ardeidae)			
Botaurus lentiginosus	American Bittern	1,5	USGS-NWHC
Ixobrychus exilis	Least Bittern	1	Brogden and Rhoades 1983
Ardea herodias	Great Blue Heron	NR	Rosen and Bischoff 1949
Ardea cinerea	Grey Heron	NR	Pedersen et al. 2003
Ardea alba	Great Egret	NR	Raggi and Stratton 1954
		1	Brogden and Rhoades 1983
Egretta thula	Snowy Egret	NR	Oddo et al. 1978
		1	Hirsh et al. 1990
Egretta caerulea	Little Blue Heron	1	Brogden and Rhoades 1983
Nycticorax nycticorax	Black-crowned Night Heron	1	Wilson et al. 1995b
Ibis and spoonbills (Threskiornithidae)			
Threskiornis aethiopicus	Sacred Ibis	NR	Crawford et al. 1992
Plegadis chihi	White-faced Ibis	1	USGS-NWHC
Flamingos (Phoenicopteridae)			
Phoenicopterus ruber	Greater Flamingo	1	Brand and Duncan 1983
Ospreys (Pandioninae)			
Pandion haliaetus	Osprey	3,4	Hindman et al. 1997
Hawks, eagles, and kites (Accipitridae)			
Haliastur indus	Brahminy Kite	NR	Steinhagen and Schellhaas 1968

(Continued)

Table 12.1. (Continued)

Scientific Name	Common Name	Serotypes Reported	Citations
Haliaeetus leucocephalus	Bald Eagle	1	Rosen 1972
		1,3,7	Wilson et al. 1995a
Haliaeetus albicilla	White-tailed Sea Eagle	NR	Steinhagen and Schellhaas 1968
Terathopius ecaudatus	Bateleur	NR	Okoh 1980
Circus cyaneus	Northern Harrier	1	Rosen and Morse 1959
Accipiter nisus	Eurasian Sparrowhawk	NR	Jaksic et al. 1964[d]
Accipiter sp.	Goshawk	NR	Woodford and Glasier 1955
Buteo lineatus	Red-shouldered Hawk	1,7	Wilson et al. 1995a
Buteo jamaicensis	Red-tailed Hawk	1	Brogden and Rhoades 1983
		1,7	Wilson et al. 1995a
Buteo buteo	Eurasian Buzzard	NR	Steinhagen and Schellhaas 1968
Buteo lagopus	Rough-legged Hawk	NR	Morishita et al. 1997
Aquila rapax	Tawny Eagle	NR	Waddington 1944
Aquila heliaca	Imperial Eagle	NR	Steinhagen and Schellhaas 1968
Aquila chrysaetos	Golden Eagle	1	Rosen et al. 1973
Falcons and caracaras (Falconidae)			
Caracara cheriway	Crested Caracara	NR	USGS-NWHC
Falco tinnunculus	Eurasian Kestrel	NR	Steinhagen and Schellhaas 1968
Falco sparverius	American Kestrel	NR	Rosen 1971
		1	Brogden and Rhoades 1983
		3	Morishita et al. 1996b
Falco rusticolus	Gyrfalcon	1,3,4	Williams et al. 1987
Falco peregrinus	Peregrine Falcon	1	Hirsh et al. 1990
		1,3,7	Wilson et al. 1995a
Falco mexicanus	Prairie Falcon	1	Brogden and Rhodes 1983
Rails, gallinules and coots (Rallidae)			
Rallus longirostris	Clapper Rail	NR	USGS-NWHC
Rallus aquaticus	Water Rail	NR	Korbel 1990
Gallinula chloropus	Common Moorhen	1	Brogden and Rhoades 1983
Fulica americana	American Coot	NR	Rosen and Bischoff 1949
		1	Heddleston et al. 1972
		3; 3,12,15; 3,4,12,15	Brogden and Rhoades 1983
Cranes (Gruidae)			
Grus canadensis	Sandhill Crane	NR	Rosen 1971
		1	Hirsh et al. 1990
Grus americana	Whooping Crane	1,15	USGS-NWHC
Plovers and lapwings (Charadriidae)			
Vanellus vanellus	Northern Lapwing	NR	Curtis 1979
		1	Macdonald et al. 1981
Charadrius semipalmatus	Semipalmated Plover	NR	USGS-NWHC
Charadrius melodus	Piping Plover	1	USGS-NWHC
Charadrius vociferus	Killdeer	NR	USGS-NWHC
Oystercatchers (Haematopodidae)			
Haematopus ostralegus	Palearctic Oystercatcher	NR	Christensen 1996
		3	Morishita et al. 1996b

Table 12.1. (Continued)

Scientific Name	Common Name	Serotypes Reported	Citations
Haematopus palliatus	American Oystercatcher	NR	Blus et al. 1978
Avocets and stilts (Recurvirostridae)			
Himantopus mexicanus	Black-necked Stilt	1	Hirsh et al. 1990
Recurvivostra americana	American Avocet	1	USGS-NWHC
Sandpipers (Scolopacidae)			
Tringa melanoleuca	Greater Yellowlegs	1	Brogden and Rhoades 1983
Calidris mauri	Western Sandpiper	NR	USGS-NWHC
Calidris minutilla	Least Sandpiper	NR	Rosen and Bischoff 1949
Limnodromus griseus	Short-billed Dowitcher	1	USGS-NWHC
Limnodromus scolopaceus	Long-billed Dowitcher	1	Brogden and Rhoades 1983
Phalaropus sp.	Phalarope	NR	Rosen and Bischoff 1949
Scolopax rusticola	Eurasian Woodcock	NR	Smit et al. 1980[e]
Gulls, jaegers, skuas, and terns (Laridae)			
Catharacta skua	Great Skua	1	Parmelee et al. 1979
Larus ridibundus	Black-headed Gull	NR	Curtis 1979
		13	Macdonald et al. 1981
Larus philadelphia	Bonaparte's Gull	1	Wilson et al. 1995b
Larus canus	Mew Gull	1; 7	Brogden and Rhoades 1983
Larus delawarensis	Ring-billed Gull	NR	Locke et al. 1970
		1	Brogden and Rhoades 1983
Larus californicus	California Gull	NR	Rosen and Bischoff 1949
		1	Wilson et al. 1995b
Larus argentatus	Herring Gull	7	Heddleston et al. 1972
		3,12; 7	Brogden and Rhoades 1983
		3; 3,4	Windingstad et al. 1988
		1; 4,7	Wilson et al. 1995b
Larus glaucescens	Glaucous-winged Gull	NR	Rosen and Bischoff 1949
Larus occidentalis	Western Gull	NR	Rosen and Bischoff 1949
Larus marinus	Great Black-backed Gull	NR	Montgomery et al. 1979
		4	Wilson et al. 1995b
Larus dominicanus	Kelp Gull	NR	Kaschula and Truter 1951
Larus spp.	Gulls	NR	Suarez and Ilazabal 1941
Sterna maxima	Royal Tern	NR	USGS-NWHC
Sterna hirundo	Common Tern	7,10	USGS-NWHC
Auks, murres, and puffins (Alcidae)			
Uria aalge	Common Murre	NR	Macdonald 1963[c]
Pigeons and doves (Columbidae)			
Columba livia	Rock Pigeon	3	Macdonald et al. 1981
		5	Brogden and Rhoades 1983
Columba palumbus	Common Wood-pigeon	NR	Smit et al. 1980[e]
Streptopelia decaocto	Collared Dove	NR	Smit et al. 1980[e]
Zenaida macroura	Mourning Dove	1	USGS-NWHC
Cockatoos (Cacatuidae)			
Nymphicus hollandicus	Cockatiel	3	Morishita et al. 1996a[e]

(*Continued*)

Table 12.1. (Continued)

Scientific Name	Common Name	Serotypes Reported	Citations
Parrots (Psittacidae)			
Melopsittacus undulatus	Budgerigar	NR	Smit et al. 1980[e]
Coracopsis nigra	Black Parrot	3; 4,7	Morishita et al. 1996a
Psittacus erithacus	Gray Parrot	4,7	Morishita et al. 1996a
Pionites leucogaster	White-bellied Parrot	3	Morishita et al. 1996a
Barn owls (Tytonidae)			
Tyto alba	Barn Owl	NR	Korbel 1990
		1,7	Wilson et al. 1995a
		3,4	Morishita et al. 1996a
Owls (Strigidae)			
Otus flammeolus	Flammulated Owl	NR	Morishita et al. 1997
Megascops kennicotti	Western Screech-owl	1	Morishita et al. 1996b
Megascops asio	Eastern Screech-owl	NR	Faddoul et al. 1967
		3	Brogden and Rhoades 1983
Megascops choliba	Tropical Screech-owl	NR	Brada and Campelo 1960[d]
Bubo bubo	Eurasian Eagle-owl	NR	Jöst 1915
Bubo scandiacus	Snowy Owl	NR	Hunter 1967
		1	Brogden and Rhoades 1983
Athene cunicularia	Burrowing Owl	3,4	Brogden and Rhoades 1983
		1,3,7	Wilson et al. 1995a
Athene noctua	Little Owl	NR	Smit et al. 1980[e]
Strix aluco	Tawny Owl	NR	Curtis 1979
		3	Macdonald et al. 1981
Strix occidentalis	Spotted Owl	3,4,7	Wilson et al. 1995a
Asio otus	Long-eared Owl	1	Wilson et al. 1995a
Asio flammeus	Short-eared Owl	NR	Rosen and Morse 1959
		1; 3	Wilson et al. 1995a
Swifts (Apodidae)			
Apus apus	Common Swift	NR	Korbel 1990
Woodpeckers (Picidae)			
Dendrocopus major	Great Spotted Woodpecker	NR	Korbel 1990[e]
Colaptes auratus	Northern Flicker	NR	Wickware 1945
Colaptes sp.	Flicker	3,4	Christiansen et al. 1992b
	Woodpecker	NR	Jaksic et al. 1964
Crows, jays and magpies (Corvidae)			
Garrulus glandarius	Eurasian Jay	NR	Jaksic et al. 1964[d]
Pica hudsonia	Black-billed Magpie	NR	Windingstad et al. 1988
Corvus frugilegus	Eurasian Rook	NR	Novikov 1954
Corvus brachyrhynchos	American Crow	1	Zinkl et al. 1977
Corvus corone	Carrion Crow	NR	Keymer 1958[f]
Corvus corax	Common Raven	1	USGS-NWHC
Swallows (Hirundinidae)			
Delichon urbica	Common House-Martin	NR	Korbel 1990
Nuthatches (Sittidae)			
Sitta europaea	Eurasian Nuthatch	NR	Korbel 1990
Sitta carolinensis	White-breasted Nuthatch	3,4	Christiansen et al. 1992b

Table 12.1. (Continued)

Scientific Name	Common Name	Serotypes Reported	Citations
Thrushes (Turdidae)			
Sialia currucoides	Mountain Bluebird	3,4	USGS-NWHC
Turdus merula	Eurasian Blackbird	NR	Keymer 1958[f]
		NR	Curtis 1979
		1,4,5	Macdonald et al. 1981
Turdus pilaris	Fieldfare	NR	Korbel 1990
Turdus philomelos	Song Thrush	NR	Smit et al. 1980[e]
Turdus migratorius	American Robin	NR	Bivins 1955
		1; 3	Heddleston et al. 1972
		3,12	Brogden and Rhoades 1983
Mockingbirds and thrashers (Mimidae)			
Mimus polyglottos	Northern Mockingbird	NR	Heddleston 1976
		5	Brogden and Rhoades 1983
Starlings (Sturnidae)			
Sturnus vulgaris	European Starling	NR	Bivins 1953
		1; 3; 3,4; 6; 8	Heddleston et al. 1972
		1,5	Macdonald et al. 1981
Acridotheres tristis	Common Myna	1	Sawada et al. 1999
Waxwings (Bombycillidae)			
Bombycilla cedrorum	Cedar Waxwing	NR	Locke and Banks 1972
Old World Flycatchers (Muscipaidae)			
Muscicapa striata	Spotted Flycatcher	NR	Curtis 1979
Erithacus rubecula	European Robin	NR	Keymer 1958[f]
Buntings, sparrows, seedeaters, and allies (Emberizidae)			
Passerculus sandwichensis	Savannah Sparrow	3,12	Brogden and Rhoades 1983
		1	Christiansen et al. 1992a
Zonotrichia leucophrys	White-crowned Sparrow	1; 3; 3,4	Snipes et al. 1988[f]
		1,11; 6	Christiansen et al. 1992a[f]
Junco hyemalis	Dark-eyed (Oregon) Junco	3,4	Christiansen et al. 1992b
Blackbirds, grackles, and orioles (Icteridae)			
Euphagus cyanocephalus	Brewer's Blackbird	3	Snipes et al. 1988[f]
Quiscalus quiscula	Common Grackle	NR	Bivins 1955
Icterus galbula	Baltimore Oriole	NR	Faddoul et al. 1967
Siskins, crossbills, and allies (Fringillidae)			
Fringilla coelebs	Common Chaffinch	NR	Sticker 1888[c]
Carduelis chloris	European Greenfinch	NR	Korbel 1990
Carduelis pinus	Pine Siskin	8	Heddleston et al. 1972
Coccothraustes vespertinus	Evening Grosbeak	NR	Faddoul et al. 1967
		3	Brogden and Rhoades 1983
		3,4	Heddleston et al. 1972

(*Continued*)

Table 12.1. (Continued)

Scientific Name	Common Name	Serotypes Reported	Citations
Old World sparrows (Passeridae)			
Passer domesticus	House Sparrow	NR	Heddleston 1976
		1; 3,4; 4,13	Snipes et al. 1988[f]
		3	Brogden and Rhoades 1983

Note: Only cases where pasteurellosis was clearly associated with a predator bite in the original report are footnoted as such.

[a] NR: serotype not reported in the first citation.

[b] Diagnostic case records, U.S. Geological Survey, National Wildlife Health Center, Madison, Wisconsin, U.S.A.; serotypes generally identified by the methods of Heddleston et al. (1972).

[c] Probable host for *P. multocida;* incomplete description of methods used to isolate and identify pasteurellae.

[d] Probable host species; bird species not definitively identified in text.

[e] Pasteurellosis associated with a cat bite.

[f] Apparently healthy bird, or died from other causes.

species, the author specified how many infections were associated with cat bites. For the other 19 species, approximately 56% of the birds had associated cat-bite lesions. Likewise, birds from rehabilitation or veterinary clinics have been reported with the acknowledgment that some pasteurellosis cases were associated with cat bites (Jennings 1954, 1955; Curtis 1979; Macdonald et al. 1981); however, the birds with cat bites were not always identified.

ETIOLOGY

Pasteurella multocida is an encapsulated Gram-negative bacterium whose shape may vary from a rod to a coccobacillus. Bipolar staining characteristic is evident with methylene blue, Wright's stain, Giemsa stain, and Gram stain (Wobeser 1981). For a while, each isolate was named according to the clinical presentation and animal group from which it was recovered, such as *P. avicida* or *P. aviseptica,* and *P. muricida* or *P. muriseptica* (Heddleston 1972). Rosenbusch and Merchant (1939) proposed the species *P. multocida* (from Latin "multo": many; "caedo": kill); this subsequently has become the accepted name (Heddleston 1972). *Pasteurella multocida* was the sole species in the genus *Pasteurella* until the 1930s, when a variety of new species and other taxa were described (Blackall and Miflin 2000). Since the 1930s, additional species, subspecies, and other, unnamed taxa of the genus *Pasteurella* have been described from birds (Piechulla et al. 1985; Blackall and Miflin 2000).

An identification system to distinguish among *P. multocida* strains by serological and biochemical characteristics includes five capsular serotypes (A, B, D, E, and F) based on a hemagglutination method (Heddleston et al. 1972; Rimler et al. 1984; Rimler and Glisson 1997), 16 somatic serotypes (1–16) based on characterization of capsular and cell wall antigens (Christensen and Bisgaard 2000), and three subspecies based on carbohydrate fermentation patterns (Mutters et al. 1985). Most avian strains have capsular antigens characteristic of type A and can react with more than one somatic serotype (Rhoades and Rimler 1989; Christensen and Bisgaard 2000). The capsule appears to be an important determinant of the virulence in type A strains (Chung et al. 2001; Borrathybay et al. 2003). Based on the application of ribotyping, outer membrane protein profiles (Omp), and polymerase chain reaction (PCR) techniques, avian strains of *P. multocida* are a genetically diverse and heterogeneous group (Petersen et al. 2001a; Davies et al. 2003). Serotype 1 is, by far, the most common serotype reported from wild birds on a worldwide basis, followed by serotypes 3 and 3,4 (Table 12.1). Most North American *P. multocida* isolates from wild waterfowl and shorebirds have been serotype 1 in the Pacific, Central, and Mississippi Flyways, with serotypes 3 and 4 predominating in the Atlantic Flyway (Wilson et al. 1995b; Friend 1999). Recently, serotype 1 has been isolated from Common Eiders in the Atlantic Flyway (National Wildlife Health Center, unpublished data).[1] Serotype 1, alone or in combination with other serotypes, has not been reported from pheasants, pigeons, or psittacine birds. Nine of the 16 known serotypes have been reported in wild birds, with at least 29 different combinations. Serotypes 2, 9, 10, 12, 14, and 15 have not been reported in wild avian species. Mutters et al. (1985) proposed a classification method that includes three subspecies of *Pasteurella multocida: P. m. multocida, P. m. gallicida,* and *P. m. septica,* based on their differential abilities to ferment several carbohydrates. To date, *P. m. multocida* appears to be the most common subspecies isolated from wild birds. Most of 295 *P. multocida* isolates from California wildfowl were classified as *P. m. multocida* (63%), followed by *P. m. gallicida* (37%), and *P. m. septica* (<1%)(Hirsh et al. 1990). Morishita et al. (1996a) found four *P. m. multocida* isolates from psittacine birds and one isolate that could not be classified according to the three subspecies (nonbiotypable). Among raptors, Morishita et al. (1996b) found seven *P. m. multocida,* three *P. m. gallicida,* and one nonbiotypable isolates. Based on ribotyping, avian *P. m. gallicida* strains clustered together, whereas *P. m. multocida* and *P. m. septica* did not appear as separate lines (Petersen et al. 2001a).

Despite the widespread use of serotyping, no consistent relationship was found between serotype, biochemical characteristics, and host species of origin (Heddleston 1976). Because only a few *P. multocida* serotypes regularly occur in wild birds, serotyping and biochemical methods lack discriminatory power for detailed epizootiologic studies, such as determining transmission among species, tracking the spread of epizootics, or determining the origin of epizootics. The stability of serologic and biochemical characteristics also has been questioned (Hunt et al. 2000) and the same serotype may have genetic differences that limit the value of serotyping in epizootiologic investigations (Christensen et al. 1998; Lee, M. D. et al. 2000). Understanding of the epizootiology of avian cholera would be increased if isolates of *P. multocida* from wild birds were typed by serologic or genotypic typing methods and pathogenicity confirmed by testing in live birds (Samuel et al. 2003b, 2005a).

Studies utilizing genotyping of avian cholera strains from wild birds have been limited. However, techniques based on genetic analysis of the bacterium hold the promise of greater sensitivity, discriminatory power, and stability to identify differences among strains. Eiders, cormorants, shorebirds, and gulls in two epizootics from different locations were infected with the same clone of *P. multocida* (Christensen et al. 1998) and isolates from diurnal raptors were genetically related and similar to those found in waterfowl (Morishita et al. 1996b). Recent molecular techniques such as pulsed field gel electrophoresis, repetitive sequence-based PCR, and amplified fragment length polymorphism have been applied to pasteurellae epizootics in domestic birds (Gunawardana et al. 2000; Amonsin et al. 2002) and show promise for investigation of avian cholera epizootics. Future development of genotypic methods remains a potentially promising area to increase our knowledge of avian cholera epizootiology. The complete genetic sequence of one common avian strain recently was completed (May et al. 2001) and may provide a template for development of genetic methods and comparison among strains.

More detailed descriptions of the biochemical and serological characteristics of *P. multocida* are reported by Rhoades and Rimler (1984), Adlam and Rutter (1989), Holmes (1998), and Christensen and Bisgaard (2000). The molecular biology and methods for genetic analysis of *P. multocida* have been reviewed in Hunt et al. (2000) and Blackall and Miflin (2000).

EPIZOOTIOLOGY

Life History

Avian cholera epizootics are usually explosive in waterfowl and other water birds, appearing with little warning (Botzler 1991). In many epizootics, birds appear to die overnight and carcasses may not be evident until healthy waterfowl leave their roost site (Vaught et al. 1967). Epizootics are commonly associated with dense concentrations of susceptible birds and can involve hundreds to thousands of birds of many species (Blanchong et al. 2006a). The pattern of rapid and unpredictable mortality affecting many species of birds suggests simultaneous exposure via a common source of infection, most likely contaminated water (Wobeser 1992). Although factors precipitating outbreaks are commonly associated with stressors, in many cases the occurrence of avian cholera has been associated with the arrival of specific species, such as Snow Geese. In the Rainwater Basin, the timing of epizootics and patterns of mortality among species are correlated with an increase in Lesser Snow Goose abundance during spring migration (Blanchong et al. 2006a). Mortality usually declines near the end of epizootics, as birds disperse from the epizootic site, and there can be an increased presence of sick birds, suggesting that *P. multocida* strains may become less virulent (Rosen and Bischoff 1949; Rosen and Morse 1959).

Although avian cholera mortality can occur at any time of the year, major epizootics are typically seasonal, taking place on major waterfowl concentration areas, primarily in winter or early spring (Friend 1987). Deaths may continue to occur in some species as they migrate north (Wobeser 1992). Summer epizootics also take place in colonial-nesting species of waterfowl such as Common Eiders, Lesser Snow and Ross's Geese, and Cape or Great Cormorants (Crawford et al. 1992; Wobeser 1992; Samuel et al. 1999a; Pedersen et al. 2003). Within North America avian cholera has been reported in every month and it appears that *P. multocida* is present in at least some waterfowl populations throughout the entire year (Samuel et al. 2005a).

In addition to highly visible epizootics, scattered low-level mortality from avian cholera may be more common than is generally accepted; such mortality usually goes undetected and seldom develops into extensive epizootics (Botzler 1991; Wobeser 1992; Botzler 2002). Single cases or small outbreaks have been reported regularly (Bivens 1953, 1955; Macdonald 1963, 1965; Rosen 1969, 1972; Blus et al. 1978; Wobeser 1981; Botzler 1991) and may occur within a single species, suggesting mortality of carrier birds or that transmission is occurring primarily through direct contact (Wobeser 1992). Any one of these small events may flare into an extensive epizootic because a single case that results from exacerbation of a carrier state might be sufficient to start an epizootic under the proper conditions (Wobeser 1981). After an epizootic starts, contamination of the environment (especially water) and dense concentrations of susceptible birds probably facilitates transmission of *P. multocida.*

Transmission

Transmission of *P. multocida* to susceptible animals has been hypothesized to occur in several ways, including inhalation, ingestion, cat bites, and arthropod bites (Botzler 1991). Transmission to susceptible birds from contaminated wetlands or from direct bird-to-bird contact are the most likely routes of transmission during epizootics.

Transmission by inhalation probably occurs through production of aerosols. Because *P. multocida* can concentrate at the water surface (Rosen and Bischoff 1949; Potter and Baker 1961), transmission can occur by inhalation of bacterial laden aerosols (droplet infection) formed when high densities of birds land, take flight, bathe, or disturb the water surface and eject high bacterial concentrations into the atmosphere (Rosen and Morse 1959; Blanchard and Syzdek 1970). *Pasteurella multocida* can enter the mucous membranes of the pharynx, upper respiratory tract (Wobeser 1992), or conjunctiva (Wilkie et al. 2000). Domestic turkeys were very susceptible to *P. multocida* by inoculation into the palatine air spaces (Donahue and Olson 1971). Waterfowl and American Coots died from avian cholera when *P. multocida* was inoculated by aerosol route, but required more bacterial inocula and longer exposure than would be expected under natural conditions (Titche 1979).

Pasteurella multocida also may be transmitted to susceptible birds by ingestion of bacteria in contaminated food or water. Water contaminated with *P. multocida* from birds or carcasses is likely of primary importance in transmitting avian cholera among waterfowl (Wobeser 1992). Quortrup et al. (1946) found that healthy ducks placed near those orally infected with *P. multocida* died after 28 hours if they had access to the same drinking water. Domestic turkeys were infected with *P. multocida* from a common water source used by experimentally infected turkeys (Pabs-Garnon and Soltys 1971). American Coots exposed to drinking water contaminated with 2.3×10^7 *P. multocida* per ml died from avian cholera within two days (Zinkl et al. 1977). Waterfowl such as American Coots and American Wigeon (*Anas americana*), which graze frequently at the water surface, were among the first species to die at avian cholera sites (Botzler 1991).

For either inhalation or ingestion, contaminated water likely plays a significant role in the transmission of *P. multocida.* Carcasses that remain in wetlands can be an important source of *P. multocida* in water, and some avian cholera epizootics have stopped when carcasses were removed and bacteria no longer were detectable in water (Price and Brand 1984). In addition to carcasses, infected birds can transmit *P. multocida* to susceptible birds by either oral or cloacal shedding (Samuel et al. 2003a). Waterfowl that die from avian cholera often produce up to 15 ml of nasal discharge as well as mucoid intestinal material containing massive numbers of *P. multocida* (Rosen 1971; Wobeser 1997). Thus, carcasses or living infected birds can provide an important source of bacteria that contaminate wetlands or directly transmit infection to other birds.

Predation or scavenging on infected animals may play a role in transmitting *P. multocida* or causing mortality in avian predators. An unusual avian cholera epizootic in California involved waterfowl and predatory scavenging by montane voles *(Microtus montanus),* gulls, Short-eared Owls *(Asio flammeus),* Northern Harriers *(Circus cyaneus),* and a weasel (Rosen and Morse 1959). American Crows (*Corvus brachyrhynchos*) scavenging infected waterfowl died from avian cholera during an epizootic in Nebraska (Zinkl et al. 1977), and a Gyrfalcon *(Falco rusticolus)* reportedly died from *P. multocida* serotype 1 after ingesting a bird during an epizootic in waterfowl and Wild Turkeys (*Meleagris gallopavo*) (Williams et al. 1987). It has been proposed that Ospreys (*Pandion haliaetus*) that contracted avian cholera either were infected by ingesting sick waterfowl or by using infected carcasses or bones as part of their nest material (Hindman et al. 1997). *Pasteurella multocida* serotype 1 has been isolated from a number of Bald Eagles (*Haliaeetus leucocephalus*) and other raptors known to prey on waterfowl during avian cholera epizootics (Wilson et al. 1995a).

Transmission of *P. multocida* by ingestion of infected invertebrates during an avian cholera epizootic is possible, but remote. Based on the low survival of *P. multocida* in snails *(Physa virginia),* Miller and Botzler (1995) argued that it is unlikely that these snails would effectively transmit *P. multocida*. However, the role of contaminated fly maggots in domestic birds (Kitt 1888) deserves further consideration. Other routes of transmission via arthropods or animal bite can also occur, but these sources are unlikely to produce epizootic mortality in wild birds. Among domestic birds, *P. multocida* can be carried or transmitted by Mallophaga (*Eomenacanthus stramineus* and *Menopon gallinae*) (Derylo 1967, 1969), the soft tick *Argas persicus* (Iovchev 1967; Petrov 1970; Glukhov and Novikov 1975), and poultry mites (*Dermanyssus gallinae*) (Bigland 1954). *Pasteurella multocida* also has been recovered from mites (*Dermanyssus* spp.) collected from wild ducks dying from avian cholera (Quortrup et al. 1946), and transmission of *P. multocida* by tabanid flies has been reported (Krinsky 1976). Pasteurellosis can be transmitted to individual birds bitten by mammals, including cats (Smit et al. 1980; Korbel 1990) and raccoons *(Procyon lotor)* (Gregg et al. 1974). However, there is no direct evidence that animal or arthropod bites play an important role in infectious transmission of avian cholera among wild birds (Botzler 1991).

Factors Affecting Epizootics

Although *P. multocida* infections have been studied in domestic birds for more than two centuries (Rimler and Glisson 1997), some aspects of the disease in wild birds are yet to be fully clarified, including the importance of host susceptibility, stress factors, and environmental conditions in initiating, maintaining, and terminating avian cholera epizootics. Our knowledge about the roles of these factors in avian cholera epizootics remains insufficient to predict mortality events. In addition, the importance of weather, bird distribution and density patterns, disease carriers, pathogen virulence, and other factors in contributing to avian cholera epizootics has received limited attention.

Susceptibility to avian cholera varies among bird species, both in the laboratory and in the field, based on differences in behavior and habitat use (Rosen 1969). For example, wild birds at greatest risk to avian cholera maintained larger flock sizes, used land areas together, and commonly grazed on land or at the water surface (Combs and Botzler 1991). In addition, virulence can be highly variable among different *P. multocida* isolates or strains (Wilkie et al. 2000; Petersen et al. 2001b; Samuel et al. 2003b).

Host density may be a predisposing factor to avian cholera epizootics. High densities of susceptible birds can exceed the threshold necessary to facilitate an epizootic. Epizootics among domestic birds have increased when their densities increased (Van Es and Olney 1940). High density or prolonged contact among wild birds because of limited habitat, drought conditions, shallow or stagnant water, and inclement weather often have been associated with epizootics of avian cholera on wintering areas (Petrides and Bryant 1951; Vaught et al. 1967; Rosen 1969; Klukas and Locke 1970; Zinkl et al. 1977). A study of avian cholera among nesting Lesser Snow Geese found that 5 to 9% of the birds died in foci scattered throughout the colony and mortality was generally associated with greater nest density (Samuel et al. 1999a). Increased density probably increases the rate of infection (Wobeser 1992), but it may also increase stress conditions that produce disease in carrier birds (Wobeser 1997).

Environmental Factors

Weather conditions including temperature, fog, and precipitation are among the factors that can play an important role in avian cholera epizootics. Cold weather can increase stress levels or crowding of birds on the remaining ice-free wetlands, conditions that appear to precipitate epizootics. Temperatures may also affect host susceptibility to avian cholera. Later disease onset and lower mortality occurred among inoculated domestic turkeys housed at 33–37°C, compared to turkeys held at 22°C or lower (Simensen et al. 1980). Two peak periods of avian cholera mortality were noted following several days of very cold temperatures in Nebraska (Windingstad et al. 1988), and cold temperatures were associated with higher mortality after an epizootic began, but snow cover, cold temperature, and number of geese were not related to the initiation of another epizootic (Windingstad et al. 1998). Because *P. multocida* has very poor survival in water at 4° C compared to 20° C (Bredy and Botzler 1989), these mortality patterns imply that cold weather may influence disease outbreaks primarily through host ecology and susceptibility. Other weather conditions such as prolonged fog may reduce the mobility of birds, increasing the period of potential infectious contact among individuals or species, as well as reduce ultra-violet radiation and thus promote survival of the *P. multocida* bacterium. A direct correlation between rainfall and avian cholera was reported in a study with domestic birds (Hoffman and Stover 1942). Although there is no apparent consistent relationship between precipitation and avian cholera epizootics among wild birds (Botzler 1991), avian cholera mortality was more common and widely distributed in the Pacific and Central Flyways during a warmer and wetter El Niño year (Samuel et al. 2003b).

A number of laboratory studies have been conducted using artificially inoculated water to determine environmental and wetland conditions that affect *P. multocida* survival. Survival of *P. multocida* in the laboratory ranged from several days to greater than a year (Hutyra et al. 1949; Bendheim and Even-Shoshan

1975; Titche 1979; Bredy and Botzler 1989). Survival is enhanced by the presence of animal organic matter (Rosen and Bischoff 1950; Olson and Bond 1968; Titche 1979), warm temperatures (18–20°C), the addition of animal protein, NaCl, and the presence of other microorganisms (Bredy and Botzler 1989). In contrast, variation in pH, clay content, and sucrose level had little effect on survival of the pasteurellae (Bredy and Botzler 1989). High concentrations of calcium and magnesium ions, singly or in combination, increased survival of *P. multocida* in waters collected from avian cholera sites in Nebraska (Price et al. 1992), but ammonium, nitrate, or orthophosphate ions had little effect. In all these cases, the conditions of the laboratory experiments were quite different than conditions occurring under natural wetland conditions. Field studies evaluating the effect of wetland water quality on avian cholera have been limited in scope and somewhat contradictory. Early reports indicated a correlation between wetland water conditions and avian cholera epizootics; however, more comprehensive studies have not demonstrated a significant relationship. Differences in specific conductance, calcium, magnesium, chloride, sulfate, and sodium levels were reported between areas affected by avian cholera, and areas not experiencing epizootics in the Rainwater Basin of Nebraska (Windingstad et al. 1984). Many of the environmental differences at these wetlands persisted over time (Gordon 1989) despite changes in the distribution of epizootics in the Rainwater Basin. In contrast, Lehr et al. (2005) found no consistent water quality differences between wetlands with avian cholera mortality or where *P. multocida* was isolated and wetlands without avian cholera or *P. multocida*, respectively. An extensive study evaluating relationships between environmental variables measured in previous laboratory or field studies was conducted at wetlands with and without avian cholera epizootics throughout the United States (Blanchong et al. 2006b). No consistent relationship between the environmental variables and occurrence of avian cholera was found. Overall it appears that early findings of association between water conditions and avian cholera epizootics, especially in the Rainwater Basin, may have been associated with bird distribution patterns rather than specific environmental conditions. However, recent studies reported a positive association between the abundance of *P. multocida* isolates recovered in wetlands with avian cholera epizootics and the concentration of nutrients typically associated with eutrophication (potassium, nitrate, phosphorus, and phosphate) (Blanchong et al. 2006b). These findings raise concern about disease implications of the increasing eutrophication of wetland ecosystems throughout North America. More research is needed to confirm these results and determine whether eutrophic nutrients enhance the survival of *P. multocida* or severity of epizootics.

There is little information evaluating avian cholera epizootiology in the context of habitat characteristics and land use, and no clear association between these factors and epizootics. Vegetation at an avian cholera site in Nebraska was characterized by low species diversity, whereas a site with little avian cholera had high species diversity (Brown et al. 1983). In contrast, no apparent pattern between the occurrence of avian cholera and variation in emergent vegetation was found (Gordon 1989). In the same area, Smith et al. (1989) found no relation between avian cholera mortality and surface water drainage among wetlands, wetland classifications, and land use. However, Smith and Higgins (1990) found that the occurrence of avian cholera epizootics was inversely related to the density of semipermanent wetland basins. It is uncertain whether some of these wetland characteristics are directly related to disease outbreaks or indirectly associated based on waterfowl distribution and use patterns.

Sources/Reservoirs of *Pasteurella multocida*

A major unknown element in the epizootiology of avian cholera has been a dependable, persistent source (reservoir) where *P. multocida* can survive year-round and produce recurring disease. Two major reservoirs have been proposed for *P. multocida* among wildfowl: ambient soil or water at enzootic wetlands and carrier birds (Botzler 1991). The importance of carrier birds among chickens and other domestic birds has been known for many years (Wobeser 1992), and *P. multocida* isolates are occasionally recovered in healthy waterfowl, but their serotype and virulence are seldom determined. In contrast, the consistent recurrence of disease in many areas (if not specific wetlands), isolation of *P. multocida* from wetland water or sediment, and survival of bacteria for considerable time periods in the laboratory have provided support for the wetland reservoir hypothesis.

To assess the hypothesis related to wetland reservoirs, *P. multocida* has been inoculated in soil and water to determine survival and growth. Depending on the environmental conditions, survival of *P. multocida* in soil ranges from 15 to 113 days (Hutyra et al. 1949; Dimov 1964; Olson and Bond 1968; Awad et al. 1976; Backstrand and Botzler 1986), whereas survival in wetland water ranges from 10 to 30 days (Rosen 1969; Titche 1979; Backstrand and Botzler 1986). Field investigations in enzootic areas have also been conducted to determine persistence of *P. multocida* in wetlands. In California, *P. multocida* could not be isolated from wetland water or sediments prior to the occurrence of avian cholera, and only sporadic isolations were made during and after the occurrence of avian cholera in the area (Lehr et al. 2005). *Pasteurella multocida* was not isolated from water or sediment samples collected in autumn from 44 wetlands in six U.S. states that experienced avian cholera epizootics the previous winter or spring, leading to the conclusion that the bacteria did not survive the summer and that wetlands are not a good reservoir (Samuel et al. 2004). An evaluation of 23 of these wetlands concluded that *P. multocida* did not persist for more than one to two months following the termination of epizootics (Blanchong et al. 2006c). In addition, there was no association between *P. multocida* persistence and water quality characteristics, virulence of isolates, or whether isolates were recovered from sediment or water samples. Overall, recent field investigations associated with avian cholera epizootics provide no evidence that wetland ecosystems (water or sediments) can serve as a year-round reservoir of *P. multocida.*

Carrier animals are the alternate hypothesized reservoir in the epizootiology of avian cholera. Among domestic birds, many recovered chickens became carriers, and it was suggested that birds surviving avian cholera from one year provided the reservoir for the next year's outbreak (Pritchett et al. 1930a, 1930b; Pritchett and Hughes 1932). Feces from established carrier birds could not maintain *P. multocida* and were unimportant sources of environmental contamination; rather, established carriers were significant sources of *P. multocida* for domestic animals only through oral and nasal discharges, especially into water (Iliev et al. 1965). Tissue samples from 578 domestic waterfowl and 240 chickens evaluated through mouse inoculation showed that birds from infected flocks most frequently carried *P. multocida* in the cloacal mucosa, whereas birds from flocks without avian cholera most frequently carried *P. multocida* in their pharynx (Muhairwa et al. 2000). In addition, it was noted that healthy poultry as well as convalescent animals could be carriers of *P. multocida.* Heddleston (1972) believed that the life of a carrier bird was the only limit to the duration of a chronic carrier state in domestic fowl.

Evaluation of potential *P. multocida* carriers in wild birds has been challenging because sensitive diagnostic tests are not available and there is uncertainty about where *P. multocida* might be sequestered in healthy birds. In some studies, apparently healthy wild birds have been found carrying *P. multocida* including American Coots, Mallards, Northern Pintails (*Anas acuta*), American Wigeon, Green-winged Teal, Common Eiders, Lesser Snow Geese, and California Gulls (*Larus californicus*) (Vaught et al. 1967; Korschgen et al. 1978; Titche 1979; Samuel et al. 1997). Six of nine California Gulls fed *P. multocida*–contaminated meat shed *P. multocida* in their feces for up to 120 hr (Titche 1979). However, *P. multocida* was not found in feces among 450 free-living waterfowl in zoological settings (Fallacara et al. 2004). Interestingly, most *P. multocida* isolates collected from wild rodents, lagomorphs, and carnivores, as well as flea pools from these animals, were serotypes 1A and 3A, the same serotypes generally found in wildfowl during avian cholera epizootics (Quan et al. 1986). In a controlled study using artificially infected Mallards, *P. multocida* was isolated from oral, nasal, and cloacal swabs and a variety of tissues of birds that survived infection (Samuel et al. 2003a).

Lesser Snow Geese historically have been proposed as a potential reservoir of *P. multocida.* Avian cholera mortality in the Central and Mississippi Flyways closely followed the migration patterns of Lesser Snow Geese, starting from Hudson Bay (Brand 1984). In addition, *P. multocida* has been isolated from dead birds during avian cholera epizootics on the wintering grounds (Rosen and Morse 1959), breeding grounds (Samuel et al. 1999a), and migratory pathways of Lesser Snow Geese (Wobeser et al. 1979). It also has been noted that avian cholera in the Sacramento Valley of California usually follows the arrival of Lesser Snow Geese (J. G. Mensik, Sacramento National Wildlife Refuge, unpublished data).[3] Lesser Snow Geese may be particularly important in the epizootiology of avian cholera because they have increased dramatically, are frequently involved in large epizootics, associate in dense aggregations that enhance disease transmission, and nest in colonies that facilitate continuation of the disease during summer (Samuel et al. 1999c). In the Rainwater Basin of Nebraska, Lesser Snow Goose was the species commonly found during avian cholera epizootics and associated with early spring epizootics; levels of Lesser Snow Goose mortality were positively associated with mortality in other species (Blanchong et al. 2006a). The potential importance of Lesser Snow Geese in the epizootiology of avian cholera, including the confirmation of carrier birds, was recently demonstrated by isolation of pathogenic *P. multocida* serotype 1 from apparently healthy birds on breeding (Samuel et al. 1997) and wintering (Samuel et al. 2005a) areas.

Ross's and Lesser Snow Geese wintering in the Central Flyway were found to be carriers of pathogenic *P. multocida* serotype 1 (Samuel et al. 2005a). Isolates were recovered from oral, cloacal, leg joint, eye, and nasal swabs collected from approximately 2% of the apparently healthy birds tested of both species. Most of these serotype 1 isolates were pathogenic to waterfowl in challenge studies (Samuel et al. 2005a). In the past, when *P. multocida* was isolated from carrier animals or soil and water, these isolates often were not serotyped or inoculated into susceptible birds to determine their virulence (Samuel et al. 2005a). Virulence testing has been an important step in resolving these discrepancies because many strains of *P. multocida* are not pathogenic in birds (Botzler 1991; Samuel et al. 2003b; Samuel et al. 2005a). These results provide the most convincing evidence to date that wild birds are carriers of *P. multocida* and therefore function as a reservoir for avian cholera. The apparent importance of Lesser Snow (and Ross's) Geese as carriers of avian cholera coupled with the dramatic increase in abundance and distribution of these two species as well as their propensity to occur in large aggregations throughout the year amplifies the potential role of these species in avian cholera epizootics (Samuel et al. 2005a). There is considerably less information on potential reservoirs among other bird species. No *P. multocida* were found among samples from the pharynx, choana, or cloaca of clinically healthy raptors or psittacine birds (Morishita et al. 1996a,b) or from 1709 free-living passerines in Ohio (Morishita et al. 1999). Among waterfowl, which appear to be the most likely carriers of avian cholera, only Greater White-fronted Geese (*Anser albifrons*) have been evaluated to determine their potential role as avian cholera carriers. Based on testing more than 600 breeding geese using serology and bacterial isolation, birds were previously infected with *P. multocida* serotype 1, but there was no evidence of *P. multocida* carriers (Samuel et al. 2005b).

Although many researchers favored the hypothesis that carrier birds were the most important reservoir for wild birds, there were many ambiguities on the respective importance of wetlands, as well as carrier animals. Current information indicates that some waterfowl species serve as reservoirs and carriers of avian cholera and likely play an important role in spreading and transmitting disease to other species. In contrast, wetland ecosystems appear to play an important role in transmitting disease to susceptible birds but are not an important reservoir of *P. multocida*. Further research is needed to determine which waterfowl species are carriers of *P. multocida* and to delineate the role of carrier birds in the epizootiology of avian cholera.

CLINICAL SIGNS

Most wild birds with avian cholera are found dead with no premonitory signs. Even in large epizootics with extensive mortality, it is uncommon to observe sick birds. Waterfowl often have been observed in apparent good health the day prior to death, and the esophagus and proventriculus of dead birds may be filled with recently ingested food, indicating acute mortality. Female Common Eiders often are found dead sitting on their clutch (Swennen and Smit 1991). In water, birds may die with their head resting on their back. Lethargic birds that can be approached closely may be more common in the late stages of prolonged epizootics among waterfowl (Friend 1999). Birds with signs suggestive of neurological involvement (erratic uncoordinated flight, circling while walking or swimming, or opisthotonos) have also been reported. Clear mucoid fluid containing large amounts of *P. multocida* bacteria may run from the nares of freshly dead waterfowl. Scavenging species (such as crows and gulls) may have a more chronic course of disease than occurs in waterfowl. American Crows were debilitated, lethargic, dyspneic, and reluctant or unable to fly; some had rapidly blinking nictitating membranes, interpreted to indicate neurological involvement (Zinkl et al. 1977; Taylor and Pence 1981).

PATHOGENESIS

Little is known about the pathogenesis of avian cholera in wild birds. By extrapolation from poultry, the pathogenesis is probably complex and variable, depending on the strain of *P. multocida,* susceptibility of the host species, how they contact each other (Rimler and Glisson 1997), and the infectious dose. Pathogenicity also may increase with bird-to-bird transmission over a short period of time (Matsumoto and Strain 1993). Bacteria probably enter the body most commonly through mucous membranes of the pharynx or upper respiratory tract. Pehlivanoglu et al. (1999) found no significant difference in mortality among ducks inoculated via intraocular, intranasal, and oral routes. Skin wounds may also serve as a portal of entry. After virulent *P. multocida* enter the body of a susceptible bird, the bacteria multiply rapidly, resulting in septicemia. To accomplish this, the bacteria must evade bacteriocidal properties of serum and the phagocytic defense system. How this occurs in wild birds has not been studied, but in other species resistance to phagocytosis is associated with capsular and outer membrane components of the bacterium (Harmon et al. 1992; Poermadjaja and Frost 2000). In the acute disease, clinical signs (fever, systemic hypotension, and shock), death, and the predominant lesions of hemorrhage and necrotic foci in the liver are attributed to endotoxin produced by the bacterium (Collins 1977). Disseminated intravascular coagulation may be seen, and consumption coagulopathy occurs in turkeys (Friedlander and Olson 1995). Chronic infections, as occur in crows and gulls, also have evidence of vascular injury and may be localized rather than generalized.

PATHOLOGY

Gross lesions vary with the duration of illness. Birds that die acutely, such as most waterfowl, cormorants, and penguins, are in good body condition. The esophagus and proventriculus may be filled with food. In some birds, or species that are highly susceptible, there may be no gross lesions that are apparent. More regularly, lesions are scattered petechial hemorrhages on the epicardium (Figure 12.2) and serosal membranes. In birds that survive slightly longer, 1 to 2 mm white to yellow foci of necrosis are present in the liver (Figure 12.2); less commonly, there may be petechial hemorrhages in the hepatic parenchyma. The spleen may be normal, or enlarged and contain pale necrotic foci. In waterfowl, the lungs are often congested and may be edematous, particularly if the bird aspirated water prior to death. The intestines are often filled with abundant mucoid material and there is copious mucoid discharge from the nares.

In birds with more chronic disease, such as crows, gulls, and raptors, there may be fibrinous pericarditis, airsacculitis, and focal pneumonia (Zinkl et al. 1977; Crawford et al. 1992). Taylor and Pence (1981) described hemorrhagic meningitis in American Crows. In individual birds, *P. multocida* may also cause a variety of localized inflammatory lesions, involving the sinuses, joints, oviduct, middle ear, and other tissues. The histopathology of acute avian cholera is not specific, except for focal hepatic necrosis and the massive numbers of small cocco-bacillary bacteria that are often visible in blood vessels and tissues throughout the body. Thus, confirmation of avian cholera diagnoses also requires isolation and identification of the *P. multocida* bacterium.

DIAGNOSIS

A history of acute deaths of many birds, with few clinical signs, together with minimal gross lesions consisting of petechial hemorrhages on serosal membranes and focal hepatic necrosis, is highly suggestive of avian cholera. The presence of many small coccobacilli in smears of heart blood is very supportive of that diagnosis. Definitive diagnosis must be based on isolation and identification of the organism. In cases of septicemia, the organism can be isolated from heart blood and all organs. Liver is usually the organ of choice for culture, but bone marrow, for example from the ulna, is suitable for culture from scavenged carcasses. *Pasteurella multocida* grows readily on a variety of media, including blood agar and trypticase soy agar, incubated at 37° C. *Pasteurella* selective media (Moore et al. 1994; Lee, C. W. et al. 2000) may increase success in isolating the organism in some situations. Isolates can be identified using the criteria proposed by Heddleston (1975).

IMMUNITY

Some of the first experiments by Pasteur in the field of immunology were conducted using avian cholera, and most subsequent immunological work on this disease has been to protect domestic animals (Rosen 1971). Today, control of avian cholera in domestic birds in some parts of the world depends largely on vaccination programs (Christensen and Bisgaard 2000) in combination with hygiene and other related biosecurity measures. Many live and inactivated vaccines have been developed to control the disease, but both types have limitations. Because live vaccines can also cause disease, most commercial vaccines are produced as killed bacteria (bacterins) (Christensen and Bisgaard 2000). Although bacterins are inexpensive to produce, they must be injected and may produce short-term (two to three months) immunity only to homologous serotypes (Rebers and Heddleston 1977). As a result, immunization of wild birds is usually viewed as impractical. However, immunization may provide a valuable tool for protecting captive populations, populations of special concern (Price 1985), or in experimental studies to determine the impact of avian cholera on bird populations (Samuel et al. 1999b). Queen and Quortrup (1946) showed the potential for immunizing wild ducks with an

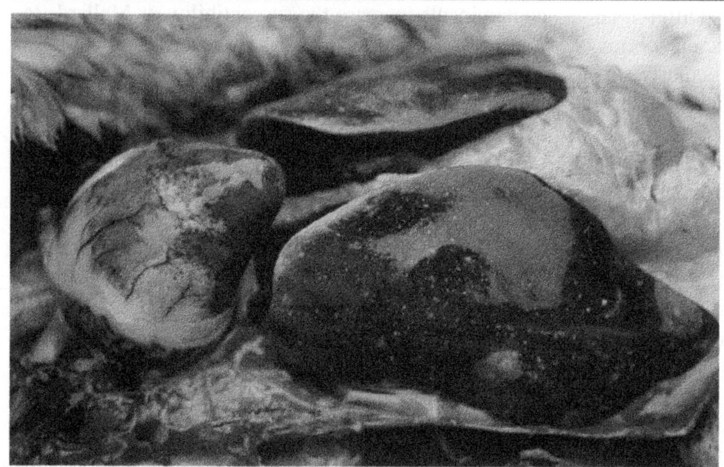

Figure 12.2. Hemorrhages of varying degrees of severity and necrosis are frequently visible on the heart and liver (respectively) of avian cholera infected birds. Pinhead-sized hemorrhages adjacent to the coronary fat bands are in evidence in this Canada Goose. Multifocal necrosis evident in the liver is also characteristic of avian cholera and typically appears as small, discrete, pale spots that vary in size and shape.

autogenous bacterin, and Price (1985) developed a serotype 1 bacterin that protected Canada Geese (*Branta canadensis*) and produced antibody response and partial protection from challenge in Pekin ducks and Redheads (El Tayeb 1993). However, this bacterin appeared to offer only limited protection when used in wild Lesser Snow Geese (El Tayeb 1993; Samuel et al. 1999b).

Early work on avian cholera in wild birds suggested that natural immunity did not occur (Rosen 1971), although there was one record of waterfowl serum containing antibody to *P. multocida* (Donahue and Olson 1969). Recent serological surveys of Lesser Snow, Ross's, and Greater White-fronted Geese (Samuel et al. 1999c; Samuel et al. 2005a; Samuel et al. 2005b) indicated that seropositive birds were present at wintering and breeding areas whether or not avian cholera epizootics were evident. At Arctic breeding areas the prevalence of seropositive geese increased in years with disease epizootics, and approximately 50% of the Lesser Snow Geese infected during breeding ground epizootics survived and seroconverted (Samuel et al. 1999c). In laboratory challenge trials in Mallards with *P. multocida* serotype 1, Samuel et al. (2003a) found that > 90% of surviving birds seroconverted, but antibody titers declined to background levels within three to four months following infection. Thus, current serological surveys likely detected only recent infection. Based on vaccination in domestic and wild birds, it appears that short-term immunity is likely for birds that survive infection. This is supported by the occurrence of antibodies in wild geese, indicating the potential for some species to develop an immune response to natural *P. multocida* infection. However, further research is needed to understand whether these survivors become disease carriers, whether they develop protective immunity against future infection, and the role of immunity in disease dynamics.

A related aspect of immunity is the differential effect of disease mortality associated with nutritional status, species, ages, or sex cohorts of birds. Differential species mortality has been reported during epizootics, with American Coots often appearing particularly susceptible (Botzler 1991; Botzler 2002); however, it is difficult to separate habitat use, bird distribution, immunity, and susceptibility issues from these reports. Most wild birds dying during avian cholera epizootics are in good physical condition (Friend 1987; McLandress 1983; Mensik and Botzler 1989), suggesting that nutritional deficiencies do not play an important role as a predisposing factor among wildfowl. Jeske et al. (1994) found that during epizootics, susceptibility to avian cholera among Mallards probably was not related to body condition of the birds.

There is limited evidence that age may affect susceptibility to avian cholera. Hunter and Wobeser (1980) reported that immature Mallards (four months old) were less susceptible than five-week-old ducklings. Windingstad et al. (1998) reported that immature Canada Geese had higher mortality rates than adults, and McLandress (1983) found that immature Lesser Snow and Ross's Geese died more frequently than did adults during the most severe stages of avian cholera epizootics. In contrast, Mensik and Botzler (1989) reported a similar age structure for American Coots that were apparently healthy and shot and those that died from avian cholera.

Host sex has been considered a predisposing factor for avian cholera, with males having a higher rate of mortality than females (Botzler 1991), although the reasons for this difference are unknown. Male Ross's Geese, Lesser Snow Geese (McLandress 1983), and Canada Geese (Windingstad et al. 1998) had higher mortality rates than females during avian cholera epizootics. However, no difference in mortality was found for male and female American Coots (Mensik and Botzler 1989). Higher prevalence of seropositive female Lesser Snow Geese than males was reported by Samuel et al. (1999c) when no avian cholera epizootics occurred, supporting the conclusion that females are more likely to survive infection. Finally, female Pekin ducks were more likely to survive challenge with *Pasteurella multocida* serotype 1 than males (Samuel et al. 2003b).

There is little information on the effects of environmental contaminants on immunity to avian cholera. Experimental studies on the relationship between avian cholera and pesticide (DDT and dieldrin) exposure were conducted by Friend (1971), but the results were inconclusive. Resistance to *P. multocida* was lower among Mallards exposed to sublethal levels of fuel oil, crude oil, and fuel oil mixed with oil dispersant (Rocke et al. 1984), but susceptibility was not affected by repeated oral exposure to sewage sludge (Goldberg and Yuill 1990). Whiteley and Yuill (1991) reported that some contaminants increase the susceptibility of Mallards to *P. multocida.* Ingested lead has also been considered as a factor affecting susceptibility to *P. multocida,* but similar tissue lead levels were found in Lesser Snow Geese dying from avian cholera compared to hunter-killed birds (Gordus 1993b). Higher levels of cadmium and lower levels of selenium and mercury were found among Long-tailed Ducks *(Clangula hyemalis)* dying from avian cholera compared to tissue metal concentrations found among apparently healthy birds collected several years earlier (Mashima et al. 1998).

PUBLIC HEALTH CONCERNS

In general, avian strains of *P. multocida* rarely infect humans (Hubbert 1970a, 1970b) and are not considered a high risk to human health. Some avian strains will cause localized abscesses in mammals if inoculated subcutaneously, and infections through skin wounds might occur in humans. To prevent potential contamination, infected birds should be handled with rubber gloves and exposed skin should be washed thoroughly after contact.

DOMESTIC ANIMAL HEALTH CONCERNS

Evidence for transmission of pasteurellae between domestic and wild birds is inconsistent. Where transmission may have occurred, it is not clear which species was the source of infections found in both domestic and wild birds. Some have expressed concern about transmission of *P. multocida* between domestic animals and wildlife and whether one group serves as a reservoir for the other. However, because *P. multocida* can be isolated from tissues, particularly the upper respiratory tract, of many animals, presence of *P. multocida* in animals from one group does not establish a risk for the other group. In assessing relationships and transmission pathways, phenotypic, genotypic, and pathogenicity features of bacterial isolates all must be considered.

The strains of *P. multocida* from birds that died from avian cholera usually cause fatal disease when inoculated into mice and rabbits. Many domestic mammals, however, are considered resistant to infection, and subcutaneous inoculation of domestic animals with avian serotypes may result in only localized abscesses. Heddleston and Watko (1963) found that *P. multocida* from avian cholera can survive and remain virulent in the nasal passages of cattle for several weeks. They proposed that *P. multocida* could transmit readily among domestic birds, wildlife, and a variety of other farm and laboratory animals. However, only one weak serotype 1 cross-reactor was found from 35 *P. multocida* isolates obtained from nasal swabs of feedlot cattle near an avian cholera epizootic in Nebraska (Windingstad et al. 1988). No *P. multocida* was recovered from cloacal or pharyngeal swabs of 20 domestic ducks and geese on a farm adjacent to the epizootic. Windingstad et al. concluded that there was little connection between domestic animals and the epizootic of avian cholera in wildfowl.

The relationship between avian cholera in wild birds and domestic poultry is also uncertain, although the two groups sometimes may share *P. multocida* strains. Sparrows, pigeons, and rats infected with *Pasteurella* sp. were able to transmit avian cholera from infected to healthy chickens in each of the chicken—wildlife—chicken sequences (Serdyuk and Tsimokh 1970), suggesting that wild birds or rodents might be a reservoir for domestic poultry. In addition, *P. multocida* was reported from a variety of wild mammals and birds on turkey farms experiencing avian cholera epizootics in the preceding two to eight months (Snipes et al. 1988). However, the serotypes of isolates from wildlife were the same as those affecting the turkeys on only two of seven premises checked, suggesting little connection between the avian cholera in turkeys and *P. multocida* in wildlife. Later, Snipes et al. (1990) found common serotypes between wildlife and domestic turkeys on the same premises in eight of 13 cases. In a study of avian cholera epizootics on three turkey farms in California, one farm had evidence that wild birds were a possible reservoir of infection, another had no evidence that wild birds were involved, and on the third farm there were several strains of *P. multocida,* including one shared by turkeys and a House Sparrow (*Passer domesticus*) (Christiansen et al. 1992b). A close genomic relationship between isolates from wild birds and back-yard poultry indicated that *P. multocida* can be exchanged between the two groups (Christensen et al. 1998), and Christensen et al. (1999) concluded that wild birds could transmit infection to domestic birds. *Pasteurella multocida* isolated from wild birds with avian cholera were highly virulent for turkeys, partridges, and pheasants, but less so for chickens (Petersen et al. 2001b). By studying DNA fingerprint patterns, Pedersen et al. (2003) found that the *P. multocida* in wild birds were also common in free-ranging domestic birds, but it was not possible to make conclusions about the direction or extent to which an exchange of isolates could occur.

WILDLIFE POPULATION IMPACTS

Although mortality during avian cholera epizootics can be substantial and highly visible to wildlife managers and to the general public, accurate determination of mortality rates and population impacts has been difficult. The impacts of avian cholera on bird populations, especially migratory waterfowl, should be considered at three levels of assessment: local wintering or breeding distributions, regional populations, and continental species abundance. Impacts can vary among species depending on their abundance, number of individuals at risk to infection, species and individual susceptibility, and behavioral characteristics that increase the risk of exposure to *P. multocida.*

Assessment of disease occurrence and magnitude of losses is complicated by the spatial and temporal variability in exposure to the agent and disease mortality, the difficulty of studying highly mobile and migratory bird populations, and the many confounding influences of predation, scavenging, and decomposition on determining disease-related mortality. Unless epizootic events are extensive and draw attention to a particular area, chronic low-level disease mortality may be easily overlooked (Zwank et al. 1985). When epizootics occur, mortality may be underestimated because sick birds may seek seclusion or are removed by predators and scavengers. Most estimates of disease mortality based on carcass counts are typically conservative because scavengers can dispose of most carcasses within three days when disease losses are at a low level (Humburg et al. 1983; Stutzenbaker et al. 1986). Chronic low-level avian cholera mortality may occur throughout the year and constitute a substantial portion of the annual losses in some populations of birds (Wobeser 1992). Even when mortality is extensive, carcasses may be difficult to find and represent less than 25–50% of the actual mortality (Humburg et al. 1983; Stutzenbaker et al. 1986).

Avian cholera can cause dramatic mortality in local bird populations, but the impact can be difficult to document unless it occurs during a relatively sedentary period of the annual cycle. Crawford et al. (1992) reported that greater than 14,500 adult Cape Cormorants died from avian cholera during the breeding season. This represented about 8% of the breeding population, but losses on individual islands ranged to approximately 16% of the breeding birds. Local epizootics have been reported in breeding Common Eiders in North America (Reed and Cousineau 1967) and Europe (Swennen and Smit 1991; Christensen 1996; Pedersen et al. 2003). Mortality at local breeding colonies varied from 17–25% in North America to greater than 80% in Denmark (Christensen 1996; Pedersen et al. 2003). Several of these epizootics are believed to have had substantial impacts on local breeding colonies. During avian cholera epizootics in northern California, American Coots appeared to be more susceptible than other waterfowl and their losses were estimated at 11.5% of the population (Botzler 2002). Lesser Snow Geese have been shown to be carriers of *P. multocida* and they nest in large aggregations that may help maintain the disease over the summer (Wobeser 1992; Samuel et al. 1999a). However, determination of avian cholera mortality at remote Arctic breeding colonies has been difficult to document. Mortality in Lesser Snow Geese breeding on Banks Island reached 30,000 and 20,000 adult geese in 1995 and 1996, respectively (Samuel et al. 1999a). Although losses amounted to 5–9% of the nesting colony, mortality did not appear to substantially hinder the recent rapid growth of this population.

Large local epizootics of avian cholera and extensive, wide-scale epizootics raise concerns about the disease impacts on regional populations of waterfowl. Typically these epizootics occur on important waterfowl concentration areas, such as wintering or staging areas, where multiple species are affected. In some cases, the magnitude of these local and regional losses has been sufficient that regional population impacts should be considered. In several key waterfowl areas in the U.S. (California and Nebraska), avian cholera mortality involving thousands of birds recurs almost annually. In these and other areas, including Maryland and Virginia, periodic epizootics can exceed tens of thousands of birds. Rosen (1971) estimated that up to 2% of the ducks and 6% of the swans wintering in California were lost to avian cholera; however, Botzler (1991) believed that these estimates were too high. To determine the impacts of avian cholera on Lesser Snow Geese wintering in California, Samuel et al. (1999b) conducted an experimental vaccination study. They reported that harvest and avian cholera were the two principal causes of mortality for these geese and that avian cholera may be one of the factors affecting the population on Wrangel Island (Russia), the only remaining Lesser Snow Goose colony in the Palearctic. In a study on Common Murres (*Uria aalge*) in the Baltic Sea, Österblom et al. (2004) reported that annual survival rates of adult birds were reduced from > 90% to < 80% due to epizootics of avian cholera at two breeding colonies.

Stout and Cornwell (1976) reported that disease mortality was the most important source of nonhunting mortality in North America during the period of 1930–1964, prior to the widespread distribution of avian cholera. Bellrose (1976) also believed that disease, including avian cholera, directly or indirectly accounted for the largest proportion of nonhunting mortality in waterfowl. However, even in years with unusually severe and widespread epizootics, there is little scientific evidence that avian cholera has substantially impacted continental populations of birds. Some species or populations with limited abundance may be affected adversely by a variety of mortality factors including disease. For example, populations that have a limited distribution during a portion of their annual cycle may be especially vulnerable to avian cholera or other infectious disease problems. For many waterfowl populations, avian cholera is one of the additional unpredictable factors including harvest, predation, other disease agents, weather conditions, accidents, and pollutants affecting annual reproduction and survival of these birds (Botzler 1991).

TREATMENT AND CONTROL

Antibacterial chemotherapy (sulfonamides and antibiotics) has been used extensively in the treatment of avian cholera in domestic birds (Rimler and Glisson 1997) and could be used in captive birds. However, against the peracute forms of the disease, drugs may be more valuable as a prophylactic than as a therapeutic agent (Rosen 1971). Vaccination is commonly used in domestic fowl to reduce the potential for disease epizootics and related mortality. A vaccination strategy has also been employed for captive Canada Geese

(Price 1985), but most vaccines have a limited duration of ≤ 1 year, require individual handling and immunization, and have varying degrees of efficacy among species. In either case, large-scale drug therapy or vaccination of wild populations is likely to be impractical, if not futile. On a limited scale, ponds have also been treated with copper sulfate mixed in hydrochloric acid (Rosen and Bischoff 1949), small puddles and water holes have been disinfected with a cresylic compound (Gershman et al. 1964), and small drinking ponds have been filled (Swennen and Smit 1991) in attempts to eradicate the disease; however, the efficacy of these techniques is unproven. All of these treatments and techniques may have beneficial application for individually valuable birds in captive flocks, zoological collections, or endangered species with a high risk of infection. In many cases involving free-ranging birds, the risks associated with capture and handling birds for treatment or vaccination may exceed the risk associated with avian cholera infection. As a general rule, treatment and prevention measures for wild birds are best focused on actions that will benefit the population at risk rather than individual birds.

Appropriate actions to control avian cholera epizootics depend on the severity and distribution of disease and the importance of the species or populations involved. Aircraft hazing of Whooping Cranes (*Grus americana*) and creation of artificial feeding sites for Bald Eagles have been used to move these species away from major epizootic areas (Friend 1999). More typically, the control strategy for wetlands with ongoing disease epizootics involves regular wetland surveillance, carcass removal, and disposal of carcasses. However, the benefits of a carcass collection program have not been rigorously tested (Botzler 1991). Under extreme conditions, wetland disinfection, depopulation, or treatment measures may be warranted. Depopulation appears to be feasible only under a limited set of conditions involving a discrete and localized epizootic that presents a high risk to other susceptible species, when complete eradication of infected birds without substantial risk of disease spread is feasible, and when eradication measures are specific to the target species (Wobeser 1997; Friend 1999). Pursglove et al. (1976) describe a successful multi-agency depopulation of American Coots at Back Bay, Virginia. However, the effectiveness of depopulation efforts for Common Eiders (Korschgen et al. 1978) and American Coots (Montgomery et al. 1979) has been questioned.

MANAGEMENT IMPLICATIONS

Efforts to control the occurrence or spread of avian cholera in waterfowl can generally be divided among overlapping approaches. The first of these strategies is to prevent the occurrence of avian cholera epizootics. Because most epizootics of avian cholera occur among dense concentrations of waterfowl and at traditional wetland areas, it is typically believed that lowering the density of birds in these high-risk areas and dispersing them over a larger area should be useful in preventing disease (Wobeser 1997). Management practices that encourage concentration of birds should be avoided in areas where avian cholera is a recurring event. In many cases, reduction in the density of birds should at least reduce the rate of transmission if disease epizootics are initiated. In addition, specific landscape management strategies should be developed that separate known carrier species such as Lesser Snow and Ross's Geese from other susceptible species (Samuel et al. 2005a). In some cases it may be necessary to prevent or severely reduce bird use on specific wetlands that seem to serve as focal areas for waterfowl infection (Friend 1999). Unfortunately, it appears that avian cholera epizootics are likely enhanced by the gregarious nature of most waterfowl species and by habitat losses that encourage dense concentrations of migratory birds, especially on wintering areas.

The second strategy is directed at early detection of epizootics to minimize environmental contamination and reduce transmission of *P. multocida* to susceptible birds. Frequent surveillance of wetland areas where migratory birds are concentrated, have a history of recurrent epizootics, and following adverse weather or stress conditions can contribute to detection of mortality at an early stage in the die-off. In the early stages, carcasses should be removed from the wetlands and submitted to a wildlife disease diagnostic laboratory for evaluation and confirmation of avian cholera. Early in the epizootic, carcass collection and disposal (typically by incineration) provides the best opportunity to prevent substantial losses. Carcass collection contributes to the control of avian cholera by removing dead birds that are heavily contaminated with *P. multocida*. These carcasses may decoy other susceptible birds to a contaminated site or attract bird scavengers that are susceptible to the disease and can spread it to other sites (Botzler 1991; Friend 1999). In some cases with low-level mortality, local mammalian predators and scavengers may substantially contribute to the removal of infected carcasses from wetlands.

Most epizootics eventually end as birds move from the area or conditions that precipitated the epizootic subside. In some cases, management activities that prevent or reduce bird use of affected wetlands, wetland drainage, or the addition of a large volume of water to dilute concentrations of *P. multocida* (Friend 1999) may be combined with carcass collection activities. However, these actions require careful evaluation to prevent infected or carrier birds from moving the disease to another location. More information is required about the epizootiology of avian cholera in waterfowl so that effective preventive measures can be developed and instituted to combat this disease.

UNPUBLISHED DATA

1. Diagnostic case records, U.S. Geological Survey, National Wildlife Health Center, Madison, Wisconsin, U.S.A.
2. Canadian Cooperative Wildlife Health Centre, Western College of Veterinary Medicine, University of Saskatchewan, Saskatoon, Saskatchewan, Canada.
3. J. G. Mensik, U.S. Fish and Wildlife Service, Sacramento National Wildlife Refuge, Willows, California, U.S.A.

LITERATURE CITED

Adlam, C., and J.M. Rutter (eds). 1989. *Pasteurella and Pasteurellosis.* Academic Press, London, England, 341 pp.

Amonsin, A., J.F.X. Wellehan, L.L.Li, J. Laber, and V. Kapur. 2002. DNA fingerprinting of *Pasteurella multocida* recovered from avian sources. *Journal of Clinical Microbiology* 40:3025–3031.

Awad, F.I., A.A. Salem, and A.A. Fayed. 1976. Studies on the viability of *Pasteurella multocida* type 1 under simulated environmental conditions in Egypt. *Egyptian Journal of Veterinary Sciences* 13:57–69.

Backstrand, J.M., and R.G. Botzler. 1986. Survival of *Pasteurella multocida* in soil and water in an area where avian cholera is enzootic. *Journal of Wildlife Diseases* 22:257–259.

Bellrose, F.C. 1976. *Ducks, Geese, and Swans of North America.* Stackpole Books, Harrisburg, PA, U.S.A., 544 pp.

Bendheim, U., and A. Even-Shoshan. 1975. Survival of *Pasteurella multocida* and *Pasteurella anatipestifer* in various natural media. *Refuah Veterinarith* 32:40–46.

Bezzel, E. 1979. *Wildenten.* BLV Verlagsgesellschaft mbH., München, Federal Republic of Germany, 156 pp.

Bigland, C.H. 1954. A rabbit infestation with poultry mites and experimental mite transmission of fowl cholera. *Canadian Journal of Comparative Medicine* 18:213–214.

Bivins, J.A. 1953. Pasteurellosis in a starling. *Cornell Veterinarian* 43:241–243.

Bivins, J.A. 1955. Pasteurellosis in feral birds. Cornell Veterinarian 45:180–181.

Blackall, P.J., and J.K. Miflin. 2000. Identification and typing of *Pasteurella multocida:* A review. *Avian Pathology* 29:271–287.

Blackburn, B.O., K.L. Heddleston, and C.J. Pfow. 1975. *Pasteurella multocida* serotyping results (1971–73). *Avian Diseases* 19:353–356.

Blanchard, D.C., and L. Syzdek. 1970. Mechanism for water-to-air transfer and concentration of bacteria. *Science* 170:626–628.

Blanchong, J.A., M.D. Samuel, and G. Mack. 2006a. Multi-species patterns on avian cholera mortality in Nebraska's Rainwater Basin. *Journal of Wildlife Diseases* 42:81–91.

Blanchong, J.A., M.D. Samuel, D.R. Goldberg, D.J. Shadduck, and L. H. Creekmore. 2006b. Wetland environmental conditions associated with the risk of avian cholera outbreaks and the abundance of *Pasteurella multocida. Journal of Wildlife Management* 70:54–60.

Blanchong, J.A., M.D. Samuel, D.R. Goldberg, D.J. Shadduck, and M. A. Lehr. 2006c. Persistence of *Pasteurella multocida* in wetlands following avian cholera outbreaks. *Journal of Wildlife Diseases* 42:33–39.

Blus, L.J., L.N. Locke, and E. Cromartie. 1978. Avian cholera and organochlorine residues in an American oystercatcher. *Estuaries* 1:128–129.

Borrathybay, E.,T. Sawada, Y. Kataoka, E. Okiyama, E. Kawamoto, and H. Amao. 2003. Capsule thickness and amounts of a 39 kDa capsular protein of avian *Pasteurella multocida* type A strains correlate with their pathogenicity for chickens. *Veterinary Microbiology* 97:215–227.

Botzler, R.G. 1991. Epizootiology of avian cholera in wildfowl. *Journal of Wildlife Diseases* 27:367–395.

Botzler, R.G. 2002. Avian cholera on north coast California: Distinctive epizootiological features. *Annals of the New York Academy of Sciences* 969:224–228.

Bougerol, C. 1967. *Essai sur la pathologie des oiseaux de chasse au vol.* Alfort, France (cited in Cooper, 1978; original not seen).

Brada, W., and J.C.F. Campelo. 1960. Isolamento de *Pasteurella multocida* em coruja (*Otus choliba choliba* Vieillot). *Arquivos do Instituto de Biologia Animal* 3:117–120.

Brand, C.J. 1984. Avian cholera in the Central and Mississippi flyways during 1979–1980. *Journal of Wildlife Management* 48:399–406.

Brand, C.J., and R.M. Duncan. 1983. Avian cholera in an American flamingo, *Phoenicopterus ruber:* A new host record. *California Fish and Game* 69:190–191.

Bredy, J., and R.G. Botzler. 1989. The effects of six environmental variables on the survival of *Pasteurella multocida* in water. *Journal of Wildlife Diseases* 25:232–239.

Brogden, K.A., and K.R. Rhoades. 1983. Prevalence of serologic types of *Pasteurella multocida* from 57 species of birds and mammals in the United States. *Journal of Wildlife Diseases* 19:315–320.

Brown, P.C., J.P. Scherz, and R.M. Windingstad. 1983. Remote sensing and avian cholera in Nebraska wetlands. In *Technical Papers of the American Congress on Surveying and Mapping. American Society of Photogrammetry,* Salt Lake City, UT, U.S.A., pp. 483–492.

Christensen, J.P., and M. Bisgaard. 2000. Fowl cholera. *Revue Scientifique et Technique de Le Office International Des Epizooties* 19:626–637.

Christensen, J.P., H.H. Dietz, and M. Bisgaard. 1998. Phenotypic and genotypic characters of isolates of *Pasteurella multocida* obtained from back-yard poultry and from two outbreaks of avian cholera in avifauna in Denmark. *Avian Pathology* 27:373–381.

Christensen, J.P., K.D. Petersen, H.C. Hansen, and M. Bisgaard. 1999. Occurrence of fowl cholera in Danish wild birds and poultry production. *Dansk-Veterinaertidsskrift* 82:342–346.

Christiansen, K.H., T.E. Carpenter, K.P. Snipes, and D.W. Hird. 1992a. Transmission of *Pasteurella multocida* on California turkey premises in 1988–89. *Avian Diseases* 36:262–271.

Christiansen, K.H., T.E. Carpenter, K.P. Snipes, D.W. Hird, and G.Y. Ghazikhanian. 1992b. Restriction endonuclease analysis of *Pasteurella multocida* isolates from three California turkey premises. *Avian Diseases* 36:272–281.

Christensen, T.K. 1996. An outbreak of pasteurellosis in Denmark in 1996. *Wetlands International Seaduck Specialist Group Bulletin* 6:44–49.

Christensen, T.K., T. Bregnballe, T.H. Andersen, and H.H. Dietz. 1997. Outbreak of pasteurellosis among wintering and breeding common eiders *Somateria mollissima* in Denmark. *Wildlife Biology* 3:125–128.

Chung, J.Y., I. Wilkie, J.D. Boyce, K.M. Townsen, A. J. Frost, M. Ghoddusi, and B. Adler. 2001. Role of capsule in the pathogenesis of fowl cholera caused by *Pasteurella multocida* serogroup A. *Infection and Immunity* 69:2487–2492.

Collins, F.M. 1977. Mechanisms of acquired resistance to *Pasteurella multocida* infections: A review. *Cornell Veterinarian* 67:103–138.

Combs, S.M., and R.G. Botzler. 1991. Correlations of daily activity with avian cholera mortality among wildfowl. *Journal of Wildlife Diseases* 27:543–550.

Cooper, J.E. 1978. Veterinary aspects of captive birds of prey. The Standfast Press, Saul, Gloucestershire, U.K., 247 pp.

Crawford, R.J. M., D.M. Allwright, and C.W. Heyl. 1992. High mortality of cape cormorants (*Phalacrocorax capensis*) off western South Africa in 1991 caused by *Pasteurella multocida. Colonial Waterbirds* 15:236–238.

Curtis, P.E. 1979. Observations on avian pasteurellosis in Britain. *The Veterinary Record* 104:471–474.

Davies, R.L., R. MacCorquodale, and B. Caffrey. 2003. Diversity of avian *Pasteurella multocida* strains based on capsular PCR typing and variation of the OmpA and OmpH outer membrane proteins. *Veterinary Microbiology* 91:169–182.

De Lisle, G.W., W.L. Stanislawek, and P.J. Moors. 1990. *Pasteurella multocida* infections in rockhopper penguins (*Eudyptes chrysocome*) from Campbell Island, New Zealand. *Journal of Wildlife Diseases* 26:283–285.

Derylo, A. 1967. Rola wszolow w przenoszeniu pasterelozy u kur. *Wiadomosci Parazytologiczne* 13:619–623.

Derylo, A. 1969. Wszoly (Mallophaga) jako wektory *Pasteurella multocida. Annales Universitatis Mariae Curie-Sklodowska, Sectio C:* 24:355–366.

Dimov, I. 1964. Survival of avian *Pasteurella multocida* in soils at different acidity, humidity and temperature. (In Russian with German summary.) *Nauchni Trudove Vissh Veterinarnomeditsinski Institute "Prof. D-r-G Pavlov"* 12:339–345.

Donahue, J.M., and L.D. Olson. 1969. Survey of wild ducks and geese for *Pasteurella* spp. *Bulletin of the Wildlife Disease Association* 5:201–205.

Donahue, J.M., and L.D. Olson. 1971. Research technique. Inoculation of *Pasteurella multocida* into the palantine air spaces as an exposure method for fowl cholera in turkeys. *Avian Diseases* 15:158–162.

El Tayeb, A.B. 1993. Preparation and evaluation of *Pasteurella multocida* vaccines in waterfowl and sandhill cranes. Ph.D. Thesis, University of Wisconsin, Madison, WI, U.S.A., 125 pp.

Faddoul, G.P., G.W. Fellows, and J. Baird. 1967. Pasteurellosis in wild birds in Massachusetts. *Avian Diseases* 11:413–418.

Fallacara, D.M., C.M. Monahan, T.Y. Morishita, C.A. Bremer, and R.F. Wack. 2004. Survey of parasites and bacterial pathogens from free-living waterfowl in zoological settings. *Avian Diseases* 48:759–767.

Friedlander, R.C., and L.D. Olson. 1995. Consumption coagulopathy in turkeys exposed to *Pasteurella multocida. Avian Diseases* 39:141–144.

Friend, M. 1971. Pesticide—infectious disease interaction studies in the mallard. Ph.D. Thesis, University of Wisconsin, Madison, WI, U.S.A., 287 pp.

Friend, M. 1981. Waterfowl diseases—changing perspectives for the future. *Proceedings International Waterfowl Symposium* 4:189–196.

Friend, M. 1987. Avian cholera. In *Field Guide to Wildlife Diseases, Vol. 1, General Field Procedures and Diseases of Migratory Birds,* M. Friend and C.J. Laitman (eds.). *Resource Publication 167,* U. S. Fish and Wildlife Service, Washington, D.C., U.S.A., pp. 69–82.

Friend, M. 1999. Avian cholera. In *Field Manual of Wildlife Diseases, General Field Procedures and Diseases of Birds,* M. Friend and J. C. Franson (eds.). U.S. Geological Survey Information and Technology Report 1999–001, pp. 75–92.

Fujihara, Y.,M. Onai, S. Koizumi, N. Satoh, and T. Sowada. 1986. An outbreak of fowl cholera in wild ducks (Rosybilled pochard) in Japan. *Japanese Journal of Veterinary Science* 48:35–43.

Gerschman, M., J.F. Witter, H.E. Spencer, Jr., and A. Kalvaitis. 1964. Case report: Epizootic of fowl cholera in the common eider duck. *Journal of Wildlife Management* 28:587–589.

Glukhov, V.F., and V.G. Novikov. 1975. Reproduction of the pathogen of poultry pasteurellosis in the body of *Argas persicus.* (In Russian.) *Nauchnye Trudy Stavropol'skii Sel'skokhozyaistvennyi Institut* 5:47–50.

Goldberg, D.R., and T.M. Yuill. 1990. Effects of sewage sludge on the immune defenses of mallards. *Environmental Research* 51:209–217.

Gordon, C.C. 1989. The relationship of wetland characteristics to avian cholera (*Pasteurella multocida*) outbreaks in the Rainwater Basin area of Nebraska. M.S. Thesis. South Dakota State University, Brookings, SD, U.S.A., 126 pp.

Gordus, A.G. 1993a. Notes on the first known avian cholera epizootic in wildfowl in North America. *Journal of Wildlife Diseases* 29:367.

Gordus, A.G. 1993b. Lead concentrations in livers and kidneys of snow geese during an avian cholera epizootic in California. *Journal of Wildlife Diseases* 29:582–586.

Gratzl, E., and H. Koehler. 1968. Pasteurellose (Geflügelcholera). In *Spezielle Pathologie und Therapie der Geflügelkrankheiten.* Ferdinand Enke Verlag, Stuttgart, Federal Republic of Germany, pp. 493–520.

Gray, H. 1913. Avian cholera. In *A System of Veterinary Medicine,* Vol. I, E.W. Hoare (ed.). Alexander Eger, Chicago, IL, U.S.A., pp. 420–432.

Green, R.G., and J.E. Shillinger. 1936. Progress report of wildlife disease studies for 1935. *Transactions of the North American Wildlife Conference* 1:469–471.

Gregg, D.A., L.D. Olson, and E.L. McCune. 1974. Experimental transmission of *Pasteurella multocida* from raccoons to turkeys via bite wounds. *Avian Diseases* 18:559–564.

Gritman, R.B., and W.I. Jensen. 1965. Avian cholera in a trumpeter swan (*Olor buccinator*). *Bulletin of the Wildlife Disease Association* 1:54–55.

Gunawardana, G.A., K.M. Townsend, and A.J. Frost. 2000. Molecular characterization of avian *Pasteurella multocida* isolates from Australia and Vietnam by REP-PCR and PFGE. *Veterinary Microbiology* 72:97–109.

Harmon, B.G., J.R. Glisson, and J.C. Nunnally. 1992. Turkey macrophage and heterophil bacteriocidal activity against *Pasteurella multocida. Avian Diseases* 36:986–991.

Heddleston, K.L. 1972. Avian pasteurellosis. In *Diseases of Poultry,* M.S. Hofstad, B.W. Calnek, C.F. Helmboldt, W. M. Reid, and H. W. Yoder, Jr. (eds.). Iowa State University Press, Ames, IA, U.S.A., pp. 219–251.

Heddleston, K.L. 1975. Pasteurellosis. In *Isolation and Identification of Avian Pathogens,* S.B. Hinchner, C.H. Domermuth, H.G. Purchase, and J.E. Williams (eds.). Arnold Printing Corp., Ithaca, NY, U.S.A., pp. 38–44.

Heddleston, K.L. 1976. Physiologic characteristics of 1,268 cultures of *Pasteurella multocida. American Journal of Veterinary Research* 37:745–747.

Heddleston, K.L., and K.R. Rhoades. 1978. Avian pasteurellosis. In *Diseases of Poultry,* M.S. Hofstad, B.W. Calnek, C.F. Helmboldt, W.M. Reid, and H.W. Yoder, Jr. (eds.). Iowa State University Press, Ames, IA, U.S.A., pp. 181–199.

Heddleston, K.L., and P.L. Watko. 1963. Fowl cholera: susceptibility of various animals and their potential as disseminators of the disease. In *Proceedings of the U.S. Livestock Association 67th Annual Meeting* pp. 247–251.

Heddleston, K.L., T. Goodson, L. Leibovitz, and C.I. Angstrom. 1972. Serological and biochemical characteristics of *Pasteurella multocida* from free-flying birds and poultry. *Avian Diseases* 16:729–734.

Hill, W.C.O. 1953. Report of the society's prosector for the year 1952. *Proceedings of the Zoological Society of London* 123:227–251, (p. 235).

Hindman, L.J., W.F.V. Harvey, G.R. Costanzo, K.A. Converse, and G. Stein, Jr. 1997. Avian cholera in ospreys: First occurrence and possible mode of transmission. *Journal of Field Ornithology* 68:503–508.

Hinshaw, W.R., and J.E. Emlen. 1943. Pasteurellosis in California valley quail. *Cornell Veterinarian* 33: 351–354.

Hirsh, D.C., D.A. Jessup, K.P. Snipes, T.E. Carpenter, D. W. Hird, and R.H. McCapes. 1990. Characteristics of *Pasteurella multocida* isolated from waterfowl and associated avian species in California. *Journal of Wildlife Diseases* 26:204–209.

Hoffman, H.A., and D.E. Stover. 1942. An analysis of thirty thousand autopsies on chickens. *California Department of Agriculture Bulletin* 31:7–30.

Holmes, B. 1998. *Actinobacillus, Pasteurella,* and *Eikenella.* In *Topley and Wilson's Microbiology and Microbial Infections,* 9th Ed., Vol. 2, G.S. Wilson, A.A. Miles, and M.T. Parker (eds.). Edward Arnold, London, U.K., pp. 1191–1215.

Hubbert, W.T. 1970a. I. Pasteurella multocida infection due to animal bite. *American Journal of Public Health* 60:1103–1108.

Hubbert, W.T. 1970b. II. Pasteurella multocida infection in man unrelated to animal bite. *American Journal of Public Health* 60:1109–1117.

Hudson, C.B. 1944. Fowl cholera in ring-necked pheasants. *Journal of the American Veterinary Medical Association* 109:211–212.

Hudson, J.R. 1959. Pasteurellosis. In *Infectious Disease of Animals,* Vol. 2, A. Stableforth and I. Galloway (eds.). Butterworths Scientific Publ., London, U.K., pp. 413–436.

Humburg, D.D., D. Graber, S. Sheriff, and T. Miller. 1983. Estimating autumn-spring waterfowl nonhunting mortality in Missouri. *Transactions of the North American Wildlife and Natural Resources Conference* 48:241–256.

Hunt, M.L., B. Adler, and K.M. Townsend. 2000. The molecular biology of *Pasteurella multocida. Veterinary Microbiology* 72:3–25.

Hunter, B.F. 1967. Isolation of *Pasteurella multocida* from a snowy owl (*Nyctea scandiaca*), a new host record. *California Fish and Game* 53:213–214.

Hunter, B., and G. Wobeser. 1980. Pathology of experimental avian cholera in mallard ducks. Avian Diseases 24:403–414.

Hutyra, F., J. Marek, and R. Manninger. 1949. *Special Pathology and Therapeutics of the Diseases of Domestic Animals,* Vol. I, 5th English Ed. J. R. Greig (ed.). Alexander Eger Inc., Chicago, IL, U.S.A., 962 pp.

Iliev, R., R. Arsov, and V. Lazarov. 1965. Can fowl, carriers of *Pasteurella,* excrete the organism in feces? (In Bulgarian with German summary.) *Nauchni Trudove Vissh Veterinarnomeditsinski Institute "Prof. D-r-G Pavlov"* 14:7–12.

Iovchev, E. 1967. Die Rolle von *Argas persicus* in der Epizootiologie der Geflügelcholera. *Angewandte Parasitologie* 8:114–117.

Jaksic, B.L., M. Dordevic, and B. Markovic. 1964. Fowl cholera in wild birds. (In Serbo-Croatian with German summary.) *Veterinarski Glasnik* 18:725–730.

Januschke, E. 1915. Geflügelcholera beim Sperber (*Accipiter nisus* sc. Nisus com.). *Wiener Tierärztliche Monatsschrift* 1915:272–273.

Jennings, A.R. 1954. Diseases in wild birds. *Journal of Comparative Pathology 64:*356–359.

Jennings, A.R. 1955. Diseases in wild birds. *Bird Study* 2:69–72.

Jeske, C.W., M.R. Szymczak, D.R. Anderson, J.K. Ringelman, and J. A. Armstrong. 1994. Relationship of body condition to survival of mallards in San Luis Valley, Colorado. *Journal of Wildlife Management* 58:787–793.

Jorde, D.G., J.R. Longcore, and P.W. Brown. 1989. Tidal and nontidal wetlands of northern Atlantic states. In *Habitat Management for Migrating and Wintering Waterfowl in North America,* L.M. Smith, R.L. Pederson, and R.M. Kaminski (eds.). Texas Tech University, Lubbock, TX, U.S.A, pp. 451–474.

Jöst, E. 1915. Avian cholera in the uhu (*Bubo maximum*) (In German) *Beitrage Tierheilkunde* 1915:11 (Original not seen).

Kaschula, V.R., and D.E. Truter. 1951. Fowl cholera in sea gulls on Dassen Island. *Journal of South African Veterinary Medical Association* 22:191–192.

Keymer, I.F. 1958. A survey and review of the causes of mortality in British birds and the significance of wild birds as disseminators of disease. *The Veterinary Record* 70:713–720.

Kitt, T. 1888. Beiträge zur Kenntniss der Geflügelcholera und deren Schutzimpfung. *Deutsche Zeitschrift für Tiermedicin und Vergleichende Pathologie* 13:1–30.

Klein, E. 1889. Ueber ein akute infektiöse Krankheit des schottischen Moorhuhnes (*Lagopus scoticus*). *Zentralblatt für Bakteriologie und Parasitenkunde* 6:36–41.

Klukas, R.W., and L.N. Locke. 1970. An outbreak of fowl cholera in Everglades National Park. *Journal of Wildlife Diseases* 6:77–79.

Korbel, R. 1990. Epizootiologie, Klinik und Therapie der *Pasteurella-multocida*-Infektion beim Vogelpatienten nach Katzenbiss. *Tierärtzliches Praxis* 18:365–376.

Korschgen, C.E., H.C. Gibbs, and H.L. Mendall. 1978. Avian cholera in eider ducks in Maine. *Journal of Wildlife Diseases* 14:254–258.

Krinsky, W.L. 1976. Animal disease agents transmitted by horse flies and deer flies (Diptera: Tabanidae). *Journal of Medical Entomology* 13:225–275.

Kwon, Y.K., and M.I. Kang. 2003. Outbreak of fowl cholera in Baikal teals in Korea. *Avian Diseases* 47:1491–1495.

Lee, C.W., I.W. Wilkie, K.M. Townsend, and A.J. Frost. 2000. The demonstration of *Pasteurella multocida* in the alimentary tract of chickens after experimental oral infection. *Veterinary Microbiology* 72:47–55.

Lee, M.D., F.T. Burch, J.J. Maurer, A. Henk, and S. Thayer. 2000. DNA fingerprinting of plasmid-containing serotype A:3,4 *Pasteurella multocida* isolated from cases of fowl cholera in chickens and turkeys. *Avian Diseases* 44:201–204.

Lehr, M.A., R.G. Botzler, M.D. Samuel, and D.J. Shadduck. 2005. Associations between water quality, *Pasteurella multocida,* and avian cholera mortality at the Sacramento National Wildlife Refuge. *Journal of Wildlife Diseases* 31:291–297.

Leotta, G.A., M. Rivas, I. Chinen, G.B. Vigo, F.A. Moredo, N. Coria, and M.J. Wolcott. 2003. Avian cholera in a southern giant petrel (*Macronectes gigantues*) from Antarctica. *Journal of Wildlife Diseases* 39:732–735.

Locke, L.N., and R.C. Banks. 1972. Avian cholera in cedar waxwings in Ohio. *Journal of Wildlife Diseases* 8:106.

Locke, L.N., V. Stotts, and G. Wolfhard. 1970. An outbreak of fowl cholera in waterfowl on the Chesapeake Bay. *Journal of Wildlife Diseases* 6:404–407.

Locke, L.N., J.A. Newman, and B.M. Mulhern. 1972. Avian cholera in a bald eagle from Ohio. *Ohio Journal of Science* 72:294–296.

Macdonald, J.W. 1963. Mortality in wild birds. *Bird Study* 10:91–108.

Macdonald, J.W. 1965. Mortality in wild birds. *Bird Study* 12:181–195.

Macdonald, J.W., D. Owen, K.G. Spencer, and P.E. Curtis. 1981. Pasteurellosis in wild birds. *The Veterinary Record* 109:58.

Matsumoto, M., and J.G. Strain. 1993. Pathogenicity of *Pasteurella multocida:* Its variable nature demonstrated by *in vivo* passages. *Avian Diseases* 37: 781–785.

Mashima, T.Y., W.J. Fleming, and M.K. Stoskopf. 1998. Metal concentrations in oldsquaw (Clangula hyemalis) during an outbreak of avian cholera, Chesapeake Bay, 1994. *Ecotoxicology* 7:107–111.

May, B.J., Q. Zhang, L.L.Li, M.L. Paustian, T.S.Whittam, and V. Kapur. 2001. Complete genomic sequence of *Pasteurella multocida,* Pm70. In *Proceedings of the National Academy of Sciences of the United States of America* 98:3460–3465.

McLandress, M.R. 1983. Sex, age, and species differences in disease mortality of Ross's and lesser snow geese in California: Implications for avian cholera research. *California Department of Fish and Game* 69:196–206.

Mensik J.G., and R.G. Botzler. 1989. Epizootiological features of avian cholera at Centerville, Humboldt County, California. *Journal of Wildlife Diseases* 25:240–245.

Miguel, B.,C. Wang, W.R. Maslin, R.W. Keirs, and J. R. Glisson. 1998. Subacute to chronic fowl cholera in a flock of Pharaoh breeder quail. *Avian Diseases* 42:204–208.

Miller, S.L., and R.G. Botzler. 1995. Recovery of *Pasteurella multocida* from experimentally-exposed freshwater snails. *Journal of Wildlife Diseases* 31: 358–363.

Montgomery, R.D., G. Stein, Jr., V.D. Stotts, and F.H. Settle. 1979. The 1978 epornitic of avian cholera on the Chesapeake Bay. *Avian Diseases* 24:966–978.

Moore, M.K., L. Cicnjak-Chubbs, and R.J. Gates. 1994. A new selective enrichment procedure for isolating *Pasteurella multocida* from avian and environmental samples. *Journal of Wildlife Diseases* 30:317–324.

Moors, P.J., D.J. Tisdall, and G.W. de Lisle. 1988. Deaths of rockhopper penguins at Campbell Island from bacterial infection by *Pasteurella multocida. Cormorant* 16:131–132.

Morishita, T.Y., L.J. Lowenstine, D.C. Hirsh, and D.L. Brooks. 1996a. *Pasteurella multocida* in psittacines: Prevalence, pathology, and characterization of isolates. *Avian Diseases* 40:900–907.

Morishita, T.Y., L.J. Lowenstine, D.C. Hirsh, and D. L. Brooks. 1996b. *Pasteurella multocida* in raptors: Prevalence and characterization of isolates. *Avian Diseases* 40:908–918.

Morishita, T.Y., L.J. Lowenstine, D.C. Hirsh, and D.L. Brooks. 1997. Lesions associated with *Pasteurella multocida* in raptors. *Avian Diseases* 41:203–213.

Morishita, T.Y., P.P. Aye, E.C. Ley, and B. S. Harr. 1999. Survey of pathogens and blood parasites in free-living passerines. *Avian Diseases* 43:549–552.

Muhairwa, A.P., J.P. Christensen, and M. Bisgaard. 2000. Investigations on the carrier rate of *Pasteurella multocida* in healthy commercial poultry flocks and flocks affected by fowl cholera. *Avian Pathology* 29:133–142.

Mullié, W.C., Th. Smit, and L. Moraal. 1979. Vogelcholera (Pasteurellosis) als oorzaak van sterfte onder watervogels in het Deltagebied in 1977. *Vogeljaar* 27:11–20.

Mullié, W.C., Th. Smit, and L. Moraal. 1980. Zwanensterfte ten gevolge van vogelcholera in het Nederlandse Deltagebied in 1979. *Watervogels* 5:142–147.

Mutters, R., P. Ihm, S. Pohl, W. Frederiksen, W. Mannheim. 1985. Reclassification of the genus Pasteurella Trevisan 1887 on the basis of deoxyribonucleic acid homology, with proposals for the new species *Pasteurella dagmatis, Pasteurella canis, Pasteurella stomatis, Pasteurella anatis,* and *Pasteurella langua. International Journal of Systematic Bacteriology* 35:309–322.

Novikov, A. 1954. Migrating rooks as carriers of fowl cholera (In Russian.) *Veterinariya* (Moscow) 31:27.

Oddo, A.F., R.D. Pagan, L. Worden, and R.G. Botzler. 1978. The January 1977 avian cholera epornitic in northwest California. *Journal of Wildlife Diseases* 14:317–321.

Okoh, A.E. 1980. An outbreak of pasteurellosis in Kano Zoo. *Journal of Wildlife Diseases* 16:3–5.

Olson, L.D., and R.E. Bond. 1968. Survival of *Pasteurella multocida* in soil, water, carcasses and in the mouths of various birds and mammals. In *Proceedings of the Annual Meeting of the Livestock Sanitation Association* 72:244–246.

Österblom, H., H.P. Van Der Jeugd, and O. Olsson. 2004. Adult survival and avian cholera in Common Guillemots Uria aalge in the Baltic Sea. *Ibis* 146:531–534.

Pabs-Garnon, L.F., and M.A. Soltys. 1971. Methods of transmission of fowl cholera in turkeys. *American Journal of Veterinary Research* 32:1119–1120.

Parmelee, D.F., S.J. Maxson, and N.P. Bernstein. 1979. Fowl cholera outbreak among brown skuas at Palmer Station. *Antarctic Journal of the United States* 14:168–169.

Pedersen, K., H.H. Dietz, J.C. Jørgensen, T.K. Christensen, T. Bregnballe, and T. H. Andersen. 2003. *Pasteurella multocida* from outbreaks of avian cholera in wild and captive birds in Denmark. *Journal of Wildlife Diseases* 39:808–816.

Pehlivanoglu, F., T.Y. Morishita, P.P. Aye, R.E. Porter, Jr., E. J. Angrick, B. S. Harr, and B. Nersessian. 1999. The effect of route of inoculation on the virulence of raptorial *Pasteurella multocida* isolates in Pekin ducks (*Anas platyrhynchos*). *Avian Diseases* 43:116–121.

Petersen, K.D., H. Christensen, M. Bisgaard, and J.E. Olsen. 2001a. Genetic diversity of *Pasteurella multocida* fowl cholera isolates as demonstrated by ribotyping and 16S rRNA and partial atpD sequence comparisons. *Microbiology* 147: 2739–2748.

Petersen, K.D., J.P. Christensen, A. Permin, and M. Bisgaard. 2001b. Virulence of *Pasteurella multocida* subsp. multocida isolated from outbreaks of fowl cholera in wild birds for domestic poultry and game birds. *Avian Pathology* 30:27–31.

Petrides, G.A., and C.R. Bryant. 1951. An analysis of the 1949–50 fowl cholera epizootic in Texas Panhandle waterfowl. *Transactions of the North American Wildlife Conference* 16:193–216.

Petrov, D. 1970. On the carriage of *Pasteurella multocida* by *Argas persicus*. *Veterinarno-Meditsinski Nauki* 7:11–16.

Phillips, J.C., and F.C. Lincoln. 1930. *American Waterfowl. Their Present Situation and the Outlook for Their Future.* Houghton Mifflin Co., Boston, MA, U.S.A., 312 pp.

Piechulla, K., M. Bisgaard, H. Gerlach, and W. Mannheim. 1985. Taxonomy of some recently described avian *Pasteurella/Actinobacillus*–like organisms as indicated by deoxyribonucleic acid relatedness. *Avian Pathology* 14:281–311.

Poermadjaja, B., and A. Frost. 2000. Phagocytic uptake and killing of virulent and avirulent strains of *Pasteurella multocida* of capsular serotype A by chicken macrophages. *Veterinary Microbiology* 72:163–171.

Potter, L.F., and G.E. Baker. 1961. The microbiology of Flathead and Rogers Lakes, Montana. II. Vertical distribution of the microbial populations and chemical analyses of their environments. *Ecology* 42:338–348.

Price, J.I. 1985. Immunizing Canada geese against avian cholera. *Wildlife Society Bulletin* 13:508–515.

Price, J.I., and C.J. Brand. 1984. Persistence of *Pasteurella multocida* in Nebraska wetlands under epizootic conditions. *Journal of Wildlife Diseases* 20:90–94.

Price, J.I., B.S. Yandell, and W.P. Porter. 1992. Chemical ions affect survival of avian cholera organisms in pondwater. *Journal of Wildlife Management* 56:274–278.

Pritchett, I.W., and T.P. Hughes. 1932. The epidemiology of fowl cholera. VI. The spread of epidemic and endemic strains of *Pasteurella avicida* in laboratory populations of normal fowl. *Journal of Experimental Medicine* 55:71–78.

Pritchett, I.W., F.R. Beaudette, and T.P. Hughes. 1930a. The epidemiology of fowl cholera. IV. Field observations of the "spontaneous" disease. *Journal of Experimental Medicine* 51:249–258.

Pritchett, I.W., F.R. Beaudette, and T.P. Hughes. 1930b. The epidemiology of fowl cholera. V. Further field observations of the "spontaneous" disease. *Journal of Experimental Medicine* 51:259–274.

Pursglove, S.R., Jr., D.F. Holland, F.H. Settle, and D.C. Gnegy. 1976. Control of a fowl cholera outbreak among coots in Virginia. *Southeastern Association of Game and Fish Commissioners* 30:602–609.

Quan, T.J., K.R. Tsuchiya, and L.G. Carter. 1986. Recovery and identification of *Pasteurella multocida* from mammals and fleas collected during plague investigations. *Journal of Wildlife Diseases* 22:7–12.

Queen, F.B., and E.R. Quortrup. 1946. Treatment of *Pasteurella multocida* (fowl cholera) infection in wild ducks with autogenous bacterin and penicillin. *Journal of the American Veterinary Medical Association* 108:94–100.

Quortrup, E.R., F.B. Queen, and L.J. Merovka. 1946. An outbreak of pasteurellosis in wild ducks. *Journal of the American Veterinary Medical Association* 108: 101–103.

Raggi, L.G., and G.S. Stratton. 1954. Pasteurellosis in coots. *Cornell Veterinarian* 42:229–230.

Rebers, P.A., and K.L. Heddleston. 1977. Fowl cholera: Induction of cross-protection in turkeys with bacterins prepared from host-passaged *Pasteurella multocida. Avian Diseases* 21:50–56.

Reed, A. 1975. Migration, homing and mortality of breeding female eiders *Somateria mollissima dresseri* of the St. Lawrence estuary, Quebec. *Ornis Scandia* 6:41.

Reed, A., and J.G. Cousineau. 1967. Epidemics involving the common eider (*Somateria mollissima*) at Ile Blanche, Quebec. *Naturaliste Canadien* 94:327–334.

Rhoades, K.R., and R.B. Rimler. 1984. Avian pasteurellosis. In *Diseases of Poultry,* 8th edition, M.S. Hofstad, H.J. Barnes, B.W. Calnek, W.M. Reid, and H.W. Yoder, Jr. (eds.). Iowa State University Press, Ames, IA, U.S.A, pp. 141–156.

Rhoades, K.R., and R.B. Rimler. 1989. Fowl cholera. In *Pasteurella and Pasteurellosis,* C. Adlam and J.M. Rutter (eds.). Academic Press, London, U.K., pp. 95–113.

Rimler, R.B., and J.R. Glisson. 1997. Fowl cholera. In *Diseases of Poultry,* 10th ed., B.W. Calnek, H.J. Barnes, C.W. Beard, L.R. McDougald, and Y. M. Saif (eds.). Iowa State University Press, Ames, IA, U.S.A, pp. 143–161.

Rimler, R.B., P.A. Rebers, and M. Phillips. 1984. Lipopolysaccharides of the Heddleston serotypes of *Pasteurella multocida. American Journal of Veterinary Research* 45:759–763.

Rocke, T.E., T.M. Yuill, and R.D. Hinsdill. 1984. Oil and related toxicant effects on mallard immune defenses. *Environmental Research* 33:343–352.

Rosen, M.N. 1969. Species susceptibility to avian cholera. *Bulletin of the Wildlife Disease Association* 5:195–200.

Rosen, M.N. 1971. Avian cholera. In *Infectious and Parasitic Diseases of Wild Birds,* J. W. Davis,

L. H. Karstad, and D. O. Trainer (eds.). Iowa State University Press, Ames, IA, U.S.A, pp. 59–74.

Rosen, M.N. 1972. The 1970–71 avian cholera epornitic's impact on certain species. *Journal of Wildlife Diseases* 8:75–78.

Rosen, M.N., and A.I. Bischoff. 1949. The 1948–49 outbreak of fowl cholera in birds in the San Francisco Bay area and surrounding counties. *California Fish and Game* 35:185–192.

Rosen, M.N., and A.I. Bischoff. 1950. The epidemiology of fowl cholera as it occurs in the wild. *Transactions of the North American Wildlife Conference* 15:147–154.

Rosen, M.N., and E.E. Morse. 1959. An interspecies chain in a fowl cholera epizootic. *California Fish and Game* 45:51–56.

Rosen, M.N., K.D'amico, and E.J.O'Neill. 1973. First record of a golden eagle death due to avian cholera. *California Fish and Game* 59:209–210.

Rosenbusch, G., and I.A. Merchant. 1939. A study of the hemorrhagic septicemia *Pasteurellae. Journal of Bacteriology* 37:69–89.

Samuel, M.D., D.R. Goldberg, D.J. Shadduck, J.I. Price, and E.G. Cooch. 1997. *Pasteurella multocida* serotype 1 isolated from a lesser snow goose: Evidence of a carrier state. *Journal of Wildlife Diseases* 33:332–335.

Samuel, M.D., J.Y. Takekawa, G. Samelius, and D.R. Goldberg. 1999a. Avian cholera mortality in lesser snow geese nesting on Banks Island, Northwest Territories. *Wildlife Society Bulletin* 27:780–787.

Samuel, M.D., J.Y. Takekawa, V.V. Baranyuk, and D.L. Orthmeyer. 1999b. Effects of avian cholera on survival of Lesser Snow Geese *Anser caerulescens:* an experimental approach. *Bird Study* 46:S239–S247.

Samuel, M.D., D.J. Shadduck, D.R. Goldberg, V. Baranyuk, L. Sileo, and J.I. Price. 1999c. Antibodies against *Pasteurella multocida* in snow geese in the western Arctic. *Journal of Wildlife Diseases* 35: 440–449.

Samuel, M.D., D.J. Shadduck, D.R. Goldberg, and W.P. Johnson. 2003a. Comparison of methods to detect *Pasteurella multocida* in carrier waterfowl. *Journal of Wildlife Diseases* 39:125–135.

Samuel, M.D., D.J. Shadduck, D.R. Goldberg, M.A. Wilson, D.O. Joly, and M.A. Lehr. 2003b. Characterization of *Pasteurella multocida* isolates from wetland ecosystems during 1996 to 1999. *Journal of Wildlife Diseases* 39:798–807.

Samuel, M.D., D.J. Shadduck, and D.R. Goldberg. 2004. Are wetlands the reservoir for avian cholera? *Journal of Wildlife Diseases* 40:377–382.

Samuel, M.D., D.J. Shadduck, D.R. Goldberg, and W.P. Johnson. 2005a. Avian cholera in waterfowl: The role of lesser snow and Ross's geese as disease carriers in the Playa Lakes Region. *Journal of Wildlife Diseases* 41:48–57.

Samuel, M.D., D.J. Shadduck, and D.R. Goldberg. 2005b. Avian cholera exposure and carriers in greater white-fronted geese breeding in Alaska, U.S.A. *Journal of Wildlife Diseases* 41:498–502.

Sawada, T.,E. Borrathybay, E. Kawamoto, T. Koeda, and S. Ohta. 1999. Fowl cholera in Japan: Disease occurrence and characteristics of *Pasteurella multocida* isolates. *Bulletin of the Nippon Veterinary and Animal Science University* 48:21–32.

Serdyuk, N.G., and P.F. Tsimokh. 1970. Role of free-living birds and rodents in the distribution of pasteurellosis (In Russian). *Veterinariya* (Moscow) 6:53–54.

Shillinger, J.E., and L.C. Morley. 1942. Diseases of upland game birds. *U.S. Fish and Wildlife Service Conservation Bulletin 21,* Fish and Wildlife Service, Washington, D. C., U.S.A, 12 pp.

Simensen, E., L.D. Olson, and G.L. Hahn. 1980. Effects of high and low environmental temperatures on clinical course of fowl cholera in turkeys. *Avian Diseases* 24:816–832.

Smit, T., L.G. Moraal, and T. Bakhuizen. 1980. *Pasteurella multocida* infecties bij vogels na een kattebeet. *Tijdschrift voor Diergeneeskunde* 105:327–329.

Smith, B.J., and K.F. Higgins. 1990. Avian cholera and temporal changes in wetland numbers and densities in Nebraska's (U.S.A) Rainwater Basin area. *Wetlands* 10:1–6.

Smith, B.J., K.F. Higgins, and C.F. Gritzner. 1989. Land use relationships to avian cholera outbreaks in the Nebraska Rainwater Basin area. *Prairie Naturalist* 21:125–136.

Snipes, K.P., T.E. Carpenter, J.L. Corn, R.W. Kasten, D. C. Hirsh, D.W. Hird, and R.H. McCapes. 1988. *Pasteurella multocida* in wild mammals and birds in California: Prevalence and virulence for turkeys. *Avian Diseases* 32:9–15.

Snipes, K.P., D.C. Hirsh, R.W. Kasten, T.E. Carpenter, D.W. Hird, and R.H. McCapes. 1990. Homogeneity of characteristics of *Pasteurella multocida* isolated from turkeys and wildlife in California (U.S.A). *Avian Diseases* 34:315–320.

Steinhagen, P. and G. Schellhaas. 1968. Pasteurellose in einer Falknerei. *Berliner und Münchener Tierärtzliche Wochenschrift* 81:72–75.

Sticker, A. 1888. Käsige Processe bei der Geflügelcholera. *Archiv für Wissenschaftliche und Praktische Tierheilkunde* 14:333–347.

Stout, I.J., and G.W Cornwell. 1976. Nonhunting mortality of fledged North American waterfowl. *Journal of Wildlife Management* 40:681–693.

Stutzenbaker, C.D., K. Brown, and D. Lobpries. 1986. Special report: An assessment of the accuracy of documenting waterfowl die-offs in a Texas coastal marsh. In *Lead poisoning in Wild Waterfowl,* J. S. Feierabend, and A. B. Russell (eds.). National Wildlife Federation, Washington, D.C., U.S.A, pp. 88–95.

Suarez, J.G., and L.L. Ilazabal. 1941. Epidemia de colera en los patos marinos. *Revista de Madicina Veterinaria* (Buenos Aires) 23:145–149.

Swennen, C., and Th. Smit. 1991. Pasteurellosis among breeding eiders *Somateria mollissima* in The Netherlands. *Wildfowl* 42:94–97.

Taylor, T.T., and D.B. Pence. 1981. Avian cholera in common crows, *Corvus brachyrhynchos,* from the central Texas Panhandle. *Journal of Wildlife Diseases* 17:511–514.

Titche, A. 1979. Avian cholera in California. *Wildlife Management Branch Administrative Report 79–2,* California Department of Fish and Game, Sacramento, CA, U.S.A, 49 pp.

Van den Hurk, C.F.G.W. 1946. Aanteekeningen bij de epizoötie van vogelcholera over Nederland in het najarr van 1945. *Tijdschrift voor Diergeneeskund* 71:361–365.

Van Es, L. and J.F. Olney. 1940. An inquiry into the influence of environment on the incidence of poultry diseases. *University of Nebraska Agricultural Experiment Station Research Bulletin* 118:17–21.

Vaught, R.W., H.C. McDougle, and H.H. Burgess. 1967. Fowl cholera in waterfowl at Squaw Creek National Wildlife Refuge, Missouri. *Journal of Wildlife Management* 31:248–253.

Waddington, F.G. 1944. Pasteurellosis in poultry and wild birds in Tanganyika territory. *Veterinary Journal* 100:187–191.

Wetzel, R., and W. Rieck. 1972. *Krankheiten des Wildes.* Verlag Paul Parey, Hamburg, Federal Republic of Germany, 256 pp.

Whiteley, P.L., and T.M. Yuill. 1991. Interactions of environmental contaminants and infectious disease in avian species. *Acta XX Congressus Internationalis Ornithologici* 4:2338–2342.

Wickware, A.B. 1945. Case reports of relatively infrequent diseases observed at the Poultry Pathology Laboratory. *Canadian Journal of Comparative Medicine* 9:151–154.

Wilkie, I.W., S.E. Grimes, D. O'Boyle, and A.J. Frost. 2000. The virulence and protective efficacy for chickens of *Pasteurella multocida* administered by different routes. *Veterinary Microbiology* 72:57–68.

Willach, R. 1895. Eine Cholera unter dem Wassergeflügel in Schwetzingen. *Deutsche Thierärztliche Wochenschrift* 3:444–445.

Williams, E.S., D.E. Runde, K. Mills, and L.D. Holler. 1987. Avian cholera in a gyrfalcon (*Falco rusticolus*). *Avian Diseases* 31:380–382.

Wilson, M.A., R.M. Duncan, G.E. Nordholm, and B.M. Berlowski. 1995a. Serotypes and DNA fingerprint profiles of *Pasteurella multocida* isolated from raptors. *Avian Diseases* 39:94–99.

Wilson, M.A., R.M. Duncan, G.E. Nordholm, and B.M. Berlowski. 1995b. *Pasteurella multocida* isolated from wild birds of North America: A serotype and DNA fingerprint study of isolates from 1978 to 1993. *Avian Diseases* 39:587–593.

Windingstad, R.M., J.J. Hurt, A.K. Trout, and J. Cary. 1984. Avian cholera in Nebraska's rainwater basin. *Transactions of the North American Wildlife and Natural Resources Conference* 49:576–583.

Windingstad, R.M., S.M. Kerr, R.M. Duncan, and C.J. Brand. 1988. Characterization of an avian cholera epizootic in wild birds in western Nebraska. *Avian Diseases* 32:124–131.

Windingstad, R.M., M.D. Samuel, D.D. Thornburg, and L.C. Glaser. 1998. Avian cholera mortality in Mississippi flyway Canada geese. In *Biology and Management of Canada Geese,* Proceedings of the International Canada Goose Symposium, D.H. Rusch, M.D. Samuel, D.D. Humburg, and B.D. Sullivan (eds.). Milwaukee, WI, U.S.A, pp. 283–290.

Wobeser, G.A. 1981. Avian cholera. In *Diseases of Wild Waterfowl.* Plenum Press, New York, NY, U.S.A, pp. 47–60.

Wobeser, G.A. 1992. Avian cholera and waterfowl biology. *Journal of Wildlife Diseases* 28:674–682.

Wobeser, G.A. 1997. *Diseases of Wild Waterfowl,* 2nd Ed. Plenum Press, New York, NY, U.S.A, 324 pp.

Wobeser, G.A., and F.A. Leighton. 1988. Avian cholera epizootic in wild ducks. *Canadian Veterinary Journal* 29:1015.

Wobeser, G.A., D.B. Hunter, B. Wright, D.J. Nieman, and R. Isbister. 1979. Avian cholera in waterfowl in Saskatchewan, Spring 1977. *Journal of Wildlife Diseases* 15:19–24.

Wobeser, G.A., F.A. Leighton, A.D. Osborne, D.J. Nieman, and J.R. Smith. 1982. Avian cholera in waterfowl in western Canada, 1978–1981. *The Canadian Field-Naturalist* 96:317–322.

Woodford, M.H., and P.E. Glasier. 1955. Sub-committee's report on disease in hawks, 1954. *The Falconer* 111:63–65.

Zinkl, J. G.,N. Dey, J.M. Hyland, J.J. Hurt, and K.L. Heddleston. 1977. An epornitic of avian cholera in waterfowl and common crows in Phelps County, Nebraska, in the spring, 1975. *Journal of Wildlife Diseases* 13:194–198.

Zwank, P.J., V.L. Wright, P.M Shealy, and J.D. Newson. 1985. Lead toxicosis in waterfowl in two major wintering areas in Louisiana. *Wildlife Society Bulletin* 13:17–26.

13
Salmonellosis

Pierre-Yves Daoust, John F. Prescott

INTRODUCTION

The genus *Salmonella* has a worldwide distribution and is one of the most common causes of bacterial diarrhea in humans and animals. It includes close to 2,500 serologically distinguishable variants (serotypes), which have been reported from a wide variety of animals, including reptiles, birds, and mammals. Most of these serotypes show little specificity for their host species. Depending on factors related to the bacterial serotype, host species, and environmental conditions, exposure of an animal to salmonellae may result in an asymptomatic carrier state, acute enteritis or septicemia, or multifocal chronic infection. In wild birds, salmonellosis is a common cause of sporadic mortality, particularly among young birds in large breeding colonies and songbirds around feeders in winter, but it has also been associated with widespread outbreaks of disease in songbirds. Based on the different manifestations of salmonellosis that are known in domestic poultry, much probably remains to be learned about the epizootiology of this disease in wild birds, including possible adaptation of the agent to wild bird species and the potential contribution of transovarian transmission to the persistence of salmonellae in wild bird populations.

SYNONYMS

Paratyphoid, pullorum disease, fowl typhoid, arizonosis.

HISTORY

Although Gaffky was the first to culture *S.* Typhi, the cause of typhoid fever, from a human patient in 1884, the genus was named in honor of Salmon, an American veterinary surgeon with the United States Department of Agriculture who, together with Smith, isolated *S.* Choleraesuis from pigs in 1886. Salmonellosis in poultry has been studied since at least 1889, when an outbreak of fowl typhoid, caused by *S.* Gallinarum, was described in a chicken flock in England. Pullorum disease, caused by *S.* Pullorum, was first described as a cause of fatal septicemia in young chicks in 1900 in the United States (Shivaprasad 1997). Fowl typhoid and pullorum disease had serious economic impacts on the commercial poultry industry, before the implementation of rigorous control measures in the middle of the twentieth century. Infection by paratyphoid salmonellae, which encompass a diverse group of other serotypes, was reported in an avian species for the first time in 1895 following an outbreak of infectious enteritis in domestic pigeons (Rock Pigeons, *Columba livia*) in the United States (Gast 1997). However, it was not until the 1930s that infection by salmonellae was recognized as a cause of disease in wild birds, with the report by Van Dorssen (1935) of isolation of *S.* Typhimurium from a renal lesion in a Mew Gull (*Larus canus*) in the Netherlands. In the United States, Faddoul et al. (1966) provided one of the first detailed reports of salmonellosis in wild birds but pointed out that *S.* Pullorum had been isolated in a very few instances from wild birds in the late 1940s. Wilson and MacDonald (1967), in Great Britain, may have been the first to use phage typing as a means of serotype identification in the study of *S.* Typhimurium in wild birds.

DISTRIBUTION

Because salmonellae are primarily enteric bacteria, their distribution follows closely that of humans and animals of a wide variety of species, including reptiles, birds, and mammals throughout the world. Also for this reason, increased amounts of untreated sewage or manure associated with large concentrations of people or their livestock favor the accumulation and dispersal of salmonellae in their immediate environment. This, in turn, increases the likelihood of free-ranging wild animals in the region being exposed to, becoming intestinal carriers of, and dispersing these bacteria. There are many examples of a direct correlation between the prevalence of salmonellae in the intestinal tract of various species of wild birds and the proximity of their habitat to that of people or livestock (Table 13.1). This is particularly true for species such as gulls and Rock Pigeons that normally benefit from a close association with human and domestic animal activities and refuse.

Table 13.1. Prevalence of *Salmonella* serotypes in asymptomatic birds of various species in different regions of the world.

Location	Species	Prevalence	Serotype (material cultured)	Reference
Hamburg, Germany	gull (unspecified)	0% in regions free from influence of sewage; 28% in city streets; 66% in city port; 78% near city's sewage disposal work	several: *S.* Typhi B most common, followed by *S.* Typhimurium (feces)	Müller 1965
	pigeon (unspecified), presumably Rock Pigeon (*Columba livia*)	30%		
	duck (unspecified)	16%		
	sparrow (unspecified)	0.2%		
	thrush (unspecified)	0.15%		
London, England	ducks: mainly Tufted Duck (*Aythya fuligula*), Common Pochard (*A. farina*), Green-winged Teal (*Anas crecca*)	4.2% on a water reservoir	several: *S.* Typhimurium most common (feces)	Mitchell and Ridgwell 1971
	gull (unspecified)	17% at Water Board's installations		
	Rock Pigeon	2.25% in the city		
Wales, England	Herring Gull (*Larus argentatus*)	7% from a colony offshore; 24.4% and 30.9% from two colonies with access to refuse dumps.	several: *S.* Bredeny most common, followed by *S.* Hadar and *S.* Typhimurium (feces)	Williams et al. 1976
Scotland	gulls (*Larus* spp.)	2.1% if access to domestic litter only; 6.5% if access to agricultural land and sewage facilities; 8.3% if access to fish processing plant and urban litter; 16.7–21.1% if access to untreated sewage outfalls	several: *S.* Agona most common, followed by *S.* Panama and *S.* Typhimurium (feces)	Fenlon 1981

(Continued)

Table 13.1. (Continued)

Location	Species	Prevalence	Serotype (material cultured)	Reference
Scotland	Lesser Black-backed Gull (*L. fuscus*)	11.4% at refuse dumps	several: *S.* Virchow and *S.* Typhimurium most common (cloacal lavage)	Girdwood et al. 1985
	Herring Gull	7.7% at refuse dumps		
	Black-headed Gull (*L. ridibundus*)	3.9% at refuse dumps and in fields		
Czech Republic	Black-headed Gull	4.2% of adults; 19.2% of nonflying young; (all caught at various locations)	several: *S.* Typhimurium most common (cloacal swab, feces)	Čižek et al. 1994
	Mew Gull (*L. canus*)	2.8% at a municipal dump	*S.* Enteritidis (cloacal swab, intestinal content, liver, spleen)	
	House Sparrow (*Passer domesticus*), European Serin (*Serinus serinus*)	26% on a farm with salmonellosis	*S.* Typhimurium PT 104 (cloacal swab, intestinal content, liver, spleen)	
	Rock Pigeon, Barn Swallow (*Hirundo rustica*), White Wagtail (*Motacilla alba*), Eurasian Blackbird (*Turdus merula*), Black Redstart (*Phoenicurus ochruros*), Great Tit (*Parus major*), Blue Tit (*Cyanistes caeruleus*), European Starling (*Sturnus vulgaris*), House Sparrow, Eurasian Tree Sparrow (*Passer Montanus*), Chaffinch (*Fringilla coelebs*), European Greenfinch (*Carduelis chloris*), European Serin, Yellowhammer (*Emberiza citrinella*)	0.5% on farms with no salmonellosis; the Rock Pigeon was the only species positive	*S.* Typhimurium var. Copenhagen (cloacal swab, intestinal content, liver, spleen)	
	Great Tit, Eurasian Jay (*Garrulus glandarius*), House Sparrow, Eurasian Tree Sparrow, Chaffinch, Yellowhammer	0% on military training grounds	(cloacal swab, intestinal content, liver, spleen)	

Eastern United States	Great Egret (*Ardea alba*), Snowy Egret (*Egretta thula*), Tricolored Heron (*E. tricolor*), Black-crowned Night-Heron (*Nycticorax nycticorax*), Glossy Ibis (*Plegadis falcinellus*)	5.4%	*S.* Newport, *S.* Typhimurium var. Copenhagen (feces from nests)	Kirkpatrick 1986
Eastern United States	Raptors with preference for mammalian prey: Northern Goshawk (*Accipiter gentilis*), Red-tailed Hawk (*Buteo jamaicensis*), Northern Harrier (*Circus cyaneus*)	28.6%	*S.* Enteritidis, *S.* Newport (cloacal swab)	Kirkpatrick and Trexler-Myren 1986
	Raptors with preference for avian and/or insect prey: Cooper's Hawk (*A. cooperii*), Sharp-shinned Hawk (*A. striatus*), Merlin (*Falco columbarius*), American Kestrel (*F. sparverius*)	0%	(cloacal swab)	
East-central United States	European Starling House Sparrow House Finch (*Carpodacus mexicanus*), Purple Finch (*C. purpureus*), American Goldfinch (*Carduelis tristis*), Song sparrow (*Melospiza melodia*)	7.1% in various habitats 1.07% in various habitats 0% in various habitats	not determined (cloacal swab)	Morishita et al. 1999
Central Canada	House Sparrow	8.3% in a suburban area; 14% in the country; 43% near a veterinary hospital	*S.* Typhimurium PT 20, 40 and 160 (brain, liver, spleen)	Tizard et al. 1979
Central Canada	Ring-billed Gull (*L. delawarensis*)	8.7%	several: *S.* Hadar most common (cloacal swab)	Quessy and Messier 1992
New Zealand	Kelp Gull (*L. dominicanus*), Red-billed Gull (*L. scopulinus*)	0% on an isolated beach; 0% near sewage ponds and a harbour; 26.5% near an abattoir and a city dump	*S.* Typhimurium (intestinal content, liver, spleen)	Robinson and Daniel 1968

This form of exposure of wild birds to salmonellae rarely seems to evolve to clinical disease, and shedding of the bacteria in their feces is often of brief duration. However, clinical salmonellosis has occurred in strictly marine coastal species, such as Little Penguins (*Eudyptula minor*) in southern Australia (McOrist and Lenghaus 1992) and Northern Gannets (*Morus bassanus*) on both sides of the north Atlantic, indicating that no avian species is sheltered from this bacterium if its normal habitat overlaps to any extent that of people and their livestock. *Salmonella* Enteritidis was isolated from feces of a Gentoo Penguin (*Pygoscelis papua*) in South Georgia, Antarctica, suggesting local contamination by discharge of sewage or wastes from ships (Olsen et al. 1996).

HOST RANGE

The potential avian host range of the genus *Salmonella* appears unlimited. Many serotypes do not have a specific target host, and wild birds that are closely associated with people and livestock are more likely than others to show a relatively high prevalence of intestinal carriers of these serotypes because of increased levels of environmental contamination by these bacteria. However, certain serotypes of *Salmonella* are preferentially, if not exclusively, found in a defined host species in which they cause disease. This phenomenon of host-adaptation is well recognized in humans and domestic animals (for example, *S.* Typhi in humans, *S.* Choleraesuis in swine, *S.* Dublin in cattle, *S.* Pullorum and *S.* Gallinarum in chickens). Host-adaptation goes beyond serotype association. Identification of individual strains of different *Salmonella* serotypes by bacteriophage typing has revealed a continuing adaptation of strains apparent within these serotypes. Serotype Typhimurium, in particular, contains numerous strains that appear to vary widely in their host range and their degree of host-adaptation (Rabsch et al. 2002). For example, *S.* Typhimurium definitive phage type (DT) 49 and DT 104 appear to have a broad host range. In contrast, in Rock Pigeons, *S.* Typhimurium var. Copenhagen is considered a specifically adapted subtype of great importance, with DT 2 and DT 99 being isolated almost exclusively from this species in Europe and North America (Rabsch et al. 2002). The frequent isolations of certain strains of *S.* Typhimurium from songbirds suggest a similar process. These strains, particularly DT 40 and DT 160, may have become adapted to certain species of songbirds, may reside in their populations in an endemic form, and may cause epizootics under appropriate conditions. *Salmonella* Typhimurium DT 40 has been associated most often with mortality in birds of the family Fringillidae (finches): Pine Siskin (*Carduelis pinus*), Common Redpoll (*Carduelis flammea*), Purple Finch (*Carpodacus purpureus*), and American Goldfinch (*Carduelis tristis*) in North America; and Eurasian Bullfinch (*Pyrrhula pyrrhula*), European Greenfinch (*Carduelis chloris*), Common Chaffinch (*Fringilla coelebs*), and Eurasian Siskin (*Carduelis spinus*) in Europe (Pennycott et al. 1998; Daoust et al. 2000). *Salmonella* Typhimurium DT 160 may be best adapted to House Sparrows (*Passer domesticus*), both in North America and Europe, and recently was identified also in this species in New Zealand (Wobeser and Finlayson 1969; ProMED-mail 2001).

Host-adaptation determines the relationship between the host and the pathogen, including the host's propensity to become a long-term asymptomatic carrier. Highly host-adapted serotypes typically cause systemic disease with high mortality rates in their respective hosts, but are generally of lesser pathogenicity to other species. Paradoxically, they must also be able to establish a long-term carrier state in some infected individuals of their adopted host species in order to ensure their transmission, because transmission by other species may be reduced. Thus, host-adapted *Salmonella* can persist in their hosts for a long time relative to nonhost-adapted *Salmonella* and will emerge to cause disease under favorable circumstances. Such circumstances are often hard to define because they relate to the complexity of the continuing interaction between host, adapted pathogen, and environment, including impaired host innate and specific immune mechanisms. *Salmonella* Pullorum and *S.* Gallinarum are highly adapted to chickens and, to a lesser extent, turkeys and cause significant disease in these two species. However, they have limited pathogenicity for most other avian species, and they show reduced virulence for mice (Bäumler et al. 1998). In the first half of the twentieth century, when pullorum disease and fowl typhoid were a serious problem in the poultry industry worldwide, the causative bacteria could be recovered occasionally from free-flying wild birds, but there was never mortality in these birds, and the infection could almost always be correlated with a local outbreak of the corresponding disease in domestic poultry. In contrast, *S.* Typhimurium, which itself includes many strains, is the serotype most often associated with disease in wild birds.

Host-adaptation is a dynamic and continuously evolving process. Infection with *S.* Typhimurium DT 104 is mostly associated with cattle. *Salmonella* Enteritidis, particularly phage type (PT) 4, is now mainly associated with poultry, but in the early 1900s, rodents were the only known animal reservoir of this serotype (Edwards and Bruner 1943). However, the apparent host adaptation of *S.* Typhimurium DT 104 and *S.* Enteritidis PT 4 to cattle and chickens, respectively, has not lessened their virulence in other species. They have become the two most common strains of *Salmonella* isolated from humans in many countries (Angulo and Swerdlow 1998; Poppe et al. 1998), and rodents continue to be important in the epidemiology of *S.* Enteritidis (Henzler and Opitz 1992).

ETIOLOGY

Salmonellosis is caused by Gram-negative, rod-shaped bacteria of the genus *Salmonella,* family *Enterobacteriaceae,* organisms whose natural habitat is the large intestine of carrier animals. There are currently 2,463 serotypes (serovars) of *Salmonella,* based on differences in lipopolysaccharide somatic "O" antigens and flagellar "H" antigens. The nomenclature of *Salmonella* is complex because it has changed many times over the years. Currently, it is recognized that virtually every *Salmonella* belongs in a single species, *S. enterica,* the only exception being *S. bongori. Salmonella enterica* is in turn divided into six subspecies, which are referred to by a Roman numeral and a name (I, subsp. *enterica;* II, subsp. *salamae;* IIIa, subsp. *arizonae;* IIIb, subsp. *diarizonae;* IV, subsp. *houtenae;* VI, subsp. *indica*) (Brenner et al. 2000). The majority (1,454) of *Salmonella* serotypes belong to subsp. *enterica* and are isolated from warm-blooded animals including humans and birds. Serotypes of the other subspecies are usually isolated from cold-blooded animals (mostly reptiles) and the environment. An exception is subsp. *arizonae,* which is isolated commonly from domestic turkeys. The Centers for Disease Control and Prevention in the United States use names for serotypes in subspecies I and antigenic formulae for unnamed serotypes described after 1966 in subspecies II, IV, and VI. To emphasize that serotypes are not separate species, the serotype name is not italicized and the first letter is capitalized (Brenner et al. 2000). Despite the large number of serotypes, a rather limited number (about 40) cause 95% of cases of salmonellosis in humans.

Phage typing distinguishes strains (clones) of individual *Salmonella* serotypes based on their susceptibility to be lysed by a set of selected bacterial viruses (bacteriophages). Because of its sensitivity and stability, this method has become an important tool to understand the epidemiology of infection by salmonellae. Standard phage typing systems, or schemes, have been described for several *Salmonella* serotypes (Jones et al. 2000). For each serotype, a unique number is given to individual phage types (PT), each number representing a specific pattern of susceptibility to the set of bacteriophages used for that serotype. Anderson et al. (1977) refined the previous phage typing system for *S.* Typhimurium and defined 207 definitive phage types (DT). Ward et al. (1987) differentiated 27 phage types of *S.* Enteritidis. The number of phage types for each of these two serotypes has since expanded (Jones et al. 2000).

Salmonella evolved as a pathogen over the last 100 million years in three distinct phases and continues to evolve. Its infection by bacteriophages may have played a vital role in this process (Figueroa-Bossi et al. 2001). The first phase in this evolution involved acquisition of *Salmonella* pathogenicity island I (SPI 1), which encodes virulence factors involved in the ability of these organisms to invade the intestine and cause diarrhea. *Salmonella enterica* then diverged from *S. bongori* by acquisition of a second pathogenicity island (SPI 2), which gives the organism its ability to invade more deeply and to survive in tissues after it has invaded the intestine. The final major phase was the process of branching into distinct phylogenetic groups, with a dramatic expansion of *S. enterica* subsp. I into warm-blooded animals (Bäumler et al. 1998). Some subsp. I serotypes further acquired the *Salmonella* virulence plasmid, which is characteristic of the major host-adapted serotypes, such as Gallinarum and Pullorum, as well as the most virulent of the nonhost-adapted serotypes, such as Enteritidis and Typhimurium. Possession of the virulence plasmid and its *spv* operon of virulence genes makes these serotypes particularly pathogenic. The *spv* locus on the virulence plasmid correlates with the ability of bacteria possessing it to cause lethal septicemic infections, probably as a result of enhanced survival in macrophages, but its exact function is unknown (Bäumler et al. 2000).

The basis of host-adaptation of certain serotypes of *Salmonella* is unclear but may relate to the relative plasticity of the *Salmonella* genome afforded by phage-mediated transfer of a small number of host-specific virulence factors (Rabsch et al. 2002). It is in part a function of the presence of different types of specific fimbrial adhesions that recognize intestinal surfaces. This phenomenon of strains partially adapting to particular hosts may have occurred in wild birds, as discussed earlier.

EPIZOOTIOLOGY

Survival in the Environment

The prevalence of salmonellae in the open environment (water, soil, feed) is a function of the degree of its contamination by fecal material from infected hosts. Most serotypes can survive for a long time in the environment. Their persistence in soil or water is influenced by several factors, including temperature, pH, humidity, presence of organic matter, composition of indigenous bacterial flora, and exposure to sunlight. *Salmonella* Typhimurium can survive for 16 months in poultry feed and litter maintained at 25°C, but being susceptible to destruction by heat, will survive for only a few weeks at 38°C (Williams and Benson 1978). *Salmonella* Typhimurium can also survive for up to six months in cold cattle manure, but for less than seven days in composted cattle manure, which can reach temperatures above 50°C (Forshell and Ekesbo 1993). It can survive for up to nine months in soil, which, in an avian breeding colony or around bird feeders, would be sufficient to maintain its presence from one year to the next (Literák et al. 1996; Refsum et al. 2003). It is unlikely that salmonellae can survive for more than three weeks in fresh water free of organic material, but they may survive for up to nine months in pond and stagnant water (Pelzer 1989). They are also capable of surviving in salt water and may therefore contaminate marine fish, molluscs, and crustaceans. Insects, such as flies and cockroaches, may contribute further to contamination of the environment with salmonellae. Cockroaches are able to excrete these bacteria in their feces for up to 20 days following experimental inoculation, and viable bacteria may be isolated from their exposed dorsal body surfaces for up to 78 days (Durrant and Beatson 1981).

Wild Birds As Carriers

Salmonella infections in wild birds are acquired largely from their environment and, with some exceptions, these birds play little part in the transmission of infection to domestic animals and humans. Surveys of the intestines or feces of wild birds have shown that carriage of *Salmonella* is uncommon (0 to <1%) in free-living, migratory or nonmigratory wild birds that do not eat food or drink water contaminated with *Salmonella* (Brittingham et al. 1988) (Table 13.1). Most *Salmonella* intestinal carriage in wild birds is not associated with clinical illness and, in the absence of reinfection, is likely to last no more than a few weeks. This and the low number of these bacteria normally excreted by infected birds (Fenlon 1981) probably limit transmission to other birds within a flock. However, because young birds are generally more susceptible to infection by salmonellae, nestlings and recently fledged birds within a breeding colony may be more likely to acquire infection from their parents.

Differences in feeding ecology among avian species in relation to the type of contaminated environment will influence the prevalence of salmonellae in these species. Gulls (*Larus* spp.), in particular, commonly carry *Salmonella*. It is likely that these are acquired largely from human sewage but may also be acquired from environments contaminated with fecal material of domestic animal species (Fenlon 1981). These birds may, in turn, contaminate nearby or distant pastures or water storage reservoirs because of their habit of feeding or roosting in large flocks and of long-distance movement for feeding purposes (Williams et al. 1977; Johnston et al. 1981; Coulson et al. 1983). The increase in populations of some species of gulls during the twentieth century, such as Herring Gulls (*L. argentatus*) in Scotland (Girdwood et al. 1985) and Ring-billed Gulls (*L. delawarensis*) in the Great Lakes region of North America (Chudzik et al. 1994), has also contributed to the prominence of this group of birds in the epidemiology of salmonellosis in humans and domestic animals. The Black-headed Gull (*L. ridibundus*), a small and agile bird, is one of the most successful gull species in Europe. Because of its large population and broad range of movements, it may be more important than other avian species as a potential secondary source of *Salmonella* infection for humans and livestock (Čižek et al. 1994).

Birds such as European Starlings (*Sturnus vulgaris*) and House Sparrows that feed in the immediate vicinity of intensive farming operations may also carry *Salmonella,* almost certainly as a result of acquisition of infection from food or other sources on the farming operations (Davies and Wray 1996; Craven et al. 2000). Both species are closely associated with human habitations, have a varied diet that includes grains and insects, and often forage on the ground (Elphick et al. 2001), factors that may increase their likelihood of being exposed to bacterial pathogens of human or livestock origin. Morishita et al. (1999) isolated salmonellae of undetermined serotype from 62 of 868 (7.1%) European Starlings and four of 373 (1.07%) House Sparrows in east central United States.

Differences in behavior between sexes may result in different levels of contamination. Monaghan et al. (1985) showed a significantly higher prevalence of salmonellae in female than male Herring Gulls and ascribed this to the dominant nature of males and the fact that they prefer to feed in more traditional areas associated with the fishing industry, leaving refuse dumps to females. In contrast, Pennycott et al. (1998) observed a higher mortality rate in male than female European Greenfinches (*Carduelis chloris*) around feeders. However, they were unsure whether this was the result of a higher proportion of males than females in the population of these birds in winter months when they are more likely to use feeding stations, of the more dominant males possibly spending more time at the feeders, or some other factors.

In wild birds exposed to salmonellae from an environment contaminated by human and agricultural activities, the intestinal carrier stage often appears short lived. Girdwood et al. (1985) caught Herring Gulls of unspecified age at refuse dumps and brought them into captivity in order to determine the duration of excretion of salmonellae by intestinal carriers. The maximum duration of excretion of these bacteria was four days, suggesting that these birds acted mainly as passive carriers of the bacteria. Most of the crows and magpies (species not specified) carrying *S.* Typhimurium originating from an epizootic in sheep in South Australia appeared to clear themselves of infection after 14–30 days (Watts and Wall 1952).

The level and duration of the fecal shedding period in wild birds infected by salmonellae are probably influenced by the same factors as in domestic poultry, including host adaptation of the bacteria, dose of the inoculum, and exposure to stressful conditions. The host-adapted *S.* Pullorum and *S.* Gallinarum typically produce a systemic infection and can persist in internal organs, including the ovary, for the duration of the bird's life, but they colonize the digestive tract poorly (Shivaprasad 1997). Within a same serotype of non-host-adapted salmonellae, more invasive strains also tend to be shed in feces for a shorter time than less invasive strains, possibly because their systemic distribution triggers a stronger immune response (Barrow et al. 1988). However, some strains of *S.* Enteritidis can persist in the intestinal tract of adult chickens for months, albeit at low levels, and also colonize internal organs, including the ovary and oviduct (Gast and Beard 1990).

The composition of the normal intestinal microflora, which can vary greatly according to the bird's age, also influences fecal shedding of salmonellae. After the first few weeks of life, a more mature intestinal microflora exerts an inhibitory effect on these bacteria. Seven weeks after experimental inoculation of *S.* Typhimurium directly into the crop of chicks, a larger proportion of birds inoculated at one day of age than those at eight days of age remained intestinal carriers of the bacterium, and the mean number of cecal salmonellae was greater in birds inoculated at a younger age (Gast and Beard 1989). Čižek et al. (1994) isolated salmonellae from feces of 4.2% and 19.2% of adult and nonflying young Black-headed Gulls, respectively. This difference may have been age related. Alternatively, it may have reflected a more recent stage of infection in the younger birds, because fecal cultures are less likely to identify chronic carriers than birds in early active stages of infection (Brown et al. 1975).

Transmission

Salmonellae are primarily enteric bacteria, and the fecal-to-oral route of exposure is the main means of transmission. In confined captive environments with high humidity, it is possible for salmonellae to be transmitted by inhalation or conjunctival inoculation, although, in either case, some of the bacteria probably reach the pharynx and are swallowed (Humphrey et al. 1992).

Egg transmission through direct infection of the ova probably represents the most important means of perpetuation and spread of *S.* Pullorum and *S.* Gallinarum in domestic poultry (Shivaprasad 1997). Transmission of infection by other salmonellae via the egg can occur either by incorporation of the bacteria directly into the ova before ovulation, by their incorporation into the egg albumen during transit in the oviduct, or through contamination of the egg surface before or during oviposition (Gast 1997). Bacterial deposition into the egg contents before oviposition is a particularly important aspect of the epidemiology of *S.* Enteritidis in chickens (Gast 1997; Angulo and Swerdlow 1998; Gast and Holt 2000). Following contamination of the outer surface of the egg, salmonellae may penetrate the shell and shell membranes and invade the developing embryo, or the latter may be exposed to the bacteria at the time of hatching when the shell structure is disrupted (Gast 1997; Battisti et al. 1998).

There is no good evidence that egg transmission represents an important method of persistence of salmonellosis in wild bird populations when the bacteria are acquired through environmental contamination from human and livestock activities. The overall prevalence of *Salmonella* carriers among adult Herring Gulls in Scotland was found to be 7.7%, but no *Salmonella* was isolated from 134 eggs and 72 hatchlings collected from a Herring Gull colony in central Scotland (Girdwood et al. 1985). However, the possibility of egg transmission has not been tested with strains of serotypes that have become well adapted to particular groups of wild birds, such as *S.* Typhimurium var. Copenhagen in Rock Pigeons or *S.* Typhimurium DT 40 in birds of the family Fringillidae.

An outbreak of embryonic and neonatal mortality caused by *S.* Havana and *S.* Virchow in captive birds of prey was traced to contamination of the adults by day-old poultry chicks used as food (Battisti et al. 1998). However, the exact method of transmission of the bacteria to the embryos and hatchlings, for example via direct ovarian transmission or through shell contamination, was not determined.

Songbirds

Although most *Salmonella* infections in wild birds can be regarded as an indication of environmental contamination from human and livestock activities, it is apparent that some phage types of *S.* Typhimurium have adapted to, or in other ways become established in, some songbird species frequenting bird feeders. The disease under these conditions is most common in winter months when large numbers of birds gather at feeding sites. Population density appears to be an important factor in the spread of infection (Kirkwood 1998). Birds of these species have also died from *Escherichia coli* O86 septicemia around feeding stations (Pennycott et al. 1998), emphasizing the importance of fecal contamination as the vehicle for spread of infection. Bird feeding supports many birds in some countries. By promoting local artificial concentrations of songbirds, feeders can provide ideal conditions for the emergence of infectious diseases, not only through increased fecal contamination of the food sources and their vicinity but also by increasing the likelihood of stress associated with enhanced social interactions. This often takes place at a time of year that imposes rigorous physiological demands on the birds, for example, winter. Contamination of the seeds prior to packaging has not been identified as a cause of these sporadic salmonellosis outbreaks around bird feeders.

Salmonella Typhimurium DT 40 is a common strain that has been associated for many years with endemic infection of certain species frequenting bird feeding stations in Great Britain (Wilson and MacDonald 1967; Kirkwood 1998). In that country, House Sparrows and ground-feeding finches such as Eurasian Bullfinch, European Greenfinch, Common Chaffinch, and Eurasian Siskin are most often affected. Another phage type, DT 160, is recognized in birds around feeders in eastern Canada (Prescott et al. 1998), being usually limited to sporadic local outbreaks of infection in House Sparrows in winter. This phage type was also recognized many years ago in House Sparrows and European Greenfinches in Great Britain (Wilson and MacDonald 1967; Wobeser and Finlayson 1969) and recently in feeder bird mortalities in New Zealand, spreading from House Sparrows into other species (ProMED-mail 2001). Whether this is the same phage type that is associated with sporadic winter bird feeder mortalities in House Sparrows in other parts of North America (Brittingham and Temple 1986) remains to be determined.

Since the late 1980s, several outbreaks of infection by *S.* Typhimurium covering very large geographic areas of North America have been observed during the winter and spring seasons (Daoust et al. 2000). These outbreaks affected mainly birds of the family Fringillidae, especially Pine Siskin and Common Redpoll, and, to a lesser extent, Purple Finch, American Goldfinch, and Evening Grosbeak (*Coccothraustes vespertinus*), with limited spill-over to other birds sharing the same feeding habitat, such as House Sparrow, Northern Cardinal (*Cardinalis cardinalis*), European Starling, and Mourning Dove (*Zenaida macroura*). Mortalities were identified mostly around bird feeders that, by encouraging artificial concentrations, may have increased the likelihood of disease and death. However, the geographic magnitude of these epizootics suggested that mortality was widespread among songbirds throughout their range, rather than being confined to the vicinity of feeders. Similar epizootics have been described in feeder birds during cold winters in Sweden (Hurvell et al. 1974; Malmqvist et al. 1995; Tauni and Österlund 2000) and Norway (Refsum et al. 2003). During two consecutive winters, cloacal swabs were collected from 1,990 apparently healthy passerine birds throughout Norway. *Salmonella* Typhimurium was isolated from 40 (2%) of these birds. The carrier species largely reflected the species most often suffering from fatal infection, with 8.8% of Eurasian Siskins, 8.0% of House Sparrows, 3.4% of Common Redpolls, and 2.8% of Eurasian Bullfinches being infected (Refsum et al. 2003).

Factors contributing to the emergence of salmonellosis among songbirds more or less simultaneously over large geographic areas remain poorly understood. It is typical for birds of the family Fringillidae to gather in large flocks during fall and winter for migrations and feeding (Elphick et al. 2001), and this would favor disease transmission. Finches also readily feed on the ground and on feeders for prolonged periods of time. This behavior may increase the likelihood of these birds coming in contact with seeds or other material contaminated by feces. In contrast, other species that are found dead less commonly around bird feeders, such as the Black-capped Chickadee (*Poecile atricapilla*), are more sedentary, and they tend to dart to a bird feeder, grab seeds, and leave (Elphick et al. 2001). For this reason, they may be less likely to become infected by contaminated seeds, or to become sick and die in the vicinity of a feeder where they would be easily found. A similar feeding behavior in tits (Paridae) in Europe may also partly explain their lesser susceptibility to infection by salmonellae as compared to finches (*Fringillidae*) and sparrows (Ploceidae, Emberizidae) (Refsum et al. 2003). A factor contributing to epizootics of salmonellosis in some cases could be an increased proportion of susceptible juvenile birds as a result of good weather conditions and abundant food supplies during the previous year. Conversely, harsh winter conditions in the form of very cold weather, heavy snow, or freezing rain could add greatly to an already stressful environment and also increase the likelihood of the birds concentrating at feeders.

During the winter 1997–98 outbreak in eastern North America, which involved primarily *S.* Typhimurium DT 40, the Common Redpoll was the species with greatest losses in the central and eastern provinces of Canada and in the northern United States (Daoust et al. 2000). Of all songbirds affected during that epizootic, it was also the most northerly species. In winter, these birds migrate as far south as is needed to find an adequate food supply, with peak numbers in southern locations typically occurring biennially (Kennard 1976). The 1997–1998 winter season coincided with one such peak year. It is possible that an unusual abundance of immigrating Common Redpolls favored the occurrence of salmonellosis in this species and that the disease then spilled over to other species sharing its habitat. Winter 1997–1998 was also a year of "superflight" of winter finches, when several species of these birds irrupted simultaneously into southern Canada and the United States from their normal wintering grounds in the north (BirdSource 1997). The Pine Siskin has been another important target in several of the major epizootics of salmonellosis in North America. As do Common Redpolls, Pine Siskins form denser flocks than other songbirds, and they also tend to show biennial irruptions (BirdSource 2003).

In winter 1998–1999, an increased number of immigrating Common Redpolls and Eurasian Siskins in Sweden, ascribed to an unusual abundance of unharvested linseed in fields during the previous fall and to increasing acres of lay-land and associated weed seeds, coincided with an outbreak of avian-associated salmonellosis in domestic cats (Tauni and Österlund 2000).

CLINICAL SIGNS

Exposure to salmonellae may result in an asymptomatic intestinal carrier stage, an acute, rapidly fatal septicemia with or without enteritis, or chronic localized infections that may or may not be clinically apparent. Clinical manifestations of acute salmonellosis are nonspecific and similar to those caused by other forms of bacterial septicemia (Gast 1997). They may consist of fluffed-out feathers in songbirds or ruffled feathers in larger birds, deep or rapid breathing, shivering, weakness, lethargy and apparent indifference of the bird to its surroundings, and eventual coma. Nervous signs, such as incoordination or tremors, may occasionally be seen. Eyelids may be swollen and stuck together by exudate. Death usually ensues within 24 hours. If enteritis develops, there may be diarrhea, causing the vent to be pasted with fluid feces and urates. Some birds may recover from either septicemia or enteritis and become asymptomatic intestinal carriers. In other birds, infection may localize to various sites in the body, with the clinical manifestations varying with the location and extent of the lesions (Gast 1997). Ocular infection may develop, with resulting blindness. Arthrosynovitis, particularly of the humero-radio-ulnar (elbow) and tibio-metatarsal (hock) joints, will interfere with flying or will cause lameness and focal swelling. Focal or multifocal airsacculitis may develop, which, depending on its extent, may be asymptomatic, decrease the bird's flying capacity, or cause gradual weight loss. In chickens, transmission of salmonellosis through the eggs may result in a high proportion of dead embryos and the rapid death of newly hatched chicks before any clinical sign can be observed.

PATHOGENESIS

The outcome of infection by salmonellae is determined by several factors, including the serotype and sometimes the phage type involved in relation to the avian species infected, the dose of the inoculum, the age of the bird, other resistance factors including heritable factors, and concurrent environmental stressors, either physical or social, that may decrease the resistance of individuals. The result may vary from a carrier state of variable duration to acute systemic infection and death. Young birds are consistently much more susceptible to disease and death from salmonellosis than adults. Although this increased susceptibility may result in part from the poorer immunologic response of very young birds to foreign antigens (Holt 2000), it is largely due to the immaturity of their intestinal flora (Gast 1997). Acquisition of normal intestinal flora from the environment protects the bird against salmonellae, either by competing for intestinal carrier sites or by producing antagonistic factors that inhibit their growth. In domestic poultry exposed to bacteria of the paratyphoid group, susceptibility to infection is highest during the first 10 days after hatching and decreases rapidly thereafter. With the poultry-adapted *S.* Pullorum, the peak of mortality usually occurs during the second or third week after hatching, whereas *S.* Gallinarum, also adapted to poultry, frequently causes morbidity and mortality in adults as well. However, exposure to a heavily contaminated environment or particularly stressful conditions can overwhelm the resistance of adult birds to any serotype and precipitate disease

Under favorable circumstances, in sufficient numbers, and in most warm-blooded animals, *Salmonella* bacteria colonize the intestine and proceed to invade the intestinal epithelium. In the early stage, they adhere preferentially to microfold (M) cells of the lymphoid follicle-associated epithelium. These cells are specialized to sample the many foreign antigens within the intestinal lumen for presentation to underlying immune cells. They are covered by a thinner glycocalyx than other cells, which facilitates this antigen capture but which may also present a lesser physical barrier for bacterial attachment. Shortly afterward, the *Salmonella* bacteria invade adjacent enterocytes and goblet cells (Meyerholz et al. 2002). They elicit a marked influx of polymorphonuclear leukocytes into the infected mucosa, with extensive inflammation, and induce watery diarrhea. Serotypes possessing the virulence plasmid, which may provide enhanced survival in macrophages, often reach the local lymph nodes and from here may enter the circulation through the thoracic ducts or reach the liver through the hepatic portal veins (Bäumler et al. 2000). They resist nonspecific host defense mechanisms such as complement but are taken up by macrophages of the liver, spleen, and elsewhere. In this intracellular location, they undergo a transient phase of growth while being protected from circulating antibodies. In the absence of specific immunity, *Salmonella* bacteria eventually kill their host macrophages and may continue to multiply in tissues, with uncontrolled proliferation and sepsis killing the host (Bäumler et al. 2000).

In songbirds, salmonellosis has an unusual presentation in that it appears to preferentially involve initial bacterial invasion of the esophagus and crop, with subsequent sepsis, rather than invasion from the intestine. The reason for the ability of *Salmonella* to cause lesions in the esophagus and crop of songbirds is not known. It may reflect a particular affinity of the bacteria for this location, in a manner similar to their affinity for the lower intestinal lumen in other species. However, it is not known whether these organs represent sites where the bacteria can reside in a latent form or whether they are preferred sites for bacterial growth after the disease has started. In chickens, the ceca and, to a lesser extent, the crop are considered to be the major sites of colonization of the digestive tract by salmonellae (Barrow et al. 1988). Feed withdrawal in chickens favors the survival of salmonellae in the crop contents by causing a decrease in the population of lactobacilli residing in the crop and a consequent rise in pH of its lumen (Corrier et al. 1999). Such a scenario might also occur in intensely hungry songbirds in winter.

The variable susceptibility of different strains of mice to *Salmonella* infection is associated with genetically controlled differences in macrophage survival. This may result in part from differences in efficiency of activation of the complement system by the bacteria and their subsequent opsonization prior to phagocytosis (Nakano et al. 1995). There are also well-recognized differences in susceptibility of different breeds of chickens to *Salmonella* infection (Guillot et al. 1995), although the basis for this has not been clarified. In chickens, breed inheritance of resistance was associated with a dominant autosomal resistance gene (Bumstead and Barrow 1993). Such innate resistance might be associated with the natural resistance-associated macrophage protein 1 (Nramp1), which affects phagosome acidification (Hackam et al. 1998). Whether or not certain wild bird species are more susceptible than others to salmonellosis has not been determined, but this could be a factor in the susceptibility of certain finches to clinical disease.

PATHOLOGY

Birds dying from acute septicemic salmonellosis have very few gross lesions, if any. These may consist only of congested lungs and kidneys and swollen, congested, mottled liver and spleen, which may have small hemorrhagic or necrotic foci. With further progression of the lesions, tan-to-white foci or nodules of necrosis and inflammation can develop in any organ or tissue, including liver and spleen, pectoral muscles (Figure 13.1), subcutis, brain, and other sites. There may be locally extensive or diffuse fibrinous or fibrinopurulent inflammation of the pericardium, peritoneum, and air sacs, and accumulation of exudate in the anterior chamber of the eyes (hypopyon) (Gast 1997; Pennycott et al. 1998; Alisantosa et al. 2000; Daoust et al. 2000). These lesions may be accompanied by various degrees of depletion of fat stores and atrophy of pectoral muscles, depending on the duration of the illness. This depletion of energy reserves can occur very rapidly in small birds because of their normally high energy demands. In young birds that have acquired the disease through egg transmission or at the time of hatching, the yolk sac, rather than containing bright yellow fluid, shows delayed resorption and has a creamy or caseous consistency (Gast 1997; Alisantosa et al. 2000). In some cases of infection by *S.* Pullorum in chickens, the accumulation of inflammatory cells in organs such as the heart, gizzard muscle, pancreas, and intestinal wall can be massive, and the large white nodules formed by these inflammatory cells may be confused with neoplastic tissue associated with Marek's disease, caused by a herpesvirus (Shivaprasad 1997).

Lesions of enteritis, which may be more common in adult birds that survive longer, often predominate in the

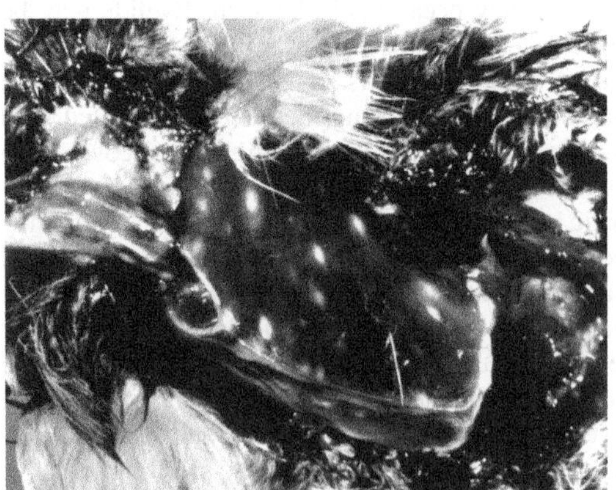

Figure 13.1. Multiple foci of acute necrosis and inflammation in the pectoral muscles of a Northern Cardinal, caused by *S.* Typhimurium.

caudal half of the intestinal tract, particularly the ceca (typhlitis), for which salmonellae have a high affinity. In the early stages, these lesions may consist mainly of congestion and ulceration. If these lesions have time to progress, necrotic material and exudate accumulate on the mucosal surface, giving it a dull, rough appearance and dark-brown color because of the presence of free blood (Figure 13.2). With further progression, the intestinal lumen, particularly in the ceca, may be filled with a core of necrotic material and exudate.

In a large proportion of songbirds with salmonellosis, the crop and esophagus contain multifocal to confluent areas of mucosal necrosis and fibrinopurulent inflammation, which, from the serosal surface, may resemble yellow to white food material or even individual seeds (Figures 13.3, 13.4) (Pennycott et al. 1998; Daoust et al. 2000). Other than depletion of fat stores and atrophy of pectoral muscles, the ingluvitis (derived from the term "ingluvies," or crop) and/or esophagitis are often the only easily noticeable lesions in songbirds that have died of salmonellosis.

The joints (particularly elbow and hock) and air sacs represent common sites of chronic localized infection caused by salmonellae. Gross lesions at these sites may include a variable amount of fibrous tissue mixed with straw-colored viscous fluid and fibrin and, in more chronic cases, sequestration of caseous necrotic material. The cavity of affected joints is not always involved, suggesting that, in some cases, the infection may instead target the articular bursae (bursitis) or tendon sheaths (tenosynovitis) (Brunett 1930). In young birds, the infection may localize to fast-growing long bones, such as the proximal growth plate of the tibia,

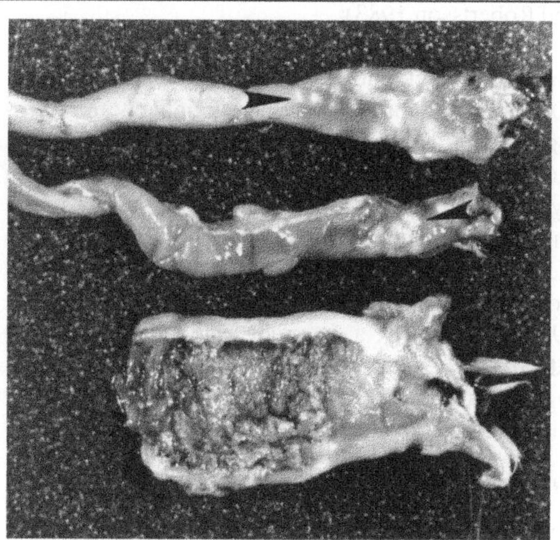

Figure 13.2. Lesions of enteritis caused by *S.* Typhimurium in a House Sparrow. Small foci of mucosal necrosis, visible from the serosal surface, resemble small seeds in the unopened segments of intestine (arrowheads). The opened portion (bottom), taken near the cloaca, shows diffuse mucosal necrosis. (Photo courtesy of Western College of Veterinary Medicine, University of Saskatchewan.)

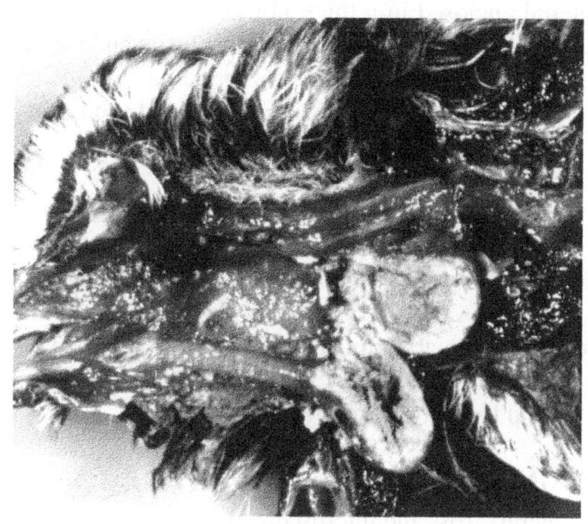

Figure 13.3. Diffuse necrosis and inflammation of the mucosal surface of the crop of a House Sparrow, caused by *S.* Typhimurium. (Photo courtesy of Western College of Veterinary Medicine, University of Saskatchewan.)

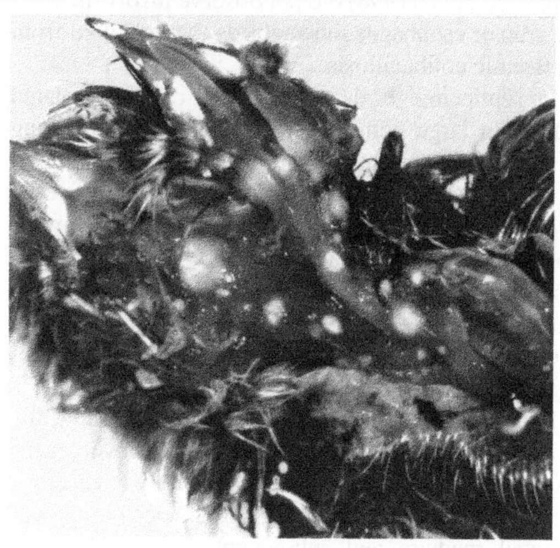

Figure 13.4. Multifocal necrosis and inflammation in the esophageal mucosa of a Common Redpoll, caused by *S.* Typhimurium. (Photo courtesy of The Canadian Veterinary Medical Association, Canadian Veterinary Journal 2000; 41:54–59.)

and cause focal or multifocal osteomyelitis (Daoust 1978). Progression of ocular lesions may result in panophthalmitis, with eventual replacement of the whole eye by a mass of caseous necrotic material. In domestic poultry affected by *S.* Pullorum or *S.* Gallinarum, the ovary of adult females may contain a few misshapen ova consisting of masses of oily or caseous material enclosed in a thick fibrous capsule; some of these abnormal ova may be only loosely attached to the ovary or even be free in the coelomic cavity. *Salmonella* Pullorum was recovered from the distorted ovary of an otherwise healthy American Coot (*Fulica americana*) (Rausch 1947).

Microscopic lesions include a combination of necrosis and inflammation, usually with abundant bacteria. The proportion of inflammatory cells within the exudate varies according to the duration of the process, with heterophils and fibrin dominating in the early stages, and histiocytes, multinucleated giant cells, and lymphocytes moving in later.

DIAGNOSIS

In general, gross and microscopic lesions of salmonellosis are comparable to those of other bacterial diseases, whether in its septicemic form or in the form of localized infections. Therefore, the diagnosis must be confirmed by bacteriological isolation and identification. However, the presence of enteritis or typhlitis and, in songbirds, of ingluvitis and esophagitis, should increase the suspicion of salmonellosis. Pennycott et al. (1998) did not observe involvement of the crop or esophagus in songbirds that had died from septicemic colibacillosis.

In septicemic birds, *Salmonella* can be isolated readily in large numbers from several organs using blood and MacConkey's agar incubated at 37°C for 24 hr. Nonlactose-fermenting colonies are identified as *Salmonella* by standard methods, such as conventional tests for Enterobacteriaceae or use of miniaturized kit systems such as API 20E (Farmer III 1999). Isolates should be serotyped by reference laboratories and, whenever possible, phage-typed for epidemiological purposes.

Detection of intestinal carriers in nonclinically affected birds takes more effort because it involves the use of a pre-enrichment broth followed by a selective-enrichment broth before plating onto a selective and differential medium and subsequent identification and serotyping (Waltman 2000). For survey purposes, examination of the entire intestine represents the most reliable method of bacterial recovery, followed in decreasing order by cloacal lavage and cloacal swab (Girdwood et al. 1985). In chickens, and probably other avian species, the ceca provide the best evidence of the presence of salmonellae in the intestinal tract. Culture of the intestinal wall yields positive results more frequently than that of intestinal contents (Brown et al. 1975).

IMMUNITY

Both humoral and cellular components of the immune system appear to play a role in protection against infection by *Salmonella,* but the importance of their respective contributions is unclear. In chicken hens infected with *S.* Pullorum or *S.* Enteritidis, which cause systemic disease, passage of specific serum agglutinating antibodies into the yolk may promote embryonic survival and protect the newly hatched chick, but, in the process, it also promotes successful transovarian transmission of the bacteria (Shivaprasad 1997; Holt 2000). Oral infection of young (four-day-old) chickens with *S.* Typhimurium triggers cell-mediated immunity and the production of serum and mucosal antibodies which can be detected within two to three weeks (Hassan et al.1991). Mucosal humoral immunity probably offers protection against enteric and early systemic infection, for example as a result of inhibition of bacterial adherence to mucosal surfaces, opsonization, and antibody-mediated cellular cytotoxicity (Holt 2000). However, cell-mediated immunity has been shown experimentally to have a more important protective role than serum antibody response against systemic infection (Lee et al. 1981; Lindberg and Robertsson 1983).

In some countries, antibody response is used to monitor herd or flock infection caused by common somatic (O) antigenic types. However, it is unlikely that serological tests could be applied to wild birds for this purpose without adequate knowledge of their sensitivity and specificity. Antibody detection does not imply an ongoing infection; antibody titers against salmonellae can persist long after bacteria have been cleared from tissues and fecal shedding has stopped (Gast 1997). Conversely, a detectable antibody response to infection may not occur in very young birds or following mild subclinical infection leading to fecal shedding without invasion of the intestinal wall (Gast 1997).

PUBLIC HEALTH CONCERNS

Salmonellae remain one of the main causes of human food-borne illness throughout much of the world, but free-flying wild birds have rarely been shown to be the source of these infections. In 26 incidents of salmonellosis in cattle and humans investigated in Scotland between 1973 and 1979 and associated with environmental contamination, only three were ascribed to gulls. Sources of contamination in the other cases included effluents from sewage, septic tanks, and abattoirs (Reilly et al. 1981). In most industrialized countries, *S.* Enteritidis became the most common cause of human salmonellosis during the last decades of the twentieth century, and contaminated domestic poultry meat and eggs have been recognized as one of the most important sources of infection.

Because the prevalence of intestinal carriers of salmonellae in wild birds and the number of these bacteria that they excrete are generally low, they may represent a potential health hazard to humans only when large numbers of them roost at the same site, such as gulls on water storage reservoirs or small birds near human dwellings. In most of these instances, however, wild birds (and other free-ranging animals such as rodents) act simply to amplify bacterial concentration in habitats already contaminated by human or livestock activities, simply by virtue of the large concentration of animals associated with some flocks.

It is notable that infection in people acquired directly from wild birds has been reported only in association with outbreaks of salmonellosis in birds at feeders, not with healthy birds. In New Zealand, an epidemic of human salmonellosis caused by *S.* Typhimurium PT 160 followed the emergence of the disease in House Sparrows; victims of the infection were 30 times more likely than healthy people to have touched wild birds within three days before their illness (ProMED-mail 2001). In Norway, infection with an unusual *S.* Typhimurium in humans (mainly children ≤ 4 years of age) coincided with fatal infections in Eurasian Bullfinches and was associated with contact with wild birds or their droppings or with eating snow, sand, or soil, although drinking untreated water was the greatest risk factor (Kapperud et al. 1998). Some years earlier, a nationwide human outbreak caused by the same strain was traced to contaminated chocolate bars, and it was hypothesized that songbirds had gained access to the factory from which the chocolate bars originated and had contaminated some part of the production line (Kapperud et al. 1990). Salmonellosis in people was reported in Sweden concurrently with an outbreak of salmonellosis in domestic cats acquired from diseased songbirds; in two of the four human cases, the patients had no direct contact with wild birds but rather had acquired infection indirectly, from their sick cats (Tauni and Österlund 2000). One large-scale study of bird feeding stations in southern Ontario, Canada, failed to isolate any Salmonella over the course of a winter, one year after an outbreak of salmonellosis in songbirds had occurred in that region (Prescott et al. 2000). This suggested either a low contamination of the environment during the year of the study or better cleaning care of the feeders by their owners due to increased awareness of the potential for disease transmission at feeders.

DOMESTIC ANIMAL HEALTH CONCERNS

As in humans, wild birds have rarely been shown to play a primary role in the epidemiology of salmonellosis in domestic animals. Focussing on endemic wild bird species as possible vectors of Salmonella for intensively reared farm animals often misses the point that Salmonella infection is commonly endemic on these farms because of acquisition from contaminated feed and recycling between farm animals through fecal contamination of their immediate environment. Wild birds that are in contact with salmonellae of human or livestock origin may increase bacterial contamination when large numbers of them roost or feed on pastures. Coulson et al. (1983) blamed Herring Gulls breeding along the east coast of Scotland for contaminating inland sheep and cattle pastures in that region with *S.* Montevideo that they had likely brought from their wintering grounds in northeast England, with subsequent abortion in sheep. Herring Gulls were also thought to be responsible for transmitting a rare serotype, *S.* Zanzibar, from a sewage outfall contaminated by a human source to nearby cattle farms in Scotland (Johnston et al. 1981). In England, *S.* Livingstone was isolated from soil of a refuse dump contaminated by material from septic tanks, from feces of Herring Gulls collected at a nearby colony, and from feces of cattle grazing in nearby fields where the gulls roosted and fed (Williams et al. 1977). An epizootic of salmonellosis caused by *S.* Anatum on a cattle farm in eastern United States was ascribed to haylage contaminated by wild birds (either blackbirds, European Starlings, or geese) and subsequently stored improperly in a silo (Glickman et al. 1981).

Salmonellosis in domestic cats has often been observed concurrently with outbreaks of the disease in songbirds (Scott 1988; Tauni and Österlund 2000). Weak or lethargic birds dying from septicemic salmonellosis represent an ideal source of infection for cats. Many of the affected cats described by Tauni and Österlund (2000) had been seen by their owners to eat a bird one to two days before the onset of disease. All affected cats were anorectic and lethargic, 57% had vomiting, and 31% had diarrhea.

WILDLIFE POPULATION IMPACTS

Salmonellosis is rarely a cause of extensive mortality in most wild avian species and, therefore, is unlikely to threaten their populations, although the situation may be different for some species of songbirds. As with other infectious diseases, salmonellosis can occasionally cause widespread mortality in avian flocks or colonies when the proper conditions are present. A large proportion of young birds in a densely populated breeding colony in relative proximity to an environment contaminated by human or agricultural activities provides such conditions. In summer 1989, approximately 5,000 Cattle Egrets (*Bubulcus ibis*) of all ages (nestlings, fledglings, adults) died at two rookeries and on a lake in California, western United States. Salmonella species, including *S.* Typhimurium and another isolate that could not be serotyped, were recovered from birds collected on all three areas. A field investigation identified possible exposure to this bacterium from drinking water in nearby canals or from feeding in irrigated agricultural fields that were fertilized with manure (K. A. Converse, unpublished data).[1] In general, however, and with the exception of songbirds, this disease is unlikely to threaten avian species on a large scale because the infection rate among wild birds is usually low.

In the late 1980s, outbreaks of salmonellosis among songbirds started to be identified on a large geographic scale in North America, specifically in northeastern United States in spring 1988 (affecting Pine Siskin), western North America in winter 1992–93 (Pine Siskin, Evening Grosbeak, Purple Finch, House Sparrow), eastern portion of the Rocky Mountains of western North America in winter-spring 1994 (Pine Siskin, American Goldfinch, Evening Grosbeak, Cassin's Finch [*Carpodacus cassinii*]), and eastern and midwestern United States and Canada in winter 1997–98 (Common Redpoll, Pine Siskin, Purple Finch, American Goldfinch) (Daoust et al. 2000). No reliable estimate of the total mortality is available for any of these outbreaks, but the magnitude of their geographic range suggests that each likely affected tens of thousands of birds. The actual impact of these outbreaks cannot be determined without proper knowledge of the total size of the North American populations of some of the species involved. However, the broad distributions and irruptive tendencies of many of these species make it difficult to arrive at even crude estimates of total numbers.

TREATMENT AND CONTROL

The only practical approach to control of outbreaks and prevention of clinical salmonellosis in songbirds depends on reducing the risk of transmission by a combination of hygienic measures and attempts to reduce densities at feeding stations, where most transmission seems to occur. A campaign in Sweden to use feeders designed so that birds defecate outside the feeding area and to regularly clean and disinfect feeders appeared to limit the spread of infection (Hurvell et al. 1974). Assuming that bird feeders are a major site of transmission of epidemic salmonellosis, feeders such as tube or squirrel-proof feeders that do not accumulate bird droppings should be used. Platform feeders are probably the worst in this regard (Brittingham and Temple 1986). Food should not be repeatedly placed in the same location on the ground. Feeders and bird tables should be regularly cleaned, depending on how dirty they become. Following cleaning, feeders can be washed or soaked in 10% hypochlorite-type bleach for a few minutes; all surfaces should be thoroughly rinsed with water after bleaching, and the feeder should be dried well before being restocked with seeds.

If songbird mortalities are observed in the immediate area, cleaning and disinfection should be done daily (Kirkwood and Macgregor 1997). The ground beneath feeders should be swept regularly and feeders moved regularly to reduce buildup of partially eaten feed (which attracts ground-feeding birds) and feces. Bird drinkers and baths should be changed daily and regularly cleaned and disinfected (Kirkwood and Macgregor 1997). Rubber gloves should be worn for self protection when cleaning and disinfecting bird feeders or drinkers. If mortality increases, the feeders should be dismantled in order to encourage the birds to disperse.

In the event of outbreaks of salmonellosis in wild birds, rapid confirmation of diagnosis is essential. The public who feed birds should be informed of the outbreak and advised on hygienic precautions, including the value of keeping cats indoors during the outbreak. Public-service announcements in the media are the best way to reach people who feed birds because most do not belong to formal birding organizations (Prescott et al. 2000).

In captive flocks, strict sanitation is essential to prevent outbreaks of salmonellosis and other infectious diseases, as well as to decrease the likelihood of transmission of these diseases to caretakers. Competitive exclusion is used as a form of prevention of salmonellosis in poultry farms. This consists of giving to young chicks an inoculum of a mixture of commensal intestinal bacteria from mature birds in order to decrease the likelihood of intestinal colonization by salmonellae (Gast 1997). Intestinal carriers should be identified and removed. This may require repeated fecal cultures because salmonellae typically are shed intermittently. Removal of adult female carriers is particularly advisable for poultry because of the possibility of transovarian transmission, which is unproven but also of concern in wild birds.

Because cell-mediated immunity may have a more important role than humoral immunity for long-term protection against salmonellosis, development of effective vaccination for domestic poultry has focussed on the use of live but virulence-attenuated Salmonella rather than bacterins that produce a good serum antibody response, but often without significant production of mucosal (secretory) antibodies or cellular immune response. A number of live attenuated vaccines are available or have been tested in poultry, and those against the host-specific *S.* Gallinarum and *S.* Pullorum are used extensively (Barrow and Wallis 2000). Subcutaneous vaccination with bacterins against *S.* Typhimurium var. Copenhagen in Rock Pigeons induced serum agglutinating antibodies and caused a reduction in fecal shedding of the bacteria following oral challenge, but it did not protect the birds against systemic disease (Vereecken et al. 2000). Vaccination usually gives protection against homologous antigens only. According to Barrow and Wallis (2000), no study has so far demonstrated a good cross-protection between different Salmonella serotypes for any significant duration after vaccination.

If treatment of individual captive birds is necessary, appropriate antibiotics should be selected on the basis of sensitivity tests. Salmonella isolates linked to food-producing animals are more likely than others to show antibiotic resistance because of the antibiotic selective pressures that these isolates may have faced through anthropogenic husbandry practices (Helmuth 2000). For example, *S.* Typhimurium DT 104, which is most commonly associated with cattle, characteristically shows multiple antibiotic resistance (Poppe et al. 1998; Helmuth 2000). Oral treatment of groups of birds with antibiotics repeatedly has proven unsuccessful in eliminating the carrier stage and may actually have favored the development of disease in some cases by altering the normal intestinal flora that competes with salmonellae. The possible development of resistance to antibiotics following such treatment, not only by salmonellae but also by other members of the intestinal flora such as *E. coli,* should also be a concern (Smith and Tucker 1978).

MANAGEMENT IMPLICATIONS

The most important message that most outbreaks of salmonellosis in wild birds should convey is that when and where they occur, environmental contamination from human or domestic animal sources may have reached a level unacceptable for the safety of livestock and human beings as well as wildlife. A close association has been made on many occasions and under many different circumstances between levels of human and agricultural activities and the prevalence of Salmonella carriers among wild birds (Table 13.1). This indicates that elimination of point sources of infection, such as refuse dumps, untreated sewage outlets, and runoffs from livestock and poultry operations, is the most appropriate way not only of lowering the potential occurrence of outbreaks of salmonellosis in wild birds but also of reducing the likelihood of carrier birds amplifying bacterial contamination in the environment.

The total amount of food provided annually at bird feeders in North America likely represents a substantial subsidy to songbirds. Whether this is sufficient to offset mortality caused by salmonellosis or whether it may in fact promote these outbreaks by maintaining artificially high populations of these birds remains to be determined. According to Kirkwood (1998), the 15,000 tons of peanuts fed annually to songbirds in Great Britain are more than enough to meet the energy requirements of the entire breeding population of European Greenfinches in that country (approximately 550,000 pairs). Although factors contributing to sporadic outbreaks of salmonellosis among songbirds at feeders in winter are well understood, large-scale epizootics in this group of birds appear to be a relatively recent phenomenon, and the details of their dynamics are still obscure. Therefore, it is not yet possible to determine the significance of these large epizootics for the populations involved or ways of curtailing their occurrence or magnitude. The possible epidemiological relationship between the occurrence of these epizootics and the current popularity of bird feeders needs more attention.

UNPUBLISHED DATA

1. Kathryn A. Converse, U.S. Geological Survey, National Wildlife Health Center, Madison, Wisconsin, U.S.A.

LITERATURE CITED

Alisantosa, B., H. L. Shivaprasad, A. S. Dhillon, O. Jack, D. Schaberg, and D. Bandli. 2000. Pathogenicity of Salmonella enteritidis phage types 4, 8 and 23 in specific pathogen free chicks. *Avian Pathology* 29: 583–592.

Anderson, E. S., L. R. Ward, M. J. de Saxe, and J. D. H. de Sa. 1977. Bacteriophage-typing designations of Salmonella typhimurium. *Journal of Hygiene* 78:297–300.

Angulo, F. J., and D. L. Swedlow. 1998. Salmonella Enteritidis infections in the United States. *Journal of the American Veterinary Medical Association* 213:1729–1731.

Barrow, P. A., J. M. Simpson, and M. A. Lovell. 1988. Intestinal colonization in the chicken by food-poisoning Salmonella serotypes; microbial characteristics associated with faecal excretion. *Avian Pathology* 17:571–558.

Barrow, P. A., and T. S. Wallis. 2000. Vaccination against Salmonella infection in food animals: rationale, theoretical basis and practical application. In *Salmonella in Domestic Animals,* C. Wray and A. Wray (eds.). CABI Publishing, Wallingford, Oxon, U.K., pp. 323–339.

Battisti, A., G. Di Guardo, U. Agrimi, and A.I. Bozzano. 1998. Embryonic and neonatal mortality from salmonellosis in captive bred raptors. *Journal of Wildlife Diseases* 34:64–72.

Bäumler, A.J., R.M. Tsolis, T.A. Ficht, and L.G. Adams. 1998. Evolution of host adaptation in Salmonella enterica. *Infection and Immunity* 66:4579–4587.

Bäumler, A.J., R.M. Tsolis, and F. Heffron. 2000. Virulence mechanisms of Salmonella and their genetic basis. In *Salmonella in Domestic Animals,* C. Wray and A. Wray (eds.). CABI Publishing, Wallingford, Oxon, U.K., pp. 57–72.

BirdSource. 1997, revised 8 September 1999. Winter finches invaded much of North America in the winter of 1997–98 in record numbers! Cornell Laboratory of Ornithology. [Online.] Retrieved from the World Wide Web: www.birdsource.org/winfin/index.html, 21 pp.

BirdSource. 2003. Biennial irruptions of pine siskins across North America. National Audubon Society, Cornell Laboratory of Ornithology. [Online.] Retrieved from the World Wide Web: www.-birdsource.org/results/irruptions.htm, 4 pp.

Brenner, F. W., R. G. Villar, F. Angulo, R. Tauxe, and B. Swaminathan. 2000. Salmonella nomenclature. *Journal of Clinical Microbiology* 38:2465–2467.

Brittingham, M. C., and S. A. Temple. 1986. A survey of avian mortality at winter feeders. *Wildlife Society Bulletin* 14:445–450.

Brittingham, M. C., S. A. Temple, and R. M. Duncan. 1988. A survey of the prevalence of selected bacteria in wild birds. *Journal of Wildlife Diseases* 24:299–307.

Brown, D. D., J. G. Ross, and A. F .G. Smith. 1975. Experimental infection of cockerels with Salmonella typhimurium. *Research in Veterinary Science* 18:165–170.

Brunett, E. L. 1930. Paratyphoid infection of pigeons. The Cornell Veterinarian 20:169–176.

Bumstead, N., and P. A. Barrow. 1993. Resistance to Salmonella gallinarum, S. pullorum, and S. enteritidis in inbred lines of chickens. *Avian Diseases* 37:189–193.

Chudzik, J. M., K. D. Graham, and R. D. Morris. 1994. Comparative breeding success and diet of ring-billed and herring gulls on South Limestone Island, Georgian Bay. *Colonial Waterbirds* 17:18–27.

Čižek, A., I. Literék, K. Hejlíček, F. Treml, and J. Smola. 1994. Salmonella contamination of the environment and its incidence in wild birds. *Journal of Veterinary Medicine* B 41:320–327.

Corrier, D. E., J. A. Byrd, B. M. Hargis, M. E. Hume, R. H. Bailey, and L. H. Stanker. 1999. Survival of Salmonella in the crop contents of market-age broilers during feed withdrawal. *Avian Diseases* 43:453–460.

Coulson, J. C., J. Butterfield, and C. Thomas. 1983. The herring gull Larus argentatus as a likely transmitting agent of Salmonella montevideo to sheep and cattle. *Journal of Hygiene* 91:437–443.

Craven, S. E., N. J. Stern, E. Line, J. S. Bailey, N. A. Cox, and P. Fedorka-Cray. 2000. Determination of the incidence of Salmonella spp., Campylobacter jejuni, and Clostridium perfringens in wild birds near broiler houses by sampling intestinal droppings. *Avian Diseases* 44:715–720.

Daoust, P.-Y. 1978. Osteomyelitis and arthritis caused by Salmonella typhimurium in a crow. *Journal of Wildlife Diseases* 14:483–885.

Daoust, P.-Y., D.G. Busby, L. Ferns, J. Goltz, S. McBurney, C. Poppe, and H. Whitney. 2000. Salmonellosis in songbirds in the Canadian Atlantic provinces during winter-summer 1997–98. *Canadian Veterinary Journal* 41:54–59.

Davies, R. H., and C. Wray. 1996. Persistence of Salmonella enteritidis in poultry units and poultry food. *British Poultry Science* 37:589–596.

Durrant, D. S., and S. H. Beatson. 1981. Salmonellae isolated from domestic meat waste. *Journal of Hygiene* 86:259–264.

Edwards, P. R., and D. W. Bruner. 1943. The occurrence and distribution of Salmonella types in the United States. *Journal of Infectious Diseases* 72:58–67.

Elphick, C., J. B. Dunning, Jr., and D. A. Sibley (eds.). 2001. *The Sibley Guide to Bird Life and Behavior.* National Audubon Society. Alfred A. Knopf, New York, NY, U.S.A., 608 pp.

Faddoul, G. P., G. W. Fellows, and J. Baird. 1966. A survey of the incidence of salmonellae in wild birds. *Avian Diseases* 10:89–94.

Farmer III, J. J. 1999. Enterobacteriaceae: introduction and identification. In *Manual of Clinical Microbiology,* 7th Ed., P. R. Murray, E. J. Baron, M. A. Pfaller, F. C. Tenover, and R. H. Yolken (eds.). American Society for Microbiology, pp. 442–458.

Fenlon, D.R. 1981. Seagulls (Larus spp.) as vectors of salmonellae: an investigation into the range of serotypes and numbers of salmonellae in gull faeces. *Journal of Hygiene* 86:195–202.

Figueroa-Bossi, N., S. Uzzau, D. Maloriol, and L. Bossi. 2001. Variable assortment of prophages provides a transferable repertoire of pathogenic determinants in Salmonella. *Molecular Microbiology* 39:260–271.

Forshell, L. P., and I. Ekesbo. 1993. Survival of salmonellas in composted and not composted solid animal manures. *Journal of Veterinary Medicine* B 40:654–658.

Gast, R.K. 1997. Paratyphoid infections. In *Diseases of Poultry,* 10th Ed., B. W. Calnek, H. J. Barnes, C.W. Beard, L. R. McDougald, and Y. M. Saif (eds.). Iowa State University Press, Ames, IA, U.S.A., pp. 97–121.

Gast, R. K., and C. W. Beard. 1989. Age-related changes in the persistence and pathogenicity of Salmonella typhimurium in chicks. *Poultry Science* 68:1454–1460.

Gast, R. K., and C. W. Beard. 1990. Isolation of Salmonella enteritidis from internal organs of experimentally infected hens. *Avian Diseases* 34:991–993.

Gast, R. K., and P. S. Holt. 2000. Deposition of phage type 4 and 13a Salmonella enteritidis strains in the yolk and albumen of eggs laid by experimentally infected hens. *Avian Diseases* 44:706–710.

Girdwood, R. W. A., C. R. Fricker, D. Munro, C.B. Shedden, and P. Monaghan. 1985. The incidence and significance of salmonella carriage by gulls (Larus spp.) in Scotland. *Journal of Hygiene* 95:229–241.

Glickman, L.T., P.L. McDonough, S. J. Shin, J.M. Fairbrother, R.L. LaDue, and S. E. King. 1981. Bovine salmonellosis attributed to Salmonella anatum-contaminated haylage and dietary stress. *Journal of the American Veterinary Medical Association* 178:1268–1272.

Guillot, J.F., C. Beaumont, F. Bellatif, C.Mouline, F. Lantier, P.Colin, and J. Protais. 1995. Comparison of resistance of various poultry lines to infection with Salmonella enteritidis. *Veterinary Research* 26:81–86.

Hackam, D.J., O D. Rotstein, W. Zhang, S. Gruenheid, P. Gros, and S. Grinstein. 1998. Host resistance to intracellular infection: mutation of natural resistance-associated macrophage protein 1 (Nramp1) impairs phagosomal acidification. *Journal of Experimental Medicine* 188:351–364.

Hassan, J.O., A.P.A. Mockett, D. Catty, and P.A. Barrow. 1991. Infection and reinfection of chickens with Salmonella typhimurium: bacteriology and immune responses. *Avian Diseases* 35:809–819.

Helmuth, R. 2000. Antibiotic resistance in Salmonella. In *Salmonella in Domestic Animals.* C. Wray and A. Wray (eds.). CABI Publishing, Wallingford, Oxon, U.K., pp. 89–106.

Henzler, D. J., and H. M. Opitz. 1992. The role of mice in the epizootiology of Salmonella enteritidis infection on chicken layer farms. *Avian Diseases* 36:625–631.

Holt, P. S. 2000. Host susceptibility, resistance and immunity to Salmonella in animals. In *Salmonella in Domestic Animals.* C. Wray and A. Wray (eds.). CABI Publishing, Wallingford, Oxon, U.K., pp.73–87.

Humphrey, T. J., A. Baskerville, H. Chart, B. Rowe, and A. Whitehead. 1992. Infection of laying hens with Salmonella enteritidis PT4 by conjunctival challenge. *The Veterinary Record* 131:386–388.

Hurvell, B., K. Borg, A. Gunnarson, and J. Jevring. 1974. Studies of Salmonella typhimurium infections in passerine birds in Sweden. *International Congress of Game Biology* 11:493–497.

Johnston, W. S., D. Munro, W. J. Reilly, and J. C. M. Sharp. 1981. An unusual sequel to imported Salmonella zanzibar. *Journal of Hygiene* 87:525–528.

Jones, Y. E., I. M. McLaren, and C. Wray. 2000. Laboratory aspects of Salmonella. In *Salmonella in Domestic Animals.* C. Wray and A. Wray (eds.). CABI Publishing, Wallingford, Oxfordshire, U.K., pp. 393–405.

Kapperud, G., S. Gustavsen, I. Hellesnes, A. H. Hansen, J. Lassen, J. Hirn, M. Jahkola, M. A. Montenegro, and R. Helmuth. 1990. Outbreak of Salmonella typhimurium infection traced to contaminated chocolate and caused by a strain lacking the 60-megadalton virulence plasmid. *Journal of Clinical Microbiology* 28:2597–2601.

Kapperud, G., H. Stenwig, and J. Lassen. 1998. Epidemiology of Salmonella typhimurium O:4-12 infection in Norway. *American Journal of Epidemiology* 147:774–782.

Kennard, J. H. 1976. A biennial rhythm in the winter distribution of the common redpoll. Bird-Banding 47:231–237.

Kirkpatrick, C.E. 1986. Isolation of Salmonella spp. from a colony of wading birds. *Journal of Wildlife Diseases* 22:162–264.

Kirkpatrick, C.E., and V.P. Trexler-Myren. 1986. A survey of free-living falconiform birds for Salmonella. *Journal of the American Veterinary Medical Association* 189:997–998.

Kirkwood, J.K. 1998. Population density and infectious disease at bird tables. *The Veterinary Record* 142:468.

Kirkwood, J.K., and S. K. Macgregor. 1997. Infectious diseases of garden birds: minimizing the risks. Universities Federation for Animal Welfare: Wheathampstead, Hertfordshire, U.K., 17 pp.

Lee, G. M., G. D. Jackson, and G. N. Cooper. 1981. The role of serum and biliary antibodies and cell-mediated immunity in the clearance of S. typhimurium from chickens. *Veterinary Immunology and Immunopathology* 2:233–252.

Lindberg, A. A., and J. Å. Robertsson. 1983. Salmonella typhimurium infection in calves: cell-mediated and humoral immune reactions before and after challenge with live virulent bacteria in calves given live or inactivated vaccines. *Infection and Immunity* 41:751–757.

Literák, I., A.Čížek, and J. Smola. 1996. Survival of salmonellas in a colony of common black-headed gulls Larus ridibundus between two nesting periods. *Colonial Waterbirds* 19:268–269.

Malmqvist, M., K-G. Jacobson, P. Häggblom, F. Cerenius, L. Sjöland, and A. Gunnarsson. 1995. Salmonella isolated from animals and feedstuffs in Sweden during 1988–1992. *Acta Veterinaria Scandinavica* 36:21–39.

McOrist S, and C. Lenghaus. 1992. Mortalities of little penguins (Eudyptula minor) following exposure to crude oil. *The Veterinary Record* 130:161–162.

Meyerholz, D.K., T.J. Stabel, M.R. Ackermann, S.A. Carlson, B.D. Jones, and J. Pohlenz. 2002. Early epithelial invasion by Salmonella enterica serovar Typhimurium DT 104 in the swine ileum. *Veterinary Pathology* 39:712–720.

Mitchell, T. R., and T. Ridgwell. 1971. The frequency of salmonellae in wild ducks. *Journal of Medical Microbiology* 4:359–361.

Monaghan, P., C. B. Shedden, K. Ensor, C. R. Fricker, and R. W. A. Girdwood. 1985. Salmonella carriage by herring gulls in the Clyde area of Scotland in relation to their feeding ecology. *Journal of Applied Ecology* 22:669–680.

Morishita, T. Y., P. P. Aye, E. C. Ley, and B. S. Harr. 1999. Survey of pathogens and blood parasites in free-living passerines. *Avian Diseases* 43:549–552.

Müller, G. 1965. Salmonella in bird faeces. *Nature* 207:1315.

Nakano, A., E. Kita, and S. Kashiba. 1995. Different sensitivity of complement to Salmonella typhimurium accounts for the difference in natural resistance to murine typhoid between A/J and C57BL/6 mice. *Microbiology and Immunology* 39:95–103.

Olsen, B., S. Bergström, D.J. McCafferty, M. Sellin, and J. Wiström. 1996. Salmonella enteritidis in Antarctica: zoonosis in man or humanosis in penguins? *The Lancet* 348:1319–1320.

Pelzer KD. 1989. Salmonellosis. *Journal of the American Veterinary Medical Association* 195:456–463.

Pennycott, T. W., H. M. Ross, I. M. McLaren, A. Park, G. F. Hopkins, and G. Foster. 1998. Causes of death of wild birds of the family Fringillidae in Britain. *The Veterinary Record* 143:155–158.

Poppe, C., N. Smart, R. Khakhria, W. Johnson, J. Spika, and J. Prescott. 1998. Salmonella typhimurium DT104: a virulent and drug-resistant pathogen. *Canadian Veterinary Journal* 39:559–565.

Prescott, J. F., C. Poppe, J. Goltz, and G. D. Campbell. 1998. Salmonella typhimurium phage type 40 in feeder birds *The Veterinary Record* 142:732.

Prescott, J.F., D.B. Hunter, and G.D. Campbell. 2000. Hygiene at winter bird feeders in a southwestern Ontario city. *Canadian Veterinary Journal* 41:699–703.

ProMED-mail. 2001, 25 December. Salmonellosis, birds, humans, New Zealand. International Society for Infectious Diseases. [Online.] Retrieved from the World Wide Web: www.promedmail.org, archive number 20011225.3113, 3 pp.

Quessy, S., and S. Messier. 1992. Prevalence of Salmonella spp., Campylobacter spp. and Listeria spp. in ring-billed gulls (Larus delawarensis). *Journal of Wildlife Diseases* 28:526–531.

Rabsch, W., H.L. Andrews, R.A. Kingsley, R. Prager, H.Tschäpe, L.G. Adams, and A.J. Bäumler. 2002. Salmonella enterica serotype Typhimurium and its host-adapted variants. *Infection and Immunity* 70:2249–2255.

Rausch, R. 1947. Pullorum disease in the coot. *Journal of Wildlife Management* 11:189.

Refsum, T., T. Vikøren, K. Handeland, G. Kapperud, and G. Holstad. 2003. Epidemiologic and pathologic aspects of Salmonella Typhimurium infection in passerine birds in Norway. *Journal of Wildlife Diseases* 39:64–72.

Reilly, W.J., G.I. Forbes, G.M. Paterson, and J.C.M. Sharp. 1981. Human and animal salmonellosis in Scotland associated with environmental contamination. *The Veterinary Record* 108:553–555.

Robinson, R.A., and M.J. Daniel. 1968. The significance of salmonella isolations from wild birds and rats in New Zealand. *New Zealand Veterinary Journal* 16:53–55.

Scott, F.W. 1988. Salmonella implicated as cause of song bird fever. *Feline Health Topics for Veterinarians* 3(3):5–6.

Shivaprasad, H.L. 1997. Pullorum disease and fowl typhoid. In *Diseases of Poultry,* 10th Ed., B.W. Calnek, H. J. Barnes, C.W. Beard, L. R. McDougald, and Y.M. Saif (eds.). Iowa State University Press, Ames, IA, U.S.A., pp. 82–96.

Smith, H.W., and J.F. Tucker. 1978. Oral administration of neomycin to chickens experimentally infected with Salmonella typhimurium. *The Veterinary Record* 102:354–356.

Tauni, M.A., and A. Österlund. 2000. Outbreak of Salmonella typhimurium in cats and humans associated with infection in wild birds. *Journal of Small Animal Practice* 41:339–341.

Tizard, I. R., N.A. Fish, and J. Harmeson. 1979. Free flying sparrows as carriers of salmonellosis. *Canadian Veterinary Journal* 20:143–144.

Van Dorssen, C.A. 1935. Salmonella typhi-murium-infectie bij een kleine zeemeeuw (Larus canus). Tijdschrift voor Diergeneeskunde 62:1263–1264.

Vereecken, M., P. De Herdt, R. Ducatelle, and F. Haesebrouck. 2000. The effect of vaccination on the course of an experimental Salmonella typhimurium infection in racing pigeons. *Avian Pathology* 29:465–471.

Waltman, W.D. 2000. Methods for the cultural isolation of Salmonella. In *Salmonella in Domestic Animals.* C. Wray and A. Wray (eds.). CABI Publishing, Wallingford, Oxon, U.K., pp. 355–372.

Ward, L.R., J.D.H. de Sa, and B. Rowe. 1987. A phage typing system for Salmonella enteritidis. Epidemiology and Infection 99:291–294.

Watts, P.S., and M. Wall. 1952. The 1951 Salmonella typhimurium epidemic in sheep in South Australia. *Australian Veterinary Journal* 28:165–168.

Williams, B.M., D.W. Richards, and J. Lewis. 1976. Salmonella infection in the herring gull (Larus argentatus). *The Veterinary Record* 98:51.

Williams, B.M., D.W. Richards, D. P. Stephens, and T. Griffiths. 1977. The transmission of S livingstone to cattle by the herring gull (Larus argentatus). The Veterinary Record 100:450–451.

Williams, J. E., and S. T. Benson. 1978. Survival of Salmonella typhimurium in poultry feed and litter at three temperatures. *Avian Diseases* 22:742–747.

Wilson, J. E., and J. W. MacDonald. 1967. Salmonella infection in wild birds. *British Veterinary Journal* 123:212–219.

Wobeser, G.A., and M.C. Finlayson. 1969. Salmonella typhimurium infection in house sparrows. *Archives of Environmental Health* 19:882–884.

14
Avian Tuberculosis

Kathryn A. Converse

INTRODUCTION

Tuberculosis occurs worldwide in birds as a contagious, chronic, bacterial disease caused principally by *Mycobacterium avium* and less frequently by *M. genavense. Mycobacterium avium* is a widely distributed species that causes infections in many vertebrate host taxa (Cromie et al. 2000). *Mycobacterium genavense* is an opportunist organism in the environment that was recognized as a cause of human infections in 1987 (Böttger 1994) and was first reported in 1993 as an avian pathogen in eight species of pet birds (Hoop et al. 1993). Less commonly, tuberculosis in birds is caused by *M. intracellulare, M. fortuitum, M. tuberculosis, M. gordonae,* and *M. nonchromogenicum* (Hoop et al. 1996; Tell et al. 2001). Although the term mycobacteriosis applies to any disease from mycobacterial infection, disease caused by *M. avium* and related mycobacteria conventionally is called avian tuberculosis, based on the tuberculated lesions caused by this infection. In this chapter the term avian tuberculosis is used broadly to refer to avian mycobacterial disease, whereas avian mycobacteriosis is used only when specifically discussing nontubercular disease, such as that caused by *M. genavense.*

Avian tuberculosis is usually a slowly developing disease that leads to anorexia, emaciation, lethargy, dyspnea, and death within months. After being established, it can persist in the environment and bird populations for years (Thoen 1997). Captive bird populations may have a high incidence of avian tuberculosis due to the greater density of birds and long-term use of an area potentially contaminated by infected birds.

Although the etiologic agent has been known for more than a century, avian tuberculosis is still a disease that is difficult to diagnose in live birds. Even when it is detected, there are few effective drugs or vaccines and they are only feasible for use in captive birds (Thoen 1997). Postmortem in many cases the causative agents are not identified because of nonspecific necropsy findings and inability to culture mycobacteria (Böttger 1996).

SYNONYMS

Avian mycobacteriosis, *M. avium* complex (MAC) disease, *M. avium-intracellulare* complex (MAIC or MAI) disease.

HISTORY

The human tubercle bacillus was discovered by Kock in 1882. By 1884, tuberculosis was reported in many zoo species including Lesser (Darwin's) Rhea (*Pterocnemia pennata*), common fowl, Common Peafowl (*Pavo cristatus*), Golden Pheasant (*Chrysolophus pictus*), guineafowl, grouse, pigeon, partridge, stork, crane, falcon, and eagle (Sutton and Gibbes 1884). Most early observations of tuberculosis in wild birds were associated with transmission studies conducted either in private aviaries or on farms with domestic fowl, swine, and cattle (Meissner and Anz 1977; MacKenzie 1988). Avian tuberculosis in free-living sparrows, blackbirds, wood-pigeons, and pheasants was attributed to their contact with farms and domestic poultry (Rankin and McDiarmid 1969). In more recent years avian tuberculosis has occurred sporadically in free-flying wild birds and remained an important disease in birds that are housed in zoos and aviaries.

Prior to 1980, mycobacterial infections in humans were rarely caused by *M. avium* complex (MAC). By 1991, the *M. avium-intracellulare* (MAIC) complex accounted for 96% of the mycobacterial infections in patients with AIDS, and 50% of HIV positive patients developed MAIC disease as a terminal event (Daborn and Grange 1993).

DISTRIBUTION

Avian tuberculosis occurs in captive and free-flying wild birds worldwide including reports from North America, Europe, Australia, India (Gale 1971; Smit et al. 1987; Hejlicek and Treml 1993), South America (Thoen 1997), Africa (Woodford 1982; Kock et al. 1999), Southeast Asia (Deng et al. 1996; Morita et al. 1997), and Russia (Fedyanina and Toropova 1975; Kovalev 1983). Between 1978 and 2004, among diagnostic cases at the U.S. Geological Survey's National Wildlife Health Center, avian tuberculosis was confirmed in 83 birds of 32 species that were collected in 18 of the United States.[1]

HOST RANGE

A wide range of free-living and captive birds in at least 15 orders have been diagnosed with avian tuberculosis (Rankin and McDiarmid 1969; Gale 1971; Panigrahy et al. 1983; Smit et al. 1987; MacKenzie 1988; Shane et al. 1993; Franson et al. 1996b; Thoen 1997; Kock et al. 1999). There are no reports of avian species that are resistant to all mycobacteria. Tuberculosis occurs in many orders of birds and susceptibility varies; incidence in captive collections appears to be highest in Anseriformes (ducks, geese, and swans), Gruiformes (cranes), and Galliformes (pheasants, chickens, and turkeys) (Tell et al. 2001). Susceptibility to mycobacteria in birds may vary with temperature, habitat use, feeding patterns, and increased stressors such as malnutrition, pinioning, crowding, and environmental extremes (Cromie et al. 1991; Tell et al. 2001). Information on the prevalence of *M. avium* in free-ranging wild birds primarily has been obtained from either extended carcass collections during mortality events caused by other diseases (Friend 1999) or reported in long-term diagnostic summaries (Table 14.1).

ETIOLOGY

The mycobacteria are a group of intracellular, rod shaped, Gram-positive bacteria with a lipid-rich, waxy cell wall. The waxy outer cell wall makes mycobacteria highly resistant to desiccation, ultraviolet light, and freezing and, therefore, they can persist in the environment for months to years.

The genus *Mycobacterium* contains many pathogenic species that can cause illness in: birds (*M. avium*), mammals (*M. tuberculosis, M. bovis, M. avium paratuberculosis*), fish (*M. marinum*), frogs (*M. fortuitum*), turtles (*M. chelonae*), and cats and rodents (*M. lepraemurium*). Within *Mycobacterium avium,* organisms are divided into four subspecies: *M. avium avium; M. avium silvaticum* (formerly wood-pigeon mycobacteria or *M. avium columbae*); *M. avium hominissuis;* and *M. avium paratuberculosis* (cause of Johne's disease in cattle)(Thorel et al. 1990; Tell et al. 2001; Thorel 2004). The first three subspecies can be virulent or partially virulent (*M. a. hominissuis*) for birds. Mycobacteria isolates were serotyped beginning in the middle 1960s using a seroagglutination technique developed by Schaefer (1965), who later along with Wolinsky (1973) proposed a numbering scheme to distinguish serotypes. Because conventional biochemical tests cannot distinguish *Mycobacteria avium avium* (*M. avium*) and *M. intracellulare,* these two species, along with several unclassified serovars, are often referred to as a complex (MAIC) of serovars 1–28: *M. avium* (serovars 1–6 and 8–11), and M. *intracellulare* (serovars 7, 12–20, 23, and 25) (Wayne et al. 1993). The dominant mycobacteria species for strains belonging to serovars 21, 22, 24, 26, 27, and 28 are not determined (Wayne et al. 1993). Avian tuberculosis is caused principally by *M. avium* serovars 1 to 3 in the United States and Europe (Tell et al. 2001; Thorel 2004), and serovars 1 and 2 appear to be most common in wild birds (Thoen 1997).

Mycobacterium avium and *M. intracellulare* can be distinguished by genetic tests using nucleic acid hybridization probes. Furthermore, pulsed-field gel electrophoresis of large DNA restriction fragments is useful to distinguish strains within a species (Thorel 2004). Restriction fragment length polymorphism (RFLP) analyses were shown to be capable of distinguishing isolates from bird infections. In one study, all of the *M. avium* complex isolates from avian species shared the same insertion sequence IS1245 genetic fingerprint and also exhibited closely related IS901 RFLP patterns associated with serovars 1, 2, and 3 (Ritacco et al. 1998). In addition, sequencing of the 16S-23S ribosomal RNA (rRNA) gene internally transcribed spacer (ITS) has been completed for a set of MAC reference strains and was shown to be useful for differentiating among strains for epizootiological studies (Frothingham and Wilson 1993).

Avian tuberculosis is usually caused by *M. avium,* but other mycobacteria are detected in wild bird species. There is increasing detection of *M. genavense* rather than *M. avium* as the cause of mycobacteriosis in pet birds (Hoop et al. 1996; Holsboer Buogo et al. 1997). Psittacines are susceptible to infection by *M. tuberculosis and M. bovis* (Ackerman et al. 1974) and are the only birds known to become infected with *M. tuberculosis* from direct contact with infected humans (Washko et al. 1998).

EPIZOOTIOLOGY

Avian tuberculosis can occur at high prevalence rates in wild bird populations and is transmitted primarily through direct and indirect contact with other wild birds as well as domestic birds (Rankin and McDiarmid 1969). Mycobacteria are opportunistic organisms that live and grow in a range of temperatures and pH's in dust and damp environments including soils, mud, water, and wetlands (Frey and Hagan 1931; Ichiyama et al. 1988; Morita et al. 1997). The organism has a

Table 14.1. Representative prevalence rates for avian tuberculosis in wild birds.

Common Name	Scientific Name	Positive/Total Examined (%)	Year(s)	Country (State)	Reference
Tundra (Bewick's) Swan	*Cygnus columbianus bewicki*	10/264 (9.9)	1951–1989	Britain	Brown et al. 1992
Mute Swan	*Cygnus olor*	4/264 (3.9)			
Lesser Flamingo	*Phoenicopterus minor*	14	1973	Kenya	Cooper and Karstad 1975
		17/42 (40)	1993		Kock et al. 1999
Whistling ducks	Tribe: Dendrocygnini	21/170 (12)	1989–1998	Britain	Cromie et al. 2000
Dabbling ducks	Tribe: Anatini	15/307 (5)			
Diving ducks	Tribe: Aythyini	10/200 (5)			
Perching ducks	Tribe: Cairinini	15/123 (12)			
Seaducks, mergansers	Tribe: Mergini	4/47 (8.5)			
Overall study	. . .	28/4052 (0.07)	1947–1976	U.S.A. (CA)	Floerke 1977
Ducks	8 spp.	23/28			
Canada Goose	*Branta canadensis*	3/28			
Sandhill Crane	*Grus canadensis*	1/28			
American Coot	*Fulica americana*	1/28			
Barnacle Goose	*Branta leucopis*	13/178 (7)	1993	Britain	Forbes et al. 1993
Red-tailed Hawk	*Buteo jamaicensis*	4/163 (2.5)	1975–1992	U.S.A. (WI, IL, CA)	Franson et al. 1996
Great Horned Owl	*Bubo virginianus*	2/132 (1.5)	1975–1993	U.S.A. (NE, NV)	Franson and Little 1996
Overall study	. . .	82/11, 664 (.07)	1975–1985	Netherlands	Smit et al. 1987
Common Buzzard	*Buteo buteo*	20/82			
Eurasian Kestrel	*Falco tinnunculus*	17/82			
Black-headed Gull	*Larus ridibundus*	11/82			
Mew Gull	*Larus canus*	34/82			
(+21 other species)					
Whooping Crane	*Grus americana*	7/18 (39)	1982–1990	U.S.A.	Lewis, J. C. cited in Synder et al. 1991
White-headed Tree Duck	*Dendrocygna viduata*	1/10 (10)	1976[a]	Nigeria	Thoen et al. 1976

a: Year published (year of occurrence not reported).

hydrophobic cell wall rich in lipids and is usually found at the interface of air and water in soils, mud, and wetlands (Cromie et al. 2000).

Transmission of *M. avium* can occur in several ways, but the most important means are direct contact with sick birds or contact with food and water contaminated with the feces from infected birds. *Mycobacterium avium* can be isolated from avian fecal samples and environmental samples in the vicinity of infected birds (Schaefer et al. 1973). Large numbers of bacilli can be released from tubercles in liver and intestine into fecal material, providing a continual source of contamination for the environment. Mycobacteria also can spread by aerosolization of bacteria from lesions in the respiratory tract of infected birds (Thoen 1997). The mycobacteria are readily available to free-living birds using these environments; highest exposure would be expected in waterfowl and other water birds. Waterfowl classified as dabblers and divers had a significantly higher incidence of tuberculosis than waterfowl classified as grazers, possibly due to their increased exposure to *M. avium* in aerosols (Cromie et al. 1991) or more constant contact with the aquatic environment. Avian tuberculosis reached epidemic proportions in free-ranging flamingos (Kock et al. 1999) and occurred in 39% of the reintroduced Rocky Mountain population of endangered Whooping Cranes (*Grus americana*) (Snyder et al. 1991).

The presence of bacilli in fecal samples, and the prolonged course of the disease in birds, increases the potential of other birds being exposed to mycobacteria that can persist in the soil, water, litter, and buried carcasses for months to years (Thoen 1997). The waxy outer cell wall makes mycobacteria highly resistant to desiccation, UV light, and freezing. *Mycobacterium avium* can persist outside of the host animal by producing mycobactin and acquiring iron, factors essential for growth and survival in the environment (Collins and Manning 2001).

The potential for vertical transmission of avian tuberculosis has been documented in domestic poultry but not in free-living wild birds. Experimentally inoculated chicken eggs may hatch and the chicks will be infected with tubercle bacilli (Thoen 1997). Culture results from eggs of naturally infected hens have been mixed. *Mycobacterium avium* was successfully cultured from a small proportion of eggs that were naturally infected in some studies but not in others (Thoen 1997). Transmission via infected eggs is not considered a common means of dissemination.

There is evidence that *M. avium* can be mechanically transmitted by arthropods. Ticks (*Argas persicus*) that were spontaneously infected in poultry yards with tuberculous hens preserved *M. avium* for more than 16 months and excreted mycobacteria in their feces (Kovalev 1983). *Mycobacterium avium* penetrated from the intestine into the hemolymph in 30% of the ticks.

Infection with *M. avium* can be influenced by other factors such as crowding, high stocking densities, genetics, and social stresses (Gross et al. 1989). A study of captive waterfowl showed that genetic and environmental factors affected the incidence of and susceptibility to mycobacteria (Cromie et al. 1991).

Knowledge of the *M. avium* serovars and strains can help determine the source of an infection, distribution in the environment and in animal populations, and the modes of transmission among individuals and within populations (Tsang et al. 1992). For example, in one study, serovars were used to investigate potential sources of *M. avium* in humans; serovars typically found in birds (serovars 1, 2, or 3) were not cultured from sawdust or insects, but other cross-reacting serovars were detected (Meissner and Anz 1977). Although the most common isolates from pigs examined during a Netherlands study were *M. avium* serotype 2 or 3, only one of 21 porcine isolates had the IS1245 RFLP pattern indicative of strains of potential avian origin (Komijn et al. 1999).

Captive birds in close confinement in moist environments are at risk of mycobacterial infections by direct contact with infected birds or mycobacteria that can accumulate and persist in water, litter, and soil (Thoen 1997). Prevalence rates can be high in captive populations of wild birds. Rates as high as 84% were reported in a captive breeding population of endangered White-winged Ducks (*Cairina columbianus scutulata*) (Cromie et al. 2000), and epidemics have occurred in aviary waterfowl flocks (Hillgarth and Kear 1979). Approximately 7% of Whooper Swans (*Cygnus cygnus*) and almost 10% of Bewick's Swan (*Cygnus columbianus bewickii*) that were winter visitors to the Wildfowl and Wetland Trust in Great Britain had avian tuberculosis (Brown et al. 1992). The prevalence of *M. avium* in mud and soil used by captive waterfowl at the Wildfowl Trust for more than 60 years may have been the source of infection for the migratory swans. The epizootiology of avian tuberculosis, even in captive flocks, may be more complex than simple bird-to-bird transmission of one mycobacterial strain. On investigating this disease in captive flocks of the endangered Lesser White-fronted Goose (*Anser erythropus*), epidemiologists found multiple *M. avium* strains in the infected geese and these were distinctly different from environmental isolates (Kauppinen et al. 2001).

CLINICAL SIGNS

Birds with avian tuberculosis usually are sick for a few weeks to several months with anorexia, progressive weight loss, dull and ruffled feathers, weakness, diarrhea, abdominal distension, and lethargy (Thoen et al. 1984). Death is the usual outcome. Dyspnea, lameness, and blindness may occur if lungs, bones, or eyes are involved. Sudden death from avian tuberculosis was reported in captive birds that appeared healthy but when examined the birds were emaciated (Hoop et al. 1996). More specific clinical signs may be observed in the late stages of the disease, but they are variable and reflect the route of exposure, duration of the infection, and particular organ systems involved. Infections by *M. avium* and *M. genavense* produce almost identical clinical signs in birds (Mendenhall et al. 2000). A wide variety of clinical signs observed in captive and free-living bird species are described in Tell et al. (2001).

PATHOGENESIS

The pathogenicity of mycobacteria is dependent on the ability of the bacteria to survive, replicate, and induce a response in the host. Mycobacteria probably enter bird hosts by penetration of the bronchial or intestinal mucosa as in human hosts (Inderlied 1993). Following ingestion, the waxy cell wall protects the bacteria from digestive acids and enzymes until they reach the intestine. *Mycobacterium avium* are bound to enterocytes in the intestinal submucosa and mucosa and eventually may migrate to the bloodstream, spleen, and liver (Inderlied 1993). Invading mycobacteria are phagocytized by macrophages and multiply intracellularly unless cytokine-facilitated bacteriostasis takes place and/or the mycobacteria are killed in the macrophages. Mycobacteria can survive phagocytosis by inhibition of the phagosome-lysosome fusion, disruption of cytokine production (Tell et al. 2001), or inactivation of intracellular superoxide radicals generated by the host cell (Thorel et al. 2001). The virulence of the mycobacteria is linked to lipids in the cell wall that contain mycosides, phospholipids, and sulpholipids that may protect the bacterium from phagocytosis and glycolipids that incite a granulomatous response from the host (Tell et al. 2001). The bacteria are isolated by this host response within activated macrophages and lymphocytes in localized granulomas (tubercles). Bacteria may persist in these granulomas for many years. If cellular immunity fails and bacteria in the granulomas escape, the infection is reactivated and can spread to other parts of the body.

PATHOLOGY

Postmortem lesions of avian tuberculosis usually consist of multiple, variably sized, gray, tan, or yellow nodules that protrude from the serosal surface of the intestine or are embedded in the parenchyma of organs (Figure 14.1). The mode of entry for the bacteria determines the organs involved and the clinical signs that are observed. Following ingestion, mycobacteria are transferred from the intestine to parenchymatous organs such as liver, spleen, and bone marrow, while inhalation of the bacteria can lead to lesions in the nasal passage, trachea, bronchi, lungs, and air sacs. Lesions in wild birds most commonly occur in the liver, spleen, and intestinal tract and less commonly in the lung and kidney. Lesions can be concentrated in one tissue or broadly disseminated due to intermittent periods of bacteremia (Thoen 1997). Granulomas in the intestinal wall may be ulcerated on the mucosal surface, providing a site for mycobacteria to be shed into the lumen. The spleen and other parenchymatous organs may be completely occupied

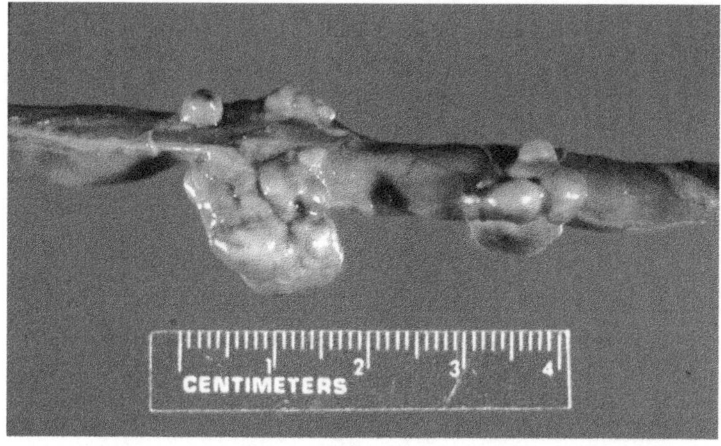

Figure 14.1. Small intestine of a Sandhill Crane with multiple nodular granulomas of avian tuberculosis protruding from the serosa.

by coalescing granulomas (Figures 14.2 and 14.3) (Sykes 1982; Thoen et al. 1984).

Unusual presentations may not be initially recognized or cultured for mycobacteria; for example, lesions may occur in a joint (Cooper et al. 1975), cervical spinal cord (Lairmore et al. 1985), the conjunctiva (Pocknell et al. 1996), or be associated with polycystic livers (Roffe 1989). In some species or individuals, most noteably psittacine and passerine caged birds, nonspecifically enlarged livers and spleens, and tubular thickened intestines may be the result of *M. avium* infection. Similarly, *M. genavense* infections in Budgerigars (*Melopsittacus undulatus*), Common Canaries (*Serinus canarius*), and several other psittacine and passerine pet birds caused enlarged livers or spleens with no grossly visible granulomatous nodules (Hoop et al. 1993; Ramis et al. 1996). The tissue distribution of avian tuberculosis lesions in a variety of avian species is provided by Tell et al. (2001). Other diseases that can produce similar gross lesions include aspergillosis, histomoniasis, and neoplasms.

Microscopic lesions of avian tuberculosis in wild birds include a variety of pathologic changes: scattered foci of epithelioid macrophages and lymphocytes in early stages of infection, sheets of large macrophages with vacuolated (foamy) cytoplasm that contain acid-fast organisms, and well-defined caseous granulomas in more advanced and disseminated stages of disease (Thoen et al. 1984; Ramis et al. 1996). Granulomas in any site usually contain a central area of necrosis surrounded by a zone of epithelioid macrophages with

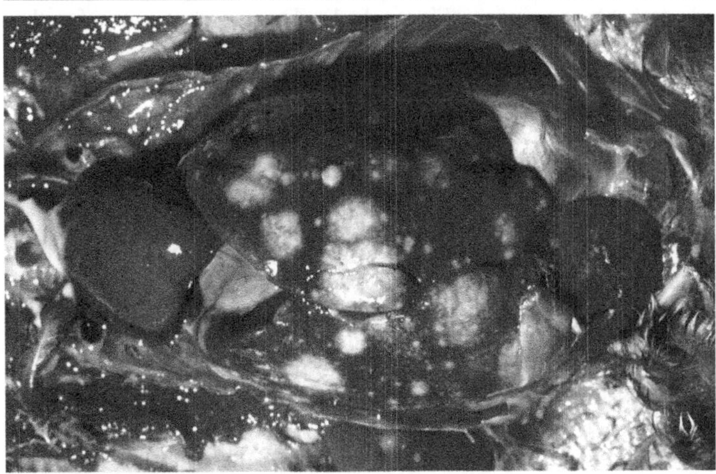

Figure 14.2. Enlarged liver of a Canvasback (*Aythya valisineria*) with pale granulomas of avian tuberculosis scattered in the liver parenchyma.

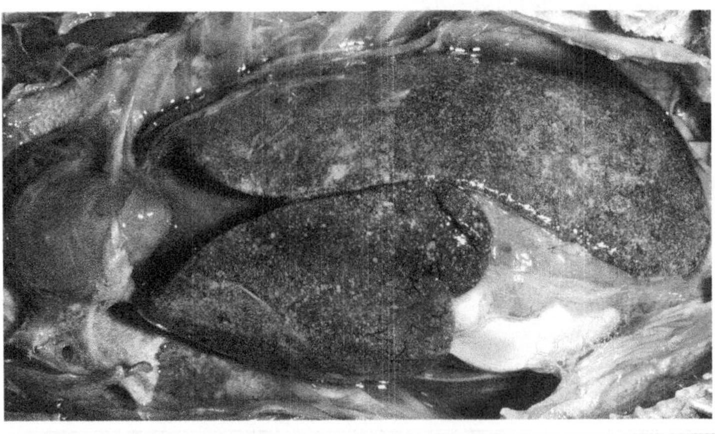

Figure 14.3. Miliary granulomas of avian tuberculosis in the enlarged liver of an American Wigeon (*Anas americana*).

occasional multinucleated giant cells, lymphocytes, and with time a capsule of connective tissue may form around the periphery. In cases in which no discrete nodules were observed grossly, microscopic lesions are characterized by histiocyte aggregations, diffusely or in nodules, in organs rather than granulomas with central necrosis (VanDerHeyden 1994). Photomicrographs of tuberculosis in multiple species and tissues can be found in Thoen et al. (1984). The most consistent finding in avian tuberculosis is the presence of acid-fast intracellular bacteria in macrophages or among necrotic debris in granulomas. *Mycobacterium avium* infected cells appear distended, and acid-fast organisms can be demonstrated in them using the Kinyoun modification of the Ziehl-Neelsen stain (Hoop et al. 1993; Thoen 1998).

DIAGNOSIS

Postmortem diagnosis of avian tuberculosis is based on the presence of typical lesions and detection of mycobacteria in blood or tissues. Avian tuberculosis is suspected in dead birds with granulomas along the intestine, in liver, spleen, and other sites. A presumptive diagnosis of tuberculosis is supported by microscopic findings of small, acid-fast, rod-shaped bacteria in smears of caseous nodules, scrapings of cut surfaces of lesions, or microscopic sections.

Unless acid-fast stains are applied, bacteria will not be found during microscopic examination. The waxy cell wall prevents mycobacteria from absorbing stain using conventional Gram stain protocols. The Ziehl-Neelsen acid-fast stain uses detergents to remove the waxy coat and allow staining with Carbol-Fuchsin red dye. Most mycobacteria can be identified using the Ziehl-Neelsen test, but it does not differentiate between species of mycobacteria. Fluorochrome (auromine O) stains can be used in conjunction with acid-fast stains (Koneman et al. 1997). The advantage of flourochrome stain is high visibility of the fluorescing bacteria against a dark background (Koneman et al. 1997; Tell et al. 2003). Not all acid-fast organisms are mycobacteria, so the diagnosis must be confirmed by isolation or identification of *M. avium* in tissues (Thorel 1994).

A procedure using the polymerase chain reaction (PCR) for the identification of *M. bovis* was adapted to identify mycobacteria of the *M. avium* complex in formalin-fixed, paraffin-embedded tissues, resulting in the determination that the 16S rRNA gene primers are the most useful for identification of *M. avium* when testing the tissues of birds and nonruminant species (Miller et al. 1999). Using this technique, samples from 16/18 (89%) birds with an *M. avium* isolate were positive. There also are PCR procedures that can be used to rapidly screen unfixed tissues with high specificity and sensitivity (Tell et al. 2003). PCR techniques may present the only means to detect *M. genavense* from tissue specimens in many cases, because culture of this fastidious organism is often unsuccessful (Hoop et al. 1996).

Culture is considered the "gold standard" for detection of mycobacterial infection. Preferred tissues for culture and isolation of avian mycobacteria are liver, spleen, or bone marrow, but any other tissues that have gross lesions may yield positive cultures. Tissues are inoculated into Lowenstein-Jensen medium, Proskauer-Beck liquid medium containing 5% serum, Herrold's medium, Middlebrook 7H10 and 7H119, or Coletsos medium supplemented with 1% sodium pyruvate (Thoen 1998; Thorel 2004). Ideally, *M. avium* cultures should be maintained in an atmosphere of 5–10% carbon dioxide at a temperature of 41°C (Thoen 1998). Cultures *of M. avium* will not produce niacin, reduce nitrate, or hydrolyze Tween 80 but will reduce tellurite (Thoen 1998). Requirements for culture media, time, substrate, nutrients, temperature, and oxygenation can vary by the species, and some fastidious species such as *M. genavense* may fail to grow (Tell et al. 2001). *Mycobacterium avium sylvaticum* does not synthesize mycobactins in *in vitro* cultures, so mycobactin must be added to the culture medium (Grange 1996). Isolation and identification of *M. avium* may require a minimum of four weeks.

A radiometric culture technique that uses liquid culture medium (BACTEC) can increase the sensitivity and speed of culturing *M. avium* from tissues and fecal material (Clark et al. 1995; Tell et al. 2001). This technique detects mycobacterial growth by production of the gas ion $^{14}CO_2$. BACTEC was reported as the superior technique for the isolation of *M. genavense* (Hoop et al. 1996). However, the equipment required for this technique is expensive and not always available at laboratories.

Reliable molecular tests that use nucleic acid hybridization probes to detect genetic fingerprints are commercially available. These tests can be used to identify the MAIC, and more specifically to distinguish between *M. avium, M. intracellare,* and *M. genavense;* they currently are validated for use only on isolates obtained by culture (Thorel 2004). Similarly, serotyping, or 16S-23S rRNA gene ITS region sequencing, which may both be particularly useful for epidemiologic tracking, is done on isolates.

The diagnosis of avian tuberculosis in live birds can be a difficult process and is based on a combination of compatible clinical signs, postmortem tests on other birds from the flock or epizootic, and a variety of additional techniques that can include blood tests, radiography, laproscopy, cytology, tuberculin and hemagglutination tests, serology, and additional molecular techniques (Tell et al. 2001). Radiography and ultrasonography may provide images of lesions, but unless laproscopy in conjunction with biopsy and culture is done, most tests on live birds are not definitive. Such tests are primarily used in captive birds of high value because anesthesia is required and these tests are expensive. Hematology can be used to screen individual birds to detect an elevated white blood cell count with marked monocytosis, heterophilia, hyperfibinogenemia, and thrombocytosis (Hawkey et al. 1990; Tell et al. 2001, 2004).

Tuberculin skin tests have been used to detect the presence of mycobacteria in live wild and domestic birds. In this test a small amount of tuberculin (avian purified protein derivative) (PPD) is injected intradermally into tissues and is monitored for an inflammatory reaction over 48 hours. In domestic poultry, injections into the wattle that produce soft swelling within 48 hours indicate exposure to avian tubercle bacilli. However, false positive and false negative reactions can occur (Thoen 1997). Tuberculin tests have been attempted in nondomestic birds. A sick Whooping Crane was injected intradermally in the featherless skin on the top of the head. After 48 hours, a punch biopsy of the indurated area contained a cellular reaction characteristic of delayed hypersensitivity (Synder et al. 1991). Tuberculin test results were unsatisfactory in raptors and waterfowl (Cromie et al. 1993). No successful results were obtained when injected into the cloacal skin of psittacines (VanDerHeyden 1994). For the tuberculin test to be used in wild birds, the birds must be trapped, injected, held for 48 hours, and reexamined before release or removal from the population.

Alternatively tests can be done on whole blood or serum to detect antibodies to mycobacteria. The rapid agglutination test uses whole blood and can be as reliable as the tuberculin test in poultry, but false positive agglutination reactions can occur in healthy birds (Thoen 1997; Tell et al. 2001). Antibodies against *M. avium* can be detected in sera with an enzyme-linked immunosorbent assay (ELISA), a rapid, simple, standardized test that requires a small amount of serum (Thoen 1997). A positive response can indicate previous exposure to mycobacteria, latent infection, or active infection. An ELISA successfully detected tuberculosis in waterfowl, even in the early stages, with no false positives (Forbes et al. 1993). In comparison with hematological analyses and agglutination tests, ELISA to detect mycobacteria in captive waterfowl was the most sensitive and specific test without the false positives and negatives that occurred with the other two tests (Cromie et al. 1993). During this study, hematological tests became positive late in the course of the disease, while the ELISA detected disease at an early stage before the birds were excreting bacilli (Cromie et al. 1993).

An apparently healthy bird can be infected for a long period of time and shed mycobacteria in its feces. A series of positive fecal cultures in an individual bird probably indicates an active infection rather than environmental mycobacteria passing through. A very rapid method for detecting low numbers of organisms and identifying species of mycobacteria uses PCR to detect genetic material of the mycobacteria. A PCR test successfully identified and differentiated *M. avium* and *M. intracellulare* in clinical specimens from humans (Yamamoto et al. 1993). However, in a diagnostic test comparison, neither a PCR procedure nor acid-fast stains were as sensitive or reliable as culture in detecting *M. avium* in feces from experimentally inoculated Japanese Quail (*Coturnix japonica*) (Tell et al. 2003).

IMMUNITY

Differences in susceptibility and immunological response to mycobacteria among wild birds species are probably as varied as differences in responses among mammal species (Cromie et al. 2000). Difficulties are presented by the complexity of the MAIC, the lack of knowledge and understanding of the mechanisms of immunological response, and differing responses in the thousands of bird species (Cromie et al. 2000). Individuals that are exposed to mycobacteria may escape infection, develop a chronic infection, or develop progressive disease and die. Pathogenic mycobacteria survive and replicate within macrophages, in contrast to nonpathogenic mycobacteria that are rapidly killed by macrophages (Inderlied 1993). However, the role of birds' immune response in facilitating protection has not been determined, and that lack of knowledge places limits on uses of sensitive diagnostic technologies to detect mycobacteria in different species of wild birds (Cromie et al. 2000; Tell et al. 2001).

Hypotheses on the important factors in birds' immunological response to *M. avium* range from primarily cellular, to humoral, or perhaps a combination of both responses. Studies were conducted in captive waterfowl to monitor antibody indices in relation to tuberculous infections, determine the efficacy of a vaccine, and evaluate cell-mediated and humoral responses to the vaccine (Cromie et al. 2000). Antibody levels in Cairinini (perching ducks) rose significantly three to six months prior to death from *M. avium,* and vaccination produced a 70% reduction in deaths from tuberculosis in these ducks. However, the vaccine did not protect ducks in seven other taxonomic tribes. During challenges with *M. avium,* cell-mediated immune response to mycobacterial antigens declined but humeral response to these antigens increased significantly. It was proposed that wildfowl mortality from pathogenic *M. avium* may increase following excessive exposure over time to environmental mycobacteria, which may reduce cellular immune response to the harmful mycobacteria (Cromie et al. 2000). However, the role of birds' immune response in protection from *M. avium* remains to be determined.

PUBLIC HEALTH CONCERNS

Since 1980, in response to infections in patients with acquired immunodeficiency syndrome (AIDS), the study of the epidemiology of MAIC disease has led to development of new molecular techniques to identify and classify the MAIC complex (Tsang et al. 1992). There is now better understanding of the genetics of antimicrobial resistance, the interaction of the MAIC with the immune system, and experimental use of combination therapies (Inderlied et al. 1993).

The potential for transmission of *M. avium* to immunocompromised patients cannot be ignored. In 1991 in the United States, tuberculosis associated with MAIC occurred as a terminal event in 50% of AIDS patients (Daborn and Grange 1993). *Mycobacterium avium* serovars 1–10 occur more frequently in patients with AIDS than *M. intracellulare* serovars. Disseminated MAI complex tuberculosis occurs late in HIV/AIDS infections. In 1993 the average life expectancy of an AIDS patient with MAIC disease was seven months compared to 13 months in AIDS patients without mycobacteriosis (Daborn and Grange 1993).

Prior to the advent of AIDS, *M. avium* complex infections in humans occurred as complications of pneumoconiosis, silicosis, rheumatoid arthritis, neoplastic disease (Thoen et al. 1984), leukemia, and congenital severe immunodeficiency diseases (Kiehn et al. 1985). Now *M. genavense* and *M. avium* complex serovars 1, 4, and 8 are commonly isolated from immunocompromised humans (Kiehn et al. 1985; Tsang et al. 1992; Böttger 1994). However, only 14% of 4,452 cultures serotyped from human and environmental sources collected from 1982 to 1991 were *M. avium* serovars 1–3 or a serovar 1 and 8 mixture (Tsang et al. 1992). The geographical distribution of *M. avium* serovars in this study suggested that the human infections were acquired from the environment and probably ingested in water. Therefore, serotyping of mycobacteria from water is important in an epidemiological investigation of mycobacterial disease (Tsang et al. 1992).

The ultimate source of human infections with serovars 1–3 would be expected to be the natural hosts, chickens and wild birds, which excrete the organism in the feces, rather than *M. avium* infections from swine or cattle, in which infections are more often sequestered in lymph nodes (Meissner and Auz 1977). Evidence of direct transmission of mycobacteria from wild birds to humans is not available. However, a Green-winged Macaw (*Ara chloroptera*) was infected with *M. tuberculosis* by taking food from the lips of an infected person (Washko et al. 1998), so it is plausible that a bird might infect a human with *M. avium* in the same manner. *Mycobacterium avium* infections have occurred in avian and mammalian species that live in close contact with humans, such as commercial Emus (*Dromaius novaehollandiae*), Greater (Common) Rheas (*Rhea americanus*), chickens (Shane et al. 1993; Sanford et al. 1994; Thoen 1997), basset and mixed-breed hounds (Shackelford and Reed 1989; Kim et al 1994), miniature schnauzers (Eggers et al. 1997), and Siamese cats (Jordon et al. 1994). In the past decade, *M. genavense* has been isolated from canaries (Ramis et al. 1996), Budgerigars, parrots, finches (Hoop et al. 1993; Ferrer et al. 1997), and many species of zoo birds (Portaels et al. 1996). The knowledge that *M. avium* and *M genavense* cause illness in birds and mammals that are frequently in close contact with humans suggests that humans at risk should not be in contact with species with avian tuberculosis and should minimize direct contact with these pet species.

DOMESTIC ANIMAL HEALTH CONCERNS

The incidence of tuberculosis in domestic poultry has been reduced by management changes, but the incidence in some wild bird populations is now five to 10 times greater than in domestic poultry (Thoen 1997; Cromie et al. 2000). This incidence in wild birds could be a risk to poultry that are free ranging or less strictly managed. An increase in commercial farming of exotic species such as ratites in the United States and Canada could lead to development of tuberculosis in these species as well as increase the risk to nearby wildlife (Sanford et al. 1994).

The occurrence of *M. avium* in domestic mammals is sporadic, and infections usually cause localized lymph node lesions rather than generalized pathology; lesions are typically detected at slaughter (Thorel et al. 2001). Birds have long been suspected as the source of MAIC infections in domestic animals. The source of tuberculosis for swine is often speculated to be exposure to large flocks of starlings and sparrows that congregate around feeding troughs. In an early study, free-living birds that were associated with piggeries were found to be positive for mycobacteria and therefore considered a source of contamination for the pig feed (Popluhár et al. 1983). However, in more recent studies that compared *M. avium* strains in wild birds and slaughtered pigs in Brazil and the Netherlands, few pig isolates were wild bird strains (Ritacco et al. 1998; Komijn et al. 1999). Cows are thought to be exposed to *M. avium* by eating grass contaminated with fecal material from infected birds. Even though cattle do not develop active tuberculosis from birds, their frequent exposure to *M. avium* can lead to sensitization to the organism and problems in interpreting tuberculin tests (Rankin and McDiarmid 1969). *Mycobacterium avium* and *M. intracellulare* infections in domestic mammals generally are environmentally acquired, and the main sources include water, soil, contaminated litter, and compost.

There are rare reports of *M. avium* infections in horses, goats, and sheep, but reports of generalized infections in cats and dogs are more frequent (Shackelford and Reed 1989; Kim et al. 1994; Jordon et al. 1994; Eggers et al. 1997). These infections also have not been linked to direct exposure to birds.

WILDLIFE POPULATION IMPACTS

Avian tuberculosis occurs sporadically in wild birds and affects individuals rather than producing group mortality events. The disease may be under-recognized because individual dead birds escape notice or are removed by predators or scavengers. Individual dead birds often are not collected or not subjected to diagnostic examination. Mycobacterial infections are more often detected during epizootics of other diseases, such as avian cholera, that cause high mortality and involve collections of many birds. However, avian tuberculosis was reported as a contributor to a large mortality event in flamingos. An epizootic of bacterial sepsis in Kenya affected 18,500 free-ranging Lesser Flamingos (*Phoenicopteras minor*). Lesions due to *M. avium* serovar 1 were found in 40% of the flamingos examined (Kock et al. 1999). The frequency and duration of contact with other birds can influence the risk of infection. As with other infectious diseases, the potential for transmission of tuberculosis may be higher within gregarious species such as flocking birds or colony nesting birds. Ground-feeding species, particularly those that use wetlands or frequent areas with domestic animals, may encounter environmental bacilli. Predatory or scavenging avian species that feed on weakened or sick birds may be at greater risk of tuberculosis. A higher prevalence of mycobacterial infections in birds that frequent farms may be associated with direct and indirect contact with domestic birds (Rankin and McDiarmid 1969).

TREATMENT AND CONTROL

Treatment of avian tuberculosis is successful only in cases that are detected before the infection is systemic and widespread. Testing and treatment of wild birds has been limited to temporarily or permanently captive birds or individuals of endangered or threatened species that are brought in for rehabilitation. Treatment for avian mycobacterial infections with isoniazid, rifampin, ethambutol, streptomycin, clofazimine, and cycloserine is infrequent because drug treatment must be continued for 18 months or more, is very expensive, and involves constant exposure of other birds and humans to a very infectious organism. Antimycobacterial chemotherapy successfully used in the treatment of psittacines over a 10-year period is summarized by VanDerHeyden (1994) relative to the action, success, complications, and side effects of six drugs used in combinations of two or three drugs.

Control of avian tuberculosis in free-living birds is not considered feasible because the organism persists in the environment, is resistant to many anti-tuberculosis drugs and disinfectants, and it is difficult to identify infected birds. It would be impossible to test and eliminate all infected birds in a wild population. As long as some infected birds remain, the infection can be transmitted to other birds. The efficacy of vaccination as a control measure is unknown in most wild bird species and is not effective in several waterfowl species (Cromie et al. 2000).

To control avian tuberculosis in domestic poultry positive birds are usually destroyed and no treatment is recommended. Disposal of poultry after the first laying season reduced the chance of exposure to infection and reduced the number of older birds that became the source of infection (Thoen 1997).

Control of tuberculosis in captive wild birds can be attempted in several ways. Infected individuals or carriers can be culled or quarantined from the flock. All cages and pens should be decontaminated; ideally, cages should have an easily disinfected or wire bottom. Contaminated soil and substrate should be removed annually. Ponds can be drained and dredged following use by birds with mycobacterial infections. Any exposure between infected birds and free-flying wild birds should be minimized (VanDerHeyden 1994; Thoen 1997). Mycobacteria can easily be transferred between sites mechanically. Vehicles, coveralls, boots, shoes, and shipping crates should be cleaned after every use and any litter destroyed. All buildings and equipment should be disinfected with cresylic or substituted phenolic compounds in a 2–8% concentration to kill the mycobacteria (Thoen et al. 1984). Unfortunately, however, complete disinfection of natural outdoor substrates and wetlands is impracticable. The importance of crowding and direct contact with other birds as well as exposure to contaminated water or food should not be minimized during control efforts.

MANAGEMENT IMPLICATIONS

Avian tuberculosis is an important disease to consider in the management of long-lived species of free-ranging wild birds (Snyder et al. 1991; Brown et al. 1992) and captive wild birds in zoos and aviaries (Montali et al. 1976; Hillgarth and Kear 1979), as well as commercial exotic and domestic fowl (Pocknell et al.

1996; Thoen 1997). In free-ranging birds, management is limited to removal or dispersal of large perching bird concentrations and avoidance of large concentrations of water birds in moist wetland habitats.

Many wildlife species are raised in captive propagation programs to supplement or reestablish wild populations or stock animals for hunting. Birds maintained as breeding stock live longer, and their close contact with other birds increases the risk of avian tuberculosis. If infected, birds released into the wild could carry avian tuberculosis to free-living populations. Despite the difficulty of detecting avian mycobacterial infections, routine screening is of great importance to detect fecal-shed *M. avium* and to assess the health of wild birds held in captivity prior to their release.

UNPUBLISHED DATA

1. Diagnostic case records, U. S. Geological Survey, National Wildlife Health, Madison, WI, U.S.A.

LITERATURE CITED

Ackerman, L., S.C. Benbrook, and B.C. Walton. 1974. Mycobacterium tuberculosis infection in a parrot (*Amasona farinose*). *American Review of Respiratory Disease* 109:388–3990.

Bottger, E.C. 1994. Mycobacterium genavense: An emerging pathogen. *European Journal of Clinical Microbiology and Infectious Diseases* 13:932–936.

Brown, M.J., E. Lipton, and E.C. Rees. 1992. Causes of mortality among wild swans in Britain. *Wildfowl* 43:70–79.

Clark, S.l., M.T. Collins, J.L. Price. 1995. New methods for diagnosis of *Mycobacterium avium* infection in birds. In *Proceedings of the Joint Conference of the American Association of Zoo Veterinarians, Wildlife Disease Association, and American Association of Wildlife Veterinarians,* East Lansing, MI, U.S.A., pp. 151–154.

Collins, M. and E. Manning. 2001. Biology. In Johne's Information Center. University of Wisconsin-School of Veterinary Medicine. [Online.] Retrieved from the World Wide Web: www.Johnes.org/biology.

Cooper, J.E., L. Karstad, and Boughton. 1975. Tuberculosis in lesser flamingoes in Kenya. *Journal of Wildlife Diseases* 11:32–36.

Cromie, R.L., M.J. Brown, D.J. Price, and J.L. Stanford. 1991. Susceptibility of captive wildfowl to avian tuberculosis: the importance of genetic and environmental factors. *International Journal of Tuberculosis and Lung Disease* 73:105–109.

Cromie, R.L., M.J. Brown, N.A. Forbes, J.Morgan, and J.L. Stanford. 1993. A comparison and evaluation of techniques for diagnosis of avian tuberculosis in wildfowl. *Avian Pathology* 22:617–630.

Cromie, R.L., N.J. Ash, M.J. Brown, and J.L. Stanford. 2000. Avian immune responses to *Mycobacterium avium:* the wildfowl example. *Developmental and Comparative Immunology* 24:169–185.

Daborn, C.J., and J.M. Grange. 1993. HIV/AIDS and its implications for the control of animal tuberculosis. *British Veterinary Journal* 149:405–417.

Deng, R.G., S.X. Zhang, X.M.Li, F.Z. Mao, R.L. Wang, J.R. Cheng, J. W. Fu, and F. X. Yin. 1996. A survey of diseases of zoo animals in Ningxia Autonomous Region. *Chinese Journal of Veterinary Medicine* 22:13–14.

Eggers, J.S., G.A. Parker, H.A. Braaf, and M.G. Mense. 1997. Disseminated *Mycobacterium avium* infection in three miniature schnauzer litter mates. *Journal of Veterinary Diagnostic Investigation* 9:424–427.

Fedyanina, T.F., and V.T. Toropova. 1975. Tuberculosis in wild birds in Kirgizia; jackdaw, hooded crow, moorhen, rail, rook. In *Infectious Diseases of Animals and Problems of Natural Nidality,* A.A. Volkova (ed). Frunze, Kirgizskaya, SSR, USSR, pp. 117–120.

Ferrer, L.,A. Ramis, H. Fernández, and N. Majó. 1997. Granulomatous dermatitis caused by *Mycobacterium genavense* in two psittacine birds. *Veterinary Dermatology* 8:213–219.

Floerke, R. 1977. Reported cases of avian tuberculosis in California waterfowl. *California Fish and Game* 63:191–192.

Forbes, N.A., R.L. Cromie, M.J. Brown, R.J. Montali, M.Bush, and J.L. Stanford. 1993. Diagnosis of avian tuberculosis in waterfowl. In *Proceedings of the Annual Conference of the Association of Avian Veterinarians,* pp. 182–186.

Franson, J.C., and S. Little. 1996. Diagnostic findings in 132 great horned owls. *Journal of Raptor Research* 30:1–6.

Franson, J.C., N.J. Thomas, M.R. Smith, A.H. Robbins, S. Newman, and P.C. McCartin. 1996. A retrospective study of postmortem findings in red-tailed hawks. *Journal of Raptor Research* 30:7–14.

Frey, C.A., and W.A. Hagan. 1931. The distribution of acid-fast bacteria in soils. *Journal of Infectious Diseases* 49:497–506.

Friend, M. 1999. Tuberculosis. In *Field Manual of Wildlife Diseases,* M. Friend and J.C. Franson (eds.). U.S. Geological Survey, Biological Resources Division Information and Technology Report, 1999–2001, 426 pp.

Frothingham, R., and K.H. Wilson. 1993. Sequence-based differentiation of strains in the *Mycobacterium avium* complex. *Journal of Bacteriology* 175:2818–2825.

Gale, N.B. 1971. Tuberculosis. In *Infectious and Parasitic Diseases of Wild Birds,* J.W. Davis, R.C. Anderson,

L. Karstad, D.O. Trainer, (eds.). The Iowa State University Press, Ames, IA, U.S.A., 344 pp.

Grange, J.M. 1996. The biology of the genus *Mycobacterium*. *Journal of Applied Bacteriology Symposium Supplement* 81:1S–9S.

Gross, W.B., J.D. Falkinham III, and J.B. Payeur. 1989. Effect of environmental-genetic interactions on *Mycobacterium avium* challenge infection. *Avian Diseases* 33:411–415.

Hawkey, C., R.A. Koch, G.M. Henderson, and R.N. Cindery. 1990. Haematological changes in domestic fowl (*Gallus gallus*) and cranes (Gruiformes) with *Mycobacterium avium* infection. *Avian Pathology* 19: 223–234.

Hejlicek, K., and F. Treml. 1993. Epidemiology and pathogenesis of avian mycobacteriosis in the house sparrow (*Passer domesticus*) and the tree sparrow (*Passer montanus*). *Veterinarni Medicina* 38:667–685.

Hillgarth, N., and J. Kear. 1979. Diseases of shelgeese and shelducks in captivity. *Wildfowl* 30:142–146.

Holsboer Buogo, C., L. Bacciarini, N. Robert, T. Bodmer, and J. Nocolet. 1997. Presence of *Mycobacterium genavense* in birds. *Schweizer Archiv für Tierheilkunde* 139:397–402.

Hoop, R.K., E.C. Böttger, P. Ossent, and M. Salfinger. 1993. Mycobacteriosis due to *Mycobacterium genavense* in six pet birds. *Journal of Clinical Microbiology* 31:990–993.

Hoop, R.K., E.C. Böttger, and G.E. Pfyffer. 1996. Etiological agents of mycobacteriosis in pet birds between 1986 and 1995. *Journal of Clinical Microbiology* 34:991–992.

Ichiyama, S., K. Shimokata, and M. Tsukamura. 1988. The isolation of *Mycobacterium avium* complex from soil, water, and dusts. *Microbiology and Immunology* 32:733–739.

Inderlied C.B., C.A. Kemper, , and L.E.M. Bermudez, et al. 1993. The *Mycobacterium avium* complex. *Clinical Microbiology Review* 6:266–310.

Jordon, H.L., L.A. Cohn, P.J. Armstrong. 1994. Disseminated *Mycobacterium avium* complex infection in three siamese cats. *American Veterinary Medical Association* 204:90–93.

Kauppinen, J., E-L. Hintikka, E. Iivanainen, and M-L. Katila. 2001. PCR-based typing of *Mycobacterium avium* isolates in an epidemic among farmed lesser white-fronted geese (*Anser erythropus*). *Veterinary Microbiology* 81:41–50.

Kiehn, T.E., F.E. Fitzroy, P. Brannon, A.Y. Tsang, M. Maio, J.W.M. Gold, E. Whimbey, B. Wong, J.K. McClatchy, and D. Armstrong. 1985. Infections caused by *Mycobacterium avium* complex in immunocompromised patients: Diagnosis by blood culture and fecal examination, antimicrobial susceptibility tests, and morphological and seroagglutination characteristics. *Journal of Clinical Microbiology* 21:168–173.

Kim, D.-Y., D.-Y. Cho, J.C. Newton, J. Gerdes, and E. Richter. 1994. Granulomatous myelitis due to *Mycobacterium avium* in a dog. *Veterinary Pathology* 31:491–493.

Kock, N.D., R.A. Kock, J. Wambua, G.J. Kamau, and K. Mohan. 1999. *Mycobacterium avium*-related epizootic in free-ranging lesser flamingos in Kenya. *Journal of Wildlife Diseases* 35:297–300.

Komijn, R.E., P.E.W. de Haas, M.M.E. Schneider, T. Eger, J.H.M. Nieuwenhuijs, R.J. van den Hoek, D. Bakker, F.G. van Zijderveld, and D. van Soolingen. 1999. Prevalence of Mycobacterium avium in slaughter pigs in the Netherlands and comparison of IS1245 restriction fragment length polymorphism patterns of porcine and human isolates. *Journal of Clinical Microbiology* 37:1254–1259.

Koneman, E.W., S.D. Allen, W.M. Janda, P.C. Schreckenberger, and W.C. Winn Jr. 1997. Color atlas and textbook of diagnostic microbiology, 5th Ed. Lippincott-Raven, Philadelphia and New York, U.S.A., pp. 1395.

Kovalev, G.K. 1983. The role of wild birds and their ectoparasites (ticks) in the circulation and distribution of *M. avium* and possible formation of natural foci of avian tuberculosis. *Journal of Hygiene, Epidemiology, Microbiology and Immunology* 27:281–288.

Lairmore, M., T. Spraker, and R. Jones. 1985. Two cases of tuberculosis in raptors in Colorado. *Journal of Wildlife Diseases* 21:54–57.

Mackenzie, J.S. 1988. Wild Bird Diseases. Australian Wildlife, In *The John Keep refresher course for veterinarians, Proceedings 104,* Post Graduate Committee in Veterinary Science, University of Sydney, Australia, 952 pp.

McGarvey, J.A., D. Wagner, and L.E. Bermudez. 2004. Differential gene expression in mononuclear phagocytes infected with pathogenic and non-pathogenic mycobacteria. *Clinical and Experimental Immunology* 136:490–500.

Meissner, G. and W. Anz. 1977. Sources of *Mycobacterium avium* complex infection resulting in human disease. *American Review of Respiratory Disease* 116:1057–1064.

Mendenhall, M.K., S.L. Ford, C.L. Emerson, R.A. Wells, L.G. Gines, and I.S. Eriks. 2000. Detection and differentiation of *Mycobacterium avium* and *Mycobacterium genavense* by polymerase chain reaction and restriction enzyme digestion analysis. *Journal of Veterinary Diagnostic Investigation* 12:57–60.

Miller, J.M., A.L. Jenny, and J.L. Ellingson. 1999. Polymerase chain reaction identification of *Mycobacterium avium* in formalin-fixed, paraffin-embedded animal tissues. *Journal of Veterinary Diagnostic Investigation* 11:436–440.

Montali, R.J., M. Bush, C.O. Thoen, and E. Smith. 1976. Tuberculosis in captive exotic birds. *Journal of the American Veterinary Medical Association* 1969: 902–927.

Morita, Y., S. Maruyama, Y. Katsube, M. Fujita, E. Yokoyama, M. Inoue, T. Tsukahara, T. Hoshino, and H. Shimizu. 1997. Distribution of atypical mycobacteria in environments and wild birds. *Journal of the Japan Veterinary Medical Association* 50:407–410.

Panigrahy, B., F.D. Clark, and C.F. Hall. 1983. Mycobacteriosis in psittacine birds. *Avian Diseases* 27:1166–1168.

Pocknell, A.M., B.J. Miller, J.L. Neufeld, and B.H. Grahn. 1996. Conjunctival mycobacteriosis in two emus (*Dromaius novaehollandiae*). *Veterinary Pathology* 33:346–348.

Popluhar, L.J. Melter, M. Zupa. 1983. The ecology of mycobacteria on piggeries with incidence of tuberculosis. Folia Veteriniaria 27:57–65.

Portaels, F., L. Realini, L. Bauwens, B. Hirschel, W.M. Meyers, and W. de Meurichy. 1996. Mycobacteriosis caused by *Mycobacterium genavense* in birds kept in a zoo: 11-year survey. *Journal of Clinical Microbiology* 34:319–323.

Ramis, A., L. Ferrer, A. Aranaz, E. Liébana, A. Mateos, L. Dominguez, C. Pascual, J. Fdez-Garayazabal, and M.D. Collins. 1996. Granulomatous dermatitis caused by *Mycobacterium genavense* in two psittacine birds. *Avian Diseases* 40:246–251.

Rankin, J.D., and A. McDiarmid. 1969. Mycobacterial infections in free-living wild animals. In *Diseases in Free-Living Wild Animals,* Symposia of Zoological Society of London, Number 24, A. McDiarmid (ed.). Academic Press, London, U.K., 332 pp.

Ritacco V, K. Kremer, T. van der Laan, J. E. M. Pijnenburg, P. E. W. de Haas, and D. van Soolingen. 1998. Use of IS901 and IS1245 in RFLP typing of *Mycobacterium avium* complex: relatedness among serovar reference strains, human and animal isolates. *International Journal of Tuberculosis and Lung Disease* 2:242–251.

Roffe, T.R. 1989. Isolation of *Mycobacterium avium* from waterfowl with polycystic livers. *Avian Diseases* 33:195–198.

Sanford, S.E., A.J. Rehmtulla, and G.K.A. Josephson. 1994. Tuberculosis in farmed rheas (*Rhea americana*). *Avian Diseases* 38:193–196.

Schaefer, W.B. 1965. Serologic identification and classification of the atypical mycobacteria by their agglutination. *American Review of Respiratory Disease* 92:85–93.

Schaefer, W.B., J.V. Beer, N.A. Wood, E. Boughton, P.A. Jenkins, and J. Marks. 1973. A bacteriological study of endemic tuberculosis in birds. *Journal of Hygiene* 71:549–557.

Shackelford, C., and W.M. Reed. 1989. Disseminated *Mycobacterium avium* infection in a dog. *Journal of Veterinary Diagnostic Investigation* 1:273–275.

Shane, S.M., A. Camus, M.G. Strain, C.O. Thoen, and T.N. Tully. 1993. Tuberculosis in commercial emus (*Dromaius novaehollandiae*). *Avian Diseases* 37:1172–1176.

Smit, T., A. Eger, J. Haagsma, and T. Bakhuizen. 1987. Avian tuberculosis in wild birds in the Netherlands. *Journal of Wildlife Diseases* 23:485–487.

Snyder, S.B., M.J. Richard, R.C. Drewien, N. Thomas, and J.P. Thilsted. 1991. Diseases of whooping cranes seen during annual migration of the Rocky Mountain flock. In *Proceedings American Association of Zoo Veterinarians Annual Meeting,* Junge, R. E. (ed.). Calgary, Canada, pp. 74–80.

Sutton, J.B., and H. Gibbes. 1884. Tuberculosis in birds. In *Transactions Pathological Society of London* 35:477–481.

Sykes, G.P. 1982. Tuberculosis in a red-tailed hawk. *Journal of Wildlife Diseases* 18:495–499.

Tell, L.A., L. Woods, and R.L. Cromie. 2001. Mycobacteriosis in birds. *Revue Scientifique et Technique de l'Office International des Epizooties* 20:180–203.

Tell, L.A., J. Foley, M.L. Needham, and R.L. Walker. 2003. Diagnosis of avian mycobacteriosis: comparison of culture, acid-fast stains, and polymerase chain reaction for the identification of Mycobacterium avium in experimentally inoculated Japanese quail (Coturnix coturnix japonica). *Avian Diseases* 47: 444–452.

Tell, L.A., S.T. Ferrell, and P.M. Gibbons. 2004. Avian mycobacteriosis in free-living raptors in California: 6 cases (1997–2001). *Journal of Avian Medicine and Surgery* 18:30–40.

Thoen, C.O. 1997. Tuberculosis. In *Diseases of Poultry,* 10th Edition, B.W. Calnek, H.J. Barnes, C.W. Beard. L.R. McDougald and Y.M. Saif, (eds.). Iowa State University Press, Ames, Iowa, pp. 167–178.

———, 1998. Tuberculosis. In *A Laboratory Manual for the Isolation and Identification of Avian Pathogens,* Fourth Edition, D.E. Swayne, J.R. Glisson, M., W. Jackwood, J.E. Pearson, and W.M. Reed, (eds.). American Association of Avian Pathologists, University of Pennsylvania, Kennett Square, Pennsylvania. pp. 69–73.

Thoen, C.O., E.H. Himes, and A.G. Karlson. 1984. *Mycobacterium avium* complex. In *The Mycobacteria: A Source Book, Part B,* G.P. Kubica and L.G. Wayne (eds.). Marcel Dekker Inc., New York, New York, pp. 1251–1275.

Thoen, C.O., E.M. Himes, and J.H. Campbell. 1976. Isolation of *Mycobacterium avium* Serotype 3 from a white-headed tree duck (*Dendrocygna viduata*). *Avian Diseases* 20:587–592.

Thorel, M-F., M. Krichevsky, and V.V. Lévy-Frébault. 1990. Numerical taxonomy of mycobactin-dependent mycobacteria, amended description of *Mycobacterium avium,* and description of *Mycobacterium avium subsp. avium subsp. nov., Mycobacterium avium subsp. paratuberculosis subsp. nov.,* and *Mycobacterium avium subsp. silvaticum subsp. nov. International Journal of Systemic Bacteriology* 40:254–260.

Thorel, M-F., H.F. Huchzermeyer, and A.L. Michel. 2001. *Mycobacterium avium* and *Mycobacterium intracellulare* infection in mammals. *Revue Scientifique et Technique de l'Office International des Epizooties* 20:204–218.

Thorel, M-F. 2004. Chapter 2.7.8: Avian tuberculosis. In *OIE Manual of Diagnostic Tests and Vaccines for Terrestrial Animals,* 5th Ed. Office International des Epizooties, Paris, France. 2:896–904; also [Online.] Retrieved from the World Wide Web: www.oie.int/eng/normes/mmanual/A_00109.htm.

Tsang, A.Y., J.C. Denner, P.J. Brennan, and J.K. McClatchy. 1992. Clinical and epidemiological importance of typing *M. avium* complex isolates. *Journal of Clinical Microbiology* 30:479–484.

VanDerHeyden, N. 1994. Update on avian mycobacteriosis. In *Proceedings of the Annual Conference of the Association of Avian Veterinarians,* Reno, NV, U.S.A., pp.53–61.

Washko, R.M., H. Hoefer, T.E. Kiehn, D. Armstrong, G. Dorsinville, and T.R. Frieden. 1998. *Mycobacterium tuberculosis* infection in a green-winged macaw (*Ara chloroptera*): report with public health implications. *Journal of Clinical Microbiology* 36:1101–1102.

Wayne, L.G., R.C. Good, A. Tsang, R. Butler, D. Dawson, D. Groothuis, W. Gross, J. Hawkins, J. Kilburn, M. Kubin, K.H. Schröder, V.A. Silcox, C. Smith, M.F. Thorel, C. Woodley, and M.A. Yakrus. 1993. Serovar determination and molecular taxonomic correlation in *Mycobacterium avium, Mycobacterium intracellulare,* and Mycobacterium scrofulaceum: a cooperative study of the International Working Group on Mycobacterial Taxonomy. *International Journal of Systematic Bacteriology* 43:482–489.

Wolinsky, E., and W.B. Schaefer. 1973. Proposed numbering system for mycobacterial serotypes by agglutination. *International Journal of Systematic Bacteriology* 23:182–183.

Woodford, M.H. 1982. Tuberculosis in wildlife in the Ruwenzori National Park, Uganda (Part II). *Tropical Animal Health and Production* 14:155–160.

Yamamoto, T., T. Shibagaki, S. Yamori, H. Saito, H. Yamada, S. Ichiyama, and K. Shimokata. 1993. Polymerase chain reaction for the differentiation of *Mycobacterium intracellulare* and *Mycobacterium avium. International Journal of Tuberculosis and Lung Disease* 74:342–345.

15
Avian Chlamydiosis

Arthur A. Andersen, J. Christian Franson

INTRODUCTION

Avian chlamydiosis is a naturally occurring contagious, systemic, and occasionally fatal disease of birds caused by the bacterium *Chlamydophila psittaci* (formerly *Chlamydia psittaci*). *Chlamydophila psittaci* is comprised of a number of strains that produce a systemic disease in birds that varies greatly in severity depending on the strain and the host. Commonly, infection in birds results in mild to moderate clinical signs with recovery from clinical disease but persistence of infection. High death losses are rarely seen and may be due to infection with an uncommon strain for the host or due to secondary bacterial or viral infections. Infections of humans and animals with avian strains can occur, but secondary spread within nonavian species is usually limited and not a problem (Smith et al. 2005).

This chapter primarily addresses avian chlamydiosis in wild birds. Isolation of Chlamydia or serologic evidence of exposure has been reported in many species of wild birds, but infection is often inapparent and there are few documented instances of mortality. Chlamydiosis is most often diagnosed in wild birds in cases of epizootic mortality, during surveillance for other diseases, or when humans become infected with avian strains. Although apparently widespread in wild birds, little is known about the effects of Chlamydia on free-ranging populations. The disease is quite similar in commercially raised poultry and pet birds, and poultry findings will be used as examples when information about wild birds is lacking. A compendium of the disease and control procedures in pet birds has been published and includes information on the disease in humans (Smith et al. 2005). Updates of the compendium are available on Web pages of the American Veterinary Medical Association (see avma.org) and the Centers for Disease Control and Prevention (see www.cdc.gov).

SYNONYNMS

Psittacosis, ornithosis, parrot fever, Bedsonia, miyagewanella.

HISTORY

This disease originally was called psittacosis, but in the 1940s the term ornithosis was introduced to differentiate the disease occurring in, or contracted from, domestic and wild fowl from the disease occurring in, or contracted from, psittacine birds (Meyer 1941). At that time the disease partition was based on the assumption that, in humans, ornithosis was a milder disease than psittacosis. Now it is evident that the disease in humans contracted from turkeys and some wild birds may be more severe than that contracted from psittacine birds. These diseases are now all considered to be similar and the term avian chlamydiosis (AC) is preferred (Andersen and Vanrompay 2003). Avian chlamydiosis gained world prominence in 1929–1930 when outbreaks in 12 countries affected 800 people. It soon became apparent that parrots from South America were the source. Strict regulations on the importation of parrots were instituted in the U.S. and many other countries to curb the pandemic. Subsequently, psittacosis was diagnosed in wild psittacine birds in Australia (Burnet 1934, 1935, 1939a, 1939b). During this time, Leventhal, Cole, and Lillie (cited in Meyer 1965) independently observed small basophilic bodies in the tissues of infected birds and humans and suggested that they were the causative agent. Bedson and Bland soon established the etiological relationship between the basophilic bodies and the disease (cited in Meyer 1965).

For years after the first isolations from parrots and human patients, researchers believed that psittacine birds were the only source of chlamydiosis. Early attempts to determine whether other wild bird species were a source of infection were unsuccessful. Bedson and Western (1930) failed to infect pigeons experimentally. Eddie and Francis (1942) found no reactions by complement fixation (CF) in a serological survey of pheasants, partridges, and wild ducks.

Interest in Chlamydia in wild and domestic birds was renewed following successful isolations of the agent from nonpsittacine species in widely separated areas.

A chlamydial strain that was of low pathogenicity to its host was isolated in 1938 from Northern Fulmars (*Fulmaris glacialis*) on the Faeroe Islands (Rasmussen 1938). The strain was detected because it caused serious illness in humans handling the fulmars. In 1939, Chlamydia was isolated from two pigeons sent to the diagnostic laboratory of South Africa by a pigeon fancier who experienced a few unexplained losses in his flock (Coles 1940). These findings drew attention to the possibility that birds other than psittacine birds could be involved. In the years from 1942 to 1964, a large number of epidemiologic studies were conducted in many parts of the world. Most of the studies were undertaken following outbreaks in domestic ducks, turkeys, geese, pigeons, and pheasants. A number of the studies were extended to include wild birds in the area in attempts to determine the reservoir of the infection (Meyer 1965, 1967; Burkhart and Page 1971). During the same period, extensive surveys of feral pigeons were made in major cities worldwide. The results showed that most species of wild birds were susceptible to natural infection with Chlamydia and indicated that the pigeon could be an important reservoir (Meyer 1967; Burkhart and Page 1971).

DISTRIBUTION AND HOST RANGE

The geographic distribution of chlamydiae in wild and domestic birds is worldwide and the organism appears in a broad spectrum of orders, genera, and species. Kaleta and Taday (2003) compiled a comprehensive listing of reported infections in 30 orders and 460 species. The order Psittaciformes contains by far the most Chlamydia-positive bird species. This reported high rate of infection likely reflects the frequency of testing and psittacines' popularity as pets. The reported incidence in other orders of birds varied greatly depending on the likelihood that they would be tested. From the reported number of infections in other wild bird species, it can be assumed that all wild birds are susceptible to chlamydiosis.

The importance and perceived incidence of avian chlamydiosis in the past were directly related to the threat to humans. Humans primarily become infected from pet birds, domestic and feral pigeons, and domestic poultry (turkeys, ducks, and geese). Pet birds (psittacines, finches, canaries, and pigeons) are still considered the primary concern (Smith et al. 2005). Infections in domestic fowl or poultry are a distant second, with concern about them depending on how well chlamydial infections in these species are being controlled. Both the use of antibiotics in feed and the strict confinement housing of poultry may have helped reduce the incidence in many countries. Feral pigeons in cities receive some attention when numbers are high. Despite this, pigeons are not of major concern as a source of human infection.

Wild birds with chlamydiosis draw attention when die-offs are noted. These mainly occurred in pigeons, doves, gulls, geese, and ducks, species in which the carcasses are more likely to be seen because of their larger size or clustering as a result of flock behavior (Burkhart and Page 1971; Brand 1989; Franson and Pearson 1995).

Wild bird chlamydiosis deaths have included Collared Doves (*Streptopelia decaocto*) found in fields adjacent to a veterinary laboratory and in gardens in England (Gough and Bevan 1983; deGruchy 1983), Rock Pigeons (*Columba livia*) in New Brunswick, Canada (Goltz and Hines 2000), and a Gray Partridge (*Perdix perdix*) (Koppel and Polony 1959). Large numbers of birds were involved in an outbreak in North Dakota where more than 400 California Gulls (*Larus californicus*) and Ring-billed Gulls (*Larus delawarensis*) died during the summer of 1986 (Franson and Pearson 1995). This die-off took place on an island where few scavengers were present to remove the carcasses. Chlamydiosis also was diagnosed in Ring-billed Gulls at a different location in North Dakota during 2001–2003 and in Mallards (*Anas platyrhynchos*) found dead in a waterfowl mortality event in Montana in 1999 (NWHC, unpublished data).[1] Chlamydia was considered responsible for a large die-off of juvenile White-winged Doves (*Zenaida asiatica*) in July 1959 and again in July 1961 in the lower Rio Grande valley area of Texas. Following the outbreaks, many of the surviving doves had below normal body weights, indicating a weakened condition (Grimes et al. 1966).

Small numbers of birds are sometimes found infected with Chlamydia during surveillance programs or while looking for other diseases, and its impact may not be measurable. In a surveillance program involving tits, four Great Tits (*Parus major*) were found to have died from chlamydiosis (Holzinger-Umlaup et al. 1997). In Canada, Rock Pigeons were found to have died from chlamydiosis when examined in the course of a West Nile virus surveillance program (Goltz and Hines 2000). Chlamydia was isolated from tissues of a Bald Eagle (*Haliaeetus leucocephalus*) found weak and unable to sustain flight, and in an American Crow (*Corvus brachyrhynchos*) with tremors (NWHC, unpublished data).[1]

There are two known instances in which avian strains may have jumped to mammalian hosts and caused major outbreaks in animals, specifically in Snowshoe Hares (*Lepus americanus*) and Muskrats (Ondatra zibethicus) in Canada (serovar M56; Spalalin et al. 1966), and in cattle from California (serovar WC; Page 1967). Although DNA sequence analyses show that these isolates are very close to the avian strains (Everett et al. 1999a), they never have been isolated from birds or animals before or after the outbreaks.

ETIOLOGY

Chlamydiae are obligately intracellular bacteria belonging to the bacterial order Chlamydiales. They multiply in the cytoplasm of eukaryotic cells, forming membrane-bound cytoplasmic inclusions. Chlamydiae rely on the host cell for energy and the majority of their nucleotide-metabolizing enzymes. The life cycle is unique, having a growth cycle consisting of two major developmental forms. The elementary body (EB) is a condensed form, 200–300 nm in diameter, and suited to survival outside the cell. The larger reticulate body (RB), 500–1000 nm in diameter, is the replicating form and predominates throughout most of the developmental cycle. Replication is by binary fission typical of other bacteria, with the exception that chlamydiae rely on the host cell for nutrients. Intermediate forms are seen, ranging in size from 300 to 500 nm. These often are called dispersing forms or condensing forms, depending on whether they are a transition from an EB to a RB, or vice versa.

The genus *Chlamydia* was recently divided into two genera, *Chlamydia* and *Chlamydophila,* with three and six species respectively (Table 15.1) (Everett et al. 1999a). The genera correspond to the former species *Chlamydia trachomatis* and *Chlamydia psittaci.* The species and known hosts are listed in Table 15.1. The terms Chlamydia, chlamydiae, and chlamydiosis and the abbreviation *C.* are retained to refer to strains of both new genera, while the new genera and species names are used to refer to specific species.

All known avian serovars are now in the species *Chlamydophila psittaci,* which contains eight known serovars (Andersen 1997). The natural primary sources along with expected natural hosts are listed in Table 15.2. Six of the serovars have been isolated from birds and appear to be relatively host specific. The M56 and WC serovars were each isolated from a single outbreak in mammals and have not been isolated since (Spalatin et al. 1966; Page 1967). The natural hosts or the origins of these two serovars still are not known.

The typing of new isolates can be done using either serological or molecular techniques. The use of monoclonal antibodies or polymerase chain reaction-restriction fragment length polymorphism (PCR-RFLP) permits the rapid typing of most avian and mammalian strains (Andersen 1991a, 1991b, 1997; Sayada et al. 1995). The PCR-sequence analysis can not only identify the strain to which an isolate belongs but also show how it is related to other known strains (Everett and Andersen 1999; Everett et al. 1999a; Everett et al. 1999b). DNA sequencing also has the potential for tracking minor sequence changes that can aid in epidemiological studies.

Not enough isolates have been serotyped from wild birds to know whether the six known avian serovars are the main serovars in the wild birds, or whether additional serovars are circulating in the wild (Andersen 2005). However, the large number of isolates reported from more than 460 avian species suggests that additional serovars are likely to be circulating in birds. Increased use of serotyping will help determine natural hosts or reservoirs and host ranges. Serotyping will also provide information on the pathogenesis and virulence of the various serovars in each host. This information can facilitate control of these strains in both wild and domestic birds.

Table 15.1. Classification of Chlamydiaceae and hosts of the species.

Genera Species	Hosts
Chlamydia	
C. trachomatis	Humans
C. suis	Swine
C. muridarum	Rodents
Chlamydophila	
C. psittaci	Birds, Cattle, Muskrats
C. abortus	Ruminants
C. caviae	Guinea pigs
C. felis	Cats
C. pneumoniae	Humans, Horses, Koalas
C. pecorum	Ruminants, Koalas, Swine

Table 15.2. Sources and natural hosts of *Chlamydophila psittaci* serovars.

Serovar	Source	Natural Host
A	Parrots, Parakeets, Budgerigars	Psittaciformes
B	Pigeons, Turkeys	Columbiformes
C	Ducks, Swans, Geese	Anseriformes
D	Turkeys, Egrets	?
E	Pigeons, Ratites, Turkeys	Columbiformes?
F	Parakeets	?
WC	Bovine	?
M56	Muskrat, Snowshoe Hare	?

EPIZOOTIOLOGY

Over the years scientists have postulated a number of hypotheses to explain why chlamydiae have been successful in so many avian species, why sporadic outbreaks occur, and where the reservoir was located. Most of these researchers assumed that all *C. psittaci* isolates were similar, varying only in virulence, that they infected a wide range of hosts, and that the host cleared the infection following infection (Meyer 1965; Page 1967; Page and Grimes 1984; Grimes and Wyrick 1991). Research results at the time supported these hypotheses because chlamydial isolates were slow and difficult to propagate in the laboratory and serovar typing methods were not available until recently (Andersen and Van Deusen 1988; Andersen 1991a; Sayada et al. 1995).

Today we can conclude that chlamydial strains are very host specific, that in the natural host they produce a mild to moderate disease that rarely causes death, and that infection results in a long recovery period or persistent infection (Ward 1999). In addition, many strains are capable of infecting or being transmitted to other hosts, in which they may vary in virulence from no infection to severe disease and death. However, in a secondary host, persistence of infection does not appear to be a significant factor following recovery.

Although knowledge about transmission of Chlamydia in wild birds is limited, the extensive studies in domestic birds, psittacines, and pigeons provide facts upon which to base a number of new hypotheses. The worldwide distribution and wide host range suggest that transmission of the infection in nature occurs by a relatively simple process and that avian chlamydial infections in wild birds usually do not cause widespread mortality (Burkhart and Page 1971; Brand 1989).

The importance of Chlamydia in mammals as a source of infection for domestic or wild birds appears to be minimal. The direction of infection has usually been from the bird to the human or other mammal. There are few documented cases of human-to-human or mammal-to-mammal spread of an avian strain.

Experimental transmission can occur by most routes, including ingestion and inhalation of aerosol, as well as inoculation via the intramuscular, intracerebral, intravenous, intraperitoneal, and intra-air sac routes (Burkhart and Page 1971; Page 1959; Page and Grimes 1984; Grimes and Wyrick 1991; Vanrompay et al. 1994a; Vanrompay et al. 1995c). In nature the primary routes would be ingestion and inhalation (Tappe et al. 1989; Vanrompay et al. 1994a; Andersen and Vanrompay 2003). Transmission via infection of the eye, via the egg, and via external parasites must also be considered (Eddie et al. 1962; Burkhart and Page 1971; Page et al. 1975).

Ingestion of infected material and/or inhalation of infectious aerosols occurs readily when susceptible birds come in contact with birds that are shedding chlamydiae, or with locations that infected birds have contaminated. Infected birds shed chlamydiae in fecal material, nasal secretions, and eye secretions (Vanrompay et al. 1995c; Andersen 1996). The infection and shedding can occur for extended periods of time. In turkeys the lateral nasal glands, which provide moisture for the nasal membranes, have been shown to remain infected for more than 70 days (Tappe et al. 1989). Persistent intestinal infections also occur.

High concentrations of chlamydiae in the crop and crop fluids have been shown experimentally in herons and egrets (Moore et al. 1959), turkeys (Page 1959), and pigeons (Meyer 1965), and may serve as a source of infection. Oral transmission from parent to young can occur in species that feed their young by regurgitation of food from their crops. This is a common practice in pigeons, cormorants, pelicans, spoonbills, ibis, egrets, herons, and woodpeckers. Some passerine species feed their young by regurgitation for a brief initial period (Burkhart and Page 1971). Niducolous species (fed by parents in the nest) would have greater opportunity for infection from parents than precocial or nidifugous species (able to feed themselves when hatched).

Oral transmission is also more likely to occur in bird species that habitually feed together in flocks. Conditions that favor transmission include the feeding by aquatic birds in warm, shallow wetlands and mud flats that are heavily contaminated by feces. Other birds, such as the Columbiformes, pheasants, and House Sparrows (*Passer domesticus*), are ground feeders that may ingest food contaminated with feces. Avian species that are predators or scavengers may become infected through consumption of infected carcasses (Brand 1989).

Pathogenesis after ingestion was studied in turkeys (Page 1959). Chlamydial organisms of the virulent turkey serovar (serovar D) were enclosed in capsules designed to be released in the gizzard. Most birds showed no response for two weeks, and the disease at that time was similar to that seen following aerosol exposure. It was thought that a few birds developed an intestinal infection and secreted chlamydial organisms in the feces, and then exposed the other birds by inhalation of aerosolized chlamydiae. This study places doubt on the ingestion of chlamydiae as a major method of transmission.

Vertical transmission through the egg is not an efficient method of transmission within a flock, as the number of infected eggs appears to be very low. However, there are a number of reports of chlamydiae isolated from eggs of turkeys, chickens, wild geese, and ducks and these may explain the introduction of an infection into commercial duck and turkey flocks (Lehnert 1962; Illner 1962a; Wilt et al. 1972; Wittenbrink et al. 1993; Lublin et al. 1996).

Ectoparasites may harbor chlamydiae, but replication of chlamydiae within the parasites has not been demonstrated (Burkhart and Page 1971). Parasites could serve as mechanical vectors but it is unlikely that they are a major method of transmission.

Infection through the respiratory tract under experimental or captive conditions results in a high infectivity rate, rapid spread, and relatively high mortality, as demonstrated in turkeys (Page 1959), pigeons (Monreal 1958), and captive psittacines (Meyer 1965). Inhalation infection may be acquired via nasal exudates, expired aerosol droplets, fecal aerosol droplets, or dry fecal particles. Dense nesting populations in an environment of accumulating feces favor inhalation transmission. Inhalation of aerosol droplets is facilitated when humid, still air favors persistence of droplets in the air (Burkhart and Page 1971).

A number of factors will affect the success and the rate of transmission of chlamydiae. These include: (1) the susceptibility of the avian host; (2) the virulence of the strain for the host; (3) the establishment of persistent infections with periods of shedding; (4) stress; and (5) the environment (Burkhart and Page 1971).

Susceptibility to infection and disease is a function of age and the immune status of the bird. In general, young birds are considered more susceptible (Meyer 1942). Morbidity and mortality are higher at this stage of life. However, transfer of maternal antibody via the egg yolk may modify the infection in the very young and reduce the severity of disease in nestlings. Establishment of a persistent infection or an immune response in young birds will also reduce the severity of disease from later infections.

Differences in the virulence of a strain for various hosts have been recognized for more than 60 years. Northern Fulmars on the Faeroe Islands were found infected with a chlamydial strain that was of low pathogenicity to the fulmars but caused severe disease in the humans handling them (Rasmussen 1938). Humans conducting necropsies on wild birds, primarily Sandhill Cranes (*Grus canadensis*) and Snow Geese (*Chen caerulescens*), became ill with chlamydiosis (Wobeser and Brand 1982) and a strain pathogenic to humans also was reported from embryonated Snow Goose eggs (Wilt et al. 1972). In laboratory studies, the highly virulent strain associated with high mortality in turkeys is relatively avirulent for pigeons and sparrows but produces severe disease in parakeets (Page 1967). In the United States, over a large area in the South and Southwest, ratites have died from *C. psittaci* serovar E (Andersen et al. 1998). Serovar E is assumed to be endemic in one or more species of wild birds. The ratites apparently were unusually susceptible to this serovar, as no other birds in the area were reported to be affected. Routine serotyping of isolates will help determine the natural hosts of the serovars and the epidemiology of new outbreaks.

Chlamydiae often establish a persistent or chronic infection that can last months or years. Persistent infections have been well documented in humans, birds, and sheep (Ward 1999; Smith 2005; Papp 1998) and are thought to occur in most animals. They are usually infections with the chlamydial strains that naturally occur in that host. Birds can be clinically normal or show only mild clinical signs. Persistent infections increase the period of time for transmission of the infection to new birds and permit the transmission from the adult to the young.

Stress can also affect the immune system, resulting in increased susceptibility to infection. When stressed, persistently infected birds may resume shedding of the organism. Psittacine birds will often break with disease and shed chlamydiae following transportation and introduction to new housing or environments. For example, chlamydiosis with high mortality was diagnosed in captive Euphonias (*Euphonia violaceas*) and Amazilla Hummingbirds (*Amazilia amazilias*) that were transported to a quarantine facility (Meteyer et al. 1992). In wild birds, stress due to weather changes, nesting, migration, and food shortages may precipitate disease (Burkhart and Page 1971; Smith et al. 2005).

Certain environmental conditions favor transfer of chlamydiae. Moist conditions facilitate the survival of the chlamydial organisms in feces and the persistence of aerosols (Brand 1989). Aerosols can also form from dried fecal material on the ground.

CLINICAL SIGNS

Chlamydiosis has been observed in most detail in domestic poultry and pet birds, in which it can be acute, subacute, or chronic. Signs are nonspecific and include lethargy, anorexia, ruffled feathers, and weight loss or failure to thrive. Serous or mucopurulent ocular and nasal discharges, diarrhea, and green to yellow-green feces may be seen. In more severe cases, anorexia is accompanied by dark green feces and followed by dehydration, emaciation, and death.

Reports of clinical signs of chlamydiosis in wild birds are limited (Burkhart and Page 1971). Wild birds generally are reported to show minimal or no direct signs. Expected common signs may include respiratory distress and sudden death in acute cases, and conjunctivitis, diarrhea, weakness, ruffled feathers, tremors, and abnormal gait in more chronic disease. On the Faeroe Islands, sickness in fulmars was noted only after it was determined that women contracted chlamydiosis while processing young fulmars (Miles and Shrivaston 1951). Conjunctivitis is often seen in one or both eyes in pigeons (Coles 1940). In a schoolyard in Australia, infected parrots were observed to fall from trees and die within minutes (Burnet 1939a). Sudden deaths have also been noted in parakeets (Meyer 1942). A Red-tailed Hawk (*Buteo jamaicensis*) with signs of respiratory distress and diarrhea was captured in a wildlife management area. The hawk died the following day with extensive systemic lesions caused by chlamydiosis (Mirande et al. 1992).

PATHOGENESIS

The pathogenesis of chlamydiosis has been studied in domestic poultry. In turkeys experimentally infected by aerosol with virulent *C. psittaci* serovar D (Page 1959), chlamydiae were found in the air sac and mesentery within four hours after infection. At 24 hours post-infection, the titers in the lung and air sac were over 10^9 organisms per gram. At 48 hours chlamydiae were found in the blood, spleen, liver, kidney, and pericardial membrane, and at 72 hours chlamydiae could be found in the bone marrow, muscle, ovaries, and testes. At death, tissues often contained greater than 10^8 organisms per gram (Page 1959).

Turkeys were experimentally inoculated by aerosol with serovar B, which is associated with pigeons and has lower virulence in turkeys. Serovar B inoculated turkeys developed the disease much more slowly than those inoculated with serovar D (Vanrompay et al. 1995a). Chlamydiae were recovered from most of the same tissues, but not until one to six days later, and the less-virulent serovar B was not isolated from the intestine, pancreas, ovaries, or testes.

Turkeys were infected with serovar A from psittacine birds, as well as serovars B and D, and followed for pathological lesions (Beasley et al. 1961; Tappe et al. 1989; Vanrompay et al. 1995b). The type and distribution of the lesions were similar with all the serovars, with a few exceptions (Tappe et al. 1989). Airsacculitis and bronchopneumonia were more severe in turkeys infected with serovar A, and pericarditis was more severe in those infected with serovar D. Interestingly, with all three serovars the lateral nasal glands were infected through day 50. These glands supply moisture for the nasal mucosa and could be a source of aerosolized chlamydiae.

PATHOLOGY

The severity and distribution of lesions found in chlamydial infection is dependent on a number of factors, including the virulence of the strain, the susceptibility of the host, the route of exposure, the exposure level, and concurrent bacterial infections (McDonald and Bayer 1981).

Fatal infections with virulent strains in highly susceptible hosts produce necrotizing lesions in the spleen, liver, pericardium, and respiratory system. One of the most common macroscopic findings is fibropurulent serositis. Splenomegaly and hepatomegaly are often pronounced. In rare cases intense splenic vascular congestion leads to subcapsular hemorrhage and rupture of the spleen and may account for the occasional reports of sudden deaths.

Histologic changes generally are similar in most species but severity may vary. Consistent findings in psittacines include multifocal hepatic and splenic necrosis (Suwa et al. 1990). Splenic lymphocytes are markedly depleted and replaced by swollen macrophages. In the periphery of necrotic foci basophilic chlamydial inclusion bodies (both elementary and reticulate bodies) (Figure 15.1) can be seen in the cytoplasm of macrophages, hepatocytes, capillary endothelia, and bile duct epithelia. Inclusion bodies also may be found in the cytoplasm of cells in serosal exudates. Immunohistochemical staining can confirm the inclusions as chlamydial, and by electron microscopy chlamydiae in various stages of development are visible. Chlamydiae may also be detected without histologic lesions in sites such as intestinal epithelium and exocrine cells of the pancreas.

Mild to severe fibrinopurulent airsacculitis usually is present and fibrinopurulent pericarditis and/or conjunctivitis may also be seen (Suwa et al. 1990). As described in turkeys, multiplication of the organism in lungs causes a severe inflammatory response with destruction of tissue and occlusion of air spaces with cellular debris and fibrinous exudate (Page 1959). The heart may enlarge due to passive congestion and be encrusted with fibrin. Death may be caused by heart failure, with gross lesions of severe pericarditis, pneumonitis, perihepatitis, peritonitis, and airsacculitis, comprising an overwhelming systemic chlamydial infection.

Proliferation of lymphoid tissue around the bile ducts occurs early. As it progresses, bile ducts become compressed and plugged, and necrosis of the duct wall may result. Hepatic necrosis then occurs as the liver cells become infiltrated with bile. Large collections of hemosiderin in liver and spleen suggest erythrocyte destruction (Mirande et al. 1992; Vanrompay et al. 1995b).

In natural settings in which a host is infected by an endemic strain, lung tissues seldom show pathologic changes. However, air-sac membranes may be thickened and contain fibrinopurulent exudate. Often, natural infection occurs along with a viral, bacterial, or

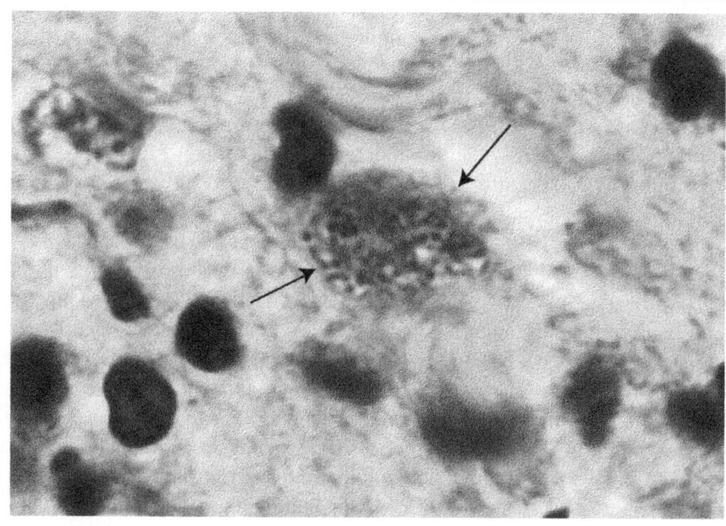

Figure 15.1. Chlamydial inclusion bodies in cell cytoplasm (arrows) in the pericardial sac of a White Pelican (*Pelecanus erythrorhynchos*) (Gimenez stain; 1000X). (Photomicrograph courtesy of Carol U. Meteyer.)

fungal infection, which increases the severity of the lesions (McDonald and Bayer 1981).

DIAGNOSIS

The diagnosis of avian chlamydiosis requires either demonstration of the organism or a four-fold rise in antibody titer along with clinical signs or pathological findings typical of the disease (Andersen 1998, 2004). Demonstration of the organism is usually the preferred method because it is more rapid and because paired acute and convalescent sera often are not available. Demonstration of the organism can be made by isolation and identification of the organism, or by histochemical or immunohistochemical staining of exudate, fecal or impression smears, or histologic preparations. Recently, enzyme linked immunosorbent assay (ELISA) and polymerase chain reaction (PCR) offer the potential of highly sensitive nonculture techniques; however, the specificity and sensitivity of these procedures need evaluation (Andersen 2004). Diagnostic test procedures and recommendations for avian chlamydiosis in domestic poultry are routinely reviewed and updated (Andersen 1998, 2004). These procedures would be the same or similar for wild birds.

Sample collection and handling will depend on the diagnostic test chosen. Samples must be collected aseptically because contaminating bacteria can interfere with some tests. In the live bird, pharyngeal and cloacal swabs are preferred. Eye swabs or scrapings should be taken when conjunctivitis is present. At necropsy the preferred tissues depend on the lesions present. Spleen, liver, air sacs, kidney, and pericardium are usually involved.

Isolation

Samples collected for isolation must be handled properly to prevent loss of infectivity of Chlamydia during shipment and processing. The preferred diluent, originally developed for Rickettsia, consists of sucrose-phosphate-glutamate (SPG). The medium recommended for Chlamydia consists of SPG buffer, which can be autoclaved or filtered (Spencer and Johnson 1983), with 10% fetal calf serum and antibiotics. In heavily contaminated samples the preferred antibiotics are streptomycin, vancomycin, and kanamycin (up to 1 mg/L each). Samples should be shipped to the laboratory on wet ice and should not be frozen if they can be processed in two to three days.

Isolation can be performed in either embryonated eggs or tissue culture. The avian strains are relatively easy to isolate and are commonly grown in McCoy, Vero, BGM, and L cell lines. Vero and BGM cells are reported to be the most sensitive for avian strains (Vanrompay et al. 1992).

During isolation of Chlamydia in cell culture, it is common to suppress cell division to allow a longer period for observation of infected cells. This also may provide increased nutrients for the growth of the organism. Suppression of cell growth is done by irradiation or, more commonly, by cytotoxic chemicals such as cycloheximide, 5-iodo-2-deoxyuridine, cytohalasin B, and emetine hydrochloride (Andersen 1998; 2004). The effects of these chemicals on growth of the Chlamydia can be variable, but they appear to enhance the growth of the avian strains.

Centrifugation of the inoculum onto the monolayer is routinely done to increase the infection rate (Andersen

1998, 2004). After incubation at 37–39°C, cultures are fixed and stained at appropriate times and repassaged if needed (Andersen 2004). When repassage is done, freeze-thawing should not be used to disrupt the cells because this will greatly reduce the Chlamydia titer.

Chicken embryos are still used for primary isolation of Chlamydia (Andersen 1998, 2004). In embryos that die from day 3 to day 10 after yolk sac inoculation, the predominant lesion is vascular congestion in the yolk sac membranes. Chlamydia must be demonstrated in dead embryos by direct staining of smears with appropriate stains, by producing an antigen and using it in a serological test, or by inoculation of tissue culture monolayers and staining with appropriate stains. If no embryos die, one or two blind passages should be performed.

Histochemical Staining and Immunohistochemistry

Chlamydia can be detected in smears of exudate and feces and in impression smears of liver and spleen using histochemical stains. More commonly used stains are Giemsa, Gimenez, Ziehl-Nielsen, and Macchiavello's. A modified Gimenez or PVK stain has been used in both smears and paraffin-embedded tissue sections (Andersen 1998). With this test the chlamydial elementary bodies (EBs) appear red with a green background. Interpreting these tests requires experience with chlamydiae because they will also stain other bacteria.

Immunohistochemical labeling is used with increasing frequency as a method to detect chlamydiae in cytological and histological preparations. The technique is more sensitive than histochemical staining, but cross-reactions with some bacteria and fungi may occur, and require that morphology be considered. The technique permits retrospective studies when formalin-fixed tissues have been saved. The selection of the primary antibody is very important because formalin will alter antigenic epitopes (Andersen 1998, 2004). With immunohistochemical labels, chlamydial antigen can be detected in liver, spleen, lung, intestine, air sac, adrenal gland, bone marrow, conjunctiva, and capillary endothelium of many organs and tissues as well as macrophages in areas of inflammation. Chlamydia also may be detected in sites without histological lesions, such as intestinal epithelium and exocrine acinar cells of the pancreas.

Enzyme-Linked Immunosorbent Assay (ELISA)

Most ELISA tests on the market detect all species of Chlamydia because they are designed to detect the lipopolysaccharide (LPS) or group-reactive antigen. The ELISA tests are rapid, require minimal experience to perform, and are relatively safe for the technician because the samples can be inactivated early in the procedure. A number of the ELISAs have been tested for use in detecting Chlamydia in birds (Vanrompay et al. 1994b); however, none are licensed for use in birds. Caution in interpretation of the results is needed because a high number of false positives can occur. Some of the Chlamydia LPS epitopes are shared with LPS epitopes in other Gram-negative bacteria. The use of monoclonal antibodies has reduced this problem in recent years; nevertheless, each ELISA test requires evaluation before use. Also, these tests lack sensitivity because a few hundred organisms are usually needed for a positive reaction. Most diagnosticians believe that a diagnosis of avian chlamydiosis can be made with an ELISA test when a strong positive reaction is obtained from birds with clinical signs or postmortem lesions of chlamydiosis, but the potential for false positive results must be considered.

Polymerase Chain Reaction (PCR)

The PCR techniques have promise as a highly specific and sensitive diagnostic test. A number of PCR techniques have been published for use in animals and birds (Hewinson et al. 1991, 1997; Takashima et al. 1996; Messmer et al. 1997; Everett et al. 1999b). Several factors must be considered when choosing a PCR test. The ribosomal DNA (23s, 16s, and intergenic spacer) and the major outer membrane protein (*omp*A) gene are the primary regions for which primers have been developed. Ribosomal DNA has multiple copies and, thus, improved sensitivity. However, cross-reactions with other microorganisms are more of a problem with ribosomal DNA. The *omp*A gene provides increased specificity, but the sensitivity is lower because the number of copies in the organism is fewer. Nested PCR procedures help increase sensitivity (Takashima et al. 1996) but require two PCR runs and increased manipulation of the DNA in the laboratory, which in turn magnify the risk of cross-contamination. Targeting a shorter DNA segment can also increase sensitivity (Hewinson et al. 1991), especially in poorer DNA preparations, because shearing of the DNA is less of a problem. A multiplex PCR has been developed that has increased specificity because it requires a match on two DNA segments (Everett et al. 1999b). However, sensitivity is limited by the least sensitive gene targeted. A TaqMan-based test has greatly increased sensitivity but requires special equipment (Everett et al. 1999b).

Serology

The complement fixation (CF) test is the most commonly used serological test in birds. It detects IgG antibody to the lipopolysaccharide antigen (group reactive antigen). Making a diagnosis of avian chlamydiosis

(AC) with the CF test requires a four-fold rise in antibody titer on serial samplings during the acute and convalescent stages of the disease. This is generally impractical with wild birds. A presumptive diagnosis of chlamydiosis can be made in a flock if the majority of the birds have high antibody titers and clinical signs typical of the disease (Grimes and Arizmendi 1996; Andersen 1998, 2004). Because of the limitations of serological tests, they are of little value in the diagnosis of AC in wild birds; however, they do have value in epidemiological studies for measuring the prevalence of infections.

Some newer serological tests will detect IgM, the antibody produced in the acute phase of infections. A presumptive diagnosis of AC can be based on a single positive reaction. These include the elementary body agglutination (EBA) (Grimes et al. 1994; Grimes and Arizmendi 1996) and the latex agglutination (LA) tests (Grimes 1986; Grimes et al. 1993; Grimes and Arizmendi 1996).

IMMUNITY

Our knowledge of protective immunity against chlamydial infections in birds is limited and must be extrapolated from other species. Excellent reviews have covered the immune response in humans and mammals (Brunham 1999; Rank 1999). Strong evidence exists that chlamydiae do induce immunity following infection. The organism elicits systemic and mucosal, humoral, and cellular immune responses. The type of immunity varies widely, depending on whether the infection is primarily at the epithelial cell level or is a systemic infection. When the infection is in epithelial cells, the immune response appears to depend on IgA and gamma interferon responses for clearance of infected cells (Rank 1999). Persistent infections normally involve the lamina propria beneath the epithelium. During persistent infection, chlamydiae may not be in a replication state and may express reduced amounts of the MOMP, which is the primary antigen to which neutralizing antibodies are produced. Instead, there appears to be increased production of antibody to the HSP60 antigen, which may be responsible for much of the chronic inflammation and fibrosis seen in persistent infections (Ward 1999).

Evidence that the MOMP is the primary antigen responsible for neutralization comes from research on *C. trachomatis* and *C. abortus*. The MOMP is approximately 40-kDa in size and has a similar structure in all chlamydiae. Sequence analysis shows that it contains four discrete regions that are highly variable and are responsible for variations in serotypes. Neutralizing monoclonal antibodies (Mabs) have been shown to be directed toward these variable domains (Rank 1999). In the case of the sheep abortion strains, the MOMP is configured as a trimer on the cell surface, which acts as a porin structure. The neutralizing Mabs are to this trimer (McCafferty et al. 1995). Cell-mediated immunity also contributes to resistance to *C. psittaci* infections, based on information from studies using the sheep abortion strain. Research shows that the level of protection following vaccination correlates well with the level of the delayed hypersensitivity response (Entrican et al. 1998).

PUBLIC HEALTH CONCERNS

The avian strains of *C. psittaci* can infect humans to cause disease that varies from mild and inapparent to potentially fatal systemic disease with severe pneumonia. Most human infection occurs through inhalation of infectious aerosols. Secondary spread of avian strains between humans is not a major problem, but has been documented (Smith et al. 2005). Precautions should be taken when handling infected birds or contaminated materials. Infectious aerosols can be readily created while handling birds or working in confined areas where dried bird droppings are present. Postmortem examination of infected birds and handling of infected cultures or eggs pose a particular human health risk (Rasmussen 1938; Wobeser and Brand 1982). Human infections can result from transient exposures such as entering rooms where infected birds had been held or cleaning infected cages. Persons working with infected birds or cleaning contaminated premises should wear protective clothing, gloves, disposable cap, and an appropriate respirator, and keep aerosols to a minimum by wetting the work area with water or disinfectant.

Because the disease is rarely fatal in properly treated patients, awareness of potential exposure and early diagnosis are important. The incubation period in humans is usually five to 14 days, but longer periods have been reported (Smith et al. 2005). Chlamydiosis symptoms in humans typically include an abrupt onset of fever, chills, headache, malaise, and myalgia. A nonproductive cough accompanied by breathing difficulty and tightness of chest are common. Although pulmonary involvement is common, auscultatory findings may appear normal or underestimate the extent of involvement. Pregnant women should be cautious because chlamydiosis can cause abortions. Tetracyclines are still the recommended antibiotics except where contraindicated, as for pregnant women and for children, for whom erythromycin appears to be satisfactory.

DOMESTIC ANIMAL HEALTH CONCERNS

It had long been believed that chlamydiae readily transfer from birds to mammals and back, and that the differences in disease severity were due to differences in virulence of the strains. With the ability to identify strains using PCR-RFLP or monoclonal antibodies, it has become apparent that transfer between birds and animals is not a major problem, although it can occur. Abortions in cattle due to Rock Pigeon–associated avian serovar B strain have been documented (Cox et al. 1998). In this case Rock Pigeons were often seen in the cattle feeding area. Clinical cases of chlamydiosis were documented in dogs that were in contact with pet birds (Gresham et al. 1996), or when the isolate was serotyped as an avian strain (Arizmendi et al. 1992). These cases were apparently self-limiting because no other animals in contact with the sick dogs were reported ill. Avian strains are not routinely isolated from animals.

The transfer of chlamydiae from wild birds to domestic poultry is assumed to occur, because the same serovars are found in both (Andersen 1991b, 1997; Vanrompay et al. 1993; Duan et al. 1999). During outbreaks of chlamydiosis in turkeys, strains with similar virulence were found in wild birds in the vicinity (Bankowski and Page 1959). Rheas that died of chlamydiosis, serovar E, were in multiple isolated flocks in a wide geographic area, making transfer between groups of rheas unlikely and transfer from local wild birds a more plausible explanation (Andersen 1998). Increased use of serotyping in the future will help determine whether there are links between infections in wild birds and domestic poultry, and also identify reservoirs of the avian serotypes.

WILDLIFE POPULATION IMPACTS

As with many infectious diseases, the impact of avian chlamydiosis on wild bird populations is poorly understood. The effects of chlamydiosis vary from being inapparent to causing severe disease and death. Inapparent or mild disease may produce signs that are subtle or difficult to measure, such as decreased fertility, weak young, impaired immune capability, or stress contributing to increased severity of other diseases (Burkhart and Page 1971; Brand 1989).

When chlamydiosis causes severe disease or death, sporadic cases involving low-level morbidity and mortality may go unnoticed because sick birds and carcasses can be rapidly removed by scavengers and diagnosis may be difficult. Recurrent outbreaks of epizootic chlamydiosis provide some of the most compelling evidence for potential population effects. For example, chlamydiosis was diagnosed in nesting gulls in three successive years in North Dakota (NWHC, unpublished data).[1] Although losses attributed to those events numbered in the thousands, the effect on the population remains unknown. Long-term surveillance and monitoring of disease and population trends in areas where chlamydiosis is frequently diagnosed may provide some insight into effects on local populations.

TREATMENT AND CONTROL

Treatment is not feasible for free-flying birds but may be indicated for individuals of rare species, groups in captivity, and during translocation or import quarantine. Treatment regimens have been described for pet birds (Smith et al. 2005). Individual birds requiring treatment should be isolated throughout the course of antibiotic therapy, which is usually 45 days. Doxycycline has been used in several formulations and by several routes in psittacines. It is recommended for use in drinking water (drug toxicity can occur) and orally in a syrup formulation. A European form of doxycycline can be given intramuscularly, and an intravenous form is available in the U.S. Chlortetracycline (1%) can be added to the feed. Poultry flocks are usually treated with chlortetracycline at 400 g per ton of feed (Page and Grimes 1984; Andersen and Vanrompay 2003). Acceptance of treated feed should be monitored carefully because chlortetracycline treated feed is unpalatable. Fowler et al. (1990) successfully treated raptors for chlamydiosis with oxytetracycline (50 mg/kg) injected into food items.

In captive flocks, control is dependent on quarantine and treatment, along with hygiene and disinfection. Incineration is advisable to decontaminate infected carcasses and waste materials. Rooms and cages should be cleaned thoroughly with water and detergent, and then disinfected with a commercial disinfectant(such as Roccal® or Zephiran®), or household products such as a 1% bleach solution, 1% Lysol®, or 70% isopropyl alchohol (Smith et al. 2005). Persons working with infected birds or cleaning contaminated premises should take biosafety precautions including the use of protective clothing and respirators and avoidance of aerosols.

In chlamydiosis outbreaks involving free-flying birds, control methods will depend on the species involved and federal and state regulations. In general, it is advisable to reduce the amount of infective material in the area by collecting and incinerating carcasses. However, on-site activities must be weighed against the likelihood of hazing infected birds away from the area and thus spreading chlamydiosis to new locations. Field personnel should wear protective gear and handle carcasses in a way to prevent contamination of the environment and avoid mechanical transmission of the organism on equipment and vehicles. The outbreak area should be closed to the public.

Because of its zoonotic potential, diagnosis of avian chlamydiosis may trigger varying degrees of governmental response, such as quarantine of birds and epidemiologic investigations, in many countries. Information on reporting requirements, recommended antibiotics, and other regulations can be obtained from animal and human health agencies for the region.

Recommendations may vary for different species or species groups. In the U.S., the Centers for Disease Control and Prevention and the American Veterinary Medical Association can be consulted for current recommendations.

MANAGEMENT IMPLICATIONS

Management actions that crowd bird populations together could be expected to increase the chances for outbreaks of chlamydiosis because stress may cause infected birds to shed the organism, and the close proximity of birds to each other will facilitate transmission. Because of the host specificity of chlamydiosis, a particular strain may be inapparent in one avain species but, when transmitted to another, may cause severe disease. Thus, programs designed for captive release or translocation of birds into the wild should incorporate quarantine, diagnostic evaluation of mortalities, and periodic testing of live birds as means to help prevent the release of birds infected with chlamydiosis. Individuals working with wild birds in the field and laboratory should be mindful of the zoonotic potential of chlamydiosis and should take reasonable biosafety precautions (such as the use of protective clothing, gloves, masks, and adequate ventilation) appropriate for handling apparently healthy birds or sick birds or for conducting necropsies.

UNPUBLISHED DATA

1. Diagnostic case records, U.S. Geological Survey, National Wildlife Health Center, Madison, Wisconsin, U.S.A.

LITERATURE CITED

Andersen, A.A. 1991a. Comparison of avian Chlamydia psittaci isolates by restriction endonuclease analysis and serovar-specific monoclonal antibodies. *Journal of Clinical Microbiology* 29:244–249.

Andersen, A.A. 1991b. Serotyping of *Chlamydia psittaci* isolates using serovar-specific monoclonal antibodies with the microimmunofluorescence test. *Journal of Clinical Microbiology* 29:707–711.

Andersen, A.A. 1996. Comparison of pharyngeal, fecal, and cloacal samples for the isolation of *Chlamydia psittaci* from experimentally infected cockatiels and turkeys. *Journal of Veterinary Diagnostic Investigation* 8:448–450.

Andersen, A.A. 1997. Two new serovars of *Chlamydia psittaci* from North America birds. *Journal of Veterinary Diagnostic Investigation* 9:159–164.

Andersen, A.A. 1998. Chlamydiosis. In *A Laboratory Manual for the Isolation and Identification of Avian Pathogens,* 4th Ed. D.E. Swayne, J.R. Glisson, M.W. Jackwood, J.E. Pearson, W.M. Reed (eds.). American Association of Avian Pathologists, University of Pennsylvania, New Bolton Center, Kennett Square, PA, U.S.A., pp. 81–88.

Andersen, A.A. 2004. Avian chlamydiosis. In *OIE Manual of Standards for Diagnostic Tests and Vaccines for Terrestrial Animals (Mammals, Birds and Bees),* 5th Ed. Office International des Epizooties (OIE), Paris, France, pp. 856–867.

Andersen, A.A. 2005. Serotyping of U.S. isolates of *Chlamydophila psittaci* from domestic and wild birds. *Journal of Veterinary Diagnostic Investigation* 17: 479–482.

Andersen, A.A., and R.A. Van Deusen. 1988. Production and partial characterization of monoclonal antibodies to four *Chlamydia psittaci* isolates. *Infection and Immunity* 56:2075–2079.

Andersen, A.A., and A. Vanrompay. 2003. Avian chlamydiosis (psittacosis, ornithosis). In *Diseases of Poultry,* 11th Ed., Y. M. Saif (ed.). Iowa State University Press, Ames, IA, U.S.A., pp. 863–879.

Andersen, A.A., J.E. Grimes, and H.L. Shivaprasad. 1998. Serotyping of *Chlamydia psittaci* isolates from ratites. *Journal of Veterinary Diagnostic Investigation* 10:186–188.

Arizmendi, F., J.E. Grimes, and R.L. Relford. 1992. Isolation of *Chlamydia psittaci* from pleural effusion in a dog. *Journal of Veterinary Diagnostic Investigation* 4:460–463.

Bankowski, R.A., and L.A. Page. 1959. Studies of two epornitics of ornithosis caused by agents of low virulence. *American Journal of Veterinary Research* 20: 935–940.

Beasley, J.N., R.W. Moore, and J.R. Watkins. 1961. The histopathologic characteristics of disease producing inflammation of the air sacs in turkeys: A comparative study of pleuropneumonia-like organisms and ornithosis in pure and mixed infections. *American Journal of Veterinary Research* 22:85–92.

Bedson, S.P., and G.T. Western. 1930. A disease of parrots communicable to man (psittacosis) aetiology—experimental observations. *Report: Public Health Medical Subjects* 61:59–107.

Brand, C.J. 1989. Chlamydial infections in free-living birds. *Journal of the Veterinary Medical Association* 195:1531–1535.

Brunham, R.C. 1999. Human immunity to chlamydiae. In *Chlamydia: Intracellular Biology, Pathogenesis, and Immunity,* R. S. Stephens (ed.). ASM Press, Washington, D.C., U.S.A., pp. 211–238.

Burkhart, R.L., and L.A. Page. 1971. Chlamydiosis (ornithosis-psittacosis). In *Infectious and Parasitic Diseases of Wild Birds,* J.W. Davis, R.C. Anderson, L. Karstad, and D.O. Trainer (eds.). Iowa State University Press, Ames, IA, U.S.A., pp. 118–140.

Burnet, F.M. 1934. Psittacosis in Australian parrots. *Medical Journal of Australia* 2:743–746.

Burnet, F.M. 1935. Enzootic psittacosis amoungst wild Australian parrots. *Journal of Hygiene* 35:412–420.

Burnet, F.M. 1939a. A note on the occurrence of fatal psittacosis in parrots living in the wild state. *Medical Journal of Australia* 1:545–546.

Burnet, F.M. 1939b. Psittacosis in Australia. In *Proceedings of the Sixth Pacific Scientific Congress* 5:349–351.

Coles, J.D.W.A. 1940. Psittacosis in domestic pigeons. *Onderstepoort Journal of Veterinary Science Animal Industry* 15:141–148.

Cox, H.U., P.G. Hoyt, R.P. Poston, T.G. Snider III, T.X. Lemarchand, and K.L. O'Reilly. 1998. Isolation of an avian serovar of *Chlamydia psittaci* from a case of bovine abortion. *Journal of Veterinary Diagnostic Investigation* 10:280–282.

deGruchy, P.H. 1983. Chlamydiosis in collared doves. *Veterinary Record* 113:327.

Duan Y.J., A. Souriau, A.M. Mahe, D. Trap, A.A. Andersen, and A. Rodolakis. 1999. Serotyping of chlamydial clinical isolates from birds with monoclonal antibodies. *Avian Diseases* 43:22–28.

Eddie, B., and T. Francis, Jr. 1942. Occurrence of psittacosis-like infection in domestic and game birds of Michigan. In *Proceedings of the Society of Experimental Biological Medicine* 50:291–295.

Eddie, B., K.F. Meyer, F.L. Lambrecht, and D.P. Furman. 1962. Isolation of ornithosis bedsoniae from mites collected in turkey quarters and from chicken lice. *Journal of Infectious Diseases* 110:231–237.

Entrican, G., J. Brown, and S. Grimes. 1998. Cytokines and the protective host immune response to Chlamydia psittaci. *Comparative Immune and Infectious Diseases* 21:15–26.

Everett, K.D.E., and A.A. Andersen. 1999. Identification of nine species of the *Chlamydiaceae* using PCR-RFLP. *International Journal of Systematic Bacteriology* 49:803–813.

Everett, K.D.E., R.M. Bush, and A.A. Andersen. 1999a. Emended description of the order *Chlamydiales*, proposal of *Parachlamydiaceae* fam. nov. and *Simkaniaceae* fam. nov., each containing one monotypic genus, revised taxonomy of the family *Chlamydiaceae*, including a new genus and five new species, and standards for the identification of organisms. *International Journal of Systematic Bacteriology* 49:415–440.

Everett, K.D.E., L.J. Hornung, and A.A. Andersen. 1999b. Rapid detection of the *Chlamydiaceae* and other families in the Order *Chlamydiales*: Three PCR Tests. *Journal of Clinical Microbiology* 37:575–580.

Fowler, M.E., T. Schulz, A. Ardans, B. Reynolds, and D. Behymer. 1990. Chlamydiosis in captive raptors. *Avian Diseases* 34:657–662.

Franson, J.C., and J.E. Pearson. 1995. Probable epizootic chlamydiosis in wild California (*Larus californicus*) and ring-billed (*Larus delawarensis*) gulls in North Dakota. *Journal of Wildlife Diseases* 31:424–427.

Goltz, J.P., and J.G. Hines. 2000. Psittacosis in Wild Rock Doves. *Canadian Co-operative Wildlife Health Centre Newsletter* 7:8.

Gough, R.E., and B.J. Bevan. 1983. Isolation and identification of *Chlamydia psittaci* from collared doves (*Streptopelia decaocto*). *Veterinary Record* 112:552.

Gresham, A.C.J., C.E. Dixon, and B.J. Bevan. 1996. Domiciliary outbreak of psittacosis in dogs: potential for zoonotic infection. *Veterinary Record* 138: 622–623.

Grimes, J.E. 1986. Chlamydia psittaci latex agglutination antigen for rapid detection of antibody activity in avian sera: Comparison with direct complement fixation and isolation results. *Avian Diseases* 30:60–66.

Grimes, J.E., and F. Arizmendi. 1996. Usefulness and limitations of three serologic methods for diagnosing or excluding chlamydiosis in birds. *Journal of the American Veterinary Medical Association* 209:747–750.

Grimes, J.E., and P.B. Wyrick. 1991. Chlamydiosis (Ornithosis). In *Diseases of Poultry*, 9th Ed., B. W. Calnek, H. J. Barnes, C. W. Beard, W. M. Reid, and H. W. Yoder, Jr. (eds.). Iowa State University Press, Ames, IA, U.S.A., pp. 311–325.

Grimes, J.E., T.D. Sullivan, and J.V. Irons. 1966. Recovery of ornithosis agent from naturally infected white-winged doves. *Journal of Wildlife Management* 30:594–598.

Grimes, J.E., D.N. Phalen, and F. Arizmendi. 1993. Chlamydia latex agglutination antigen and protocol improvement and psittacine bird anti-chlamydia immunoglobulin reactivity. *Avian Diseases* 37: 817–824.

Grimes, J.E., T.N. Tully, Jr., F. Arizmendi, and D.N. Phalen. 1994. Elementary body agglutination for rapidly demonstrating chlamydial agglutins in avian serum with emphasis on testing cockatiels. *Avian Diseases* 38: 822–831.

Hewinson, R.G., P.C. Griffiths, B.J. Bevan, S.E.S. Kirwan, M.E. Field, M.J. Woodward, and M. Dawson. 1997. Detection of *Chlamydia psittaci* DNA in avian clinical samples by polymerase chain reaction. *Veterinary Microbiology* 54:155–166.

Hewinson, R.G., S.E.S. Rankin, B.J. Bevan, M. Field, and M. J. Woodward. 1991. Detection of *Chlamydia psittaci* from avian field samples using the PCR. *Veterinary Record* 128:129–130.

Holzinger-Umlauf, H.A.M., R.E. Marschang, M. Gravendyck, and E.F. Kaleta. 1997. Investigation on the frequency of *Chlamydia sp.* infections in tits (Paridae). *Avian Pathology* 26:779–789.

Illner, F. 1962a. Zur Frage der Übertragung des Ornithosevirus durch das Ei. *Monatshefte für Veterinärmedizin* 17:116–117.

Kaleta, E.F., and E.M.A. Taday. 2003. Avian host range of *Chlamydophila* spp. based on isolation, antigen detection and serology. *Avian Pathology* 32: 435–462.

Koppel, Z., and R. Polony. 1959. Ornithosis in partridges (*Perdix perdix*). *Veterinary Casopis* 8:452–454.

Lehnert, C. 1962. Zur Frage der Uebertragung des Ornithose Virus ueber das Bruter bei Enten. *Berliner und munchener Tierarztliche Wochenschrift* 75:151–152.

Lublin, A.,G. Shudari, S. Mechani, and Y. Weisman. 1996. Egg transmission of *Chlamydia psittaci* in turkeys. *Veterinary Record* 139:300.

McCafferty, M.C., A.J. Herring, A.A. Andersen, and G.E. Jones. 1995. Electrophoretic analysis of the major outer membrane protein of Chlamydia psittaci reveals multimers which are recognized by protective monoclonal antibodies. *Infection and Immunity* 63: 2387–2389.

McDonald, S.E., and E.V. Bayer. 1981. Psittacosis in pet birds. *California Veterinarian* 4:6–17.

Messmer, T.O., S.K. Skelton, J.F. Moroney, H. Daugharty, and B.S. Fields. 1997. Application of a nested, multiplex PCR to psittacosis outbreaks. *Journal of Clinical Microbiology* 35:2043–2046.

Meteyer, C.U., R.P. Chin, A.E. Castro, L.W. Woods, and R.P. Gentzler. 1992. An epizootic of chlamydiosis with high mortality in a captive population of euphonias (*Euphonia violaceas*) and hummingbirds (*Amazilia amazilias*). *Journal of Zoo and Wildlife Medicine* 23:222–229.

Meyer, K.F. 1941. Phagocytosis and immunity in psittacosis. *Schweizerische Mediainische Wochenschrift* 71:436–438.

Meyer, K.F. 1942. The ecology of psittacosis and ornithosis. *Medicine* 21:175–206.

Meyer, K.F. 1967. The host spectrum of psittacosis-lymphogranuloma venereum (PL) agents. *American Journal of Ophthalmology* 63:1225–1246.

Meyer, K.F. 1965. Ornithosis. In *Diseases of Poultry,* 5th Ed. H.E. Biester and L.H. Schwarte (eds.). Iowa State University Press, Ames, IA, U.S.A., pp. 670–675.

Miles, J.A.R. and J.B. Shrivaston. 1951. Ornithosis in certain sea birds. *Journal of Animal Ecology* 20:195–200.

Mirande, L.A., E.W. Howerth, and R.P. Poston. 1992. Chlamydiosis in a red-tailed hawk (*Buteo jamaicensis*). *Journal of Wildlife Diseases* 28:284–287.

Monreal, G. 1958. Untersuchungen und Bcobachtungen zur Verbreitung und Klinik der Ornithose der Tauben. *Zentralblatt fur Veterinarmedizin* 14:78–80.

Moore, R.W., J.R. Watkins, and J.R. Dixon. 1959. Experimental ornithosis in herons and egrets. *American Journal of Veterinary Research* 20:884–886.

Page, L.A., and J.E. Grimes. 1984. Avian Chlamydiosis (Ornithosis). In *Diseases of Poultry,* 8th Ed. M.S. Hofstad, H.J. Barnes, B.W. Calnek, W.M. Reid, and H.W. Yoder, Jr., (eds.). Iowa State University Press, Ames, IA, U.S.A., pp. 283–308.

Page, L.S., W.T. Derieux, and R.C. Cutlip. 1975. An epornitic of fatal chlamydiosis (ornithosis) in South Carolina turkeys. *Journal of the American Veterinary Medical Association* 166:175–178.

Page, L.A. 1967. Comparison of "pathotypes" among chlamydial (psittacosis) strains recovered from diseased birds and mammals. *Bulletin of Wildlife Disease Association* 3:166–175.

Page, L.A. 1959. Experimental ornithosis in turkeys. *Avian Diseases* 3:51–66.

Papp, J.R., P.E. Shewen, C.E. Thorn, and A.A. Andersen. 1998. Immunocytologic detection of *Chlamydia psittaci* from cervical and vaginal samples of chronically infected ewes. *Canadian Journal of Veterinary Research* 62(1):72–4.

Rank, R.G. 1999. Models of Immunity. In *Chlamydia: intracellular biology, pathogenesis, and immunity,* R.S. Stephens (ed.). ASM Press, Washington, D.C., U.S.A., pp. 239–295.

Rasmussen, R.F. 1938. Ueber eine durch Sturmovogel ubertragbare Lungenerkrankung auf den Faroern. *Zentralblatt fur bakteriologie und Parasitenkunde. Abt.* I. Originale. 143:89–93.

Sayada, C.H., A.A. Andersen, C.H. Storey, A. Milon, F. Eb, N. Hashimoto, N. Hirai, J. Elion, and E. Denamur. 1995. Usefulness of *ompA* restriction mapping for avian *Chlamydia psittaci* isolate differentiation. *Research in Microbiology* 146:155–165.

Smith, K.A., K.K. Bradley, M.G. Stobierski, and L.A. Tengelsen. 2005. Compendium of measures to control *Chlamydophila psittaci* (formerly *Chlamydia psittaci*) infection among humans (psittacosis) and pet birds, 2005. *Journal of the American Veterinary Medical Association* 226: 532–39.

Spalatin, J., C.E. Fraser, R. Connell, R.P. Hanson, and D.T. Berman. 1966. Agents of psittacosis-lymphogranuloma venereum group isolated from muskrats and snowshoe hares in Saskatchewan. *Canadian Journal of Comparative Medicine and Veterinary Science* 30:260–264.

Spencer, W.N., and F.W.A. Johnson. 1983. Simple transport medium for the isolation of Chlamydia psittaci from clinical material. *Veterinary Record* 113:535–536.

Suwa, T., A. Touchi, K. Hirai, and C. Itakura. 1990. Pathological studies on chlamydiosis in parakeets (*Psittacula krameri manillensis*). *Avian Pathology* 19:355–370.

Takashima I., Y. Imai, H. Kariwa, and N. Hashimoto. 1996. Polymerase chain-reaction for the detection of *Chlamydia psittaci* in the feces of budgerigars. *Microbiology and Immunology* 40:21–26.

Tappe, J.P., A.A. Andersen, and N.F. Cheville. 1989. Respiratory and pericardial lesions in turkeys infected with avian or mammalian strains of *Chlamydia psittaci. Veterinary Pathology* 26:386–395.

Vanrompay, D., R. Ducatelle, and F. Haesebrouck. 1992. Diagnosis of avian chlamydiosis: specificity of the modified Gimenez staining on smears and comparison of the sensitivity of isolation in eggs and three different cell cultures. *Zentralblatt Veterinarmedizin* B 39:105–112.

Vanrompay, D., A.A. Andersen, R. Ducatelle, and F. Haesebrouck. 1993. Serotyping of Europe and isolates of Chlamydia psittaci from poultry and other birds. *Journal of Clinical Microbiology* 31:134–137.

Vanrompay, D., R. Ducatelle, and F. Haesebrouck. 1994a. Pathogenicity for turkeys of *Chlamydia psittaci* strains belonging to the avian serovars A, B, and D. *Avian Pathology* 23:247–262.

Vanrompay, D., A. Van Nerom, R. Ducatelle, and F. Haesebrouck. 1994b. Evaluation of five immunoassays for detection of Chlamydia psittaci in cloacal and conjunctival specimens from turkeys. *Journal of Clinical Microbiology* 32:1470–1474.

Vanrompay, D., J. Mast, R. Ducatelle, F. Haesebrouck, and B. Goddeeris. 1995a. *Chlamydia psittaci* in turkeys; pathogenesis of infections in avian serovars A, B, and D. *Veterinary Microbiology* 47:245.

Vanrompay, D., R. Ducatelle, and F. Haesebrouck. 1995b. Pathology of experimental chlamydiosis in turkeys. *Vlaams Diergeneeskundig Tijdschrift* 60: 19–24.

Vanrompay, D., R. Ducatelle, F. Haesebrouck. 1995c. *Chlamydia psittaci* infections: a review with emphasis on avian chlamydiosis. *Veterinary Microbiology* 45:93–119.

Ward, M. E. 1999. Mechanisms of chlamydia-induced disease. In *Intracellular Biology, Pathogenesis, and Immunity,* R.S. Stephens (ed.). American Society for Microbiology, Washington, D.C., U.S.A., pp. 171–210.

Wilt, P.C., N. Kordova, and J.C. Wilt. 1972. Preliminary characterization of a chlamydial agent isolated from embryonated snow goose eggs in northern Canada. *Canadian Journal of Microbiology* 18:1327–1332.

Wittenbrink, M.M., M. Mrozek, and W. Bisping. 1993. Isolation of Chlamydia psittaci from a chicken egg: Evidence of egg transmission. *Journal of Veterinary Medicine, Series B* 40:451–452.

Wobeser, G., and C.J. Brand. 1982. Chlamydiosis in 2 biologists investigating disease occurrences in wild waterfowl. *Wildlife Society Bulletin* 10:170–172.

16
Mycoplasmosis

Page Luttrell, John R. Fischer

INTRODUCTION

Twenty-three species of *Mycoplasma* have been described in avian hosts (Bradbury 1998). Most of these are found in domestic poultry, particularly chickens and turkeys, but 17 species also have been identified in wild hosts (Table 16.1). Five of these species have been isolated from wild birds only: *M. buteonis, M. corogypsi, M. falconis, M. gypis,* and *M. sturni. Mycoplasma gallisepticum* (MG), *M. synoviae,* and *M. meleagridis* are well-known pathogens in commercial poultry, causing substantial economic losses. *Mycoplasma gallisepticum* has been isolated from Wild Turkeys (*Meleagris gallopavo*) with sinusitis and from wild fringillids with conjunctivitis, most notably House Finches (*Carpodacus mexicanus*). This agent is the main focus of this chapter, but other avian mycoplasmas also are discussed. For additional reviews of mycoplasmal diseases of wild birds, see Friend (1999) and Wobeser (1997).

Mycoplasma gallisepticum

SYNONYMS

Disease due to MG is known as "mycoplasmal conjunctivitis" or "finch conjunctivitis" in passerines and as "infectious sinusitis" in Wild Turkeys.

HISTORY

Mycoplasmosis was first described as a respiratory disease in domestic poultry in 1905, but the causative agent, MG, was not successfully cultivated until nearly 50 years later (Ley 2003). Known as chronic respiratory disease in chickens and infectious sinusitis in turkeys, this disease is characterized by coughing, rales, sinus exudate, swollen sinuses (in turkeys), and airsacculitis. Serious economic losses occur from carcass condemnations, reduced feed and egg production, and retarded growth in juveniles. Prevention strategies include medication, live and killed vaccines, and farm hygiene and biosecurity. Prior to an outbreak of mycoplasmal conjunctivitis in finches in the 1990s, MG rarely had been isolated from free-flying wild birds, and the incidence of clinical disease was restricted to Wild Turkeys.

Wild Turkeys

In the early 1980s, MG was isolated from Wild Turkeys with infectious sinusitis in Georgia (Davidson et al. 1982), California (Jessup et al. 1983) and Colorado (Adrian 1984). All three cases were attributed to domestic sources that involved the intermingling and close contact between Wild Turkeys and domestic poultry during feeding activities. The organism also was cultured from a clinically healthy Wild Turkey tested during a disease survey in Texas (Fritz et al 1992). Health surveys conducted in western and eastern populations occasionally detected MG antibodies in clinically normal Wild Turkeys (Rocke and Yuill 1987; Cobb et al. 1992; Fritz et al. 1992; Hoffman et al. 1997). These incidents of overt disease and seropositive turkeys led to an increased awareness of mycoplasmosis in wild populations and to health monitoring protocols in Wild Turkey restoration programs that continue to be followed by state wildlife agencies (Davidson et al. 1988).

House Finches

In the winter of 1994, an epidemic of mycoplasmal conjunctivitis caused by MG began in House Finches in the mid-Atlantic states (Ley et al. 1996; Luttrell et al. 1996) and subsequently spread to the entire eastern population of House Finches within a few years (Fischer et al. 1997). Unlike the upper respiratory disease typical in domestic poultry and Wild Turkeys, MG caused conjunctivitis in House Finches that was distinguished by periocular swelling, crusty eyelids, and sinus exudate (Ley et al. 1996; Luttrell et al. 1996). Molecular analysis of MG isolates from finches demonstrated that a novel strain was involved in the epizootiology of conjunctivitis and that it

Table 16.1. *Mycoplasma* species isolated from wild birds.

Wild Avian Host	*Mycoplasma* Species Isolated	Associated Disease	Reference
Anseriformes			
Northern Shoveler (*Anas clypeata*)	*Anatis*	None reported	Poveda et al. 1990a
Mallard (*Anas playtrhynchos*)	*anatis*	Reduced hatchling size/growth	Goldberg et al. 1995; Samuel et al. 1995
	cloacale	None reported	Goldberg et al. 1995
Canvasback (*Aythya valisineria*)	*cloacale*	None reported	Goldberg et al. 1995
Black Duck (*Anas rubripes*)	*anatis*	None reported	Goldberg et al. 1995
	cloacale	None reported	Goldberg et al. 1995
Gadwall (*Anas strepera*)	*anatis*	None reported	Goldberg et al. 1995
Ciconiiformes			
Black Vulture (*Coragyps atratus*)	*corogypsi*	Footpad abscess	Panangala et al. 1993
Falconiformes			
Common Buzzard (*Buteo buteo*)	*buteonis*	Respiratory	Poveda et al. 1994
Peregrine Falcon (*Falco peregrinus*)	*columborale*	None reported	Poveda et al. 1990b
	gallinarum	None reported	Poveda et al. 1990a
	gallinaceum	None reported	Poveda et al. 1990a
	gallisepticum	Respiratory	Poveda et al. 1990a
	iners	None reported	Poveda et al. 1990a
Saker Falcon (*Falco cherrug*)	*anatis*	None reported	Poveda et al. 1990b
	buteonis	Respiratory	Forsyth et al. 1996
	falconis	Skeletal deformity	Erdelyi et al. 1999
Cinereous Vulture (*Aegypius monachus*)	*gallinarum*	None reported	Poveda et al. 1990b
Griffon Vulture (*Gyps fulvus*)	*gypis*	Respiratory	Poveda et al. 1994
Galliformes			
Chukar (*Alectoris chukar*)	*gallisepticum*	Respiratory	Cookson and Shivaprasad 1994
Ring-necked Pheasant (*Phasianus colchicus*)	*gallisepticum*	Respiratory	Cookson and Shivaprasad 1994; Osborn and Pomeroy 1985

Wild Turkey (*Meleagris gallopavo*)	*gallinaceum*	None reported	Hoffman et al. 1997
	gallinarum	None reported	Hoffman et al. 1997
	gallisepticum	Respiratory	Adrian 1984; Davidson et al. 1982; Fritz et al. 1992; Jessup et al. 1983
	gallopavonis	None reported	Luttrell et al. 1992b
	pullorum	None reported	Hoffman et al. 1997
	synoviae	Respiratory	Fritz et al. 1992; Luttrell et al. 1992a
Northern Bobwhite (*Colinus virginianus*)	*gallisepticum*	Respiratory	Madden et al. 1967
Gruiformes			
Common Coot (*Fulica atra*)	*anatis*	None reported	Poveda et al. 1990a
Columbiformes			
Rock Pigeon (*Columba livia*)	*columborale*	Respiratory	Kleven 1997
	columbinasale	None reported	Kleven 1997
	columbinum	Respiratory	Kleven 1997
	gallinaceum	None reported	Poveda et al. 1990a
	iners	None reported	Poveda et al. 1990a
	pullorum	None reported	Poveda et al. 1990a
Dove (*Streptopelia* sp.)	*gallisepticum*	None reported	Jain et al. 1971
Passeriformes			
Blue Jay (*Cyanocitta cristata*)	*sturni*	Conjunctivitis	Ley et al. 1998
Northern Mockingbird (*Mimus polyglottos*)	*sturni*	Conjunctivitis	Ley et al. 1998
European Starling (*Sturnus vulgaris*)	*sturni*	Conjunctivitis	Forsyth et al. 1996
House Finch (*Carpodacus mexicanus*)	*gallisepticum*	Conjunctivitis	Ley et al. 1996; Luttrell et al. 1996
Purple Finch (*Carodacus purpureus*)	*gallisepticum*	Conjunctivitis	Hartup et al. 2000
American Goldfinch (*Carduelis tristis*)	*gallisepticum*	Conjunctivitis	Fischer et al. 1997; Ley et al. 1997
Evening Grosbeak (*Coccothraustes vespertinus*)	*gallisepticum*	Conjunctivitis	Mikaelian et al. 2001
Pine Grosbeak (*Pinicola enucleator*)	*gallisepticum*	Conjunctivitis	Mikaelian et al. 2001
House Sparrow (*Passer domesticus*)	*gallisepticum*	None reported	Jain et al. 1971
	synoviae	None reported	Poveda et al. 1990a
Tree Sparrow (*Passer montanus*)	*gallisepticum*	None reported	Shimizu et al. 1979

differed from poultry strains (Ley et al. 1997). The source of this epidemic in free-flying finches remains unknown.

DISTRIBUTION

Wild Turkeys

Clinical disease caused by MG is rare in free-ranging Wild Turkeys in the United States. Isolated cases have occurred in Georgia (Davidson et al. 1982), California (Jessup et al. 1983), Colorado (Adrian 1984), and Texas (Fritz et al.1992). Serologic surveys conducted in Wild Turkeys from the eastern United States have shown little MG activity (Davidson et al. 1988; Hopkins et al. 1990). In contrast, clinically normal Wild Turkeys from western states often have been seropositive for MG and *M. synoviae* (Rocke and Yuill 1987; Fritz et al. 1992; Hoffman et al. 1997), and these organisms occasionally have been isolated during surveys of Wild Turkeys (Fritz et al. 1992).

House Finches

Mycoplasmal conjunctivitis has been reported in House Finches from every state in their eastern population range. Although not confirmed by culture in every state, clinical signs of conjunctivitis have been observed in House Finches from Maine to Georgia and westward to include states in the Great Plains from Texas to North Dakota (Fischer et al. 1997; Hartup et al. 2001a). Mycoplasmal conjunctivitis also has been reported in clinically ill finches from the Canadian provinces of Quebec and Ontario (Fischer et al. 1997; Mikaelian et al. 2001). In 2002, mycoplasmosis was observed in House Finches in Montana, and MG was confirmed by PCR and culture (Duckworth et al. 2003). This case marks the first time MG has been isolated from House Finches in their native range and indicates that the eastern and western populations may overlap in certain locations.

HOST RANGE

Mycoplasma gallisepticum primarily occurs in gallinaceous birds, particularly domestic chickens, wild and domestic turkeys, and pen-raised game birds (Ley 2003). Prior to the epidemic of finch conjunctivitis, reports of MG in wild passerines were rare (Jain et al. 1971; Shimizu et al 1979). In the 1990s, MG emerged as a new pathogen in free-ranging finches and now appears to be endemic in many eastern populations of House Finches and apparently is continuing a westward spread (Duckworth et al. 2003). Since the spread of MG through eastern House Finches, the organism also has been isolated from small numbers of other fringillid species with conjunctivitis. These include the American Goldfinch (*Carduelis tristis*) (Fischer et al. 1997; Ley et al. 1997), Purple Finch (*Carpodacus purpureus*) (Hartup et al. 2000), Pine Grosbeak (*Pinicola enucleator*), and Evening Grosbeak (*Coccothraustes vespertinus*) (Mikaelian et al. 2001).

ETIOLOGY

Mycoplasma gallisepticum belongs to the family Mycoplasmataceae in the class Mollicutes ("soft skin," from Latin), recognized as the smallest self-replicating prokaryotes (Razin 1992). Distinctive characteristics include the lack of cell walls, highly variable surface proteins, and a very small genome. This group of bacteria infects a broad range of hosts, including humans, animals, plants, and insects. Mycoplasmas generally are host and tissue specific and primarily infect muscosal surfaces of the respiratory, urinary, and reproductive systems. Most species exist commensally in their hosts as asymptomatic or mild infections. Pathogenic mycoplasmas can cause a range of conditions from mild to acute symptoms and usually form a synergistic complex in conjunction with other bacteria, viruses, or environmental stresses affecting the host.

As with many mycoplasmas, MG is a fastidious organism that requires a complex selective medium enriched with 10–15% animal serum, dextrose, and a yeast source. It is typically grown in liquid media with a phenol red growth-indicator and then plated on agar for identification. Growth occurs at an optimum temperature of 37°C. Although highly pleomorphic, MG colonies grown on agar plates typically appear as smooth, rounded translucent masses about 0.2–0.3 mm in diameter, with dense raised, centers, sometimes described as "fried eggs" (Ley 2003).

Mycoplasma gallisepticum is capable of rapid changes in its major surface proteins, a characteristic that contributes to the production of a wide range of strain variability and pathogenicity (Levisohn and Kleven 2000; Ley 2003). The MG strains may exhibit a range of host and tissue trophism and vary in levels of immunogenicity and modes of transmission. For example, the finch strain differs from most poultry strains by its proclivity for the orbital and sinus regions in fringillid hosts (Ley et al. 1997; Luttrell et al. 1998). Atypical strains that are characterized by low immunogenicity and transmissibility may cause very mild reactions and can be difficult to isolate. Some of these variant strains, such as ts-11 and F strain, have been used to produce live vaccines for use in commercial poultry (Ley 2003). The possible adaptation of mycoplasmas to new hosts may to lead to specific genotypic changes that could generate new strains or variants of pathogens. This may have been a factor in the emergence of the finch strain of MG.

The advent of molecular techniques has aided in the ability to identify species of mycoplasmal isolates from domestic and wild birds and to distinguish strains, thereby determining the sources of outbreaks. Detection of MG may be accomplished by use of species-specific DNA probes or by polymerase chain reaction (PCR) techniques (Ley et al. 1997; Lauerman 1998). Strain differentiation may be achieved with serologic techniques, electrophoretic separation of proteins or molecular procedures such as restriction fragment length polymorphism, arbitrary primed PCR, and DNA sequencing (Razin 1992; Levisohn and Kleven 2000; Liu et al. 2001). In a molecular typing study that targeted an adhesin protein of MG, some discrepancies were detected between a House Finch isolate from Texas and those from several eastern states (Liu et al. 2001). This study suggests that additional MG strains could be circulating in wild House Finches, but it is also possible that the finch strain is evolving since its adaptation to a new host and spread through wild populations (Roberts et al. 2001b; Hartup et al. 2001b).

EPIZOOTIOLOGY

The primary modes of MG transmission are horizontal, through direct contact or aerosol droplets between a carrier and a susceptible bird, and vertical, via eggs in chickens and turkeys (Ley 2003). Infection of the reproductive tract occurs through the proximity of the oviduct to abdominal air sacs (Levisohn and Kleven 2000). Field studies indicate that transmission occurs between infected adult House Finches and their offspring (Hartup and Kollias 1999; Luttrell, unpublished data), but in ovo transmission among finches has not been documented.

Mycoplasma gallisepticum is maintained primarily through avian reservoirs; domestic birds in commercial or backyard flocks as well as individuals in free-flying populations may serve as foci of infection or act as nonclinical carriers of MG. Although a fragile organism, MG can exist for short periods of time on substrates such as dust, litter, feathers, rubber boots, and clothing, so mechanical transfer also may be possible (Christensen et al. 1994). Contaminated litter and feathers may pose risks of transmission to free-ranging wild birds that visit poultry farms for feeding or nesting opportunities (Stallknecht et al. 1982; Luttrell et al. 2001). House finches and other wild birds could be exposed to MG via contaminated feeders. An evaluation of several types of backyard bird feeders indicated that tube-style feeders promote direct contact between birds competing for access and may provide contaminated feeding surfaces (Hartup et al. 1998).

Transmission of mycoplasmas is largely dependent on contact between infected and susceptible hosts and therefore is facilitated by situations in which birds are living in concentrated numbers. Under such conditions, MG can spread rapidly and infect a high proportion of exposed birds. In studies involving natural infections of MG in captive House Finches, conjunctivitis spread to 60 to 90% of flocks within two weeks (Luttrell et al. 1998; Roberts et al. 2001a). MG-related declines of House Finch populations have occurred predominantly in areas where their densities were high, such as some northeastern and mid-Atlantic states. In contrast, House Finch numbers have remained stable in locations where the initial population levels were lower and more dispersed, suggesting that transmission is population density dependent (Hochachka and Dhondt 2000).

Avian mycoplasmosis can occur at any time of the year but generally has a higher prevalence in the winter among domestic flocks (Ley 2003) and possibly Wild Turkeys (Jessup et al. 1983; Adrian 1984). Seasonal fluctuations in the prevalence of MG in House Finches may vary in different regions. Peaks in conjunctivitis are observed in late summer and early fall in southeastern states (Roberts et al. 2001b), but northeastern states report a higher prevalence in the winter months (Hartup et al. 2001b). Factors relating to these patterns are increases in susceptible juveniles after the breeding season, stress from molting, migratory behavior, social interactions, and unfavorable environmental conditions (Hartup et al. 2001b; Roberts et al. 2001b). Clinically affected birds of both sexes have been observed, although nonbreeding males appear to experience a higher level of infection during the breeding season (Hartup et al. 2001b). Plumage coloration in male House Finches may be negatively affected by MG infections (Brawner et al. 2001).

Various surveys of eastern and western populations of Wild Turkeys have revealed some differences in the prevalence of MG antibodies. Serologic surveys of western Wild Turkeys show a greater prevalence of seropositive birds (Fritz et al. 1992; Hoffman et al. 1997) than those of eastern populations (Davidson et al. 1988; Hopkins et al. 1990). This may be due to their propensity to gather in large winter flocks and mingle with domestic fowl on ranches or private property to take advantage of available food supplies (Adrian 1984; Rocke and Yuill 1987; Hoffman et al. 1997).

The infrequent occurrences of MG in Wild Turkeys have been associated with a domestic source, particularly backyard poultry, but there are no published descriptions of DNA fingerprinting of Wild Turkey isolates. The source of MG in the eastern population of House Finches is unknown. Unless there is a possible wild reservoir, House Finches may have received exposure to MG via direct contact with infected domestic birds or through MG-contaminated litter (Stallknecht et al. 1982).

CLINICAL SIGNS

Wild Turkeys

Wild Turkeys exhibit clinical signs similar to those of domestic turkeys with MG infections (Ley 2003). Periorbital sinuses on one or both sides of the head may become swollen, and vision may be impaired if swelling is severe. Other symptoms include nasal discharge, sneezing, moist rales, and difficulty in breathing. Depression and weight loss also may occur.

House Finches

In House Finches, MG causes mild to severe eyelid swelling, conjunctivitis, and watery discharge from one or both eyes and/or nares (Figure 16.1) (Ley et al. 1996; Luttrell et al. 1996; Kollias et al. 2004). Crusty lesions typically form on eyelids and nares, probably due to dried discharge. Impaired vision or blindness may develop as a result of these lesions. In severe cases, general debilitation, depression, and weight loss may occur (Luttrell et al. 1998). Upper respiratory signs such as coughing, sneezing, and rales usually are not present. Birds may become more susceptible to trauma or predation and be reluctant to fly from feeders.

PATHOGENESIS

Mycoplasma gallisepticum causes acute or chronic disease in birds and often works synergistically with other pathogenic mycoplasmas, bacteria, or viruses to create more severe clinical disease (Kleven 1998; Ley 2003). Lack of adequate nutrition, extreme temperatures, and environmental stresses also may play a role in increasing the pathogenic effects on the host.

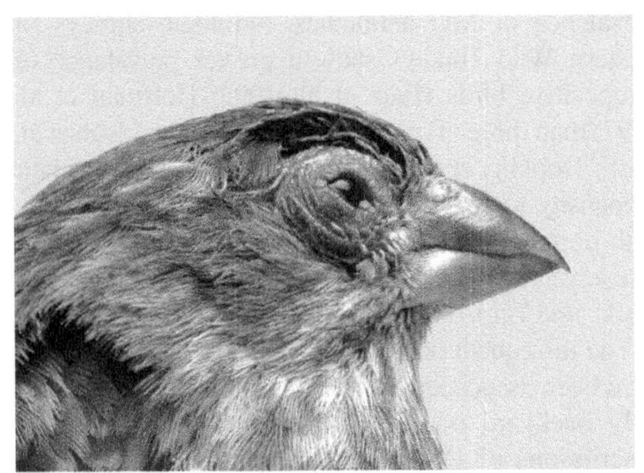

Figure 16.1. Eyelid swelling, ocular and nasal exudates, and periorbital alopecia are common in finches with mycoplasmal conjunctivitis.

The pathogenesis of mycoplasmas is complex and incompletely understood, but a primary event is the adherence of the organism to the host cell surface. One important and specialized feature in some species, including MG, is a tip structure that enables attachment to host epithelial cells and causes cell damage. Following attachment, mycoplasmas may cause cell injury directly via pathogenic mechanisms, such as inhibition of ciliary activity and production of cytotoxic substances, or indirectly via the host's response to the infection (Simecka et al. 1992). In the case of MG, the organism attaches to epithelial cells of the respiratory tract, and the resulting cell damage and host inflammatory response contribute to the development of clinical disease. Other mechanisms contributing to the pathogenicity of MG include rapid antigenic changes in surface proteins and evasion of host immune responses (Simecka et al. 1992).

Asymptomatic or chronic infections may result through the ability of MG to change its surface antigens and to immunoregulate host response (Tyron and Baseman 1992; Razin et al. 1998). Research on cell invasion by MG indicates that it is capable of penetrating and sequestering in eukaryotic cells (Winner et al. 2000), and this characteristic most likely aids in the development of a carrier state in its avian hosts.

PATHOLOGY

Wild Turkeys

Infections of MG in Wild Turkeys are characterized by unilateral or bilateral periocular swelling, infraorbital sinusitis with serous, catarrhal, or fibrinous exudate, and airsacculitis (Davidson et al. 1982). Microscopically, chronic inflammatory changes consist of mononuclear cellular infiltrates, mucosal gland hyperplasia, and submucosal lymphoid hyperplasia of affected tissues (Ley 2003).

House Finches

In House Finches, gross lesions of MG infection consist of unilateral or bilateral conjunctival swelling with serous to mucoid ocular and nasal discharge, crusts of dried exudate at the eyes and nares, and periocular alopecia. Microscopic lesions are characterized by chronic inflammation of the ocular tissues and upper respiratory system (Fischer et al. 1997; Luttrell et al. 1998). Conjunctival lesions consist of mild to severe lymphoplasmacytic inflammation of the mucosa and submucosa with epithelial and lymphoid hyperplasia (Figure 16.2). Mild to moderate keratitis may be observed in some cases. Rhinitis, characterized by mucosal necrosis, lymphoplasmacytic infiltrates, and hyperkeratosis of nasal turbinates, frequently is present

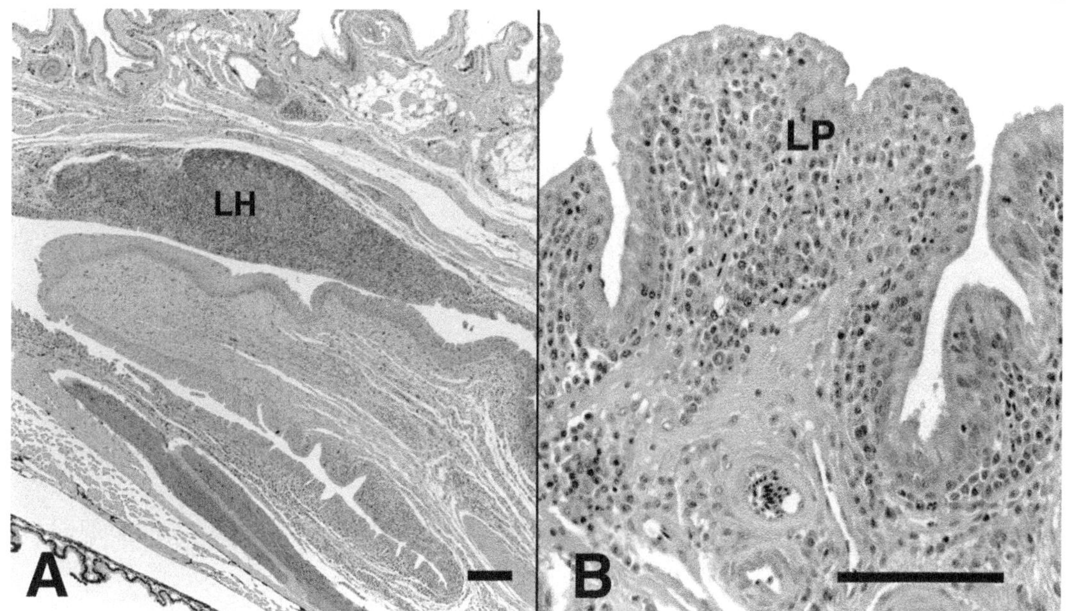

Figure 16.2. Photomicrographs of a House Finch with mycoplasmal conjunctivitis. A. Lymphoid hyperplasia (LH) and lymphoplasmacytic inflammation of the palpebral conjunctiva are present and there is epithelial hyperplasia with lymphoplasmacytic inflammation of the bulbar conjunctiva and nictitating membrane. B. Epithelium of the bulbar conjunctiva is hyperplastic and there is diffuse lymphoplasmacytic inflammation (LP). Bars = 100 μm, hematoxylin and eosin stain.

(Figures 16.3, 16.4). Chronic, lymphoplasmacytic tracheitis is observed in a small number of cases. Transmission electron microscopy of affected tissues reveals adherent mycoplasmas on the surface of affected epithelial cells (Figure 16.5).

DIAGNOSIS

A diagnosis of MG in live birds is based on clinical signs, history, and detection of the organism by culture or molecular techniques. Serologic testing can support the diagnosis. Other respiratory diseases to eliminate include avian influenza, chlamydiosis, Newcastle disease, and infectious bronchitis (Kleven 1998). In passerines, head trauma or other bacterial infections can cause ocular swelling, and avian poxvirus may create crusty lesions around eyes that could be mistaken for mycoplasmal conjunctivitis (SCWDS, unpublished data).[1] For more extensive coverage of laboratory procedures, see Kleven (1998), Bradbury (1998), and Tully and Razin (1983).

Culture

Swabs taken from the trachea, conjunctiva, choanal cleft, or sinus, or tissue suspensions made from lung or brain are placed into broth media at a pH of 7.8 and incubated at 37°C for up to two to three weeks (Bradbury 1998; Kleven 1998). Aerobic incubation is adequate although an atmosphere of 5% CO_2 is recommended by some. All MG strains ferment dextrose with acid production and agglutinate avian erythrocytes. After a color-indicated pH change or at one-week intervals, cultures can be plated onto solid (agar) media that also are incubated at 37°C in a moist atmosphere. Colonies typically appear in three to seven days or may take up to 10 to 14 days, as do some more fastidious strains such as the finch strain. Colonies are viewed with a standard light microscope and identified by various procedures including growth inhibition, direct or indirect immunofluorescence, and polymerase chain reaction (PCR) (Kleven 1998).

There are many media formulations for MG isolation, but one of the most widely used is Frey's medium with swine serum (FMS) (Kleven 1998). Other media used with success include SP4 (Whitcomb 1983), PPLO (Kleven 1998), and Edward-type (Bradbury 1998). Both broth and agar can be prepared with these various formulations. Penicillin and thallium acetate usually are added to media to inhibit growth of bacterial and fungal contaminants.

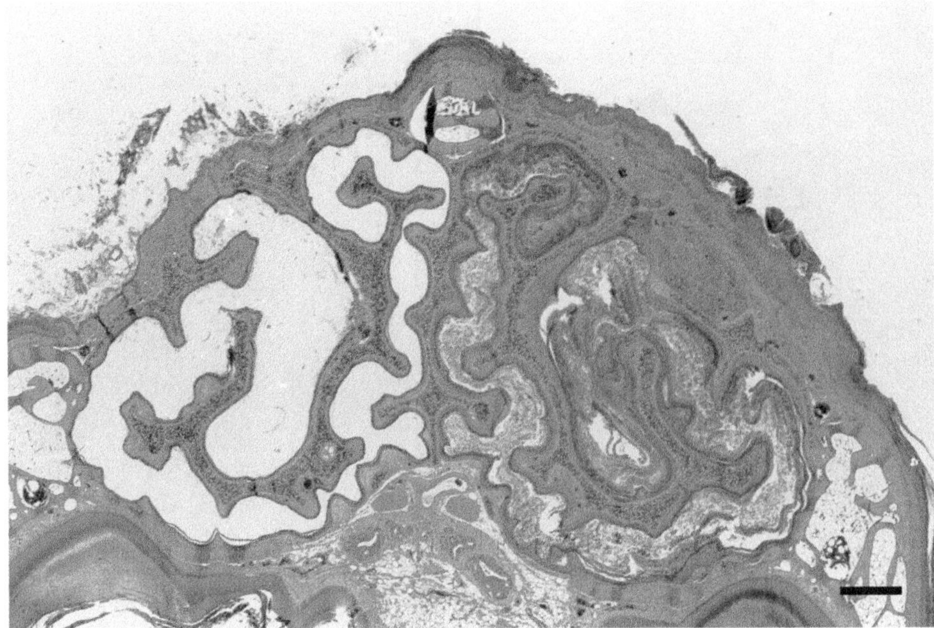

Figure 16.3. Photomicrograph of a House Finch with mycoplasmal conjunctivitis. There is unilateral rhinitis with extensive hyperkeratosis in nasal turbinates. Bar = 500 μm. Hematoxylin and eosin stain.

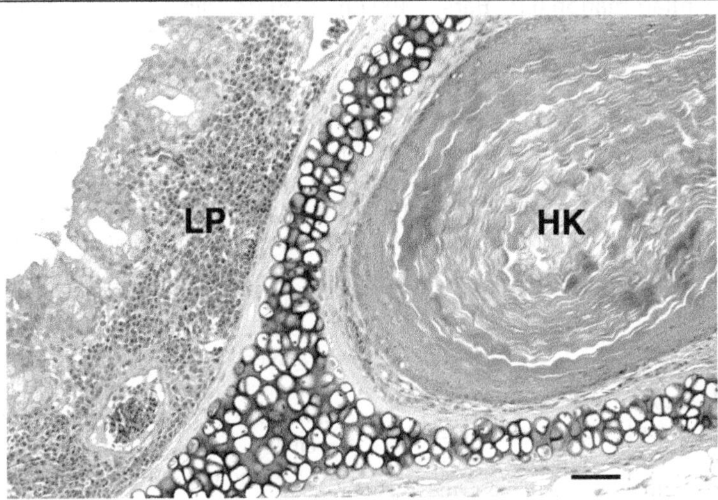

Figure 16.4. Photomicrograph of a House Finch with mycoplasmal conjunctivitis. Goblet cell hyperplasia, lymphoplasmacytic inflammation (LP), and marked hyperkeratosis (HK) are present in the nasal turbinates. Bar = 50 μm. Hematoxylin and eosin stain.

Molecular Techniques

Polymerase chain reaction techniques offer sensitive and time-efficient alternatives to culture for diagnosing pathogenic mycoplasmas, such as MG. Specific oligonucleotide primers are used to amplify small amounts of nucleic acid to detectable levels (Lauerman 1998). Random amplification of polymorphic DNA (RAPD) or arbitrary primed PCR techniques generate DNA fingerprints that are used for molecular typing of strains and also are valuable for epidemiological studies (Ley et al. 1997; Luttrell et al. 1998).

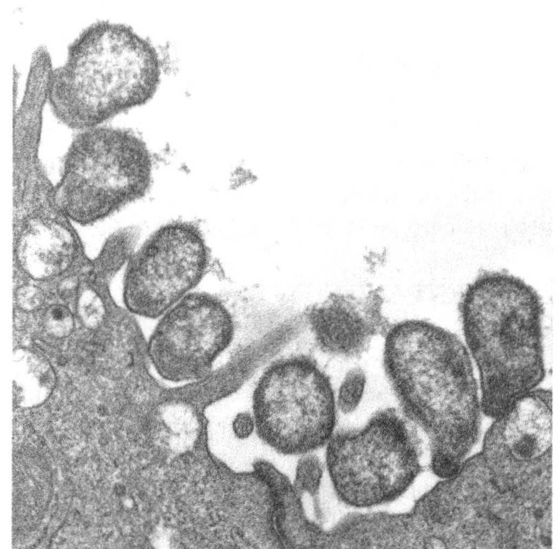

Figure 16.5. This transmission electron micrograph shows adherent *Mycoplasma gallisepticum* organisms on the tracheal epithelium of a House Finch. Mycoplasmas lack a cell wall, are pleomorphic, and often have a terminal bleb at the attachment site. Magnification = 42,000X. Uranyl acetate and lead citrate stain.

Serology

The easiest, most sensitive serologic test for screening birds for MG is the serum plate agglutination (SPA) test (Kleven 1998). It is simple, inexpensive, and applicable to many different avian hosts. The SPA test detects the earliest class of antibodies produced (IgM) and continues to be sensitive for several months or more by measuring IgG antibodies. Its main disadvantage is low specificity or the occurrence of false positives. Positive SPA tests may reflect exposure to the infectious agent, a chronic infection, an infection that has been cleared, or a nonspecific reaction. The cause of nonspecific SPA reactions in wild birds is not well understood, but possible causes are infections with other bacteria or mycoplasmas and variations in individual or species immunity (Luttrell et al. 2001).

Serologic tests with higher specificity, such as the hemagglutination inhibition (HI) test and enzyme-linked immunosorbent assay (ELISA), are recommended to confirm SPA-positive samples (Kleven 1998). However, there are problems in the direct application of these tests to wild birds, such as difficulties in test interpretations and disparities in reagents. Baseline data on positive thresholds and ranges for serologic reactions in most species of wild birds are not available, and the alternate strategy of sequential sampling to detect rising titers is usually not possible because individuals can be tested only once. The HI test utilizes avian erythrocytes as agglutination indicators, and cell incompatibility may occur if a heterologous blood cell suspension is used (Luttrell et al. 2001). Commercially available ELISAs are developed for use with domestic poultry, and reagents such as species-specific conjugates may not be suitable for a wide range of avian hosts.

IMMUNITY

Information on immunity to MG in wild birds is limited. Domestic birds that recover from MG infections develop a humoral immune response that protects them from severe clinical disease in a subsequent infection (Ley 2003), and wild birds may be similarly protected. Humoral antibodies to MG can be detected in Wild Turkeys and House Finches within two weeks after exposure to MG and last for several months or more (Rocke and Yuill 1988; Luttrell et al. 1998). Birds that are chronically infected or infected with atypical strains of low virulence may produce low or nondetectable humoral responses. This has created problems in diagnosing mycoplasmosis in domestic poultry flocks and may account for poor detectability in wild birds (Hoffman et al. 1997; Luttrell et al. 2001).

PUBLIC HEALTH CONCERNS

None known.

DOMESTIC ANIMAL HEALTH CONCERNS

Until recently, mycoplasmosis was considered a disease of primarily domestic poultry. The occurrence of MG in Wild Turkeys usually was associated with a domestic source, and its spread from wild to domestic turkeys has not been documented. However, the emergence of MG in free-flying wild passerines has created new dilemmas for both poultry farmers and wildlife managers. Biosecurity measures that prevent direct contact between free-flying wild birds and commercial poultry are essential in minimizing transmission of MG between species.

Currently, the strain of MG isolated from House Finches appears to be restricted to those birds and other fringillids (Ley et al. 1997; Luttrell et al. 1998; Hartup et al. 2000). Transmission from wild birds to commercial poultry flocks has not been documented. Chickens and turkeys experimentally inoculated with the finch strain of MG via aerosol became infected but developed only mild clinical lesions (O'Connor et al. 1999). In a related study, contact transmission of MG from naturally infected finches to chickens was documented, although clinical signs were not apparent in chickens for the 12-week co-housing period (Stallknecht et al.

1998). In both studies, seroconversion in infected birds was detected primarily by the SPA test, and results were often inconsistent or delayed.

During an epidemiological investigation of a MG outbreak in commercial turkeys, MG antibodies were detected in wild passerines captured in the farm vicinity, but no mycoplasmas were isolated (Stallknecht et al. 1982). In this instance, wild birds probably became exposed via contaminated litter and feathers on the premises, but they were not considered to be instrumental in MG transmission.

WILDLIFE POPULATION IMPACTS

Population impacts directly related to MG infections in Wild Turkeys are difficult to assess due to diagnostic difficulties and the potential for subtle long-term effects (Adrian 1984; Rocke and Yuill 1987; Hoffman et al. 1997). Although mycoplasmosis and other infectious diseases have been suspected to be factors relating to population declines in some Wild Turkey populations, there are no definitive data to indicate that MG has become a chronic, debilitating health problem for free-ranging Wild Turkeys.

House Finch populations have declined dramatically in many eastern states since the advent of the MG epidemic (Hochachka and Dhondt 2000). Through monitoring programs such as the Audubon Society's North American Christmas Bird Count and Cornell Laboratory of Ornithology FeederWatch Surveys, researchers tracked the spread of mycoplasmal conjunctivitis in eastern House Finches (Dhondt et al. 1998; Hochachka and Dhondt 2000). The expansion of MG conjunctivitis from the initial locus of infection in the mid-Atlantic states was facilitated by the seasonal migration and dispersal behavior of this species. House Finch populations were significantly reduced in many areas where high densities of birds occurred prior to the initial outbreak, but populations of lower densities experienced smaller declines (Hochachka and Dhondt 2000). More than five years after the initial outbreak of MG in mid-Atlantic House Finches, MG remained endemic in eastern House Finches but appeared to be subsiding in intensity based on a decline in observations of clinically ill finches (Hartup et al. 2001b; Roberts et al. 2001b). Field data suggest an evolving host-parasite relationship in which some populations are evolving resistance to MG or the organism is changing as it adapts to a new host (Luttrell et al. 1998; Hartup et al. 2001b; Roberts et al. 2001b).

Other species in which MG has been confirmed in association with conjunctivitis, such as the American Goldfinch or Purple Finch, currently do not show declines in conjunction with this disease. Field studies using observation of clinical signs (Hartup et al. 2001a) or positive SPA results (Hartup et al. 2000; Luttrell et al. 2001) have reported presumptive cases of MG infections in other passerine species. Of particular interest in one of these studies were clinically healthy Tufted Titmice (*Baeolophus bicolor*) that tested positive for MG by PCR (Luttrell et al. 2001). These birds may be asymptomatic carriers or have transient infections of MG. Future impacts of MG on these and other wild passerine populations are unknown.

TREATMENT AND CONTROL

The lack of cell walls in mycoplasmas renders many antibiotics, such as penicillin, ineffective in treatment of avian mycoplasmosis. Tylosin and tetracycline have been used successfully for treating clinical disease in domestic poultry (Ley 2003) and House Finches (Mashima et al. 1997; Nolan et al. 2000). However, although clinical signs were resolved in House Finches with the use of oral enrofloxacin in combination with opthalmic gentamicin in one study, treated birds remained culture or PCR positive for MG up to six months after antibiotic therapy was ended (Wellehan et al. 2001a).

Wildlife rehabilitators should avoid bringing birds suspected of having MG infections into their facilities because of possible MG transmission to other sick or injured birds (Ley et al. 1996). Although clinical signs can be resolved with the use of antibiotics, keeping treated birds in captivity for long periods of time is unfeasible for most rehabilitators, and retesting with culture and PCR is expensive. Most important, there is risk associated with releasing wild birds that have been treated for MG. Birds that recover from acute disease may become asymptomatic carriers in spite of antibiotic therapy (Wellehan et al. 2001a), and most wildlife caretakers will be unable to verify that the birds they release are no longer carrying the infectious agent.

MANAGEMENT IMPLICATIONS

Wild Turkeys

In response to concerns of disease transmission in Wild Turkeys during state relocation programs in the 1980s, protocols for the health monitoring of Wild Turkeys were recommended by state wildlife agencies, the United States Animal Health Association, and the Wildlife Disease Association (Wildlife Disease Association 1985; Davidson et al. 1988). These protocols specify that Wild Turkeys captured for interstate restocking efforts be clinically normal and seronegative for pathogenic mycoplasmas by the SPA test. The turkeys can be held temporarily while blood samples are being processed and screened. Although false positives can occur, the SPA is the easiest, most cost-efficient way to assess birds for the presence of this organism. Alternatively, determining the status of the source population can take place prior to translocation rather than testing individual birds during the relocation process. Wild turkey flocks that live in close proximity with domestic poultry and pen-raised stock are unsuitable candidates for relocation regardless of test reactions (Schorr et al. 1988; Hoffman et al. 1997).

House Finches and Other Passerines

Basic recommendations designed to reduce potential disease risks at bird feeders apply to the control of mycoplasmosis in passerines. These include maintaining sanitary feeding stations and water baths, spacing feeders to reduce crowding, and using clean and unspoiled feed (Luttrell 1997; Friend 1999). Use of tube-style feeders and crowded conditions may increase risk of transmission between passerines with conjunctivitis (Hartup et al. 1998). If a local outbreak of mycoplasmosis occurs, temporary cessation of feeding may help to disperse healthy birds before they become exposed. Due to the tendencies of MG to become a chronic, asymptomatic disease, treatment and release of individuals is not a valid option for disease control in wild populations. Although MG does not easily spread from finches to poultry (Stallknecht et al. 1998), physical contact between backyard or commercial domestic poultry and finches and other wild birds should be avoided.

Pen-Raised Birds

Pathogenic mycoplasmas have been associated with disease outbreaks in various species of pen-raised or captive wild birds. Birds maintained in close confinement, whether they are domestic or wild, are at increased risk for contagious diseases, especially mycoplasmosis. *Mycoplasma gallisepticum* has been isolated from pen-raised game birds such as Wild Turkeys (Schorr et al. 1988), Northern Bobwhites (*Colinus virginianus*) (Madden et al. 1967), Chukars (*Alectoris chukar*) (Cookson and Shivaprasad 1994), and Ring-necked Pheasants (*Phasianus colchicus*) (Cookson and Shivaprasad 1994; Osborn and Pomeroy 1985). The release of pen-raised game birds or rehabilitated wild birds that are antibody positive for MG is not recommended. Due to the possibility of a carrier state, released captive birds represent potential reservoirs for the transmission of MG to those of the same species or to other free-ranging wild birds and commercial poultry.

Other Mycoplasmal Infections in Wild Birds

Unlike MG, little is known about other mycoplasmas that infect wild birds. Some, such *as M. sturni* and *M. buteonis,* have been associated with disease in their wild hosts but have not been verified experimentally as causative disease agents. Other avian mycoplasmas are considered nonpathogenic microflora in apparently healthy birds. For example, *M. gallopavonis* has been isolated from clinically normal Wild Turkeys (Luttrell et al. 1992b), and field surveys have demonstrated the presence of *M. anatis* in several species of waterfowl that had no obvious signs of disease (Poveda et al. 1990a; Goldberg et al. 1995). *Mycoplasma synovia* (MS) and *M. meleagridis* (MM) cause airsacculitis and other problems in domestic poultry, especially in combination with other respiratory pathogens (Ley 2003). However, clinical disease or population declines specifically attributed to MS or MM have not been reported in Wild Turkeys or in any other wild avian species. Antibodies to MS and MM have been detected in health surveys of clinically normal Wild Turkeys, especially in populations in western states (Rocke and Yuill 1987; Fritz et al 1992; Hoffman et al. 1997). *Mycoplasma synovia* has been isolated from clinically ill pen-raised Wild Turkeys (Schorr et al. 1988; Luttrell et al. 1992a) and from one flock of free-ranging Wild Turkeys (Fritz et al. 1992). *Mycoplasma meleagridis* has been confirmed in several species of European raptors without clinical signs (Lierz et al. 2003).

Mycoplasma gallopavonis is the most frequently isolated mycoplasma from Wild Turkeys (Rocke and Yuill 1987; Cobb et al. 1992; Fritz et al. 1992; Luttrell et al. 1992b; Hoffman et al. 1997). This agent generally is considered nonpathogenic for wild and domestic turkeys. Because of its rapid growth and nonfastidious nature, it usually out-competes pathogenic mycoplasmas in culture, thereby complicating diagnosis in clinically ill birds. Although *M. gallopavonis* appears to be lethal for domestic turkey and chicken embryos (Rocke and Yuill 1987), its potential for pathogenicity in synergistic complexes with other microorganisms has not been determined for wild birds.

Mycoplasma sturni is a new mycoplasma that has recently emerged in North America in association with disease in passerines. First described as a cause of conjunctivitis in a European Starling (Forsyth et al. 1996), it also has been isolated from Northern Mockingbird, Blue Jay (*Cyanocitta cristata*) (Ley et al. 1998), and American Crow (*Corvus brachyrhyncos*) (Wellehan et al. 2001b), all with conjunctivitis. In starlings, *M. sturni* was associated with clinical signs similar to those caused by MG in House Finches. However, the microscopic lesions consisted of acute conjunctivitis with focal mucosal ulceration in contrast to the chronic lesions of lymphoplasmacytic inflammation and epithelial hyperplasia in House Finches with MG (Frasca et al. 1997). As does MG, *M. sturni* also ferments glucose, but it grows more rapidly in culture, usually within a few days. Although *M. sturni* has not been verified experimentally as the cause of conjunctivitis in these birds, it should be considered in making differential diagnosis of this illness in passerines. *Mycoplasma sturni* also has been isolated from clinically normal European Starlings (Luttrell et al. 2001), American Crows, and American Robins (*Turdus migratorius*) (Wellehan et al. 2001b) in the U.S., and as an incidental postmortem finding from wild Eurasian Blackbirds (*Turdus merula*), Rook (*Corvius frugilegus*), Carrion Crow (*Corvus corone*), Black-billed Magpie (*Pica pica*), and European Starling in Scotland (Pennycott et al. 2005).

Mycoplasma anatis and *M. cloacale* have been isolated from tracheas and lungs of clinically healthy wild ducks (Poveda et al. 1990a; Goldberg et al. 1995). Both mycoplasmas have been associated with disease, embryo mortality, and reduced growth in domestic ducks and geese, but the pathogenicity of these organisms for wild waterfowl is unclear (Wobeser 1997). An experimental inoculation of Mallard (*Anas platyrhynchos*) eggs with *M. anatis* resulted in reduced hatching success, hatchling size, and duckling growth (Samuel et al. 1995). Similarly to many other mycoplasmas, *M. anatis* may be carried by healthy birds but work synergistically with other microorganisms or environmental stresses to cause disease. Serologic surveys indicate variable exposure to *M. anatis* among different species of water birds. A study in North America using an ELISA test reported high rates of exposure in Mallards and American Black Ducks (*A. rubripes*) but none in Canvasbacks (*Aythya valisineria*) (Samuel et al. 1996). In a serologic survey conducted in Spain (Astorga et al. 1994), low levels of antibodies to *M. anatis* were detected in several species of waterfowl as well as in Little Egret (*Egretta garzetta*), White Spoonbill (*Platalea leucorodia*), and Pied Avocet (*Recurvirostra avosetta*).

Three species of mycoplasma have been isolated from free-flying Rock Pigeons (*Columba livia*), and all appear to be specific for this group of birds. *Mycoplasma columborale, M. columbinum,* and *M. columbinasale* have been isolated from swabs taken from trachea and oropharnyx of clinically normal Rock Pigeons as well as those with respiratory disease (Kleven 2003). *Mycoplasma columborale* also was isolated from the air sacs of a Peregrine Falcon (*Falco peregrinus*) with respiratory illness, but the infection was attributed to a diet of Rock Pigeons (Poveda et al. 1990b). Pathogenicity of these organisms for any avian host has not been verified experimentally.

Three novel species of mycoplasmas have been isolated from European raptors with respiratory disease: *M. buteonis* from a Common Buzzard (*Buteo buteo*); *M. falconis* from a Saker Falcon (*Falco cherrug*); and *M. gypis* from a Griffon Vulture (*Gyps fulvus*) (Poveda et al. 1994). *Mycoplasma buteonis* has been cultured in association with skeletal deformities in a Saker Falcon nestling (Erdelyi et al. 1999). All three of these agents also have been isolated from clinically normal raptors (Lierz et al. 2000). Another newly described species, *M. corogypsi,* was isolated from the footpad abscess of a Black Vulture (*Coragyps atratus*) (Panangala et al. 1993). Mycoplasmas normally associated with domestic poultry, such as MG, MM, *M. gallinarum, M. gallinaceum,* and *M. iners,* also have been isolated from raptors. These infections probably derive from chicken carcasses used for feeding captive birds (Poveda et al. 1990a; Lierz et al. 2000). Reported infections of *M. anatis* and *M. columborale* in raptors also probably derive from ingestion of infected prey (Poveda et al. 1990b).

UNPUBLISHED DATA

1. Southeastern Cooperative Wildlife Disease Study, College of Veterinary Medicine, University of Georgia, Athens, Georgia, U.S.A.

LITERATURE CITED

Adrian, W.J. 1984. Investigation of disease as a limiting factor in a wild turkey population. Ph.D. dissertation, Colorado State University, Fort Collins, Colorado, 61 pp.

Astorga, R.J., M.J. Cubero, L. Leon, A. Maldonado, A. Arenas, M.C. Tarradas, and A. Perea. 1994. Serological survey of infections in waterfowl in the Guadalquivir Marshes (Spain). *Avian Diseases* 38:371–375.

Bradbury, J.M. 1998. Recovery of mycoplasmas from birds. In *Mycoplasma Protocols, Methods in Molecular Biology,* Vol. 104, R. J. Miles and R.A.J. Nicholas (eds.). Humana Press, Totowa, New Jersey, NJ, U.S.A., pp. 45–51.

Brawner, W.R., III, G.E. Hill, and C.A. Sundermann. 2000. Effects of coccidial and mycoplasmal infections on carotenoid-based plumage pigmentation in male house finches. *The Auk* 117:952–963.

Christensen, N.H., C.A Yavari, A.J. McBain, and J.M. Bradbury. 1994. Investigations into the survival of *Mycoplasma gallisepticum, Mycoplasma synoviae* and *Mycoplasma iowae* on materials found in the poultry house environment. *Avian Pathology* 23:127–143.

Cobb, D.T., D.H. Ley, and P.D. Doerr. 1992. Isolation of *Mycoplasma gallopavonis* from free-ranging wild turkeys in coastal North Carolina seropositive and culture-negative for *Mycoplasma gallisepticum. Journal of Wildlife Diseases* 28:105–109.

Cookson, K.C., and H.L. Shivaprasad. 1994. *Mycoplasma gallisepticum* infection in chukar partridges, pheasants, and peafowl. *Avian Diseases* 38:914–921.

Davidson, W.R., V.F. Nettles, C.E. Couvillion, and H.W. Yoder, Jr. 1982. Infectious sinusitis in wild turkeys. *Avian Diseases* 26:402–405.

Davidson, W.R., H.W. Yoder, M. Brugh, and V.F. Nettles. 1988. Serological monitoring of eastern wild turkeys for antibodies to *Mycoplasma* spp. and avian influenza viruses. *Journal of Wildlife Diseases* 24:348–351.

Dhondt, A.A., D.L. Tessaglia, and R.L. Slothower. 1998. Epidemic mycoplasmal conjunctivitis in house finches from eastern North America. *Journal of Wildlife Diseases* 34:265–280.

Duckworth, R.A, A.V. Badyaev, K.L. Farmer, G.E. Hill, and S.R. Roberts. 2003. First case of *Mycoplasma gallisepticum* infection in the western range of the house finch (*Carpodacus mexicanus*). *The Auk* 120:528–530.

Erdelyi, K., M. Tenk, and A. Dan. 1999. Mycoplasmosis associated perosis type skeletal deformity in a saker falcon nestling in Hungary. *Journal of Wildlife Diseases* 35:586–590.

Fischer, J.R., D.E., Stallknecht, M.P. Luttrell, A.A. Dhondt, and K.A. Converse. 1997. Mycoplasmal conjunctivitis in wild songbirds: the spread of a new contagious disease in a mobile host population. *Emerging Infectious Diseases* 3:69–72.

Forsyth, M.H., J.G. Tully, T.S. Gorton, L. Hinckley, S. Frasca, Jr., H.J. Van Kruiningen, and S.J. Geary. 1996. *Mycoplasma sturni* sp. nov., from the conjunctiva of a European starling (*Sturnus vulgaris*). *International Journal of Systematic Bacteriology* 46:716–719.

Frasca, S., Jr., L. Hinckley, M.H. Forsyth, T.S. Gorton, S.J. Geary, and H.J. Van Kruiningen. 1997. Mycoplasmal conjunctivitis in a European starling. *Journal of Wildlife Diseases* 33:336–339.

Friend, M. 1999. Mycoplasmosis. In *Field Manual of Wildlife Diseases: General Field Procedures and Diseases of Birds,* M. Friend and J.C. Franson (eds.). United States Department of Interior, Biological Resources Division, Information and Technology Report 1999–001, pp. 115–119.

Fritz, B.A., C.B. Thomas, and T.M. Yuill. 1992. Serological and microbial survey of *Mycoplasma gallisepticum* in wild turkeys (*Meleagris gallopavo*) from six western states. *Journal of Wildlife Diseases* 28:10–20.

Goldberg, D.R., M.D. Samuel, C.B. Thomas, P. Sharp, G.L Krapu, J.R. Robb, K.P. Kenow, C.E. Korschgen, W.H. Chipley, M.J. Conroy, and S.H. Kleven. 1995. The occurrence of mycoplasmas in selected wild North American waterfowl. *Journal of Wildlife Diseases* 31:378–385.

Hartup, B.K., and G.V. Kollias. 1999. Field investigation of *Mycoplasma gallisepticum* infections in house finch (*Carpodacus mexicanus*) eggs and nestlings. *Avian Diseases* 43:572–576.

Hartup, B.K., H.O. Mohammed, G.V. Kollias, and A.A. Dhondt. 1998. Risk factors associated with mycoplasmal conjunctivitis in house finches. *Journal of Wildlife Diseases* 34:281–288.

Hartup, B.K., G.V. Kollias, and D.H. Ley. 2000. Mycoplasmal conjunctivitis in songbirds from New York. *Journal of Wildlife Diseases* 36:257–264.

Hartup, B.K., A.A. Dhondt, K.V. Sydensticker, W.M. Hochachka, and G.V. Kollias. 2001a. Host range and dynamics of mycoplasmal conjunctivitis among birds in North America. *Journal of Wildlife Diseases* 37:72–81.

Hartup, B.K., J.M Bickal, A.A. Dhondt, D.H. Ley, and G.V. Kollias. 2001b. Dynamics of conjunctivitis and *Mycoplasma gallisepticum* infections in house finches. *The Auk* 118:327–333.

Hochachka W.M., and A.A. Dhondt. 2000. Density-dependent decline of host abundance resulting from a new infectious disease. *Proceedings of National Academy of Science* 97:5303–5306.

Hoffman, R.W., M.P. Luttrell, W.R. Davidson, and D.H. Ley. 1997. Mycoplasmas in wild turkeys living in association with domestic fowl. *Journal of Wildlife Diseases* 33:526–535.

Hopkins, B.A., J.K. Skeeles, G.E. Houghten, D. Slagle, and K. Gardner. 1990. A survey of infectious diseases in wild turkeys (*Meleagridis gallopavo silvestris*) from Arkansas. *Journal of Wildlife Diseases* 26:468–472.

Jain, N.C., N.K. Chandiramani, and I.P. Singh. 1971. Studies on avian pleuro-pneumonia-like organisms. 2. Occurrence of mycoplasma in wild birds. *Indian Journal of Animal Sciences* 41:301–305.

Jessup, D.A., A.J. DaMassa, R. Lewis, and K.R. Jones. 1983. *Mycoplasma gallisepticum* infection in wild-type turkeys living in close contact with domestic fowl. *Journal of American Veterinary Medical Association* 183:1245–1247.

Kleven, S.H. 1997. Other mycoplasmal infections. In *Diseases of Poultry,* 10th Ed. B.W. Calnek, H.J. Barnes, C.W. Beard, L.R. McDougald, and Y.M. Saif (eds.). Iowa State University Press, Ames, Iowa, pp. 232–234.

Kleven, S.H. 1998. Mycoplasmosis. In *A Laboratory Manual for the Isolation and Identification of Avian Pathogens,* 4th Ed., D.E. Swayne, J.R. Glisson, M.W. Jackwood, J.E. Pearson, and W.M. Reed (eds.). American Association of Avian Pathologists, Kennett Square, Pennsylvania, pp. 74–80.

Kleven, S.H. 2003. Other mycoplasmal infections. In *Diseases of Poultry,* 11th Ed., Y.M. Saif (ed.). Iowa State University Press, Ames, Iowa, IA, U.S.A., pp. 772–773.

Kollias, G.V., K.V. Sydenstricker, H.W. Kollias, D.H. Ley, P.R. Hosseini, V. Connolly, and A.A. Dhondt. 2004. Experimental infection of house finches with *Mycoplasma gallisepticum. Journal of Wildlife Diseases* 40:79–86.

Lauerman, L.H. 1998. Mycoplasma PCR assays. In *Nucleic Acid Amplification Assays for Diagnosis of Animal Diseases,* L.H. Lauerman (ed.). American

Association of Veterinary Laboratory Diagnosticians, Turlock, California, CA, U.S.A., pp. 41–42.

Levisohn S. and S. H. Kleven. 2000. Avian mycoplasmosis (*Mycoplasma gallisepticum*). *Revue Scientifique et Technique Office International des Epizooties* 19: 425–442.

Ley, D.H. 2003. *Mycoplasma gallisepticum* infection. In *Diseases of Poultry,* 11th Ed., Y.M. Saif (ed.). Iowa State University Press, Ames, IA, U.S.A., pp. 722–744.

Ley, D.H., J.E. Berkhoff, and J.D. McLaren. 1996. *Mycoplasma gallisepticum* isolated from house finches (*Carpodacus mexicanus*) with conjunctivitis. *Avian Diseases* 40:480–483.

Ley, D.H., J.E. Berkhoff, and S. Levisohn. 1997. Molecular epidemiological investigations of *Mycoplasma gallisepticum* conjunctivitis in songbirds by random amplified polymorphic DNA (RAPD) analyses. *Emerging Infectious Diseases* 3:375–380.

Ley, D.H., S.J. Geary, J.E. Berkhoff, J.M. McLaren, and S. Levisohn. 1998. *Mycoplasma sturni* from blue jays and northern mockingbirds with conjunctivitis in Florida. *Journal of Wildlife Diseases* 34:403–406.

Lierz, M., R. Schmidt, L. Brunnberg, and M. Runge. 2000. Isolation of *Mycoplasma meleagridis* from free-ranging birds of prey in Germany. *Journal of Veterinary Medicine* B 47:63–67.

Liu, T., M. Garcia, S. Levisohn, D. Yogev, and S. H. Kleven. 2001. Molecular variability of the adhesin-encoding gene *pvpA* among *Mycoplasma gallisepticum* strains and its application in diagnosis. *Journal of Clinical Microbiology* 39:1882–1888.

Luttrell, M.P. 1997. Disease prevention at bird feeders. In *Field Manual of Wildlife Diseases in the Southeastern United States,* W.R. Davidson and V.F. Nettles (eds.). Southeastern Cooperative Wildlife Disease Study, The University of Georgia, Athens, GA, U.S.A., pp. 349–351.

Luttrell, M.P., S.H. Kleven, and G.M. Mahnke. 1992a. *Mycoplasma synoviae* in a released pen-raised wild turkey. *Avian Diseases* 36:169–171.

Luttrell, M.P., T.H. Eleazer, and S.H. Kleven. 1992b. *Mycoplasma gallopavonis* in eastern wild turkeys. *Journal of Wildlife Diseases* 28:288–291.

Luttrell, M.P., JR. Fischer, D.E. Stallknecht, and S.H. Kleven. 1996. Field investigation of *Mycoplasma gallisepticum* infections in house finches (*Carpodacus mexicanus*) from Maryland and Georgia. *Avian Diseases* 40:335–341.

Luttrell, M.P., D.E. Stallknecht, J.R. Fischer, C.T. Sewell, and S. H Kleven. 1998. Natural *Mycoplasma gallisepticum* infection in a captive flock of house finches. *Journal of Wildlife Diseases* 34:289–296.

Luttrell, M.P., D.E. Stallknecht, S.H. Kleven, D.M. Kavanaugh, J.L. Corn, and J.R. Fischer. 2001. *Mycoplasma gallisepticum* in house finches (*Carpodacus mexicanus*) and other wild birds associated with poultry production facilities. *Avian Diseases* 45:321–329.

Madden, D.L., W.H. Henderson, and H.E. Moses. 1967. Isolation of *Mycoplasma gallisepticum* from bobwhite quail (*Colinus virginiana*). *Avian Diseases* 11:378–380.

Mashima, T.Y., D.H. Ley, M.K. Stoskopf, E.A. Miller, S.C. Welte, J. E Berkhoff, L.A. Degernes, and W.J. Fleming. 1997. Evaluation of treatment of conjunctivitis associated with *Mycoplasma gallisepticum* in house finches (*Carpodacus mexicanus*). *Journal of Avian Medicine and Surgery* 11:20–24.

Mikaelian, I., D.H. Ley, R. Claveau, M. Lemieux, and J. Berube. 2001. Mycoplasmosis in evening and pine grosbeaks with conjunctivitis in Quebec. *Journal of Wildlife Diseases* 37:826–830.

Nolan, P.M., R.A. Duckworth, G.E. Hill, and S.R. Roberts. 2000. Maintenance of a captive flock of house finches free of infection by *Mycoplasma gallisepticum. Avian Diseases* 44:948–952.

O'Connor, R.J., K.S. Turner, J.E. Sander, S.H. Kleven, T.P. Brown, L. Gomez, Jr., and J.L. Cline. 1999. Pathogenic effects on domestic poultry of a *Mycoplasma gallisepticum* strain isolated from a wild house finch. *Avian Diseases* 43:640–648.

Osborn, O.H., and B.S. Pomeroy. 1985. Isolation of the agent of infectious sinusitis of turkeys from naturally-infected pheasants. *Avian Diseases* 2:370–372.

Panangala, V.S., J.S. Stringfellow, K. Dybvig, A. Woodard, R. Sun, D.L. Rose, and M.M. Gresham. 1993. *Mycoplasma corogypsi* sp. nov., a new species from the footpad abscess of a black vulture, *Coragyps atratus. International Journal of Systematic Bacteriology* 43:585–590.

Pennycott, T.W., C.M. Dare, C.A. Yavari, and J.M. Bradbury. 2005. *Mycoplasma sturni* and *Mycoplasma gallisepticum* in wild birds in Scotland. *Veterinary Record* 156:513–515.

Poveda, J.B., J. Carranza, A. Miranda, A. Garrido, M. Hermoso, A. Fernandez, and J. Domenech. 1990a. An epizootiological study of avian mycoplasmas in southern Spain. *Avian Pathology* 19:627–633.

Poveda, J.B., J. Giebel, H. Kirchhoff, and A. Fernandez. 1990b. Isolation of mycoplasmas from a buzzard, falcons, and vultures. *Avian Pathology* 19:779–783.

Poveda, J.B., J. Giebel, J. Flossdorf, J. Meier, and H. Kirchhoff. 1994. *Mycoplasma buteonis* sp. nov., *Mycoplasma falconis* sp. nov., and *Mycoplasma gypis* sp. nov., three species from birds of prey. *International Journal of Systematic Bacteriology* 44:94–98.

Razin, S. 1992. Mycoplasma taxonomy and ecology. In *Mycoplasmas:* Molecular biology and pathogenesis, J. Maniloff, R.N. McElhaney, L.R. Finch, and J.B.

Baseman (eds.). American Society for Microbiology, Washington, D.C., U.S.A., pp. 3–22.

Razin, S,D. Yogev, and Y. Naot. 1998. Molecular biology and pathogenicity of mycoplasmas. *Microbiology and Molecular Biology Reviews* 62:1094–1156.

Roberts, S.R., P.M. Nolan, and G.E. Hill. 2001a. Characterization of *Mycoplasma gallisepticum* infection in captive house finches (*Carpodacus mexicanus*) in 1998. *Avian Diseases* 45:70–75.

Roberts, S.R., P.M. Nolan, L.H. Lauerman, L.Li, and G.E. Hill. 2001b. Characterization of the mycoplasmal conjunctivitis epizootic in a house finch population in the southeastern U.S.A. *Journal of Wildlife Diseases* 37:82–88.

Rocke, T.E., and T.M. Yuill. 1987. Microbial infections in a declining wild turkey population in Texas. *Journal of Wildlife Management* 51:778–782.

Rocke, T.E., and T.M. Yuill. 1988. Serologic response of Rio Grande Wild Turkeys to experimental infections of *Mycoplasma gallisepticum. Journal of Wildlife Diseases* 24:668–671.

Samuel, M.D., D.R. Goldberg, C.B. Thomas, and P. Sharp. 1995. Effects of *Mycoplasma anatis* and cold stress on hatching success and growth of mallard ducklings. *Journal of Wildlife Diseases* 31:172–178.

Samuel, M.D., D.R. Goldberg, C.B. Thomas, P. Sharp, J.R. Robb, G.L. Krapu, B.N. Nersessian, K.P. Kenow, C.E. Korschgen, W.H. Chipley, and M.J. Conroy. 1996. Exposure of wild waterfowl to *Mycoplasma anatis. Journal of Wildlife Diseases* 32:331–337.

Schorr, L.F., W.R. Davidson, V.F. Nettles, J.E. Kennamer, P. Villegas, and H.W. Yoder, Jr. 1988. A survey of parasites and diseases of pen-raised wild turkeys. *Proceedings of the Annual Conference of Southeastern Association of Fish and Wildlife Agencies* 42:315–328.

Shimizu, T.K. Numano, and K. Uchida. 1979. Isolation and identification of mycoplasmas from various birds: an ecological study. *Japanese Journal of Veterinary Science* 41:273–282.

Simecka, J.W., J.K. Davis, M.K. Davidson, S.E. Ross, C.T.K-H. Stadtlander, and G.H. Cassell. 1992. Mycoplasma diseases of animals. In *Mycoplasmas: Molecular Biology and Pathogenesis,* J. Maniloff, R.N. McElhaney, L.R. Finch, and J.B. Baseman (eds.). American Society for Microbiology, Washington, D.C., U.S.A., pp. 391–415.

Stallknecht, D.E., D.C. Johnson, W.H. Emory, and S.H. Kleven. 1982. Wildlife surveillance during a *Mycoplasma gallisepticum* epornitic in domestic turkeys. *Avian Diseases* 26:883–890.

Stallknecht, D.E., M.P. Luttrell, J.R. Fischer, and S.H. Kleven. 1998. Potential for transmission of the finch strain of *Mycoplasma gallisepticum* between house finches and chickens. *Avian Diseases* 42:352–358.

Tryon, V.V. and J.B. Baseman. 1992. Pathogenic determinants and mechanisms. In *Mycoplasmas: Molecular Biology and Pathogenesis,* J. Maniloff, R.N. McElhaney, L.R. Finch, and J. B. Baseman (eds.), pp. 457–471.

Tully, J.G., and S. Razin (eds.). 1983. *Methods in Mycoplasmology: Diagnostic Mycoplasmology,* Vol. 2. Academic Press, New York, NY, U.S.A.

Wellehan, J.F. X., M.S. Zens, M. Calsamiglia, P.J. Fusco, A. Amonsin, and V. Kapur. 2001a. Diagnosis and treatment of conjunctivitis in house finches associated with mycoplasmosis in Minnesota. *Journal of Wildlife Diseases* 37:245–251.

Wellehan, J.F. X., M. Calsamiglia, D.H. Ley, M.S. Zens, A. Amonsin, and V. Kapur. 2001b. Mycoplasmosis in captive crows and robins from Minnesota. *Journal of Wildlife Diseases* 37:547–555.

Whitcomb R.F. 1983. Culture media for spiroplasmas. In *Methods in Mycoplasmology,* Vol. 1, S. Razin and J.G. Tully (eds.). Academic Press, New York, NY, U.S.A., pp. 147–158.

Wildlife Disease Association. 1985. Advisory statement on disease monitoring wild turkeys. Wildlife Disease Newsletter (Supplement), *Journal of Wildlife Diseases* 21:1–3.

Winner, F., R. Rosengarten, and C. Citti. 2000. In vitro cell invasion of *Mycoplasma gallisepticum. Infection and Immunity* 68:4238–4244.

Wobeser, G.A. 1997. Mycoplasma infections. In *Diseases of Wild Waterfowl,* 2nd Ed. Plenum Press, New York, NY, U.S.A., pp. 87–88.

17
Erysipelas

Mark J. Wolcott

INTRODUCTION

Erysipelas is a septic disease of birds and mammals resulting from infection by bacteria in the genus *Erysipelothrix.* The disease is probably under-recognized and under-reported in wild birds. The genus *Erysipelothrix* currently contains only two species, *E. rhusiopathiae* and *E. tonsillarum.*

Erysipelothrix rhusiopathiae is the species of importance in relation to avian disease. Infection can produce mortality with few concomitant signs of illness. In wild birds the disease seems to occur sporadically, and the organism is responsible only for occasional reports of mortality. During approximately a 20-year period, the U.S. Geological Survey's National Wildlife Health Center (NWHC), Madison, Wisconsin, recovered about 35 isolates of *Erysipelothrix* from wild birds, representing 20 cases out of the more than 13,000 avian cases since the mid-1980s. In only three of those 19 cases was erysipelas considered the cause or part of the cause of mortality (NWHC, unpublished data).[1] In domestic animals, including turkeys, the organism is a primary pathogen and cause of substantial disease, but in wild birds the disease typically appears to be a secondary pathogen affecting individuals and not flocks, although some literature is contradictory. Principally as a result of vaccination programs, the poultry disease does not have as great an economic impact as it had historically (Bricker and Saif 1997).

HISTORY, DISTRIBUTION, AND HOST RANGE

Erysipelothrix was one of the first organisms isolated and studied under the new science of microbiology. Koch identified and studied it as the "bacillus of mouse septicemia" in 1878. Numerous reports of bacteria similar to Koch's mouse septicemia bacillus were reported in the ensuing years and are now considered to be variants of Koch's original organism. Buchanan (1918) proposed the name combination of *Erysipelothrix rhusiopathiae* that has since been conserved. Jarmai (1919) is credited with the first report of the infection in wild birds. In a Hungarian zoological park, he isolated the organism from thrush, quail, and parrots.

Since those first reports, *Erysipelothrix* has been found to have worldwide distribution and to affect a wide variety of animals and birds, domestic and wild. The organism is apparently present in all the states within the United States. Occurrences in wild birds have taken place in many states without regard for a particular geographic region. It is an important disease-producing organism in swine and poultry, an opportunistic pathogen of humans, and is readily isolated in association with fish and marine mammals (Leighton 2001).

The host range of *Erysipelothrix,* outside of domestic animals, has been documented through reports of naturally occurring incidents. In wild bird species, those incident records include mortality reports from diagnostic laboratories and infections in captive wild birds (that is, in zoological parks). Unfortunately, the differentiation between an "infection" and a "disease" state is often unclear in these reports. The species of free-living wild birds with *Erysipelothrix* isolations are listed in Table 17.1, and records of captive wild bird species are listed in Table 17.2. The significance of *Erysipelothrix* isolations from captive wild bird species is even less clear than those from free-ranging birds because housing and rearing conditions are highly variable.

The host range for erysipelas in wild birds includes well over 60 species that were reported to have been infected, but reports of mortality events in free-ranging birds are sporadic and relatively few in the literature. Erysipelas is, however, a well-documented bird disease that can affect large numbers of birds or individuals of threatened or endangered species. The largest wild bird mortality event due to *Erysipelothrix* occurred at the Great Salt Lake, Utah, U.S.A., where more than 10,000 Eared Grebes (*Podiceps nigricollis*) were estimated to have died (Jensen and Cotter 1976). A similar event reoccurred in the same location and

Table 17.1. Free-ranging wild bird species with *Erysipelothrix* infections.

Common Name	Scientific Name	Reference
Mallard	*Anas platyrhynchos*	Keymer 1958
Pheasants	not specified	Keymer 1958
Willow Ptarmigan	*Lagopus lagopus*	McDiarmid 1962
Wood grouse (possible Capercaillie)	not specified (possible *Tetrao* sp.)	Zhukova et al. 1966
Quail	not specified	Keymer 1958
Common Loon	*Gavia immer*	NWHC[a]
Eared Grebe	*Podiceps nigricollis*	Jensen and Cotter 1976
Galapagos (Dark-rumped) Petrel	*Pterodroma phaeopygia*	NWHC
Shearwater	*Puffinus* sp.	NWHC
American White Pelican	*Pelecanus erythrorhynchos*	NWHC
Brown Pelican	*Pelecanus occidentalis*	NWHC
White stork	*Ciconia ciconia*	Keymer 1958
Bald Eagle	*Haliaeetus leucocephalus*	NWHC
Red-tailed Hawk	*Buteo jamaicensis*	NWHC
Golden Eagle	*Aquila chrysaetos*	Bigland 1957
Eurasian Coot	*Fulica atra*	Keymer 1958
California Gull	*Larus californicus*	NWHC
Herring Gull	*Larus argentatus*	Keymer 1958 McDiarmid 1962
Pigeons	not specified	Keymer 1958
Wood Pigeon	*Columba palumba*	McDiarmid 1962
European Turtle-Dove	*Streptopelia turtur*	Urbain 1947
Budgerigar	*Melopsittacus undulatus*	Urbain 1947
Little Swift	*Apus affinis*	Van Vuuren and Brown 1990
Hawaiian crow	*Corvus hawaiiensis*	Work et al. 1999
Wood Thrush	*Hylocichla mustelina*	McDiarmid 1962
Eurasian Blackbird	*Turdus merula*	Urbain 1947
American Robin	*Turdus migratorius*	NWHC
European Starling	*Sturnus vulgaris*	Faddoul et al. 1968
Finches	not specified	Keymer 1958
European Goldfinch	*Carduelis carduelis*	Urbain 1947
European Greenfinch	*Carduelis chloris*	Urbain 1947

[a] Diagnostic Microbiology Laboratory, U.S. Geological Survey, National Wildlife Health Center, Madison, Wisconsin, U.S.A.

affected Eared Grebes and California Gulls (*Larus californicus*) in winter 2001 (R. Sohn, NWHC, unpublished data).[2] In another mass mortality event, an estimated 600 Brown Pelicans (*Pelicanus occidentalis*) died from erysipelas in California from October 1987 through March of 1988 (K. Converse, unpublished data).[3] Although fish eating habits may be a predisposing condition for acquiring the disease, even insectivorous Little Swifts (*Apus affinis*) nesting on the walls of high-rise buildings in South Africa underwent high mortality (Van Vuuren and Brown 1990). The death of only one Hawaiian Crow (*Corvus hawaiiensis*) due to erysipelas was considered highly significant to this critically endangered species (Work et al. 1999).

ETIOLOGY

Erysipelothrix organisms are small, Gram-positive rods or pleomorphic rods. They are nonsporeforming and facultatively anaerobic. Optimal growth occurs at 30°C to 37°C but they can grow at temperatures from 5°C to 42°C. Previous nomenclature applied to *Erysipelothrix* includes *Bacillus erysipelatus-suis (Bacterium erysipelatos-suum), Bacillus insidiosus, Bacterium rhusiopathiae, Bacillus rhusiopathie-suis, Erysipelothrix erysipeloides, Erysipelothrix insidiosa, Erysipelothrix murisepticus,* and *Erysipelothrix porci.*

Serotyping was the first method used in an attempt at strain differentiation (Dédié 1949). By detection of heat-stable somatic antigens, 26 serotypes have been

Table 17.2. Captive wild bird species with *Erysipelothrix* infections.

Common Name	Scientific Name	Reference
Emu	*Dromaius novaehollandiae*	Griffiths and Buller 1991; Morgan et al. 1994
Geese	Not specified	Bailie et al. 1970; Karstad and Sileo 1971
Black Swan	*Cygnus atratus*	Ungureanu et al. 1966
Ducks	Not specified	Graham et al. 1939; Karstad and Sileo 1971
Wood Duck	*Aix sponsa*	Decker et al. 1976
Mallard	*Anas platyrhynchos*	Ungureanu et al. 1966
Malleefowl	*Leipoa ocellata*	Blyde and Woods 1999
Chukar	*Alectoris chukar*	Butcher and Panigrahy 1985
Red-legged Partridge	*Alectoris rufa*	Blackmore and Gallagher 1964
Pheasants	not specified	Nowak 1957; Richter et al. 1964
Silver Pheasant	*Lophura nycthemerus*	Blackmore and Gallagher 1964
Ring-necked Pheasant	*Phasianus colchicus*	Hennig et al. 2002
Golden Pheasant	*Chrysolophus pictus*	Blackmore and Gallagher 1964
Quail	not specified	Mutalib et al. 1995
Guineafowl	not specified	Goret and Joubert 1947
Little Blue Penguin	*Eudyptula minor*	Boerner 2004
Jackass Penguin	*Spheniscus demersus*	Prot-Lassalle and Nouvel 1964
Red-throated Loon	*Gavia stellata*	Blackmore and Gallagher 1964
Arctic Loon	*Gavia arctica*	Blackmore and Gallagher 1964
Little Grebe	*Tachybaptus ruficollis*	Brack and Stoll 1967
Great Crested Grebes	*Podiceps cristatus*	Blackmore and Gallagher 1964
Great Cormorant	*Phalacrocorax carbo*	Ungureanu et al. 1966
Roseate Spoonbill	*Platalea ajaja*	Blackmore and Gallagher 1964
King Vulture	*Sarcoramphus papa*	Ramsay and Baumeister 1986
Bald Eagle	*Haliaeetus leucocephalus*	Franson et al. 1994
Common Moorhen	*Gallinula chloropus*	Blackmore and Gallagher 1964
Eurasian Coots	*Fulica atra*	Blackmore and Gallagher 1964
Crane (NOS)	not specified	Keymer 1958
South African Crowned Crane	*Balearica regulorum gibbericeps*	Nowak 1957; Decker et al. 1976
Pheasant-tailed Jacana	*Hydrophasianus chirurgus*	Brack and Stoll 1967
Eurasian Oystercatcher	*Haematopus ostralegus*	Brack and Stoll 1967
Common Greenshank	*Tringa nebularia*	Brack and Stoll 1967
Great Black-backed Gull	*Larus marinus*	Blackmore and Gallagher 1964
Common Murre	*Uria aalge*	Blackmore and Gallagher 1964
Rock Pigeon	*Columba livia*	Blackmore and Gallagher 1964
European Turtle Dove	*Streptopelia turtur*	Blackmore and Gallagher 1964
Rosy-faced Lovebird	*Agapornis roseicollis*	Jadin and Beckers 1965
Little Owl	*Athene noctua*	Blackmore and Gallagher 1964
Laughing Kookaburra	*Dacelo novaguineae*	Opriessnig et al. 2005
Eurasian Jackdaw	*Corvus monedula*	Blackmore and Gallagher 1964
Bullfinch	not specified	Keymer 1958

recognized, 19 belonging to *E. rhusiopathiae* and seven belonging to *E. tonsillarum*. Until 1987, *E. tonsillarum* was known as *Erysipelothrix rhusiopathiae* serovar 7 (Takahashi et al. 1987), and later, serovars 3, 10, 14, 20, 22, and 23 were also added to the taxon *E. tonsillarum* (Takahashi et al. 1992). The two species are very similar morphologically and in their biochemical reactions but are genetically distinct by DNA-DNA homology.

In addition to serotyping, protein analyses have been used to differentiate *Erysipelothrix*. Tamura et al. (1993) used whole-cell protein electrophoresis to study the taxonomy of the genus. Chooromoney et al. (1994) used multilocus enzyme electrophoresis to assess the genetic diversity of *E. rhusiopathiae* and *E. tonsillarum* and demonstrated the ability to differentiate the two species. Bernath et al. (1997) used autoradiography and gel protein electrophoresis to study 12 strains of *Erysipelothrix* and found them all to be different, with no relationship between protein fractions and serotype.

More recently, investigators have turned to DNA analysis methods for strain differentiation tasks. Takahashi et al. (1992) used DNA-DNA hybridization analysis to firmly establish the two species of *Erysipelothrix*. Ahrne et al. (1995) used restriction fragment length polymorphisms to classify *Erysipelothrix* based on nine ribotyping patterns. Okatani et al. (2000) differentiated strains of the same serovar and identified genetic variations within strains using a randomly amplified polymorphic DNA method and later using pulsed-field gel electrophoresis (Okatani et al. 2001).

Erysipelothrix tonsillarum was first identified as a saprophyte from swine tonsils. It is considered nonpathogenic for chickens, but its occurrence and effects have not been sufficiently established or discounted in wildlife, especially in wild bird populations. At present, although *E. tonsillarum* can be isolated from many animals, it seems to be pathogenic only in dogs (Takahashi et al. 1993).

EPIZOOTIOLOGY

Although transmission of *Erysipelothrix* under natural conditions is not well understood, the most widely accepted hypotheses suggest that transmission occurs through ingestion or wound infection.

Erysipelothrix has been isolated from a wide variety of sources, but only one report suggests natural infections as a potential reservoir (Timofeeva et al. 1975). A soil association or the possibility of a carrier mammal or bird was postulated in the deaths of captive wild birds, but conclusive evidence was not presented (Blackmore and Gallagher 1964). Several studies of *Erysipelothrix* survival in soil concluded that there was little to no persistence beyond 35 days under the best conditions (Wood 1973; Chandler and Craven 1980). However, within carcasses or other highly organic matter and protected from sunlight, viability could be maintained for at least several months (Jensen and Cotter 1976; Reboli and Farrar 1989).

There is significant literature associating *Erysipelothrix* with fish and fish products, especially concerning isolations from mucus on fish skin. From this, several authors have speculated on food sources being responsible for *Erysipelothrix* transmission. Grenci (1943) isolated *Erysipelothrix* from two samples of fish meal although turkeys were not able to become infected through the feed. More recently, Franson et al. (1994) hypothesized that a diet of fish may have been the source of the organism and contributed to the death of a captive Bald Eagle (*Haliaeetus leucocephalus*). The suspected source of *Erysipelothrix* that killed Brown Pelicans in California was fish offal with protruding sharp bones that abraded or punctured gastrointestinal tissue as it was eaten (K. Converse, NWHC, unpublished data).[3]

Wellmann (1954) was able to experimentally infect doves through feeding them the organism. Richter et al. (1964) reported on cannibalism in pheasants that were fed improperly as a potential cause. Although cannibalism and oral infectivity is a concern in domestic flocks, predation and carrion ingestion should not be ruled out as a route of natural transmission in wild birds.

To more accurately assess the genetic diversity of organisms, determine differences in host predilection or virulence, and track epizootics, investigators have attempted to address strain differences in *Erysipelothrix* organisms. Kucsera (1971) was the first to apply serotyping in studying isolates in a zoological park outbreak involving wild birds. Although others have applied serotyping to studies involving wild bird strains (Kucsera 1979; Eamens 1988), some investigators have determined that serotyping of *Erysipelothrix* is unreliable for use as an epidemiological tool (Bisgaard et al. 1980; Chooromoney et al. 1994). In domestic animals, no relationship has been found between serotype and other epidemiological information such as host predilection, virulence, or seasonal distribution. Differences exist among strain differentiation by serotypes, protein fractions, and DNA-based analyses, but none of these methods has been applied extensively to isolates of *Erysipelothrix* from wild birds. The DNA-based methods, such as pulsed-field gel electrophoresis, are particularly promising. With the second species having been established only in 1987 and with the difficulty in biochemically distinguishing the species, the prevalence of *E. tonsillarum* as well as the diversity of *Erysipelothrix* strains in wild birds are not truly known.

CLINICAL SIGNS

In wild birds there are typically no specific signs associated with *Erysipelothrix* infection. Occasionally lethargy may be noted, but the death of one or more birds is usually the first sign of this acute septicemic disease in wild birds.

PATHOGENESIS

Pathogenesis in wild birds has not been well studied but should be considered similar to that seen in domestic animals. Neuraminidase is produced by most pathogenic strains and is considered an important virulence factor (Kovalev 1982; Nakato et al. 1986). Neuraminidase cleaves sialic acid, leading to vascular damage and hyaline thrombus formation. Most strains also produce hyaluronidase and coagulase, both typically associated with virulence in other organisms but not apparently a virulence factor with *Erysipelothrix* (Tesh and Wood 1988). In addition, *Erysipelothrix* capsules probably play a role in resistance to phagocytosis and may represent a significant factor in chronic infections (Shimoji et al. 1994).

PATHOLOGY

On gross examination, lesions may be subtle or unapparent. Lesions suggesting septicemia, such as generalized congestion or petechial or ecchymotic hemorrhages in pericardial fat, pleura, or skeletal muscle, can sometimes be present (Blyde and Woods 1999; Work et al. 1999; Opriessnig et al. 2005). The liver and spleen can be swollen. Arthritis is common in domestic poultry and mammals with chronic infections, but *Erysipelothrix* arthritis has not been reported in wild birds.

Microscopic lesions are also typically subtle. Intravascular clumps of small, Gram-positive rods can occasionally be noted. Fibrin thrombi may be seen in small pulmonary blood vessels, renal glomerular capillaries, hepatic sinusoids, or other sites, sometimes accompanied by acute parenchymal damage (Bricker and Saif 1997; Work et al. 1999; Boerner et al. 2004; Opriessnig et al. 2005).

DIAGNOSIS

Diagnosis of erysipelas in wild birds depends on isolation or detection of the organism. In sick birds, aerobic culturing of blood may yield success. Typically, however, necropsy specimens of internal organs (liver, spleen, heart, and kidney) are most appropriate. Culture attempts on standard sheep's blood agar yield nonhemolytic or alpha-hemolytic pinpoint colonies, resembling streptococci, after 18 to 24 hours at 37°C. Although *Erysipelothrix* grows well aerobically, growth is enhanced with slight carbon dioxide increase (5–10%). Selective media have been employed to improve the recovery but are often not needed (Harrington and Hulse 1971; Bratberg 1981). Nutrient media for neuraminidase production or high bacterial yields have also been described (Abrashev and Velcheva 1988), as well as several media for vaccine production. Embryonated chicken eggs (Cooper and Bickford 1998) and mouse inoculation can be used to purify the bacteria from mixed cultures.

In culture, *Erysipelothrix* is Gram-positive but decolorizes easily and appears as straight or curved rods, often in clumps. Colony morphology progresses from convex, circular, smooth colonies to rough colonies with undulate edges upon serial passage. The bacterium is catalase and oxidase negative and nonmotile. Inoculation of triple sugar iron agar (TSIA) shows an acid over acid reaction, with hydrogen sulfide production being a key reaction. Use of abbreviated identification schemes may lead to misidentification if the hydrogen sulfide reaction is omitted (Dunbar and Clarridge 2000). Fermentation reactions are typically weak but positive for glucose, lactose, and galactose. Carbohydrate fermentation reactions can be variable, and quality control of media and reactions with known strains is advised (White and Shuman 1961). *Erysipelothrix tonsillarum* usually ferments saccharose, whereas *E. rhusiopathiae* does not, but DNA testing is usually required for species differentiation.

Commercial test kits that do an adequate job of identifying the organism to genus are available, but most do not include or differentiate *E. tonsillarum* (Soto et al. 1994). Analysis of cellular fatty acids has been used to identify the organism (Takahashi et al. 1994) and is available commercially. Polymerase chain reaction (PCR) methods, based on amplification of a portion of either the 16S or 23S rRNA gene (Makino et al. 1994; Takeshi et al. 1999), and fluorescent antibody methods have been developed for detection of the organism (Harrington et al. 1974). The PCR methods have been applied to formalin-fixed tissue for identification of the organism when culture was negative (Hennig et al. 2002; Boerner et al. 2004). No relationship between host species and serotype has been recognized (Nørrung and Molin 1991), so serotyping is not routinely done, but other protein analyses and DNA-based strain differentiation methods appear promising for epidemiologic tracking.

IMMUNITY

Immunity to *Erysipelothrix* has not been studied in wild birds, but similarities to domestic species may exist. Young domestic poultry and stressed poultry are more likely to be infected than older or less stressed birds, suggesting that immunity may play a role (Graham et al. 1939). Studies with domestic animals show that *Erysipelothrix* can produce a chronic infection that manifests itself in an arthritic condition resulting from an incomplete immune response. Without protective antibodies, the organism is capable of evading phagocytosis, and even if phagocytized, they are able to reproduce intracellularly (Shimoji 2000). In domestic poultry, primarily turkeys, vaccination produces a degree of protection although multiple vaccinations with annual boosters are required for complete protection. Vaccines have been used to protect commercial pheasant flocks and captive emus

(Swan and Lindsey 1998). No vaccine use has been reported for wild birds.

PUBLIC HEALTH CONCERNS

Erysipelothrix infection is a zoonotic disease of relatively low pathogenicity for humans. Although there is a human disease termed erysipelas, it is due to group A streptococci and needs to be differentiated from the zoonotic disease. Typically, occupational exposure is the source of *Erysipelothrix* infection, occurring principally as a result of contact with animals and their products or wastes, although human cases without occupational exposure occasionally have been reported (Abedini and Lester 1997) (Sheng et al. 2000). Infections in humans may take one of three forms: a mild cutaneous infection known as erysipeloid; a diffuse cutaneous form; and a rare systemic complication with septicemia and endocarditis. Individuals in contact with potential *Erysipelothrix* mortality in wild birds should take precautions, such as use of protective gloves, to avoid accidental infection via skin wounds or mucous membranes.

DOMESTIC ANIMAL HEALTH CONCERNS

Erysipelothrix is the etiologic agent of swine erysipelas and causes economically important diseases in domestic turkeys, chickens, ducks, and emus. Improved animal husbandry and vaccination programs have limited the organism's impact in recent times, but the threat is still present. Although often cited as a potential source or reservoir of the organism, transmission from wild birds to domestic animals has been only hypothesized and not established (Keymer 1958; Mackenzie 1988). It is most likely that the organism exists only transiently in the wild bird population, both as an occasional saprophyte and an occasional pathogen.

WILDLIFE POPULATION IMPACTS

Based on the current prevalence of the disease in wild birds, the impact to populations is considered inconsequential. Occasional large outbreaks in Eared Grebes, such as those at the Great Salt Lake (Jensen and Cotter 1976), are rare and not known to have a significant or lasting impact on wild bird populations.

TREATMENT AND CONTROL

Specific information on treating wild birds is not well documented nor published, due predominately to the acute nature of the disease. However, *E. rhusiopathiae* is susceptible to many antibiotics including penicillin, cephalosporin, cefotaxime, clindamycin, and the fluoroquinolones. Penicillin administered by subcutaneous injection or via drinking water has successfully treated or controlled mortality in domestic poultry (Mutalib et al. 1995). Resistance to erythromycin, oxytetracycline, sulfonamides, vancomycin, and the aminoglycosides has been reported (Venditti et al. 1990). Resistance to antimicrobial agents does not seem to be plasmid mediated although plasmids are present in some strains (Takahashi et al. 1984).

During outbreaks, carcass removal (using appropriate personal protection) and incineration will reduce exposure of unaffected birds and help limit the mortality event. Natural sunlight will effectively reduce viable organisms after carcass removal has been accomplished. In captive bird management, preventive actions such as adequate sanitation, stress reduction, and health monitoring are probably more effective than attempts at disease eradication.

UNPUBLISHED DATA

1. Diagnostic Microbiology Laboratory, U.S Geological Survey, National Wildlife Health Center (USGS-NWHC), Madison, Wisconsin, U.S.A.
2. Rex Sohn, USGS-NWHC, Madison, Wisconsin, U.S.A.
3. Kathryn A. Converse, USGS-NWHC, Madison, Wisconsin, U.S.A.

LITERATURE CITED

Abedini, S., and A. Lester. 1997. *Erysipelothrix rhusiopathiae* bacteremia after dog bite. *Ugeskr Laeger* 159:4400–4401.

Abrashev, I., and P. Velcheva. 1988. A nutrient medium for the culturing and neuraminidase biosynthesis of *Erysipelothrix rhusiopathiae. Acta Microbiologica Bulgarica* 23:49–51.

Ahrné, S., I.M. Stenström, N.E. Jensen, B. Pettersson, M. Uhlén, and G. Molin. 1995. Classification of *Erysipelothrix* strains on the basis of restriction fragment length polymorphisms. *International Journal of Systematic Bacteriology* 45:382–385.

Bailie, W.E., R.J. Bury, E.J. Bicknel, and W.U. Knudtso. 1970. Case report: Erysipelothrix infection in goslings. *Avian Diseases* 14:555–556.

Bernath, S., G. Kucsera, I. Kadar, G, Horvath, and G. Morovjan. 1997. Comparison of the protein patterns of *Erysipelothrix rhusiopathiae* strains by SDS-PAGE and autoradiography. *Acta Veterinaria Hungarica* 45:417–425.

Bigland, C.H. 1957. Isolation of *Erysipelothrix rhusiopathiae* from a golden eagle. *Canadian Journal of Comparative Medicine* 21:290–291.

Bisgaard, M., V.Nørrung and N. Tornoe. 1980. Erysipelas in poultry: Prevalence of serotypes and epidemiological investigations. *Avian Pathology* 9:355–362.

Blackmore, D.K. and G.L. Gallagher. 1964. An outbreak of erysipelas in captive wild birds and mammals. *Veterinary Record* 76:1161–1164.

Blyde, D.J., and R. Woods. 1999. R. Erysipelas in malleefowl. *Australian Veterinary Journal* 77:434–435.

Boerner, L.K., R. Nevis, L.S. Hinckley, E.S. Weber, and S. Frasca Jr. 2004. *Erysipelothrix* septicemia in a little blue penguin (*Eudyptula minor*). *Journal of Veterinary Diagnostic Investigation* 16:145–149.

Brack, M., and L. Stoll. 1967. Erysipelotlirix bei Zoovögeln. *Kleintier-Praxis* 12:109–111.

Bratberg, A.M. 1981. Observations on the utilization of a selective medium for the isolation of *Erysipelothrix rhusiopathiae*. *Acta Veterinaria Scandinavica* 22:55–59.

Bricker, J.M., and Y.M. Saif. 1997. Erysipelas. In *Diseases of Poultry,* 10th Ed., B.W. Calnek University (ed.). Iowa State University Press, Ames, Iowa, U.S.A., pp. 303–313.

Buchanan, R.E. 1918. Studies in the nomenclature and classification of bacteria. *Journal of Bacteriology* 3:27–61.

Butcher, G., and B. Panigrahy. 1985. An outbreak of erysipelas in chukars. *Avian Diseases* 29:843–845.

Chandler, D.S., and J.A. Craven. 1980. Persistence and distribution of *Erysipelothrix rhusiopathiae* and bacterial indicator organisms on land used for disposal of piggery effluent. *Journal of Applied Bacteriology* 48:367–375.

Chooromoney, K.N., D.J. Hampson, G.J. Eamens, and M. Turner. 1994. Analysis of *Erysipelothrix rhusiopathiae* and *Erysipelothrix tonsillarum* by multilocus enzyme electrophoresis. *Journal of Clinical Microbiology* 32:371–376.

Cooper, G.L., and Bickford, A.A. 1998. Erysipelas. In *A Laboratory Manual for the Isolation and Identification of Avian Pathogens,* D.E. Swayne, J.R. Glisson, M.W. Jackwood, J.E. Pearson, and W.M. Reed (eds.). American Association of Avian Pathologists, Inc. Kennett Square, PA, U.S.A., pp. 47–50.

Decker, R.A., R. Lindauer, and G.W. Archibald. 1976. *Erysipelothrix* infection in two East African crowned cranes (*Balearica regulorum gibbericeps*) and a wood duck (*Aix sponsa*). *Avian Diseases* 21:326–327.

Dunbar, S.A., and J.E. Clarridge. 2000. Potential errors in recognition of *Erysipelothrix rhusiopathiae. Journal of Clinical Microbiology* 38:1302–1304.

Dédié, K. 1949. Diesäurelöslichen antigene von *Erysipelothrix rhusiopathiae. Monatshefte für Veterinärmedizin* 4:7–10.

Eamens, G.J. 1988. Pathogenicity of field isolates of *Erysipelothrix rhusiopathiae* in mice, rats and pigs. *Australian Veterinary Journal* 65:280–284.

Faddoul, G.P., G.W. Fellows, and J. Baird. 1968. *Erysipelothrix* infection in starlings. *Avian Diseases* 12:61–66.

Franson, J.C., E.J. Galbreath, S.N. Wiemeyer, and J.M. Abell. 1994. *Erysipelothrix rhusiopathiae* infection in a captive bald eagle (*Haliaeetus leucocephalus*). *Journal of Zoo and Wildlife Medicine* 25:446–448.

Goret, P., and L. Joubert. 1947. Isolement du bacille du rouget chez une pintade. *Bulletin de l'Academie Veterinaire de France* 20:463–466.

Graham, R., N.D. Levine, and H.R. Hester. 1939. *Erysipelothrix rhusiopathiae* associated with a fatal disease in ducks. *Journal of the American Veterinary Medical Association* 95:211–216.

Grenci, C.M. 1943. The isolation of *Erysipelothrix rhusiopathiae* and experimental infection in turkeys. *Cornell Veterinarian* 33:56–60.

Griffiths, G.L., and N. Buller. 1991. *Erysipelothrix rhusiopathiae* infection in semi-intensively farmed emus. *Australian Veterinary Journal* 68:121–122.

Harrington, R.J., and D.C. Hulse. 1971. Comparison of two plating media for the isolation of *Erysipelothrix rhusiopathiae* from enrichment broth culture. *Applied Microbiology* 22(1):141–142.

Harrington Jr., R., R.L. Wood, and D.C. Hulse. 1974. Comparison of a fluorescent antibody technique and cultural method for the detection of *Erysipelothrix rhusiopathiae* in primary broth cultures. *American Journal of Veterinary Research* 35:461–462.

Hennig, G.E., H.D. Goebel, J.J. Fabis, and M.I. Khan. 2002. Diagnosis by polymerase chain reaction of Erysipelas septicemia in a flock of ring-necked pheasants. *Avian Diseases* 46:509–14.

Jadin, J.M., and A. Beckers. 1965. *D'Erysipelothrix rhusiopathiae* chez *Agapornis roseicollis. Bulletins de la Société Royale de Zoologie d'Anvers* 36:17–23.

Jarmai, K. 1919. Orbanczbaczillusok elofordulasa madarakban. *Allatorvosi Lapok (Veterinarius)* 42: 57–58.

Jensen, W.I., and S.E. Cotter. 1976. An outbreak of erysipelas in eared grebes (*Podiceps nigricollis*). *Journal of Wildlife Diseases* 12:583–586.

Kaneene, J.B., R.F. Taylor, J.G. Sikarskie, T.J. Meyer, and N.A. Richter. 1985. Disease patterns in the Detroit Zoo (Royal Oak, Michigan, U.S.A.): A study of the avian population from 1973 through 1983. *Journal of the American Veterinary Medical Association* 187:1129–1131.

Karstad, L., and L. Sileo. 1971. Causes of death in captive wild waterfowl in the Kortright Waterfowl Park, 1967–1970. *Journal of Wildlife Diseases* 7:236–241.

Keymer, I.F. 1958. A survey and review of the causes of mortality in British birds and the significance of wild birds as dissemination of disease. I. A survey of the causes of mortality. *Veterinary Record* 70: 713–720.

Kovalev, G.K. 1982. Biological problems of *Erysipelothrix rhusiopathiae* (review of the literature). *Zhurnal Mikrobiologii, Epidemiologii i Immunobiologii* 3:11–18.

Kucsera, G. 1971. Detection of new serotypes among *Erysipelothrix rhusiopathiae* strains of different origin. *Acta Veterinaria Academiae Scientiarum Hungaricae* 21:211–219.

Kucsera, G. 1979. Serological typing of *Erysipelothrix rhusiopathiae* strains and the epizootiological significance of the typing. *Acta Veterinaria Academiae Scientiarum Hungaricae* 27:19–28.

Leighton, F.A. 2001. *Erysipelothrix* infection. In *Infectious Diseases of Wild Mammals,* 3rd Ed., E.S. Williams and I. K. Barker (eds.). Iowa State University Press, Ames, Iowa, U.S.A., pp. 491–493.

Mackenzie, J.S. 1988. Prokaryotic and viral diseases transmitted by wild birds. In *Australian Wildlife: The John Keep Refresher Course for Veterinarians,* Proceedings No. 104. Post Graduate Committee in Veterinary Science, University of Sidney, Sidney, Australia, pp. 657–702.

Makino, S., Y. Okada, T. Maruyama, K. Ishikawa, T. Takahashi, M. Nakamura, T. Ezaki, and H. Morita. 1994. Direct and rapid detection of *Erysipelothrix rhusiopathiae* DNA in animals by PCR. *Journal of Clinical Microbiology* 32:1526–1531.

McDiarmid, A. 1962. Diseases of free-living wild animals. *Food and Agricultural Organization: Agriculture Studies* 57:34.

Morgan, M.J., J.O. Britt, J.M. Cockrill, and M.L. Eiten. 1994. *Erysipelothrix rhusiopathiae* infection in an emu (*Dromaius novaehollandiae*). *Journal of Veterinary Diagnostic Investigation* 6:378–379.

Mutalib, A., R. Keirs, and F. Austin. 1995. Erysipelas in quail and suspected erysipeloid in processing plant employees. *Avian Diseases* 391:191–193.

Nakato, H., K. Shinomiya, and H. Mikawa. 1986. Possible role of neuraminidase in the pathogenesis of arteritis and thrombocytopenia induced in rats by *Erysipelothrix rhusiopathiae. Pathology, Research and Practice* 181(3):311–319.

Nørrung, V., and G. Molin. 1991. A new serotype of *Erysipelothrix rhusiopathiae* isolated from pig slurry. *Acta Veterinaria Hungarica* 39: 137–138.

Nowak, B. 1957. Rozyca u ptakou. *Medycyna Weterynaryjna* 13:272–275.

Okatani, A.T., H. Hayashidani, T. Takahashi, T. Taniguchi, M. Ogawa, and K. I. Kaneko. 2000. Randomly amplified polymorphic DNA analysis of *Erysipelothrix* spp. *Journal of Clinical Microbiology* 38:4332–4336.

Okatani, A.T., T. Uto, T. Taniguchi, T. Horisaka, T. Horikita, K. Kaneko, and H. Hayashidani. 2001. Pulsed-field gel electrophoresis in differentiation of *Erysipelothrix* species strains. *Journal of Clinical Microbiology* 39:4032–4036.

Opriessnig, T., R.K. Vance, and P.G. Halbur. 2005. *Erysipelothrix rhusiopathiae* septicemia in a Laughing Kookaburra (*Dacelo novaeguineae*). *Journal of Veterinary Diagnostic Investigation* 17:497–499.

Prot-Lassalle, J., and J. Nouvel. 1964. Septicemie a bacille du rouget chez des manchots en captivite. *Recueil de Medecine Veterinaire* 140:33–36.

Ramsay, E.C., and B.M. Baumeister. 1986. Isolation of *Erysipelothrix rhusiopathiae* from lesions of distal extremity necrosis in a captive king vulture. *Journal of Wildlife Diseases* 22:430–431.

Reboli, A.C., and W.E. Farrar. 1989. *Erysipelothrix rhusiopathiae:* an occupational pathogen. *Clinical Microbiology Reviews* 2:354–359.

Richter, S., M. Karlovic, and P. Grmovsek. 1964. Prikaz epizootije vrbanca u fazana. *Veterinarski Arhiv* 34: 101–106.

Sheng, W.H., P.R. Hsueh, C.C. Hung, C.T. Fang, S.C. Chang, and K.T. Luh. 2000. Fatal outcome of *Erysipelothrix rhusiopathiae* bacteremia in a patient with oropharyngeal cancer. *Journal of the Formosan Medical Association* 99:431–434.

Shimoji, Y. 2000. Pathogenicity of *Erysipelothrix rhusiopathiae:* virulence factors and protective immunity. *Microbes and Infection* 2:965–972.

Shimoji, Y., Y. Yokomizo, T. Sekizaki, Y. Mori, and M. Kubo. 1994. Presence of a capsule in *Erysipelothrix rhusiopathiae* and its relationship to virulence for mice. *Infection and Immunity* 62(7):2806–2810.

Soto, A., J. Zapardiel, and F. Soriano. 1994. Evaluation of API Coryne system for identifying coryneform bacteria. *Journal of Clinical Pathology 47:*756–759.

Swan, R.A., and M.J. Lindsey. 1998. Treatment and control by vaccination of erysipelas in farmed emus (*Dromaius novohollandiae*). *Australian Veterinary Journal* 76:325–327.

Takahashi, T., T. Sawada, K. Ohmae, N. Terakado, M. Muramatsu, K. Seto, T. Maruyama, and M. Kanzaki. 1984. Antibiotic resistance of *Erysipelothrix rhusiopathiae* isolated from pigs with chronic swine erysipelas. *Antimicrobial Agents and Chemotherapy* 25:385–386.

Takahashi, T., T. Sawada, M. Muramatsu, Y. Tamura, T. Fujisawa, Y. Benno, and T. Mitsuoka. 1987. Serotype, antimicrobial susceptibility, and pathogenicity of *Erysipelothrix rhusiopathiae* isolates from tonsils of apparently healthy slaughter pigs. *Journal of Clinical Microbiology* 25:536–539.

Takahashi, T., T. Fujisawa, Y. Tamura, S. Suzuki, M. Muramatsu, T. Sawada, Y. Benno, and T. Mitsuoka. 1992. DNA relatedness among *Erysipelothrix rhusiopathiae* strains representing all twenty-three serovars and *Erysipelothrix tonsillarum. International Journal of Systematic Bacteriology* 42:469–473.

Takahashi, T., Y. Tamura, H. Yoshimura, N. Nagamine, M. Kijima, M. Nakamura, and L.A. Devriese. 1993. Erysipelothrix tonsillarum isolated from dogs with endocarditis in Belgium. *Research in Veterinary Science* 54:264–265.

Takahashi, T., Y. Tamura, Y.S. Endoh and N. Hara. 1994. Cellular fatty acid composition of *Erysipelothrix rhusiopathiae* and *Erysipelothrix tonsillarum. Journal of Veterinary Medical Science* 56:385–387.

Takeshi, K., S. Makino, T. Ikeda, N. Takada, A. Nakashiro, K. Nakanishi, K. Oguma, Y. Katoh, H. Sunagawa, and T. Ohyama. 1999. Direct and Rapid Detection by PCR of *Erysipelothrix* sp. DNAs Prepared from Bacterial Strains and Animal Tissues. *Journal of Clinical Microbiology* 37: 4093–4098.

Tamura, Y., T. Takahashi, K. Zarkasie, M. Nakamura, and H. Yoshimura. 1993. Differentiation of *Erysipelothrix rhusiopathiae* and *Erysipelothrix tonsillarum* by sodium dodecyl sulfate-polyacrylamide gel electrophoresis of cell proteins. *International Journal of Systematic Bacteriology* 43:111–114.

Tesh, M.J., and R.L. Wood. 1988. Detection of coagulase activity in *Erysipelothrix rhusipathiae. Journal of Clinical Microbiology* 26:1058–1060.

Timofeeva, A.A., R.D. Shcherbina, T.I. Evseeva, N.G. Olsuf'ev, and I.S. Meshcheriakova. 1975. Erysipeloid on the islands of the Sea of Okhotsk. I. The sources and vectors of the causative agent of erysipeloid. *Zhurnal Mikrobiologii Epidemiologii i Immunobiologii* 9:119–126.

Ungureanu, C., A. Jordache, N. Ghitescu, and A. Danescu. 1966. Izolorea unor tulpini de *Erysipelothrix rhusiopathiae* de la pasari Salbatice tinute in captivitatae. *Lucrarile Institutului de Cercetari Veterinare, si Biopreparate Pasteur* 3:219.

Urbain, A. 1947. Infection spontanee d'oiseaux de voliere par le bacille du roget. *Bulletin de l'Academie Veterinaire de France* 20:201–203.

Van Vuuren, M., and J.M. Brown. 1990. Septicaemic *Erysipelothrix rhusiopathiae* infection in the Little Swift (*Apus affinis*). *Journal of the South African Veterinary Association* 61:170–171.

Venditti, M., V. Gelfusa, A. Tarasi, C. Brandimarte, and P. Serra. 1990. Antimicrobial susceptibilities of *Erysipelothrix rhusiopathiae. Antimicrobial Agents and Chemotherapy* 34(10):2038–2040.

Wellmann, G. 1954. Rotlaufinfektionsversuche an wilden Mauesen, Sperlingen, Huelineen, und Puten. *Tierarztliche Umschau* 9/10:269–273.

White, T.G., and R.D. Shuman.1961. Fermentation reactions of *Erysipelothrix rhusiopathiae. Journal of Bacteriology* 82:595–599.

Wood, R.L. 1973. Survival of *Erysipelothrix rhusiopathiae* in soil under various environmental conditions. *Cornell Veterinarian* 63:390–410.

Work, T.M., D. Ball and M. Wolcott. 1999. Erysipelas in a free-ranging Hawaiian crow (*Corvus hawaiiensis*). *Avian Diseases* 43:338–341.

Zhukova, L.N., T.A. Konshina, and V.M. Popugailo. 1966. Listeriosis and erysipeloid infection of rodents in the Sverdlovsk region. *Zhurnal Mikrobiologii, Epidemiologii i Immunobiologii* 43:18–23.

18
Borrelia

Björn Olsen

INTRODUCTION

Borrelias are bacteria in the order Spirochaetales, large motile helical organisms, not free living, and transmitted by arthropods from the vertebrate reservoirs. Spirochetes within the genus *Borrelia* can be divided into different pathogenic groups: Lyme disease *Borrelia,* relapsing fever *Borrelia,* and the animal spirochetosis agents *Borrelia anserina* and *Borrelia coriaceae.* Besides *B. anserina,* the disease-causing agent of domestic and feral poultry in tropical and subtropical regions, other *Borrelia* have minor or little significance as a disease agent of wild birds. On the other hand, it has been shown that birds play a role in transmission, maintenance, and long-distance movement of Lyme disease *Borrelia.*

This chapter focuses on the role of birds in the epidemiology and maintenance of enzootic cycles of *Borrelia* and the emerging role of birds in Lyme borreliosis. Avian borreliosis is summarized at the chapter's end.

Lyme Borreliosis

INTRODUCTION

Lyme borreliosis, the most prevalent tick-borne zoonoses in humans in North America, Europe, and the temperate region of Asia, is a multisystemic disorder caused by the spirochete *Borrelia burgdorferi* sensu lato (s.l., meaning "in the broad sense"). Many mammals and birds act as reservoirs for the spirochete, which is transmitted among wildlife, domestic animals, and humans, primarily by ticks of the *Ixodes ricinus* complex.

Lyme borreliosis is described as a "great imitator" because it can mimic many other diseases, which makes diagnosis difficult. In humans, a rash can appear several days after infection, forming a round ring with central clearing at the site of the tick bite. Untreated, the infection can progress into more disseminated stages and imitate other conditions, such as rheumatoid arthritis and disorders of the central and peripheral nervous system. Lyme borreliosis is treatable with antibiotics, but the best way to prevent it is to check frequently for attached ticks and remove them. For a review of the role of wild mammals in the ecology and epidemiology of Lyme borreliosis, see Brown and Burgess 2001. The interaction between wild birds and *B. burgdorferi* s.l. appears to be benign, based on the results of challenge studies. Several bird species, primarily passerines but also certain seabirds, act as competent reservoirs of *B. burgdorferi* s.l. and are capable of transmitting the spirochete to host-seeking ticks. From an epizootiological and epidemiological view, there appear to be two mechanisms for the spread of *B. burgdorferi* s.l. by birds and its maintenance in enzootic foci: (i) During migration and other long-distance movements, birds can transport infected ticks to new areas where local mammalian or avian reservoir hosts can contribute to the establishment of new foci for Lyme borreliosis. (ii) Several species of birds play a role, not just as tick carriers but as spirochetal reservoirs infective to ticks.

SYNONYMS

In humans: Lyme disease, erythema chronicum migrans, erythema migrans, acrodermatitis chronica atrophicans, lymphadenosis benigna cutis, Bannwarth's syndrome, Garin-Bujadoux syndrome, chronic lymphocytic meningoradiculoneuritis, tick borne meningoradiculoneuritis.

HISTORY

In October 1975, two mothers living in Lyme, Connecticut, whose children had recently been diagnosed with juvenile rheumatoid arthritis, notified the Connecticut State Health Department about several cases of arthritis in the area. The epidemiological investigation revealed an incidence of arthritis much higher than might be expected. The uneven distribution of the cases was puzzling, with most victims living in wooded areas and only a few in town centers. The disease was obviously not contagious and individuals of the same family often contracted the disease in different years. About 25% of the patients remembered having a strange skin rash prior to the onset of the arthritis. On the basis of these findings, it was concluded that the disease was caused by an unknown virus or bacteria transmitted by an unknown arthropod (Habicht et al. 1987). However, testing sera from Lyme disease patients for the presence of antibodies against a number of arthropod borne diseases gave no positive results. The rash, or erythema, of the Lyme migrans was reminiscent of that described by the Swedish dermatologist Arvid Afzelius in 1909 (Afzelius 1910). Afzelius named it erythema chronicum and suspected that it was caused by a tick bite.

A possible vector was identified, *Ixodes dammini,* a tick species closely related to *I. ricinus.* Despite the determination of a possible vector, no Lyme disease–causing pathogen was found until 1981, when Willy Burgdorfer examined *I. dammini* ticks collected on Shelter Island, New York. By phase contrast microscopy, he found spirochete-like bacteria in some of the ticks and realized that these spirochetes could be the causative agent of the disease (Steere et al. 1983). Alan G. Barbour of the Rocky Mountain Laboratories was able to grow the spirochetes in a special medium, BSKII (Barbour 1984). Sera from Lyme disease patients showed a pronounced antibody response to the bacteria. The etiologic agent of Lyme borreliosis was thereby discovered and the spirochete was named *Borrelia burgdorferi* (Steere et al. 1983).

ETIOLOGY

Spirochetes are long, thin, helical bacteria, with multiple bipolar endoflagella that make them highly motile and easily viewed in wet smears using a dark field or phase contrast microscope. All members of the genus *Borrelia* have an obligate parasitic lifestyle, with no free-living stages known.

Borrelia burgdorferi s.l., is a group consisting of at least ten species, including *B. burgdorferi* sensu stricto (s.s.), *B. afzelii, B. garinii, B. japonica, B. andersonii, B. valaisiana, B. lusitaniae, B. bissettii, B. tanukii, B. turdi,* and several unnamed variants (Baranton et al. 1992; Canica et al. 1993; Postic et al. 1993; Postic et al. 1998). *Borrelia burgdorferi* s.s., *B. afzelii,* and *B. garinii* are the currently known human pathogens but there are also unknown types of *B. burgdorferi* s.l. isolated from Lyme disease patients (Picken et al. 1996; Strle et al. 1997). The taxonomy and phylogenetic relationships of the different *B. burgdorferi* s.l. species is extensive and complicated. Some genospecies are strongly associated with single tick species and narrow ecosystems, whereas others are more plastic in vector and reservoir preference. For example, *B. garinii* has been isolated from at least five tick species: *I. ricinus, I. persulcatus, I. ovatus, I. hexagonus,* and *I. uriae* (Aeschlimann et al. 1986; Gern et al. 1991; Kawabata et al. 1993; Olsen et al. 1993).

Borrelia burgdorferi s.l. can be up to 30 μm long and have a diameter of 0.2–0.5 μm, with multiple bipolar endoflagella. *Borrelia burgdorferi* s.l. show chemotaxis (Shi et al. 1998) and are especially motile in viscous medium (Kimsey and Spielman 1990). Cultivation is possible at 20–37°C in the rabbit serum–supplemented BSKII medium that is a rich and complex medium (Barbour 1984). In the periplasmic space, 7 to 11 flagella attached to the poles are wrapped around the cell cylinder, giving the bacterium its characteristic flat wave shape (Barbour and Hayes 1986). The outer membrane is fluid filled with unusually high lipoprotein content (Brandt et al. 1990). Several lipoproteins, notably the outer surface proteins OspA-F, show a differential pattern of expression in ticks and vertebrate hosts (Ohnishi et al. 2001). The functions of OspA and OspC have been thoroughly studied and have been shown to be important in the tick. OspA is expressed by the spirochete in the unfed tick's midgut and mediates adhesion to the midgut epithelium (Pal et al. 2000). OspC expression is induced 36–48 hours into the blood meal and probably mediates escape of the spirochete from the tick midgut via hemolymph to the salivary glands, from where it enters the new vertebrate host (Schwan and Piesman 2000). Antibodies against OspA in the blood of vertebrate hosts kill spirochetes in the tick midgut before dispersal to the salivary glands and thereby block transmission to the vertebrate host (de Silva et al. 1999). Antibodies against OspC are also efficient, probably blocking the transmission by preventing migration of spirochetes to the salivary glands (Gilmore and Piesman 2000). Even if immunization with OspA and OspC confer protective immunity in animal studies, the use of these as vaccines may, however, be limited by the apparent variability of these proteins (Wilske et al. 1996).

Detection and Identification Methods

The diagnosis of Lyme disease in humans and domestic animals must be based on clinical symptoms and a history of exposure to ticks (Stanek et al. 1996) and confirmed by detection of the organism. Because it appears that wild birds do not show clinical signs of an ongoing infection, avian investigations focus on detection. The ultimate confirmation is cultivation of *Borrelia* spirochetes from a biopsy specimen. It is, however, difficult to perform, with a success rate of 0–70% depending on the type of specimen inoculated and stage of the disease (Wilske and Preac-Mursic 1993). Because the number of spirochetes in tissues is low, direct observation of spirochetes in samples is rarely possible, but polymerase chain reaction (PCR) amplification of *Borrelia* DNA is useful and sometimes performed in clinical diagnosis (Priem et al. 1997; Lebech et al. 2000).

Both phenotypic and genotypic typing methods have been applied to the *B. burgdorferi* s.l. strains isolated. Among the phenotypic methods, serotyping using monoclonal antibodies against OspA (Wilske et al. 1993) and OspC (Wilske et al. 1995) is the simplest and most commonly performed. It is important to note that these methods do not provide any information about whether the isolate is from a human, a bird, or a tick.

Genotypic methods are applicable not only to cultivated strains but also to PCR-amplified DNA. Methods based on PCR include species specific PCR, randomly amplified polymorphic DNA (RAPD) fingerprinting or arbitrary primed (AP-) PCR, Restriction Fragment Length Polymorphism of PCR amplified fragments (PCR-RFLP), and nucleotide sequencing (Wang et al. 1999). Methods requiring cultivation of the spirochetes are, for example, ribotyping by hybridization with rRNA-directed probes to RFLP generated fragments of genomic DNA, pulse field gel electrophoresis (PFGE), and the labor-intensive DNA-DNA reassociation analyses. Many methods have high congruence but differing resolution at the species and subspecies levels (Wang et al. 1999).

In humans, serology is commonly used to support the diagnosis although a large proportion of people do not develop antibodies against *Borrelia,* especially in early Lyme disease (Aguero-Rosenfeld et al. 1996). Enzyme-linked immunosorbent assay (ELISA) is the most common method used but there are problems with false positives due to, for example, other spirochetal infections, rheumatoid arthritis, or Epstein-Barr virus infection (Magnarelli 1995). Interpretation of the results depends on the strain used as the source of antigens as well as on the immunological background of the population in the particular geographical area (Hauser et al. 1997). Despite attempts and a few descriptions of using serology in avian studies (Olsen et al. 1996; Gauthier-Clerc et al. 1999), there has not been any development of a reliable serological method to diagnose Lyme disease *Borrelia* infections in wild birds.

When studying birds under laboratory conditions, xenodiagnosis (feeding uninfected ticks on a host and subsequently examining for tick infection) is the optimal method for assessment of reservoir competence in a specific species. During field studies, when it is virtually impossible to use xenodiagnostic methods, the evaluation of host infectivity is often based on the rate of infected larvae collected from a specific bird. If the prevalence of the infection in attached larvae exceeds that in unfed, host-seeking larvae, it is likely that the bird transmits the spirochete and serves as a competent reservoir. Another used but notoriously difficult method is to grow spirochetes from blood or body fluid samples in BSKII medium. The difficulties arise from several areas. First, during field conditions the medium is easily contaminated. Second, since the spirochetemia in birds appears to be short and transient, a negative result may just be a reflection of being in the nonspirochetemic phase. Third, birds may be infective to ticks by transmitting *B. burgdorferi* s.l. from skin or subcutanous fluid, rather than blood. To what extent birds are infective to ticks by this route is unknown. To evaluate this, studies based on cultivation from subcutaneous fluids or tissue need to be performed.

EPIZOOTIOLOGY

Terrestrial Enzootic Cycle

An enzootic cycle of infection is maintained by the passage of *B. burgdorferi* s.l. back and forth between ticks and their hosts. The main vectors for Lyme disease *Borrelia* spirochetes are the slow-feeding hard ticks (Ixodidae). Ticks are arthropods that have several life stages, and each transformation requires a blood meal from a vertebrate host. Ixodid ticks undergo three life stages, larva, nymph, and adult, in 1–3 years depending on the climate (Sonenshine 1993).

Borrelia burgdorferi s.l. is transmitted by ticks within the *Ixodes ricinus* complex. In Eurasia, *I. persulcatus* is distributed from Eastern Europe to Japan and *I. ricinus* from Eastern Europe to the Atlantic coast (Sonenshine 1993). In North America, six species of *Ixodes* ticks are involved in the transmission of *B. burgdorferi* s.l., including *I. scapularis* in the north and east and *I. pacificus* in the west (Sonenshine 1993).

Ixodid ticks feed on a broad range of vertebrate hosts. Larva mainly feed on small rodents but also on birds and lizards. Spirochete transmission during larval feeding depends on the access of infected reservoir-competent animals in a specific area, which influences the prevalence of spirochete-infected nymphs (Donahue et al. 1987). Nymphs use the same hosts as larvae and, in addition, larger mammals. The adult female needs approximately 0.7 ml of blood to be able to lay eggs. Therefore, larger mammals such as deer and rabbits are important for tick reproduction (Sonenshine, 1993). *Borrelia* can persist in the tick through the different life stages, but transovarial transmission to larvae is rare and the main source of infection is vertebrate blood (Matuschka et al. 1992; Sonenshine 1993).

In Europe, the Yellow-necked Field Mouse (*Apodemus flavicollis*), Wood Mouse (*A. sylvaticus*), and Bank Vole (*Clethrionomys glareolus*) are the main larval tick hosts and reservoirs (meaning animals that can become infected with *Borrelia* and be infectious to ticks) of *B. burgdorferi* s.l., whereas in eastern

North America, the main reservoir of *B. burgdorferi* s.s. is the White-footed Mouse (*Peromyscus leucopus*) (Aeschlimann et al. 1986; Donahue et al. 1987; Lane et al. 1991; Tälleklint and Jaenson 1994). Of importance for the population of ticks are various species of large mammals that serve as blood hosts for adult ticks but not as reservoirs for the spirochetes. The Roe Deer (*Capreolus capreolus*) of Eurasia and the White-tailed Deer (*Odocoileus virginianus*) of North America are examples of such blood hosts (Tälleklint and Jaenson 1994).

Birds' Role in the Terrestrial Enzootic Cycle. *Borrelia burgdorferi* s.l. may infect certain birds, and these birds may subsequently infect numerous vector ticks, but the avian reservoir range still remains to be defined (Table 18.1). It is not fully clear whether avian reservoir competence/incompetence is dependent on the species of *Borrelia,* species of bird, or both. The importance of passerine birds to the epidemiology of *B. burgdorferi* s.l. has been revealed in several studies.

Spirochete-infected larval ticks have been found at various frequencies on wild birds depending on locality, detection method, and season (Anderson et al. 1986; Anderson et al. 1990; Magnarelli et al. 1992; Nakao et al. 1994; Olsen et al. 1995; Smith et al. 1996; Rand et al. 1998; Humair et al. 1998). The frequency of infected tick larvae collected from birds in these studies was higher than would be expected by transovarial transmission of spirochetes to ticks (<1%) (Mejlon and Jaenson 1993), therefore the ticks are believed to have acquired infection from their avian hosts. In addition, ground foraging species such as various thrushes (*Catharus* spp.) and American Robins (*Turdus migratorius*) showed the highest frequency of attached infected ticks (Magnarelli et al. 1992; Battaly and Fish 1993). This association of infected ticks with Turdidae species has been found in Europe and Asia as well as North America (Olsen et al. 1995; Miyamoto et al. 1997; Humair et al. 1998).

Many migratory passerines are associated with long-distance dispersal of vector ticks (Olsen et al. 1995a; Smith et al. 1996; Rand et al. 1998; Ishiguro et al. 2000), and the geographic distribution of *B. burgdorferi* s.l. is sometimes thought to reflect bird migration patterns. For example, in North America, the distribution of Lyme borreliosis seems to parallel known bird migration routes (Anderson et al. 1986). A common strategy of migrating birds is to use different stopover sites where birds feed and rest. At these locations ticks and other ectoparasites may attach and later detach further along the migration routes or in breeding and wintering areas. New foci of tick-borne diseases may be created this way.

A more direct proof of birds as avian reservoirs of Lyme disease *Borrelia* is that *B. burgdorferi* s.l. has been isolated from the liver of a Veery (*Catharus fuscescens*) (Anderson et al. 1986) and from the blood of a Song Sparrow (*Melospiza melodia*) (McLean et al. 1993). In both field and experimental studies, several other species of birds seem to be reservoir competent for *B. burdorferi* s.l. (Table 18.1) (Anderson et al. 1986; Isogai et al. 1994; Olsen et al. 1995a; Stafford et al. 1995; Olsen et al. 1996; Piesman et al. 1996; Kurtenbach et al. 1998a; Richter et al. 2000). *Borrelia valaisiana* have been isolated from the Eurasian Blackbird (*Turdus merula*) (Humair et al. 1998) and *B. garinii* from the Red-bellied Thrush (*Turdus chrysolaus*) in Japan (Miyamoto et al. 1997). Also, the nonpasserine species Ring-necked Pheasant (*Phasianus colchicus*) has been found to be reservoir competent for certain strains of *B. garinii* and of *B. valaisiana* (Kurtenbach et al. 1998 a, b). Conversely, both Eurasian Blackbirds and Ring-necked Pheasants are considered reservoir incompetent for *B. afzelii* (Humair et al. 1998; Humair et al. 1999; Kurtenbach et al. 1998b), the genospecies readily transmitted by Eurasian rodents to ticks. Furthermore, *B. afzelii* has been detected only occasionally in bird-derived ticks anywhere in the world. Experimental and field-derived data suggest that *B. afzelii* is killed in ticks feeding on birds, possibly by avian complement ingested by the feeding tick (Kurtenbach et al. 2002). Further indication that not all birds seem to have the capacity to act as reservoirs is that Gray Catbirds (*Dumetella carolinensis*) did not infect vector ticks (Mather et al. 1989). It is not known whether birds are reservoir competent for *B. lusitaniae,* a genospecies that occurs predominantly in southwestern Europe and Northern Africa (De Michelis et al. 2000).

Because *B. burgdorferi* s.l. has its *in vitro* growth optimum at 33–40°C, (Hubálek et al. 1998), the high body temperature of passerine birds, 39–42°C, (Welty and Baptista 1988), was thought to rule out their importance as amplification hosts and *Borrelia* reservoirs. However, the body temperature in birds is not uniform. Some parts, such as the skin and air sacs, have lower temperatures than internal organs (Welty and Baptista 1988). Of the different *B. burgdorferi* s.l. species, *B. garinii* has the highest temperature growth optimum and is, together with *B. valaisiana,* the Lyme disease *Borrelia* species most often found in birds. This is an indication, which needs experimental confirmation, that these *Borrelias* are adapted to the higher body temperature of birds (Hubálek et al. 1998; Humair et al. 1998).

The impact of *B. burgdorferi* s.l. on individual birds or bird populations is almost unknown. In contrast to what is found in humans and many other mammals, the host parasite interaction between birds and

Table 18.1. A checklist of the reported *Borrelia burgdorferi* s.l. isolates from wild bird species.

Borrelia Species	Location	Avian Host (Scientific Name)	Tick Vector(s)	Reference
Borrelia burgdorferi s.l.	North America	American Robin (*Turdus migratorius*)	*Ixodes scapularis*	Magnarelli et al. 1992
	North America	Thrushes, various species	*I. scapularis*	Battaly and Fish 1993
B. burgdorferi s.s.	North America	Veery (*Catharus fuscescens*)	*I. scapularis*	Anderson et al. 1986
		Song Sparrow (*Melospiza melodia*)	*I. scapularis*	McLean et al. 1993
B. garinii[a]	Europe	Eurasian Blackbird (*Turdus merula*)	*I. ricinus*	Humair et al. 1998
	Japan	Rufous-bellied Thrush (*Turdus rufiventris*)	*I. persulcatus*	Miyamoto et al. 1997
	Europe	Ring-necked Pheasant (*Phasianus colchicus*)	*I. ricinus*	Kurtenbach et al. 1998a,b
	Europe	Razorbill (*Alca torda*)	*I. uriae*	Olsen et al. 1995
	Europe	Common Puffin (*Fratercula arctica*)	*I. uriae*	Gylfe et al. 1999
B. valasiana[a]	Europe	Eurasian Blackbird	*I. ricinus*	Humair et al. 1998
	Japan	Rufous-bellied Thrush	*I. persulcatus*	Miyamoto et al. 1997
	Europe	Ring-necked Pheasant	*I. ricinus*	Kurtenbach et al. 1998a,b

Note: Entries include only direct isolates from blood, skin, or organs of wild birds.

[a] Found most often in birds.

B. burgdorferi s.l. appears to be benign. It should be noted, however, that the apparent lack of symptoms might be the result of our inability to recognize and interpret symptoms in birds. In the few challenge studies performed, *B. burgdorferi* infection per se had no negative impact on birds and was often transient. For example, Japanese Quail (*Coturnix japonica*), Northern Bobwhite (*Colinus virginianus*), and Common Canaries (*Serinus canaria*) were infected by syringe-inoculated spirochetes. Spirochetal DNA was detected by PCR in the viscera, and viable spirochetes were cultured from these tissues, but without any clinical signs of disease or detectable gross or histopathological lesions (Bishop et al. 1994; Isogai et al. 1994; Olsen et al. 1996). In another study, experimentally inoculated chickens (*Gallus gallus*) became transiently infectious to ticks only when they were about a week old (Piesman et al. 1996). This transient and asymptomatic course of infection was also seen in American Robins, when nymphal ticks infected the birds and the infection was transmitted to subsequently attached larval ticks (Richter et al. 2000). Virtually all larvae became infected after feeding on these birds throughout the following month. However, infectivity declined after approximately three months.

The immune system is suppressed by stress, especially strenuous exercise (Råberg et al. 1998). Hormonal regulation, particularly increased circulating levels of glucocorticoids, may adversely affect immunocompetence (Besedovsky et al. 1996) and can reactivate latent infection (Mackowiak et al. 1984). Because the basal level of stress hormones, especially corticosteroids, are elevated in birds during migration (Holberton et al. 1996), it is possible that the stress of migration itself impairs defense against *B. burgdorferi* s.l. and increases the degree of spirochetemia. In a challenge experiment, previously infected Redwings (*Turdus iliacus*) reactivated a *B. garinii* infection during simulation of a normal stress-producing event in the life of the birds, the migration (Gylfe et al. 2000). This was the first indication that latent infections of *B. garinii* occur in birds and infection control mechanisms in the avian host may be impaired under certain conditions. The mechanisms of reactivation of *B. burgdorferi* s.l. infection in migratory birds are still unclear but the effect may be that anywhere along a migration route, ticks feeding on migrants with reactivated infections can become infected and, in turn, pass the disease along to other organisms.

At a local level, mammals may be a more significant actor than birds in maintaining the enzootic cycle of Lyme disease *Borrelia*. Birds are, on the other hand, crucial for long distance dispersal of Lyme disease *Borrelia*. The mechanism for that may be either a transportation of infected ticks or having a spirochetal infection available for questing ticks.

The Marine Enzootic Cycle

Seabirds often congregate in large colonies numbering several thousands to millions of individuals. During the breeding season, close contact between seabirds favors the exchange of endo- and ectoparasites. The tick *I. uriae* is a common ectoparasite of seabirds and has a unique circumpolar distribution in both hemispheres. More than 50 species of seabirds from both the north and south Polar Regions are infested by this tick (Eveleigh and Threlfall 1974; Mehl and Traavik 1983; Olsen et al. 1993; Olsen et al. 1995b; Bergström et al. 1999). In addition, *I. uriae* may attack other vertebrates with which it comes in contact, including various species of passerine birds, seals, River Otters (*Lutra lutra*), sheep, and humans (Mehl and Traavik 1983).

In 1993, a marine enzootic cycle involving *B. garinii, I. uriae* ticks, and a seabird species was described (Olsen et al. 1993). On a mammal-free island, *B. garinii* was isolated from *I.uriae,* and *Borrelia* DNA was detected from the foot web (palm) of a tick-infested Razorbill (*Alca torda*). In several subsequent studies, it has become evident that *B. garinii* is infecting *I. uriae* ticks in circumpolar regions of both the northern and southern hemisphere (Olsen et al. 1995; Gylfe et al. 1999). On the Faeroe Islands *B. garinii* was isolated from *I. uriae* ticks and from the blood of Common (Atlantic) Puffins (*Fratercula arctica*) (Gylfe et al. 1999). An indirect indication that Lyme disease *Borrelia* is present in the Southern Hemisphere is that *Borrelia burgdorferi* s.l. antibodies were detected in 14% of *I. uriae*–infested King Penguins (*Aptenodytes patagonicus*) on the Crozet Islands in the Southern Atlantic Ocean (Gauthier-Clerc et al. 1999).

In contrast to the terrestrial enzootic cycles of *B. garinii,* the circulation of this *Borrelia* seems to be restricted to a wide variety of colonial seabirds and the seabird-associated *I. uriae* tick. The reservoir competency of some seabird species seems to be good because a high proportion of *I. uriae* ticks at certain sites are infected (Olsen et al. 1995b). Identical *B. garinii* sequences in ticks from localities in both Polar Regions point at a trans-hemispheric dispersal of *B. garinii* by seabirds. It has been speculated that this transfer can be either indirect via transportation of infected ticks or more direct by reactivation of latent infections in the avian hosts (Olsen et al. 1995b; Gylfe et al. 2000). The former is unlikely because *I. uriae* attach to their seabird host for approximately one week (Barton et al. 1995), whereas migration between Arctic and Antarctic areas takes several weeks or months (del Hoyo et al. 1992). Seabirds rarely go ashore during migration and therefore a continual attachment and detachment of *I. uriae* at stopover sites is unlikely. All ticks attached at the breeding site will be lost and there are no opportunities to acquire new ticks during migration.

The only likely explanation as to why identical *B. garinii* is found in both hemispheres is that the spirochete is transported by the bird itself. Birds infectious to ticks are probably more efficient in spreading *B. burgdorferi* s.l. than the unlikely event of introduction of a few infected ticks (Gylfe et al. 2000). The infected seabirds per se may thus be important in long-distance dispersal and transequatorial transport of *B. burgdorferi* s.l.

There is little information about the impact of *B. garinii* on the seabirds themselves. Infestation by *I. uriae* may sometimes affect the population dynamics of seabirds (Boulinier and Danchin 1996; Haemig et al. 1999), but the importance of *B. garinii* in this context is unknown.

Avian Spirochetosis

INTRODUCTION

Avian (fowl) spirochetosis is an acute septicemic disease caused by the spirochete *Borrelia anserina*. Avian spirochetosis occurs worldwide but most commonly is a problem of domestic poultry in tropical and subtropical regions. This disease has not been reported in free-living wild birds.

SYNONYMS

Fowl spirochetosis.

HISTORY, DISTRIBUTION, AND HOST RANGE

The agent of avian spirochetosis was first described by Sakharoff in Russia in 1891 as the cause of "goose septicemia." The primary hosts are gallinaceous birds such as chickens, turkeys, and pheasants, but the disease has also been reported from natural infections in ducks, geese, grouse, canaries, and a Gray Parrot (*Psittacus erithacus*). Rock Pigeons (*Columba livia*) are relatively resistant (Cooper and Bickford 1993; Barnes 1997).

Avian spirochetosis occurs primarily in tropical and subtropical regions where fowl ticks of the genus *Argus* are distributed. The disease is especially common in such areas of Europe, Africa, India, Indonesia, Australia, and Central and South America. It is rare in North America, but outbreaks in captive birds have occurred in California and southwestern U.S.A. as recently as 1993 (Cooper and Bickford 1993).

ETIOLOGY

Borrelia anserina is a helically coiled bacterium, 9–21 μm long and .22–.26 μm wide with an approximate wavelength of 1.7 μm and seven or eight flagella (Hovind-Hougen 1995). Previous scientific names include *Borrelia gallinarum, Spirochaeta anserina, Spirochaeta gallinarum,* and *Spironema gallinarum.* Antigenically distinct strains occur, and strains differ in virulence, but no strain classification scheme has been developed (Barnes 1997).

EPIZOOTIOLOGY

Argas ticks, such as *A. persicus, A. sanchezi,* and *A. arboreus,* are the main vectors of the spirochete and serve as reservoirs. The spirochete survives in the tick through transstadial molts from larva to adult and also is transmitted transovarially in suitable reservoir tick species. Adult and nymphal *Argus* ticks are intermittent nocturnal feeders. They live in cracks and crevices of poultry houses or under tree bark. The tick can survive up to four years without a blood meal and remain infective with *B. anserina* for more than one year. Mites and mosquitoes can also transmit the disease. Feces, fluids, and tissues from infected birds are infective, so their ingestion or inoculation may spread the disease. Virulent strains of *B. anserina* can penetrate unbroken skin; however, the organism cannot survive long free in the environment (Mathey and Siddle 1955; DaMassa and Adler 1978; Barnes 1997).

CLINICAL SIGNS AND PATHOLOGY

Morbidity and mortality may vary depending on strain virulence, host species, and immunity, but mortality as high as 100% can occur. The main clinical signs are weakness, inactivity, green diarrhea, anorexia, elevated temperature, and anemia. The cause of anemia is unclear but an association with cold agglutinins and soluble immune complexes suggest that those factors enhance erythrophagocytosis by tissue macrophages (Barnes 1997).

The predominant gross finding in most species is enlargement and mottling of the spleen. Hepatomegaly and swollen kidneys may also be present. Intestinal contents are often green and mucoid, and hemorrhage may be present at the junction of the proventriculus and ventriculus. Fibrinous pericarditis is uncommon.

Microscopically, hyperplasia of the mononuclear phagocyte system, erythrophagocytosis, and hemosiderosis in the spleen are characteristic lesions (Bandopadhyay and Vegad 1983). Hemosiderosis and erythrophagocytosis may also be evident in liver. Spirochetes can be seen in blood vessels, intercellular spaces, and bile canaliculi in silver-stained tissue sections (Barnes 1997).

DIAGNOSIS

A presumptive diagnosis of avian spirochetosis is based on clinical signs, compatible gross and/or microscopic lesions, and demonstration of spirochetes in blood smears, blood buffy coat, or tissue sections (Barnes 1997). Evidence of tick bites and/or ticks in the birds' environment is supportive. The motile spirochetes can be seen in fresh wet smears using darkfield or phase contrast microscopy. The organism stains well most aniline and Romanowsky stains, as well as with Giemsa, in dry blood or tissue impression smears. Confirmation is dependent on identification of *B. anserina* antigen by serologic techniques such as immunodiffusion or immunoflourescence (Barnes 1997). The organism can be cultured in embryonated chicken eggs or BSK medium (Barbour 1984; Barnes 1997).

IMMUNITY, TREATMENT, AND CONTROL

B. anserina is susceptible to a variety of antibiotics. Penicillin or oxytetracycline is used most commonly. Birds that recover from infection are immune to the homologous strain of *B. anserina* but may be susceptible to other strains. Protective maternal antibody is transferred to chicks in yolk. Vaccination with attenuated or low virulence strains is common where the disease is most prevalent. Prevention is directed primarily toward tick control (Barnes 1997).

LITERATURE CITED

Aguero-Rosenfeld, M.E., J. Nowakowski, S. Bittker, D. Cooper, R.B. Nadelman, and G.P. Wormser. 1996. Evolution of the serologic response to *Borrelia burgdorferi* in treated patients with culture-confirmed erythema migrans. *Journal of Clinical Microbiology* 34:1–9.

Aeschlimann, A., E. Chamot, F. Gigon, J.-P. Jeanneret, D. Kesseler, and C. Walther. 1986. *Borrelia burgdorferi* in Switzerland. *Zentralblatt für Bakteriologie* 263:450–458.

Afzelius A. 1910. Verhandlungen der dermatologischen gesellschaft zu Stockholm. *Archichves Dermatologia Syphilitis* 101:404.

Anderson, J.F., R.C. Johnson, L.A. Magnarelli, and F.W. Hyde. 1986. Involvement of birds in the epidemiology of the Lyme Disease agent *Borrelia burgdorferi. Infection and Immunity* 51:394–396.

Anderson, J.F., L.A. Magnarelli, and K.C. Stafford III. 1990. Bird-feeding ticks transstadially transmit *Borrelia burgdorferi* that infect Syrian Hamsters. *Journal of Wildlife Diseases* 26:1–10.

Bandopadhyay, A.C., and J.L. Vegad. 1983. Enteritis and green diarrhoea in experimental avian spirochaetosis. *Research in Veterinary Sciences* 35:138–144.

Barbour, A.G. 1984. Isolation and cultivation of Lyme disease spirochetes. Yale. *Journal of Biology and Medicine* 57:521–525.

Barbour, A.G., and S.F. Hayes. 1986. Biology of *Borrelia* species. *Microbiological Reviews* 50:381–400.

Baranton, G., D. Postic, I. Saint Girons, P. Boerlin, J.C. Piffaretti, M. Assous, and P.A. Grimont. 1992. Delineation of *Borrelia burgdorferi* sensu stricto, *Borrelia garinii* sp. nov., and group VS461 associated with Lyme borreliosis. *International Journal of Systematic Bacteriology* 42:378–383.

Barnes, H.J. 1997. Spirochetosis. In: *Disease of Poultry,* 10th Ed., B.W. Calnek, H.J. Barnes, C.W. Beard, L.R. McDougald, and Y.M. Saif (eds.). Iowa State University Press, Ames, IA, U.S.A., pp. 318–324.

Barton, T.R., M.P. Harris, and S. Wanless. 1995. Natural attachment duration of nymphs of the tick *Ixodes uriae* (*Acari:* Ixodidae) on kittiwake *Rissa tridactyla* nestlings. *Experimental and Applied Acarology* 19:499–509.

Battaly, G.R., and D. Fish. 1993. Relative importance of bird species as hosts for immature *Ixodes dammini* (*Acari:* Ixodidae) in a suburban residential landscape of southern New York State. *Journal of Medical Entomology* 30:740–747.

Bergström, S., P.D. Haemig, and B. Olsen B. 1999. Distribution and abundance of the tick Ixodes uriae in a subantarctic seabird and mammal community. *Journal of Parasitology* 85:25–27.

Besedovsky, H.O., and A. del Rey. 1996. Immunoneuro-endocrine interactions: facts and hypotheses. *Endocrinological Reviews* 17:64–102.

Bishop, K.L., M.I. Khan, and S.W. Nielsen. 1994. Experimental infection of northern bobwhite quail with *Borrelia burgdorferi. Journal of Wildlife Diseases* 30:506–513.

Bouilinier, T., and E. Danchin. 1996. Populations trend in kittiwake *Rissa tridactyla* colonies in relation to tick infestation. *Ibis* 138:326–334.

Brandt, M.E., B.S. Riley, J.D. Radolf, and M.V. Norgard. 1990. Immunogenic integral membrane proteins of *Borrelia burgdorferi* are lipoproteins. *Infection and Immunity* 58:983–991.

Brown, R.N., and E.C. Burgess. 2001. Lyme Borreliosis. In *Infectious Diseases of Wild Mammals,* 3rd Ed., E. S. Williams and I.K. Barker (eds.). Iowa State University Press, Ames, IA, U.S.A., pp. 435–454.

Canica, M.M., F. Nato, L. du Merle, J.C. Mazie, G. Baranton, and D. Postic. 1993. Monoclonal antibodies for identification of *Borrelia afzelii* sp. nov. associated with late cutaneous manifestations of Lyme borreliosis. *Scandinavian Journal of Infectious Diseases* 25:441–448.

Cooper, G.L, and A.A. Bickford. 1993. Spirochetosis in California Game Chickens. *Avian Diseases* 37: 1167–1171.

DaMassa, A.L., and H.E. Adler. 1978. Avian spirochetosis: natural transmission by Argas (persicargas) sanchezi (Ixodoidea: Argasidae) and existence of different serologic and immunologic types of *Borrelia anserina* in the United States. *American Journal of Veterinary Research* 40:154–157.

del Hoyo, J., A. Elliott, and J. Sargatal (eds.). 1992. *Handbook of the Birds of the World: Ostrich to Ducks,* Vol. 1. Lynx Edicions, Barcelona, Spain.

De Michelis, S., H.S. Sewell, M. Collares-Pereira, M. Santos-Reis, L.M. Schouls, V. Benes, E.C. Holmes, and K. Kurtenbach. 2000. Genetic diversity of *Borrelia burgdorferi* sensu lato in ticks from mainland Portugal. *Journal of Clinical Microbiology* 38:2128–2133.

de Silva, A.M., N.S. Zeidner, Y. Zhang, M.C. Dolan, J. Piesman, E. Fikrig. 1999. Influence of outer surface protein A antibody on *Borrelia burgdorferi* within feeding ticks. *Infection and Immunity* 67:30–35.

Donahue, J.G., J.Piesman, and A. Spielman. 1987. Reservoir competence of white-footed mice for Lyme disease spirochetes. *American Journal of Tropical Medicine and Hygiene* 36:92–96.

Eveleigh, E.S., and W. Threlfall. 1974. The biology of *Ixodes* (Ceratixodes) *uriae,* White, 1852, in Newfoundland. *Acarologia* 16:621–635.

Gauthier-Clerc, M., B. Jaulhac, Y. Frenot, C. Bachelard, H. Monteil, Y. Le Maho, and Y. Handrich. 1999. Prevalence of *Borrelia burgdorferi* (the Lyme disease agent) antibodies in king penguin *Aptenodytes patagonicus* in Crozet Archipelago. *Polar Biology* 22:141–143.

Gern L., L.N. Toutoungi, C.M. Hu, and A. Aeschlimann. 1991. *Ixodes (Pholeoixodes) hexagonus,* an efficient vector of *Borrelia burgdorferi* in the laboratory. *Medical and Veterinary Entomology* 5:431–435.

Gilmore, R.D., and J. Piesman. 2000. Inhibition of *Borrelia burgdorferi* migration from the midgut to the salivary glands following feeding by ticks on OspC-immunized mice. *Infection and Immunity* 68: 411–414.

Gylfe, Å., B. Olsen, N. Marti Ras, D. Strasevicius, L. Noppa, Y. Östberg, P. Weihe, and S. Bergström. 1999. Isolation of Lyme disease *Borrelia* from Puffins (*Fratercula arctica*) and seabird ticks (*Ixodes uriae*) on Faeroe Islands. *Journal of Clinical Microbiology* 37:890–896.

Gylfe, Å., S. Bergström, J. Lundström, and B. Olsen. 2000. Reactivation of *Borrelia* infection in birds. *Nature* 403:724–725.

Habicht G.S., G. Beck, and J.L. Benach. 1987. Lyme disease. *Scientific American* July:60–65.

Hauser, U., G. Lehnert, R. Lobentanzer, and B. Wilske. 1997. Interpretation criteria for standardized Western blots for three European species of *Borrelia burgdorferi* sensu lato. *Journal of Clinical Microbiology* 35:1433–1444.

Haemig, P., S. Bergström, and B. Olsen. 1999. Survival and mortality of Grey-headed Albatross chicks in relation to infestation by the tick *Ixodes* uriae. *Colonial Waterbirds* 21:452–453.

Hovind-Hougen, K. 1995. A morphological characterization of *Borrelia anserina. Microbiology* 141:79–83.

Holberton, R.L., J.D. Parrish, and J.C. Wingfield. 1996. Modulation of the adrenocortical stress response in neotropical migrants during autumn migration. *The Auk* 113:558–564.

Hubálek, Z., J. Halouzka, and M. Heroldová. 1998. Growth temperature ranges of *Borrelia burgdorferi* sensu lato strains. *Journal of Medical Microbiology* 47:929–932.

Humair, P.F., D. Postic, R. Wallich, and L. Gern. 1998. An avian reservoir (*Turdus merula*) of the Lyme borreliosis spirochetes. *Zentralblatt für Bakteriologie* 287:521–538.

Ishiguro F., N. Takada, T. Masuzawa, and T. Fukui. 2000. Prevalence of Lyme Disease *Borrelia* spp. in ticks from migratory birds on the Japanese mainland. *Applied and Environmental Microbiology* 66:982–986.

Isogai, E., S. Tanaka, I.S. Braga III, C. Itakura, H. Isogai, K. Kimura, and N. Fujii. 1994. Experimental *Borrelia garinii* infection of Japanese Quail. *Infection and Immunity* 8:3580–3582.

Kawabata, M., T. Masuzawa, and Y. Yanagihara. 1993. Genomic analysis of *Borrelia japonica* sp. nov. isolated from *Ixodes ovatus* ticks in Japan. *Microbiology and Immunology* 37:843–848.

Kimsey, R.B., and A. Spielman.1990. Motility of Lyme disease spirochetes in fluids as viscous as the extracellular matrix. *Journal of Infectious Diseases* 162: 1205–1208.

Kurtenbach, K., D. Carey, A.N. Hoodless, P.A. Nuttall, and S.E. Randolph. 1998a. Competence of pheasants as reservoirs for Lyme disease spirochetes. *Journal of Medical Entomology* 35:77–81.

Kurtenbach, K., M. Peacey, S.G.T. Rijpkema, A.N. Hoodless, P.A. Nuttall, and S.E. Randolph. 1998b. Differential transmission of the genospecies of *Borrelia burgdorferi* sensu lato by game birds and small rodents in England. *Applied and Environmental Microbiology* 64:1169–1174.

Kurtenbach K, S.M. Schafer, H.S. Sewell, M. Peacey, A. Hoodless, P.A. Nuttall, and S.E. Randolph. 2002. Differential survival of Lyme borreliosis spirochetes in ticks that feed on birds. *Infection and Immunity* 70:5893–5895.

Lane, R.S., J. Piesman, and W. Burgdorfer. 1991. Lyme borreliosis: Relation of its causative agent to its vectors and hosts in North America and Europe. *Annual Review of Entomology* 36:587–609.

Lebech, A.M., K. Hansen, F. Brandrup, O. Clemmensen, and L. Halkier-Sorensen. 2000. Diagnostic value of PCR for detection of *Borrelia burgdorferi* DNA in clinical specimens from patients with erythema migrans and Lyme neuroborreliosis. *Molecular Diagnosis* 5:139–150.

Mackowiak, P.A. 1984. Microbial latency. *Reviews of Infectious Diseases* 6:649–668.

Magnarelli, L.A. 1995. Current status of laboratory diagnosis for Lyme disease. *American Journal of Medicine* 98:10S–14S.

Magnarelli, L.A., K.C. Stafford III, and V.C. Bladen. 1992. *Borrelia burgdorferi* in *Ixodes dammini* (Acari: Ixodidae) feeding on birds in Lyme, Connecticut, U.S.A. *Canadian Journal of Zoology* 70:2322–2325.

Mather, T.N., S.R. Telford III, A.B. MacLachlan, and A. Spielman. 1989. Incompetence of catbirds as reservoirs for the Lyme disease spirochete (*Borrelia burgdorferi*). *Journal of Parasitology* 75:66–69.

McLean, R.G., S.R. Ubico, C.A. Norton Hughes, S.M. Engstrom, and R.C. Johnson. 1993. Isolation and characterization of *Borrelia burgdorferi* from blood of a bird captured in the Saint Croix River Valley. *Journal of Clinical Microbiology* 31:2038–2043.

Mehl, R., and T. Traavik. 1983. The tick *Ixodes uriae* (Acari:Ixodides) in seabird colonies in Norway. *Fauna Norvegica Ser B* 30:94–107.

Mejlon, H.A., and T.G.T, Jaenson. 1993. Seasonal prevalence of *Borrelia burgdorferi* in *Ixodes ricinus* (Acari: Ixodidae) in different vegetation types in Sweden. *Scandinavian Journal of Infectious Diseases* 25:449–456.

Miyamoto, K., Y. Sato, K. Okada, M. Fukunaga, and F. Sato. 1997. Competence of a migratory bird, red-bellied thrush (*Turdus chrysolaus*), as an avian reservoir for the Lyme disease spirochetes in Japan. *Acta Tropica* 65:43–51.

Nakao, M., K. Miyamoto, and M. Fukunaga. 1994. Lyme disease spirochetes in Japan: enzootic transmission cycles in birds, rodents, and *Ixodes persulcatus* ticks. *Journal of Infectious Diseases* 170:878–882.

Olsen, B.T., G.T. Jaenson, J. Bunikis, L. Noppa, and S. Bergström 1993. A Lyme Borreliosis cycle in seabirds and *Ixodes uriae* ticks. *Nature* 362:340–342.

Olsen B., T.G.T. Jaenson, and S. Bergström. 1995a. Prevalence of *Borrelia burgdorferi* sensu lato-infected ticks on migrating birds. *Applied and Environmental Microbiology* 61:3082–3087.

Olsen, B., D.C. Duffy, T.G.T. Jaenson, Å. Gylfe, J. Bonnedahl, and S. Bergström. 1995b. Transhemispheric exchange of Lyme disease spirochetes by seabirds. *Journal of Clinical Microbiology* 33:3270–3274.

Olsen B., Å. Gylfe,, and S. Bergström. 1996. Canary finches (*Serinus canaria*) as an avian infection model for Lyme borreliosis. *Microbial Pathogenesis* 20:319–324.

Ohnishi, J., J. Piesman, and A.M. de Silva. 2001. Antigenic and genetic heterogeneity of *Borrelia burgdorferi* populations transmitted by ticks. In *Proceedings of the National Academy of Science, U.S.A.* 98:670–675.

Pal, U., A.M. de Silva, R.R. Montgomery, D. Fish, J. Anguita, J.F. Anderson, Y. Lobet, and E. Fikrig. 2000. Attachment of *Borrelia burgdorferi* within *Ixodes scapularis* mediated by outer surface protein A. *Journal of Clinical Investigations* 106:561–569.

Picken, R.N., Y. Cheng, F. Strle, and M.M. Picken. 1996. Patient isolates of *Borrelia burgdorferi* sensu lato with genotypic and phenotypic similarities of strain 25015. *Journal of Infectious Diseases* 174:1112–1115.

Piesman, J., M.C. Dolan, M.E. Schriefer, and T.R. Burkot. 1996. Ability of experimental infected chickens to infect ticks with the Lyme disease spirochete, *Borrelia burgdorferi. American Journal of Tropical Medicine and Hygiene* 54:294–298.

Postic, D., J. Belfaiza, E. Isogai, I. Saint Girons, P.A.D. Grimont, and G. Baranton. 1993. A new genomic species in *Borrelia burgdorferi* sensu lato isolated from Japanese ticks. *Research in Microbiology* 144:467–473.

Postic, D., N.M. Ras, R.S. Lane, M. Hendson, and G. Baranton. 1998. Expanded diversity among Californian *Borrelia* isolates and description of *Borrelia bissettii* sp. nov. (formerly *Borrelia* group DN127). *Journal of Clinical Microbiology* 36: 3497–3504.

Priem, S., M.G. Rittig, T. Kamradt, G.R. Burmester, and A. Krause. 1997. An optimized PCR leads to rapid and highly sensitive detection of *Borrelia burgdorferi* in patients with Lyme borreliosis. *Journal of Clinical Microbiology* 35:685–690.

Rand, P. W., E.H. Lacombe, R.P. Smith, and J. Ficker. 1998. Participation of birds in the emergence of Lyme disease in southern Maine. *Journal of Medical Entomology* 35:270–276.

Richter D., A. Spielman, N. Komar, and F-R. Matuschka. 2000. Competence of American Robins as Reservoir Hosts for Lyme Disease Spirochetes. *Emerging Infectious Diseases* 6:133–138.

Råberg, L., M. Grahn, D. Hasselquist, and E. Svensson. 1998. On the adaptive significance of stress-induced immunosuppression. *Proceedings of the Royal Society of London,* B 265:1637–1641.

Schwan, T. G., and J. Piesman. 2000. Temporal changes in outer surface proteins A and C of the lyme disease-associated spirochete, *Borrelia burgdorferi,* during the chain of infection in ticks and mice. *Journal of Clinical Microbiology* 38:382–388.

Shi, W., Z. Yang, Y. Geng, L.E. Wolinsky, and, M.A. Lovett. 1998. Chemotaxis in *Borrelia burgdorferi. Journal of Bacteriology* 180:231–235.

Smith, R.P., P.W. Rand, E.H. Lacombe, S.R. Morris, D. W. Holmes, and D.A. Caporale. 1996. Role of bird migration in the long distance dispersal of *Ixodes dammini,* the vector of Lyme disease. *Journal of Infectious Diseases* 174:221–224.

Sonenshine, D.E. 1993. *Biology of Ticks,* Vol.1. Oxford University Press New York, U.S.A., 412 pp.

Stafford, K.C., V.C. Bladen, and L.A. Magnarelli. 1995. Ticks (Acari: Ixodidae) infesting wild birds (Aves) and white-footed mice in Lyme, CT. *Journal of Medical Entomology* 32:453–466.

Stanek, G., S. O'Connell, M. Cimmino, E. Aberer, W. Kristoferitsch, M. Granstrom, E. Guy, and J. Gray. 1996. European Union Concerted Action on Risk Assessment in Lyme Borreliosis: clinical case definitions for Lyme borreliosis. *Klinikal Wochenschrift* 108:741–747.

Steere, A.C., R.L. Grodzicki, A.N. Kornblatt, J.E. Craft, A.G. Barbour, W. Burgdorfer, G.P. Schmid, S.E. Johnson, and S.E. Malawista. 1983. The spirochetal etiology of Lyme disease. *New England Journal of Medicine* 308:733–740.

Strle, F., R.N. Picken, Y. Cheng, J. Cimperman, V. Maraspin, S. Lotric-Furlan, E. Ruzic-Sabljic, and M. M. Picken. 1997. Clinical findings for patients with Lyme borreliosis caused by *Borrelia burgdorferi* sensu lato with genotypic and phenotypic similarities to strain 25015. *Clinical Infectious Diseases* 25:273–280.

Tälleklint, L. and T. G. T. Jaenson. 1994. Transmission of *Borrelia burgdorferi s.l.* from mammal reservoirs to the primary vector of Lyme borreliosis, *Ixodes ricinus* (Acari: Ixodidae), in Sweden. *Journal of Medical Entomology* 31:880–886.

Wang, G., A.P. van Dam, I. Schwartz, and J. Dankert. 1999. Molecular typing of *Borrelia burgdorferi* sensu lato: taxonomic, epidemiological, and clinical implications. *Clinical Microbiology Reviews* 12: 633–653.

Welty, J.C., and L. Baptista. 1988. *The Life of Birds.* Saunders College Publishing, New York, NY, U.S.A., pp. 319–346.

Wilske, B., and V. Preac-Mursic. 1993. Microbial diagnosis of Lyme borreliosis. In *Aspects of Lyme Borreliosis,* K. Weber and W. Burgdorfer (eds.). Springer-Verlag, Berlin, Germany, pp. 270–272.

Wilske, B., V. Preac-Mursic, U.B. Gobel, B. Graf, S. Jauris, E. Soutschek, E. Schwab, and G. Zumstein. 1993. An OspA serotyping system for *Borrelia burgdorferi* based on reactivity with monoclonal antibodies and OspA sequence analysis. *Journal of Clinical Microbiology* 31:340–350.

Wilske, B., S. Jauris-Heipke, R. Lobentanzer, I. Pradel, V. Preac-Mursic, D. Rössler, E. Soutschek, and R.C. Johnson. 1995. Phenotypic analysis of outer surface protein C (OspC) of *Borrelia burgdorferi* sensu lato by monoclonal antibodies: relationship to genospecies and OspA serotype. *Journal of Clinical Microbiology* 33:103–109.

Wilske, B., U. Busch, V. Fingerle, S. Jauris-Heipke, V. Preac Mursic, D. Rössler, and G. Wil. 1996. Immunological and molecular variability of OspA and OspC. Implications for *Borrelia* vaccine development. *Infection* 24:208–212.

19
Tularemia

Torsten Mörner

INTRODUCTION

Tularemia is an infectious disease caused by the Gram-negative bacterium *Francisella tularensis.* The disease occurs only in the Northern hemisphere and is seen in wild animals, domestic animals, and humans. *Francisella tularensis* can infect a wide range of animals and has been reported in more than 250 species, including mammals, birds, amphibians, invertebrates, and protozoans (Jellison 1974; Bell and Reilly 1981; Pfahler-Jung 1989; Abd et al. 2003). Tularemia is primarily a disease of rodents and lagomorphs, but naturally occurring infections with *F. tularensis* have been reported in several different bird species. Although individual cases of avian tularemia have been reported, birds do not seem to play an important role in the epidemiology of the disease other than harboring ticks that may act as vectors for mammal outbreaks. This chapter summarizes what is known about birds and tularemia. For a review of tularemia in wild mammals, see Mörner and Addison 2001.

HISTORY

Tularemia was first recognized in California ground squirrels (*Spermophilus beecheyi*) in Tulare County, California, U.S.A., in 1911 (McCoy 1911). The causative organism was isolated in 1912 (McCoy and Chapin 1912) and named *Bacterium tularense* (now *Francisella tularensis*) for Tulare County, in which the disease was first observed. Francis (1921) proposed the name tularemia for the disease. During the 1920s to 1930s in North America, anecdotal accounts of declines in game bird populations coincident with tularemia outbreaks in rabbits stimulated investigations into the effects of tularemia on game birds that share habitat and ticks with rabbits. Public health scientists experimentally demonstrated susceptibilities to *F. tularensis* in several game bird species and documented natural infections in Northern Bobwhite (*Colinus virginianus*), Ruffed Grouse (*Bonasa umbellus*), Sharp-tailed Grouse (*Tympanuchus phasianellus*), and Greater Sage-Grouse (*Centrocercus urophasianus*) (Green and Wade 1929; Green and Shillinger 1932; Parker et al. 1932). However, the only reported epizootic appears to have been a localized outbreak of tularemia in Montana, U.S.A., in which dead Greater Sage-Grouse and rabbits were both infected (Parker et al. 1932). Natural infection with *F. tularensis* has since been reported in wild birds in North America, Europe, and the former USSR.

DISTRIBUTION AND HOST RANGE

In North America tularemia has been reported in Canada, the United States including Alaska, and Mexico (Bell and Reilly 1981). In the Old World tularemia is found in almost all parts of the former USSR and in most countries in central Europe, but apparently does not occur naturally in Spain, Portugal, Ireland, and Great Britain (Pfahler-Jung 1989). In Asia, tularemia is known in Turkey, Burma, China, Japan, Iran, Afghanistan, and Lebanon (Bell and Reilly 1981; Pfahler-Jung 1989). In Africa, tularemia has been reported from Tunisia and Senegal (Jusatz 1961).

Francisella tularensis has one of the broadest host ranges of all bacteria, having been reported from 190 species of mammals, 26 species of birds, three species of amphibians, and 88 species of invertebrates up to 1989 (Hopla 1974; Jellison 1974; Pfahler-Jung 1989). Most species of mammals known to be infected up to 1980 are tabulated by Bell and Reilly (1981).

Pfahler-Jung (1989) reports that tularemia has been found in 23 different species of birds from the U.S.A., Canada, Sweden, and Austria. Natural infections in birds with *F. tularensis* have been reported in game birds and waterfowl, as well as predatory and scavenging species (Table 19.1). Rehbinder and Karlsson (1979) found Common Ravens (*Corvus corax*) to be infected, but considered the infections to have been incidental. Mörner and Mattsson (1983) found acute infection with *F. tularensis* in a Rough-legged Hawk (*Buteo lagopus*) and an Ural Owl (*Strix uralensis*) and assumed that the organism was the cause of death in these birds. Experimental infections with *F. tularensis*

Table 19.1. Natural infections in birds with *Francisella tularensis.*

Bird Species	Scientific Name	Location	Method of Identification	Reference
Northern Bobwhite	*Colinus virginianus*	U.S.A.	Isolation	Green and Wade 1929
Ruffed Grouse	*Bonasa umbellus*	U.S.A.	Isolation	Green and Shillinger 1932
Sharp-tailed Grouse	*Tympanuchus phasianellus*	U.S.A.	Isolation	Green and Shillinger 1932
Greater Sage-Grouse	*Centrocercus urophasianus*	U.S.A.	Isolation	Parker et al. 1932
Ring-necked Pheasant	*Phasianus colchicus*	U.S.A.	Isolation	Kursban and Foshay 1946
Canada Goose	*Branta canadensis*	U.S.A.	Isolation	Stahl et al. 1969
Franklin's Gull	*Larus pipixcan*	U.S.A.	Isolation	Ozburn 1944
Common Raven	*Corvus corax*	Sweden	Flourescent antibody test	Rehbinder and Karlsson 1979
Great Horned Owl	*Bubo virginianus*	U.S.A.	Isolation	Green et al. 1938
Red-tailed Hawk	*Buteo jamaicensis*	U.S.A.	Isolation	Nakamura 1950
Rough-legged Hawk	*Buteo lagopus*	Sweden	Flourescent antibody test	Mörner and Mattsson 1983
Ural Owl	*Strix uralensis*	Sweden	Isolation	Mörner and Mattsson 1983

in birds have shown that there is wide variation in susceptibility to the bacterium; inoculation is fatal in some species, whereas others survive with no apparent clinical signs; however, the bacterial subspecies used in early studies was undetermined (Table 19.2). Predatory and scavenging species appear more likely to be resistant.

ETIOLOGY

Francisella tularensis is a Gram-negative, pleomorphic rod, 0.2 × 0.2–0.7 μm in size (Eigelsbach and McGann 1984). At various times in the past it has been classified in the genera *Bacterium, Pasteurella, Brucella,* and others (Jellison 1974). *Francisella tularensis* is a facultative intracellular organism, which can multiply and survive within macrophages and hepatocytes (Conlan and North 1992; Fortier et al. 1994).

The genus *Francisella* has two species, *F. tularensis* and *F. philomiragia* (Hollis et al. 1989). *Francisella philomiragia* is less common and associated with water. *Francisella tularensis* has four subspecies: *F. tularensis* subspecies *tularensis* (syn. *nearctica,* also known as Type A); *F. tularensis* subspecies *palaearctica* (syn. *holarctica,* Type B), *F. tularensis* subspecies *mediasiatica;* and *F. tularensis* subspecies *novicida* (Farlow et al. 2001). The last two subspecies are uncommon and have limited, localized distributions.

Francisella t. tularensis is harbored primarily in mammalian hosts and is highly virulent for humans and domestic rabbits. Until recently this subspecies was considered to be present only in North America. *Francisella t. tularensis* in culture ferments glycerol and is citruline ureidase positive. *Francisella t. palaearctica* is mainly waterborne and is less virulent than *F. t. tularensis* for humans and domestic rabbits; it is found in both Eurasia and North America (Jellison 1974; Farlow et al. 2001). *Francisella t. palaearctica* in culture does not ferment glycerol and is citruline ureidase negative.

EPIZOOTIOLOGY

In general, most birds seem to be relatively resistant to infection with *F. tularensis,* and their epidemiological role generally is minor. Individual birds may die from *F. tularensis* septicemia, but some isolations from birds appear to be incidental and epizootic outbreaks

Table 19.2. Experimental infections in birds with *Francisella tularensis.*

Bird Species	Scientific Name	Location	Susceptibility	Reference
Ring-necked Pheasant	*Phasianus colchicus*	U.S.A.	Low	Green et al. 1928
Gray Partridge	*Perdix perdix*	U.S.A.	High	Green and Wade 1928b
Northern Bobwhite	*Colinus virginianus*	U.S.A.	High	Parker 1929
Blue Grouse	*Dendragapus obscurus*	U.S.A.	High	Parker and Spencer 1927 as cited in Green and Shillinger 1932
Ruffed Grouse	*Bonasa umbellus*	U.S.A.	Moderate	Green and Wade 1928a
Green-winged Teal	*Anas crecca*	U.S.A.	High	Parker 1934
Mallard	*Anas platyrhynchos*	U.S.A.	High	Parker 1934
Brown Noddy	*Anous stolidus*	U.S.A.	High	Cabelli et al. 1964b
Lesser Noddy	*Anous tenuirostris*	U.S.A.	High	Cabelli et al. 1964b
White Tern	*Gygis alba*	U.S.A.	High	Cabelli et al. 1964b
Sooty Tern	*Sterna fuscata*	U.S.A.	High	Cabelli et al. 1964b
Pigeon (presumed Rock Pigeon)	*(presumed Columba livia)*	U.S.A.	Low	Green and Wade 1928b; McCoy 1911 as cited in Simpson 1929
Mourning Dove	*Zenaida macroura*	U.S.A.	Moderate	Cabelli et al. 1964a
Eurasian Buzzard	*Buteo buteo*	France	Resistant	Alonso et al. 1975
Eurasian Buzzard	*Buteo buteo*	Sweden	Resistant	Mörner and Mattsson 1988
Rough-legged Hawk	*Buteo lagopus*	Sweden	Resistant	Mörner and Mattsson 1988
Northern Goshawk	*Accipiter gentilis*	Sweden	Resistant	Mörner and Mattsson 1988
Eurasian Sparrowhawk	*Accipiter nisus*	Sweden	Resistant	Mörner and Mattsson 1988
Tawny Owl	*Strix alucio*	Sweden	Resistant	Mörner and Mattsson 1988
Carrion Crow	*Corvus corone cornix*	Sweden	Resistant	Mörner and Mattsson 1988

of tularemia in birds, or bird populations, have not been confirmed. However, birds may act as important hosts for some of the major tick vectors of tularemia.

Francisella tularensis is a highly infectious agent that can enter the body in several ways: inoculation by blood-feeding arthropod vectors directly into the blood or tissues of the host; by penetration through intact or lacerated skin or through ocular mucous membranes after contact with blood or tissues of infected animals; by inhalation of infected aerosols or particles; or by ingestion of contaminated water or meat (Jellison 1974). Birds' exposure most likely occurs through feeding on infected prey or by sharing parasitic arthropods with infected mammals.

Blood-feeding arthropods that may act as vectors include mosquitoes, fleas, tabanid flies (mainly deer-flies *Chrysops* spp.), and ticks (Hopla 1974; Jellison 1974; Hopla and Hopla 1994). The species of tick vectors vary geographically. In North America these are principally *Dermacentor variabilis, D. andersoni, D. parumpertis,* and *D. occidentalis; Haemaphysalis leporis-palustris; Amblyomma americanum;* and *Ixodes dentatus,* though others may be implicated (Hopla 1974; Jellison 1974). *Haemaphysalis leporis-palustris* and *I. dentatus* are highly associated with lagomorphs and birds, and probably play a major role in transmission among wildlife (Bell 1980). Hopla (1960) removed rabbit ticks from Willow Ptarmigan (*Lagopus lagopus*), which were later found to be infected with *F. tularensis* (as described in Hopla 1974). *Francisella tularensis* infected ticks transported by migrating birds were believed to be the origin of endemic tularemia in mountain hares (*Lepus timidus*) on an island in the Baltic Sea (Mörner and Krogh 1984). This island is located approximately seven kilometers from the mainland, and no animals are transported to the island from the mainland. The island has a large population of hares but no rodents or other mammals. Migrating birds rest in large numbers on the island and it was believed that birds from Finland, where an outbreak of tularemia had occurred, were carrying infected ticks that introduced the disease.

Dobrokhotov and Mescheryakova (1969) demonstrated *F. tularensis* in feces from raptors in an area where there was an outbreak of tularemia among small rodents, indicating that bird droppings are a possible means for spreading the organism. However, they reported no cases of tularemia in the birds.

CLINICAL SIGNS

There are no reports of the clinical course in naturally infected birds, and clinical signs in wild animals are poorly documented, primarily due to the acute character of tularemia in most species. Experimental infections have been performed in several different species of birds. No significant clinical signs were reported in susceptible species such as Ruffed Grouse and Gray Partridge (*Perdix perdix*) in which the inoculation in general was fatal (Green and Wade 1928a, 1928b; Simpson 1929). Nor did Cabelli et al. (1964a, 1964b) report any clinical signs in the Mourning Dove (*Zenaida macroura*), Brown Noddy (*Anous stolidus*), Lesser Noddy (*Anous tenuirostris*), White Tern (*Gygis alba*), or Sooty Tern (*Sterna fuscata*). Alonsos et al. (1975) observed no clinical signs in their challenge experiment in Eurasian Buzzards (*Buteo buteo*), and neither did Mörner and Mattsson (1988) in their studies of resistant species experimentally infected with *F. tularensis* biovar *palaearctica:* Northern Goshawk (*Accipiter gentilis*), European Sparrowhawk (*A. nisus*), Eurasian Buzzard, Rough-legged Hawk, Tawny Owl (*Strix aluco*) or Carrion Crow (*Corvus corone*).

PATHOGENESIS

The pathogenesis of tularemia in birds is not known. Tularemia is in many mammalian species an acute infectious disease, although the outcome is affected by factors such as innate host susceptibility or acquired immunity as well as dose and virulence of the infecting bacteria (Moe et al. 1975). The virulence mechanism of *F. tularensis* has not yet been described. *Francisella tularensis* does not seem to produce potent exotoxins (Skrodzki, 1968). The presence of endotoxin is uncertain but has been reported (Finegold et al. 1969).

In mammals, the organism gains entrance to the body or bloodstream, multiplies locally, where it may cause local necrosis and ulceration, and then invades small vessels, spreads along the superficial and deep lymphatics, and causes inflammation and necrosis in lymph nodes as well as scattered foci of coagulation necrosis in liver, spleen, bone marrow, and lungs (Lillie and Francis 1936a; Meyer 1965). The organism can survive and multiply in macrophages and hepatocytes (Conlan and North 1992; Fortier et al. 1994).

PATHOLOGY

The pathological findings in birds differ from the findings in mammals. In mammals, tularemia is normally characterized by evidence of septicemia that produces gross and microscopic foci of necrosis randomly distributed in the liver, bone marrow, and spleen (Mörner and Addison 2001). In some peracute cases an enlarged spleen may be the only observed lesion.

Multifocal necrosis is usually absent in naturally occurring tularemia in birds, and the only lesion, if any, may be splenic enlargement. No lesions were found in Northern Bobwhite or Greater Sage-Grouse naturally infected with *F. tularensis* (Green and Wade 1929; Parker et al. 1932; Lillie et al. 1936), and necrotic hepatic foci were seen in only one of eight Ruffed Grouse and one of three Sharp-tailed Grouse (Green et al. 1938). Mörner and Mattsson (1983) found no necrotic lesions in a Rough-legged Hawk or Ural Owl from which they cultured *F. tularensis;* the only observed lesion was an enlarged spleen in the Rough-legged Hawk. Nakamura (1950) reported no lesions in a Red-tailed Hawk from which *F. tularensis* was isolated from the liver. However, in some experimentally inoculated Northern Bobwhite, scattered necrotic foci were visible grossly in liver; by light microscopy, individual necrotic hepatocytes, hyaline thrombi, and infected hepatocytes, Kupffer cells, and splenic reticuloendothelial cells were seen (Parker 1929; Lillie and Francis 1936b).

DIAGNOSIS

The post mortem diagnosis of tularemia is based on demonstrating the causative agent in conjunction with pathological lesions (Office International des Epizooties 1996). In wild birds a presumptive diagnosis has been based on demonstration of the organism and lack of evidence of other causes of death.

In mammals dying with acute infection with *F. tularensis,* the bacteria can be demonstrated in impression smears of liver, spleen, bone marrow, kidney, or lung, or in tissue sections. Large numbers of bacteria usually are seen in blood or in necrotic foci, if present. In birds, bacteria have also been detected in a variety of tissues including liver, spleen, blood, skeletal muscle, heart, and lung (Green and Wade 1928a, 1929; Green and Shillinger 1932; Parker et al. 1932; Mörner and Mattsson 1983, 1988). Gram stained smears contain Gram-negative bacteria that are normally numerous but may be overlooked because of their very small size and resemblance to stain precipitate. They can be demonstrated more specifically by direct or indirect fluorescent antibody staining, a safe and rapid diagnostic tool (Karlsson et al. 1970; Mörner and Mattsson 1988). Bacteria also can be demonstrated in tissue sections using immunofluorescent or immunohistochemical methods (Mörner 1981).

Francisella tularensis grows poorly on most ordinary bacterial culture media, although it may occasionally be isolated on blood agar. However, it grows on glucose cystine blood agar or other media containing sufficient cystine or cysteine, such as Francis medium, McCoy and Chapin medium, modified Thayer-Martin agar, glucose cysteine agar with thiamine (Eigelsbach and McGann 1984; Office International des Epizooties 1996), or chocolate agar (Reary and Klotz 1988). Heart blood, liver, spleen, and bone marrow should be cultured. *Francisella tularensis* is slow growing and often outnumbered by *E. coli* and other bacteria in carcasses, making it more difficult to demonstrate in culture (Mörner et al. 1988). The bacteria are nonmotile, nonsporulating, and bipolar staining uniform coccobacilli in young cultures but pleomorphic in older cultures. Criteria for the identification of *F. tularensis* include growth on special media, distinctive cellular morphology, and specific fluorescent antibody (Office International des Epizooties, 1996) and slide agglutination reactions. Type A can be distinguished from type B by fermentation of glycerol.

If *F. tularensis* is difficult to isolate on primary culture, it may be isolated (under appropriate animal utilization protocols and conditions of high biosafety) following inoculation of tissue suspensions from suspect cases into laboratory animals, such as mice or guinea pigs, which are highly sensitive to infection (Weaver and Hollis 1980; Office International des Epizooties 1996). The organism then can be cultured from tissues such as spleen and liver, in which it will be numerous.

The bacteria can also be identified in culture or specimens by hybridization with probes specific to the 16S rRNA gene of *F. tularensis,* and types A and B can be distinguished by this method (Forsman et al. 1990; Petersen and Schriefer 2005). Immunoelectron microscopic identification also has been described (Geisbert et al. 1993). A variety of polymerase chain reaction (PCR) methods can detect the organism in clinical or environmental samples, and some PCR methods are reported to distinguish all four subspecies; advances have also been made in molecular techniques for strain differentiation, which is potentially important in epidemiological studies (Long et al. 1993; Fulop et al. 1996; Petersen and Schriefer 2005).

Specific antibodies against *F. tularensis* may be detected in the serum of birds recently exposed to the bacterium. A tube-agglutination test and indirect fluorescent antibody test have been described (Mörner and Mattsson 1988; Mörner et al. 1988). Serology is primarily used in epidemiological surveillance.

IMMUNITY

Some avian species are resistant to infection by *F. tularensis,* but the basis of that resistance is unknown. No studies have investigated birds' immune response to *F. tularensis.* During experimental infections of Eurasian Buzzard, Northern Goshawk, and Carrion Crow some birds produced antibodies to *F. tularensis,* but titers began to decline in 53–58 days (Alonso et al. 1975; Mörner and Mattsson 1987; Mörner et al. 1988). The effectiveness of avian antibody in neutralizing the organism is unknown.

PUBLIC HEALTH CONCERNS

Hunter-harvested birds, particularly gallinaceous species such as grouse and quail, have on some occasions been suspected as the source of human infection (Parker 1929; Parker et al. 1932; Stahl et al. 1969; Jellison 1974; Hopla and Hopla 1994). Transmission from bird to human was proven to have occurred from a pheasant (Kursban and Foshay 1946). The greatest risk for humans to acquire tularemia from birds may be through *F. tularensis*–infected ticks that birds can carry.

DOMESTIC ANIMAL HEALTH CONCERNS

Although tularemia is primarily a disease of wild lagomorphs and rodents and only occasionally observed in birds, it occurs sporadically in domestic animals and in zoological gardens. Domestic animals normally contract the disease from infected food (for example, dead rabbits), or from infected vectors such as ticks, mosquitoes, or deer flies (Jellison 1974) and could, of course, contract the disease from an infected bird. Tularemia has been seen in domestic cats (Capellan and Fong 1993; Woods et al. 1998), sheep (Jellison 1974), dogs (Jellison 1974), and horses (Gustafson and DeBowes 1996). Tularemia has not been reported in domestic birds, although Jellison (1974) mentions disease outbreaks in turkeys and chickens in which tularemia was suspected but not proven to be the cause of mortality.

LITERATURE CITED

Abd, H., T. Johansson, I. Golovliov, G. Sandström, and M. Forsman. 2003. Survival and growth of *Francisella tularensis* in *Acanthamoeba castellanii. Applied and Environmental Microbiology* 69:600–606.

Alonso, J.M., H. Bercovier, M. Bourdin and H. Mollaret. 1975. Inoculation experimentale de *Francisella tularensis* à certains carnivores et oiseaux: Deductions epidemiologiques. *Medicine et Maladies Infectieuses* 5:39–48.

Bell, J.F. 1980. Tularemia. In *CRC Handbook Series in Zoonoses.* Section A: Bacterial, rickettsial and mycotic diseases, Vol. 2. J.H. Steele (ed.). CRC Press, Boca Raton, FL, U.S.A., pp. 161–193.

Bell, J.F., and J.R. Reilly. 1981. Tularemia. In *Infectious Diseases of Wild Mammals,* 2nd Ed. J.W. Davies, L.H. Karstad and D.O. Trainer (eds). Iowa State University Press, Ames, IA, U.S.A., pp. 213–231.

Cabelli, V.J., R.A. Hodapp, E.W. Ferguson, and M. Peacock. 1964a. Tularemia: Experimental Infection in the Mourning Dove. *Zoonoses Research* 3:93–98.

Cabelli, V.J., R.A. Hodapp, E.W. Ferguson, and M. Peacock. 1964b. Tularemia: Potential for transmission by birds. *Zoonoses Research* 3:99–124.

Capellan, J., and I.W. Fong. 1993. Tularemia from a cat bite: case report and review of feline-associated tularemia. *Clinical Infectious Diseases* 16:472–475.

Conlan, J.W. and R.J. North. 1992. Early pathogenesis of infection in the liver with the facultative intracellular bacteria *Listeria monocytogenes, Francisella tularensis,* and *Salmonella typhimurium* involves lysis of infected hepatocytes by leukocytes. *Infection and Immunity* 60:394–396.

Dobrokhotov, B.P., and I.S. Meshcheryakova. 1969. A new method used for detection of Tularemia Epizootics. *Zhurnal Mikrobiologii Epidemiologii i Immunobiologii* 46:38–43. [In Russian.]

Eigelsbach, H.T., and V.G. McGann. 1984. Gram-negative aerobic cocci, genus Francisella Dorofe'ev 1947. In *Bergey's Manual of Systematic Bacteriology,* Vol. 1. N.R. Krieg and J.G. Holts (eds.). Williams & Wilkins, Baltimore, MD, U.S.A., pp. 394–399.

Finegold, M.J., J.D. Pulliam, M.E. Landay, and G.G. Wright. 1969. Pathological changes in rabbits injected with *Pasteurella tularensis* killed by ionizing radiation. *Journal of Infectious Diseases* 119:635–640.

Forsman, M., G. Sandström, and B. Jaurin. 1990. Identification of *Francisella* species and discrimination of type A and type B strains of *F. tularensis* by 16S rRNA analysis. *Applied and Environmental Microbiology* 56:949–955.

Fortier, A.H., S.J. Green, T. Polsinelli, T.R. Jones, R.M. Crawfford, D.A. Leiby, K.L. Elkins, M.S. Meltzer and C.A. Nacy. 1994. Life and death of an intracellular pathogen: *Francisella tularensis* and the macrophage. *Immunology and Serology* 60:349–361.

Francis, E. 1921. The occurrence of tularemia in nature as a disease of man. *Public Health Reports* 36:1731–1738.

Fulop, M., D. Leslie, and R. Titball. 1996. A rapid, highly sensitive method for the detection of *Francisella tularensis* in clinical samples using the polymerase chain reaction. *American Journal of Tropical Medical Hygiene* 54:364–366.

Geisbert, T.W., P.B. Jahrling, and J. W. Ezzell, Jr. 1993. Use of immunoelectron microscopy to demonstrate *Francisella tularensis. Journal of Clinical Microbiology* 31:1936–1939.

Green, R.G., and J.E. Shillinger. 1932. A natural infection of the sharp-tailed grouse and the ruffed grouse by *Pasteurella tularensis. Proceedings of the Society for Experimental Biology and Medicine* 30:284–287.

Green, R.G., and E.M. Wade. 1928a. Ruffed grouse are susceptible to tularemia. *Proceedings of the Society for Experimental Biology and Medicine* 25:515–517.

Green, R.G., and E.M. Wade. 1928b. Experimental tularemia in birds. *Proceedings of the Society for Experimental Biology and Medicine* 25:637.

Green, R.G., and E.M. Wade. 1929. A natural infection of quail by *B. tularense. Proceedings of the Society for Experimental Biology and Medicine* 26:626–627.

Green, R.G., E.M. Wade, and W. Kelly. 1928. Experimental tularemia in ring-necked pheasant. *Proceedings of the Society for Experimental Biology and Medicine* 26:260–263.

Green, R.G., C.A. Evans, J.F. Bell, and C.L. Larson. 1938. Comparative pathology of tularemia. *Minnesota Wildlife Disease Investigations* Feb 1938:7–11.

Gustafson, B.W., and L.J. DeBowes. 1996. Tularemia in a dog. *Journal of the American Animal Hospital Association* 32:339–341.

Hopla, C.E. 1960. Epidemiology of tularemia in Alaska. Technical Report of the Arctic Aeromedical Laboratory US 59:1–42.

Hopla, C.E. 1974. The ecology of tularemia. *Advances in Veterinary Science and Comparative Medicine* 18:25–53.

Hopla, C.E., and A.K. Hopla. 1994. Tularemia. *In Handbook of Zoonoses,* 2nd. Ed., G.W. Beran (ed.). CRC Press, Boca Raton, FL, U.S.A., pp. 113–125.

Jellison, W.L. 1974. Tularemia in North America 1930–1974. University of Montana, Missoula, Montana, 276 pp.

Jusatz, H.J. 1961. The geographical distribution of tularemia throughout the world, 1911–1959. In *World Atlas of Epidemic Diseases.* E. Rodenwaldt (ed.). Falk Verlag, Hamburg, DEU, pp. 23–28.

Karlsson, K.A., S. Dahlstrand, E. Hanko, and O. Soderlind. 1970. Demonstration of *Francisella tularensis* in sylvan animals with the aid of fluorescent antibodies. *Acta Pathologica et Microbiologica Scandinavia,* Section B 78:647–651.

Kursban, N.J. and L. Foshay. 1946. Tularemia acquired from the pheasant. *Journal of American Medical Association* 131:1493–1494.

Lillie, R.D. and E. Francis. 1936a. The pathology of tularaemia in the Belgian hare (*Oryctolagus cuniculus*); The pathology of tularaemia in the Black-tailed rabbit (*Lepus sp.*); The pathology of tularaemia in the Cottontail rabbit (*Sylvilagus floridanus*). In *The Pathology of Tularaemia,* R.D. Lillie, 1937, National Institute of Health, U.S. Government Printing Office, Washington, D.C., U.S.A., Bull No. 167:83–126.

Lillie, R.D., and E. Francis. 1936b. The pathology of tularemia in the quail (*Colinus virginianus*). In *The Pathology of Tularaemia,* R.D. Lillie, 1937, National Institute of Health, U.S. Government Printing Office, Washington, D.C., U.S.A., Bull No. 167:203–207.

Lillie, R.D., E. Francis, and R.R. Parker. 1936. The pathology of tularaemia in other birds. In *The Pathology of Tularaemia,* R.D. Lillie, 1937, National Institute of Health, U.S. Government Printing Office, Washington, D.C., U.S.A., Bull No. 167:209–211.

Long, G.W., J.J. Oprandy, R.B. Narayanan, A.H. Fortier, K.R. Porter, and C.A. Nacy. 1993. Detection of *Francisella tularensis* in blood by polymerase chain reaction. *Journal of Clinical Microbiology* 31:152–154.

McCoy, G.W. 1911. A plague-like disease of rodents. *Public Health Bulletin* 43:53–71

McCoy, G.W., and C.W. Chapin. 1912. *Bacterium tularense* the cause of a plague-like disease of rodents. *U.S. Public Health and Marine Hospital Bulletin* 53:17–23.

Meyer K.F. 1965. *Pasteurella* and *Francisella.* In *Bacteria and Mycotic Infections of Man,* 4th Ed. R. J. Dubos and J.G. Hersch (eds.). Lippincott, Philadelphia, PA, U.S.A., pp. 681–697.

Moe, J.B., P.G. Canonico, J.L. Stookey, M.C. Powanda, and G. L. Cockerell. 1975. Pathogenesis of tularemia in immune and nonimmune rats. *American Journal of Veterinary Research* 36:1505–1510.

Mörner, T. 1981. The use of FA technique for detecting *Francisella tularensis* in formalin fixed material. A method useful in routine post mortem work. *Acta Veterinaria Scandinavia* 22:296–306.

Mörner, T., and E. Addison. 2001. Tularemia. In *Infectious Diseases of Wild Mammals,* E.S. Williams and I.K. Barker (eds.). Iowa State University Press, Ames, IA, U.S.A., pp. 303–313.

Mörner, T. and G. Krogh. 1984. An endemic case of tularemia in the mountain hare (*Lepus timidus*) on the island of Stora Karlsö. *Nordisk Veterinärmedicin* 36:310–313.

Mörner T. and R. Mattsson. 1983. Tularemia in a rough-legged buzzard (*Buteo lagopus*) and a Ural owl (*Strix uralensis*). *Journal of Wildlife Diseases* 19:360–361.

Mörner, T and R. Mattsson. 1988. Experimental infection of five species of raptors and of hooded crows with *Francisella tularensis* biovar *palaearctica. Journal of Wildlife Diseases* 24:15–21.

Mörner, T., G.Sandström, and R. Mattsson. 1988. Comparison of serum and lung extracts for surveys of wild animals for antibodies to *Francisella tularensis* biovar *palaearctica. Journal of Wildlife Diseases* 24:10–14.

Nakamura, M. 1950. Tularemia in the red-tailed hawk, *Buteo jamaicensis calurus. The Auk* 67:383–384.

Office International des Epizooties. 1996. Tularemia. In *Manual of Standards for Diagnostic Tests and Vaccines.* OIE, Paris, FR, pp. 584–588.

Ozburn, R.H. 1944. Problems of medical entomology of military importance in Canada. *Journal of Economic Entomology* 37:455–459.

Parker, R.R. 1929. Quail as a possible source of tularaemia infection in man. Public Health Reports 44:999–1000.

Parker, R.R. 1934. Recent studies of tick-borne diseases made at the United States Public Health Service Laboratory at Hamilton, Montana. *Proceedings 5th Pacific Scientific Congress* 5:3367–3374.

Parker R.R., and R.R. Spencer. 1927. Tularemia and its occurrence in Montana. Sixth Biennial Report, Montana State Board of Entomology, Helena, Montana U.S.A., p. 30–41.

Parker, R.R., C.B. Philip, and G.E. Davis. 1932. Tularemia: Occurrence in the sage hen *Centrocercus urophasianus,* also report of additional cases following contacts with quail Colinus virginianus. *Public Health Reports* 47:479–487.

Petersen, J.M., and M.E. Schriefer. 2005. Tularemia: emergence/re-emergence. *Veterinary Research* 36:455–467.

Pfahler-Jung, K. 1989. Die globale verbreitungen der Tularemie. Dissertation Justus–Liebig–Univertsitessen, DEU, 244 pp.

Reary, B.W., and S.A. Klotz. 1988. Enhancing recovery of *Francisella tularensis* from blood. *Diagnostic Microbiology and Infectious Disease* 11:117–119.

Rehbinder C. and K.A. Karlsson. 1979. Tularemia in the raven. *Nordisk Veterinärmedicin* 31:339.

Simpson, W.M. 1929. Tularemia-History, Pathology, Diagnosis, and Treatment. Paul B. Hoeber, Inc. New York, NY, U.S.A., 162 pp.

Skrodzki, E. 1968. Investigations of the pathogenesis of tularemia. VII. Attempts to discover *F. tularensis* toxins. *Biuletyn Instytutu Medycyny Morskiej w Gdansku* 19:69–76.

Stahl, I W., P.R. Schnurrenberger and R.J. Martin. 1969. Water related cases of Tularemia in Illinois. *Illinois Medical Journal* 136:276–277.

Weaver, R.E., and D. Hollis. 1980. Gram-negative fermentative bacteria and *Francisella tularensis*. In *Manual of Clinical Microbiology,* E. Lenette, A. Balows, W. Hausler, Jr., and J. P. Traunt (eds.). American Society for Microbiology, Washington, D.C., U.S.A., pp. 242–262.

Woods, J.P., M.A. Crystal, R.J. Moton, and R.J. Panciera. 1998. Tularemia in two cats. *Journal of the American Veterinary Medical Association* 212:81–83.

20
Aspergillosis

Kathryn A. Converse

INTRODUCTION

Aspergillosis is a noncontagious disease caused by inhalation of spores of ubiquitous, saprophytic fungi of the genus *Aspergillus*. *Aspergillus* spp. are associated with soil, decomposing organic matter, agricultural waste grains, ensilage, litter, and moldy feed. The three most common species of this genus are *A. fumigatus* and *A. niger*, which cause aspergillosis, and *A. flavus*, which produces a mycotoxin (aflatoxin) (Chute et al. 1965). *Aspergillus fumigatus* is the most pathogenic species affecting wild birds (Ainsworth and Rewell 1949) and poultry (Chute and O'Meara 1958), and is the most frequently isolated pathogenic fungus in immunocompromised humans (Schneemann and Schaffner 1999). Aspergillosis usually is an infection of the respiratory tract caused by inhalation of *A. fumigatus* spores, but infections also can occur in the skin, bone, eye, gastrointestinal tract, and central nervous system (Chute and Richard 1997). Aspergillosis can occur as an acute epizootic involving hundreds of wild birds or present as a chronic infection in individual birds. Usually birds are infected by inhaling large numbers of spores while feeding on moldy grains in agricultural areas or possibly at bird feeders (Adrian et al. 1978; Bowes 1990; Machin 1993). Aspergillosis is a common sequela in birds with other diseases and often occurs after wild birds are held in captivity.

SYNONYMS

Brooder pneumonia, mycotic pneumonia, mycosis, cytomycosis.

HISTORY

The genus *Aspergillus* was described in 1729 by Micheli, who observed fungal conidiophores and named them *Aspergillus* (rough head) based on their appearance (Thom and Raper 1945). Thousands of papers written between 1729 and the early twentieth century dealt with physiological morphology and biochemistry of the organism (Thom and Raper 1945).

The history of aspergillosis in wild birds dates back to the early 1800s, when it was described in a Greater Scaup (*Aythya marila*) in 1813 by Montague and in a captive flamingo by Owen in 1832 (Austwick 1968). Published reports of aspergillosis in free-living birds were rare prior to the 1940s and 1950s, when several mortality events occurred. Early reports of aspergillosis in the United States include an outbreak in Illinois in 180 Wood Ducks (*Aix sponsa*) that were feeding on moldy corn (Bellrose et al. 1945), and in 1949 an estimated 1,000 Mallards (*Anas platyrynchos*) died after eating rotten silage (Neff 1955). In Great Britain, there were early reports of this disease in free-living Thayer Gulls (*Larus thayeri*), puffins, Manx Shearwaters (*Puffinus puffinus*), Black Grouse (*Tetrao tetrix*), Mallards, pheasants, and Wood Pigeons (*Columba palumbus*) as summarized by McDiarmid (1955). Aspergillosis was common in chickens, turkeys, and captive quail and occurred most frequently as a severe mycotic pneumonia in young birds (Olson 1969; Chute and Richard 1997).

There are extensive reviews of aspergillosis in captive wild birds (Ainsworth and Rewell 1949; Reavill 1996) and free-living wild birds (McDougle and Vaught 1968; O'Meara and Witter 1971; Wobeser 1997). The history and identification of the fungal genus *Aspergillus* is described by Thom and Raper (1945), Raper and Fennell (1965), and Chute and Richard (1997).

DISTRIBUTION

Fatal *Aspergillus* spp. infections of wild birds have been reported in a wide variety of species on many continents (Table 20.1). With the exception of Antarctica, *Aspergillus* spp. have a worldwide distribution, which suggests that free-living or captive wild birds in most countries are exposed to the spores of this agent (O'Meara and Witter 1971). Studies of microfungi from Antarctic rocks and soils and examinations of carcasses of wild Antarctic species including the Brown Skua (*Catharacta antartica lonbergi*) and

Table 20.1. Aspergillosis in free living birds, as epizootics or mortality surveys reported in scientific literature.

Common Name	Scientific Name	Epizootics # Died	# with Aspergillosis / Total Died (%)	Year(s)	Country (State or Province)	Literature Citation
Mallard	*Anas platyrhynchos*	. . .	2/173 (1.2)	1937–40	U.S.A. (UT)	Quortrup and Shillinger 1941
Mallard	*Anas plaryrhynchos*	350	. . .	1941	U.S.A. (CA)	Herman 1943
Mallard	*Anas platyrhynchos*	1,100	. . .	1949	U.S.A. (CO)	Neff 1955
Mallard	*Anas platyrhynchos*	387	. . .	1975–76	U.S.A. (CO)	Adrian et al. 1978
Mallard	*Anas platyrhynchos*	200	. . .	1985	U.S.A. (SD)	Bair et al. 1988
Mallard	*Anas platyrhynchos*	150	. . .	1989	Canada (B. C.)	Bowes 1990
Northern Pintail	*Anas acuta*	. . .	17/623 (2.7)	1937–40	U.S.A. (UT)	Quortrup and Shillinger 1941
Northern Pintail	*Anas acuta*	. . .	1	1989	Canada (B. C.)	Bowes 1990
Northern Shoveler	*Anas clypeata*	. . .	10/117 (8.5)	1937–40	U.S.A. (UT)	Quortrup and Shillinger 1941
Green-winged Teal	*Anas crecca*	. . .	10/409 (2.4)	1937–40	U.S.A. (UT)	Quortrup and Shillinger 1941
Cinnamon Teal	*Anas cyanoptera*	. . .	2 /20 (10.0)	1937–40	U.S.A. (UT)	Quortrup and Shillinger 1941
American Wigeon	*Anas americana*	. . .	1/78 (1.3)	1937–40	U.S.A. (UT)	Quortrup and Shillinger 1941
Wood Duck	*Aix sponsa*	230	. . .	1943	U.S.A. (IL)	Bellrose 1945
Canvasback	*Aythya valisineria*	28	. . .	1961	U.S.A. (CA)	Rosen 1964
Lesser Scaup	*Aythya affinis*	. . .	1	1961	U.S.A. (CA)	Rosen 1964
Canada Goose	*Branta canadensis*	2000	. . .	1966	U.S.A. (MO)	McDougle and Vaught 1968
Canada Goose	*Branta canadensis*	12	. . .	1981	U.S.A. (WI)	Stroud and Duncan 1982
Canada Goose	*Branta canadensis*	. . .	2/10 (20.0)	1981–82	U.S.A. (NY)	Brand et al. 1988
Ashy-headed Goose	*Chloephaga poliocephala*	. . .	1	1984	Chile	Ulloa et al. 1987
Tundra Swan	*Cygnus columbianus*	1250	. . .	1962	U.S.A. (CA)	Rosen 1964
Tundra Swan	*Cygnus columbianus*	. . .	2/35 (5.7)	2000–02	U.S.A. (WA)	Souza and Degernes 2005
Mute Swan	*Cygnus olor*	. . .	7/193 (3.6)	1951–89	Great Britain	Brown et al. 1992
Mute Swan	*Cygnus olor*	. . .	6/41 (14.6)	1995–96	Scotland	Pennycott 1999
Bewick's Swan	*Cygnus columbianus Bewicki*	. . .	7/150 (4.6)	1951–89	Great Britain	Brown et al. 1992
Whooper Swan	*Cygnus cygnus*	. . .	1/7 (5.4)	1951–89	Great Britain	Brown et al. 1992
Trumpeter Swan	*Cygnus buccinator*	. . .	1	~1997	Canada (Ont.)	Atkinson and Brojer 1998
Trumpeter Swan	*Cygnus buccinators*	. . .	62/365 (16.9)	2000–02	U.S.A. (WA)	Souza and Degernes 2005
Sharp-tailed Grouse	*Tympanushus phasianellus*	. . .	1 (at least)	1993–96	Canada (Que.)	Mikaelian et al. 1997
Ruffed Grouse	*Bonasa umbellus*	. . .	2/18 (11.1)	1924	U.S.A. (ME)	Gross 1925
Sage Grouse	*Centrocercus urophasianus*	. . .	1	1949	U.S.A. (WY)	Honess and Winter 1956
Capercaillae	*Tetrao urogallus*	. . .	1 (at least)	~1941	Sweden	Hülphers et al. 1941
Black Grouse	*Lyrurus tetrix*	. . .	1 (at least)	~1941	Sweden	Hülphers et al. 1941

(*Continued*)

Table 20.1. (Continued)

Common Name	Scientific Name	Epizootics # Died	# with Aspergillosis / Total Died (%)	Year(s)	Country (State or Province)	Literature Citation
Willow Ptarmigan	*Lagopus lagopus*	. . .	1	1950	Norway	O'Meara and Witter 1971
Wild Turkey	*Meleagris gallopavo*	. . .	1/ 108 (0.9)	1972–84	U.S.A. (southeast)	Davidson et al. 1985
Gambel's Quail	*Callipepla gambelii*	. . .	1	~1957	U.S.A. (NV)	Gullion 1957
Common Loon	*Gavia immer*	. . .	31/434 (7.1)	1970–94	U.S.A. (FL)	Forrester et al. 1997
Common Loon	*Gavia immer*	. . .	5/31 (16.1)	1992–96	Canada (NB, NS, PEI)	Daoust et al. 1998
Common Loon	*Gavia immer*	. . .	24/105 (22.8)	1972–99	U.S.A. (NY)	Stone and Okoniewski 2001
Arctic Loon	*Gavia arctica*	. . .	1	1990–92	Belgium	Jauniaux and Coignoul 1994
Albatross, Grey-headed	*Diomedea chrysostoma*	. . .	1	1973	Australia	Tham et al. 1974
Manx Shearwater	*Puffinus puffinus*	. . .	1	~1948	Wales	Dane 1948
Great Blue Heron	*Ardea herodias*	. . .	1	1968	U.S.A. (OH)	O'Meara and Witter 1971
Bald Eagle	*Haliaeetus leucocephalus*	. . .	1	1967	U.S.A. (MO)	Coon and Locke 1968
African Fish Eagle	*Haliaeetus vocifer*	. . .	1	1970–73	East Africa	Cooper 1973
White-tailed Eagle	*Haliaeetus albicilla*	. . .	1	1981	Poland	Falandysz and Szefer 1983
Red-tailed Hawk	*Buteo jamaicensis*	. . .	9/163 (5.5)	1975–92	U.S.A.	Franson et al. 1996
Osprey	*Pandion haeliaetus*	. . .	1 (at least)	1993–96	Canada (Que.)	Mikaelian et al. 1997
Cooper's Hawk	*Accipter cooperi*	. . .	1 (at least)	1993–96	Canada (Que.)	Mikaelian et al. 1997
Northern Goshawk	*Accipiter gentilis*	3	. . .	1972	U.S.A. (MN)	Redig et al. 1980
Northern Goshawk	*Accipiter gentilis*	. . .	1 (at least)	1993–96	Canada (Que.)	Mikaelian et al. 1997
Falcon (presumed Western Marsh Harrier)	*Falco rufus* (presumed *Circus aeroginosus*)	. . .	1 (at least)	~1842	Germany	O'Meara and Witter 1971
American Coot	*Fulica americana*	. . .	3/48 (6.3)	1949–50	U.S.A. (CA)	Gullion 1952
American Coot	*Fulica americana*	40	. . .	1961	U.S.A. (CA)	Rosen 1964
Herring Gull	*Larus argentatus*	80	. . .	1939	U.S.A. (MA)	Davis and McClung 1940
Herring Gull	*Larus argentatus*	36	. . .	1971	Netherlands	Smeenk 1972
Herring Gull	*Larus argentatus*	. . .	9/86 (10.5)	1981–82	U.S.A. (NY)	Brand et al. 1988
Great Black-backed Gull	*Larus marinus*	. . .	3/8 (37.5)	1981–82	U.S.A. (NY)	Brand et al. 1988
Laughing Gull	*Larus atricilla*	. . .	1/2 (50.0)	1981–82	U.S.A. (NY)	Brand et al. 1988
Glaucous Gull	*Larus hyperboreus*	. . .	1	1943	U.S.A. (CA)	Herman and Bolander 1943
Thayer Gull	*Larus thayeri*	. . .	1	~1945	U.S.A. (FL)	Cowan 1945

Royal Tern	*Sterna maxima*	...	1	~1979	U.S.A. (FL)	Jacobson et al. 1980
Razorbill	*Alca torda*	...	1	1990–92	Belgium	Jauniaux and Coignoul 1994
Common Murre	*Uria aalge*	...	7	1990–92	Belgium	Jauniaux and Coignoul 1994
Wood Pigeon	*Columba palumbus*	14	...	1943–53	Great Britain	McDiarmid, 1955
Rock Pigeon	*Columba livia*	...	2/40 (5.0)	~1971	India	Monga 1972
Parrot (presumed parakeet)	*Psittacula sp.*	...	1/8 (12.5)	~1971	India	Monga 1972
Great-horned Owl	*Bubo virginianus*	...	1	~1985	U.S.A. (TX)	Clark et al. 1987
Great-horned owl	*Bubo virginianus*	...	1	~1997	Canada (Ont.)	Atkinson and Brojer 1998
Snowy Owl	*Nyctea scandiaca*	...	1	1941	U.S.A. (NY)	Meade and Stoner 1942
Snowy Owl	*Nyctea scandiaca*	...	1 (at least)	1993–96	Canada (Que.)	Mikaelian et al. 1997
Barn Owl	*Tyto alba*	...	1 (at least)	~1842	Germany	O'Meara and Witter 1971
Barn Owl	*Tyto alba*	...	2/81 (2.5)	1992–94	U.S.A. (HI)	Work and Hale 1996
Stitchbird	*Notiomystis cincta*	...	6/31 (19.4)	~1999	New Zealand	Alley et al. 1999
Blue Jay	*Cyanocitta cristata*	...	1	1998	U.S.A. (GA)	Young et al. 1998
Stellar's Jay	*Cyanocitta stelleri*	...	9/27 (33.3)	1992	Canada (B.C.)	Machin 1993
Eurasian Jackdaw	*Corvus monedula*	...	1	1953	England	McDiarmid 1955
American Crow	*Corvus brachyrhynchos*	1500	...	1974	U.S.A. (NE)	Zinkl et al. 1977
Common Raven	*Corvus corax*	...	1 (at least)	1968	U.S.A. (ME)	O'Meara and Witter 1971
Audubon's Warbler	*Dendroica auduboni*	3	...	1961	U.S.A. (CA)	Rosen 1964
American Robin	*Turdus migratorius*	15	...	1961	U.S.A. (CA)	Rosen 1964
Varied Thrush	*Ixoreus naevius*	...	1	1961	U.S.A. (CA)	Rosen 1964
White-crowned Sparrow	*Zonatrichia leucophrys*	...	1	1961	U.S.A. (CA)	Rosen 1964
Song Sparrow	*Melospiza melodia*	...	1	1951	U.S.A. (NY)	Manwell 1954
House Sparrow	*Passer domesticus*	10	...	1964	U.S.A. (MD)	Locke 1965
House Sparrow	*Passer domesticus*	...	3/70 (4.3)	~1971	India	Monga 1972
Sparrow	unspecified	...	6/55 (10.9)	~1971	India	Monga 1972
Common Grackle and Brown-headed Cowbird	*Quiscalus quiscula* *Molothrus ater*	283	...	1958–59	U.S.A. (MD, PA)	Clark 1960
Little Penguins	*Eudyptula minor*	...	2/48 (4.2)	1977–78	Australia	Obendorf and McColl 1980

South Polar Skua (*Stercorarius maccormicki*) did not yield any isolates of *Aspergillus* spp. (Onofri et al. 2000; Leotta et al 2002).

HOST RANGE

Data on the frequency of aspergillosis in wild birds is fragmentary and may represent studies of a particular species or geographic area or specific research results rather than the actual incidence in the wild. Aspergillosis has occurred in a wide range of wild birds representing many families, both as acute epizootics and as infections in individual birds (Table 20.1). Waterfowl, raptors, and gulls represent the majority of the free-living hosts reported to have aspergillosis. O'Meara and Witter (1971) stated that the higher prevalence of aspergillosis reported in waterfowl and game birds might represent the higher likelihood of people detecting this disease in birds that are handled and processed for food. No avian species are considered resistant to infection by *Aspergillus* spp.

Aspergillosis is described in captive wild birds of 35 species in 13 orders (Ainsworth and Rewell 1949). Waterbirds including penguins (Spheniscidae), pelicans (Pelecanidae), flamingos (Phoenicopteridae), loons (Gaviidae), petrels (Hydrobatidae), and shorebirds (Chradadriiformes) are especially susceptible to aspergillosis when held in captivity (Hillgarth and Kear 1979). This susceptibility is demonstrated by the results of examinations of 641 captive sea ducks and confirmation of aspergillosis as the cause of death in 17% of the adults, 31% of juveniles, and 27% of nestlings (Hillgarth and Kear 1979). Water birds in captivity are considered more susceptible to aspergillosis than land-dwelling birds (Hillgarth and Kear 1979). Presumably, marine species are equally susceptible when free living, but this hypothesis has not been tested.

ETIOLOGY

The genus *Aspergillus* is within the family Trichocomaceae, order Eurotiales, class Eurotiomycetes, phylum Ascomycota (CABI Bioscience 2004). The genus *Aspergillus* includes 185 species; 20 species are pathogenic to plants or animals. The vegetative form of *Aspergillus* spp. fungi is the mycelium, which is a network of branching, septate filaments called hyphae. Mycelia produce enzymes and some produce mycotoxins. Growth is initiated at the apical tip of the hypha, which grows radially across surfaces and penetrates substrates. *Aspergillus* spp. reproduce asexually by forming an aerial fruiting body: Sections of hyphae enlarge and become foot cells; a branch arises perpendicular to the foot cells, develops into a conidiophore with a swollen head (vesicle), and becomes fertile by bearing conidia (conidiospores or spores) (Al-Doory and Wagner 1985). The fruiting body of *A. fumigatus* bears radiating chains of conidia arising up to 400 μm from a flask-shaped, 20–30 μm diameter vesicle at the end of the smooth aerial stalk (Chute and Richard 1997). The conidia are very small (2.5 to 3.0 μ), detach readily, and can be easily inhaled into lungs and air sacs. *Aspergillus* spp. are tolerant of a wide temperature range of 18° to 30°C. In the laboratory, the majority of the species will grow and sporulate at 23° to 26°C (Raper and Fennell 1965).

Aspergillus fumigatus is the most pathogenic species causing aspergillosis in wild birds. Other species of *Aspergillus* that are infrequently identified in wild birds include *A. flavus, A. niger, A. nidulans,* and *A. flavus-oryzae* (Austwick 1968; Tham et al. 1974; Wobeser and Saunders 1975; Katz et al. 1996). In the laboratory, *Aspergillus* spp. grow rapidly on blood agar, Sabourad's dextrose agar, potato dextrose agar, and in Czapek's solution (Chute and Richard 1997). The color, growth rate, and marginal appearance of the colonies depend on the species and growth conditions (Al-Doory and Wagner 1985). Generally, initial flat, white colonies of short, branching, septate fungal hyphae develop distinguishing characteristics as the conidial heads mature (Kunkle and Richard 1998). Conidial heads of *A. fumigatus* are light blue-green to very dark green, and color darkens to gray-green as they age; conidia are 2–3 μm and grow at 25° to 37°C. Conidial heads *of A. flavus* range from light to deep yellow-green, shifting to olive-brown and then brown, have 3–6 μm conidia, and grow at 24° to 26°C; and *A. niger* conidial heads occur in shades of olive brown to brown and age to black, have larger, 4.0 to 5.0 μm conidia, and grow at 24° to 26°C (Raper and Fennell 1965).

EPIZOOTIOLOGY

Aspergillus spp. are ubiquitous saprophytes found in soil, decaying vegetation, and agricultural wastes such as spilled grain and corn ensilage. Generally, the *Aspergilli* readily grow in moist environments and sporulate at temperatures of 23° to 26°C.

Primary transmission is through inhalation of airborne *Aspergillus* spp. spores. Spores are released when fungal fruiting bodies are shattered by birds' movements (Bellrose 1945). An estimated six million inhaled spores were needed to produce fatal infections in day-old chickens and an even greater 17 million spores were necessary to cause a fatal infection in adult chickens (Austwick 1968). In contrast, many wild bird species are reported to be very susceptible to fungal infection and may require fewer spores to become infected (Hillgarth and Kear 1979; Brand et al. 1988; Pokras 1996; Forrester et al. 1997). In an experimental study of 21-day-old quail, all birds that received intratracheal inoculation of 2.7 million spores developed clinical signs after two days and died (Gumussoy et al. 2004). In another study, all the starlings given an intratracheal inoculation of 1.35 million spores became infected and died (Atasever and Gumussoy 2004).

Oral exposure appears to be an unlikely route of transmission. Experimental feeding of wheat cultures containing *A. fumigatus* and *A. flavus* to unvaccinated broiler chicks resulted in typical lesions of mycotoxicosis including extensive epithelial hyperplasia of the bile ducts, but no respiratory disease of aspergillosis (Chute et al. 1965). Transmission can occur via puncture wounds contaminated with hyphal fragments or spores, especially wounds that enter air sacs (O'Meara and Witter 1971). *Aspergillus* spp. spores are capable of penetrating egg shells, which may result in embryo death before hatching, or birds hatched with aspergillosis (Olsen et al. 1990). In two studies in which eggs were experimentally exposed to *A. fumigatus,* 42/44 (91%) of the hatched chicks had lesions of aspergillosis, or 36/36 (100%) were infected (O'Meara and Chute 1959).

There are acute and chronic forms of aspergillosis (O'Meara and Witter 1971; Redig et al. 1980). The acute form develops rapidly within days; the affected birds are in good body condition and there usually are no other underlying disease problems. In acute cases, birds die rapidly from severe respiratory compromise due to generalized lung infection. Large epizootics of acute aspergillosis occur in wild bird species, especially gregarious species. Birds that flock and feed together in the same areas may be exposed simultaneously to *Aspergillus* spp. spores, or natural concentrations of large numbers of birds may allow detection of mortality that might go unnoticed in well-dispersed species.

With chronic aspergillosis, birds develop a slowly progressing disease and may become debilitated before succumbing to the infection. There are well-developed lesions of aspergillosis, usually consisting of firm nodules and sometimes including colored conidospores in the respiratory tract. Chronic aspergillosis is more likely to result in individual bird deaths than group mortality events. Birds with chronic aspergillosis may have evidence of trauma, parasitism, or other concurrent diseases, or possibly a history of recent capture, captivity, or rehabilitation. Aspergillosis is commonly detected in birds that are also stressed by malnutrition, other disease, oiling, or capture and captivity (Wobeser 1997). In addition, minor localized, non-lethal *Aspergillus* spp. infections may be an incidental finding in wild birds that die from other causes.

Two hypotheses for the development of aspergillosis were presented by Friend and Trainer (1969): Either the initial dose of spores is so high that it exceeds the natural resistance of the host, or birds may be carriers of the fungi but become sick when stress occurs. Sublethal lead toxicity (liver lead concentrations of 0.4–2.4 ppm, wet weight) was considered significant in 15 Mallards with aspergillosis and may have predisposed the birds to disease (Bair et al. 1988). However, lead levels were not stated for Mallards that did not die of aspergillosis in this epizootic. Other species reported to have died of aspergillosis in association with lead poisoning include Trumpeter Swans (*Cygnus buccinator*), Canada Geese (*Branta canadensis*), and an Andean Condor (*Vultur gryphus*) (Locke et al. 1969; Souza and Degernes 2005). Aspergillosis in Mute Swans (*Cygnus olor*) was diagnosed secondarily to heavy tracheal trematode infestations (Pennycott 1999). Thiamine deficiency caused by an exclusive diet of alewives (*Alosa pseudoharengus*), a fish known to be high in thiaminase, may have increased the susceptibility of captive Herring Gulls (*Larus argentatus*) to aspergillosis (Friend and Trainer 1969). A study of migrating raptors provides additional support for the hypothesis that birds carry *Aspergillus* spp. and can succumb to infections when stressed (Redig et al. 1980). *Aspergillus* spp. was cultured from 26 of 49 (53%) clinically healthy Northern Goshawks (*Accipiter gentilis*) trapped during the 1972 fall migration, but only 4/56 (7%) of the Northern Goshawks trapped during 1973 fall migration. The differences in the prevalence of *Aspergillus* spp. during fall surveillance corresponded with higher aspergillosis mortality in Northern Goshawks submitted for necropsy during the winter of 1972 (11/15, 67%) in comparison with 1973 (2/17, 11.7%). Many of the 13 birds that died during winter 1972 had been captured, brought into captivity for falconry purposes, and died within six weeks of capture.

Changing environmental conditions are often associated with aspergillosis losses. Increases in temperature and moisture can enhance development of molds and fungus on waste grains left in agricultural fields after harvest. Harsh weather or unfavorable conditions may cause birds to feed on moldy foodstuffs. Epizootics of aspergillosis in Colorado that involved an estimated 1,000 Mallards in 1949 and 270 Mallards in 1975 were probably initiated when waterfowl fed on discarded moldy ensilage; normal feed in agricultural fields was not available during heavy snow cover (Neff 1955; Adrian et al. 1978). On Vancouver Island, Canada, more than 150 waterfowl died over a 10-day period in late October after feeding on moldy corn cobs left in fields after harvest (Bowes 1990). In South

Dakota, Mallards that fed on piles of moldy corn during three severe snowstorms died of aspergillosis 8–13 days after the storms (Bair et al. 1988). Although a specific source was not identified, it was postulated that the high prevalence of aspergillosis in 80/200 (40%) Herring Gulls in Boston, Massachusetts, was related to their habits of feeding in garbage dumps and scavenging along the shore in decaying vegetation (Davis and McClung 1940). Rosen (1964) and Zinkl et al. (1977) suggested that aspergillosis outbreaks follow dry weather and excessive dust that compromise the mucosa of the respiratory epithelium and allow proliferation of *Aspergillus* spp. spores.

Captive wild birds may encounter high densities of *Aspergillus* spp. spores in situations in which birds are overcrowded and/or stressed or have poor ventilation, contaminated or damp bedding, or moldy food (Atkinson and Brojer 1998). Outbreaks of aspergillosis in captive sea ducks were attributed to stressful conditions such as transportation, new pens, different food, nest defense, and parental demands (Hillgarth and Kear 1979). Aspergillosis may become a problem when trapping and temporarily holding wild birds. In one experiment, a proportion (7/36) of wild, trapped Canvasbacks (*Aythya valisineria*) that were held in wire enclosures died of aspergillosis 21–158 days after confinement, whereas all Canvasbacks (14) that were released on larger ponds survived (Kocan and Perry 1976).

Aspergillosis mortality may disproportionately involve young of the year birds. During gull mortality in Jamaica Bay, New York, 96% of the Herring Gulls with aspergillosis were young of the year birds (Brand et al. 1988). Chickens are known to be vulnerable to *Aspergillus* spp. infections from day 20 of incubation until between two and seven days after hatching (O'Meara and Chute, 1959). If wild birds have the same susceptibility pattern, the types of nesting materials, reuse of nests, population density at the nesting site, humidity, and temperature during nesting season potentially play a role in the incidence of aspergillosis in free-flying birds (O'Meara and Witter 1971). Colony nesting birds may be placed at risk in crowded nesting situations. Certainly wild bird species reared in captivity and hatcheries for relocation or release programs may be subjected to similar levels of humidity, warm temperatures, and *Aspergillus* spp. exposure. Morbidity from aspergillosis in young wild birds is difficult to assess, but in hatchery-acquired infections, up to 100% of domestic chicks can be affected, resulting in variable mortality. Mortality is highest in domestic chicks during the first week to 10 days of age and is influenced by the severity and duration of exposure and the stress from concurrent viral, bacterial, and protozoan diseases (O'Meara and Witter 1971).

CLINICAL SIGNS

Clinical signs of aspergillosis in wild birds vary with the severity of the disease and the organ systems that are involved. Wild birds with acute aspergillosis may become lethargic or dehydrated or both, isolate themselves from other birds, and display gasping, bill opening and closing, dyspnea, and cyanosis leading to death (Wobeser 1997; Atkinson and Brojer 1998). Acutely affected wild birds may also be found dead with no apparent premonitory signs. In chronic forms of aspergillosis, clinical signs may occur only in the later stages of infection and include emaciation, reduced activity and stamina, inability to fly, dyspnea or tachypnea, vomiting and diarrhea, and, if infections have invaded the nervous system, ataxia, torticollis, and other neurological signs (Redig 1998; Atkinson and Brojer 1998).

PATHOGENESIS AND PATHOLOGY

Inhalation is considered the usual means of exposure to *Aspergillus* spp. After inhalation, spores germinate in the aerobic environment of the respiratory tract and produce plaques of hyphae. Fungal hyphae incite a strong inflammatory cell response, predominantly in the form of macrophages and multinucleated giant cells as well as heterophils, that surrounds radiating hyphae to form a firm, pale nodule within the lung or a pale, rubbery plaque on the surface of air sacs or other airways (O'Meara and Witter 1971). In some avian tissues (presumably under appropriately aerobic conditions), the hyphae may produce conidia, which are carried to other sites in the respiratory tract and germinate, producing more lesions. Lungs and air sacs most commonly are involved, but trachea, syrinx, and bronchi may be affected as well. After there is a respiratory tract focus, any internal organ can become infected by the fungus via the vascular system, through pneumatized bones, or by direct extension to the peritoneum and abdominal organs (Jacobson et al.1980). Hematogenous dissemination of *A. fumigatus* may occur by hyphal penetration of blood vessels in the lung followed by intravascular transport of hyphae, spores, or fungal elements contained within macrophages (Hasegawa 1971; Richard and Thurston 1983). Macrophages successfully engulfed spores of *A. fumigatus* within 15 minutes of experimental exposure, indicating that very little time was needed for spores to move from the alveolus into lymphatics and blood (Richard and Thurston 1983). It has been demonstrated in studies in humans that the first defense against *Aspergillus* spp. is alveolar macrophages that ingest, inhibit, and kill the spores, and the second line of defense is neutrophil granulocytes that kill the hyphae (which are not ingested) by oxidative and nonoxidative mechanisms. Both defense systems must fail for disease to occur (Schneemann and Schaffner 1999).

Gross lesions of acute and chronic aspergillosis in birds usually differ, but lesions are not exclusive to one presentation or the other and may occur in the same bird. In acute aspergillosis, the lungs are often dark red, edematous, and contain multiple, small, white to tan nodules disseminated on the serosal surface and throughout the pulmonary parenchyma (Adrian et al. 1978; Bair et al. 1988) (Figure 20.1). In addition to lung nodules, 70% of the Mallards in a Colorado epizootic had cotton-like to firm, flat, yellow plaques in the interclavicular, anterior and posterior thoracic, and abdominal air sacs (Adrian et al. 1978).

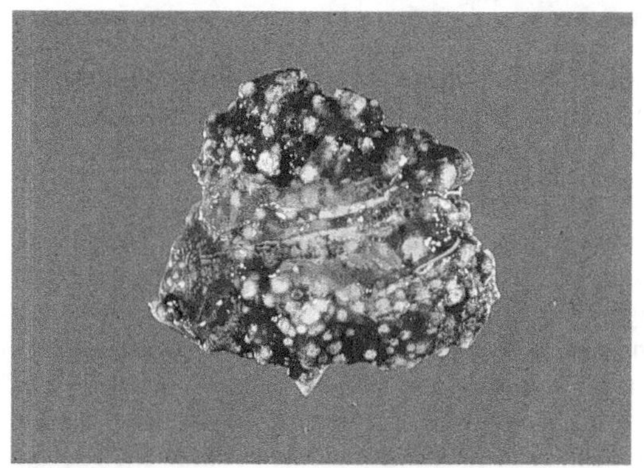

Figure 20.1. Acute aspergillosis in an immature Ring-billed Gull (*Larus delawarensis*). The lung contains numerous pale, 2–3 mm nodular granulomas.

In chronic aspergillosis, caseonecrotic plaques in the air sacs generally predominate (Ainsworth and Rewell 1949) (Figure 20.2). Plaques may appear blue-green, olive green, brown, or black, and velvety if conidia develop. In chronic cases, aspergillosis can extend from the respiratory tract to other tissues. For example, a caseous tract of aspergillosis in lung tissue in a Royal Tern (*Sterna maxima*) extended into the abdominal air sac, adhered to the kidney, and penetrated the intestinal wall (Jacobson et al. 1980).

Even if lesions remain localized in one area of the respiratory tract, aspergillosis can be fatal if it occludes a vital air passage (Figure 20.3). Three Canada Geese in Wisconsin died of asphyxiation due to complete occlusion of the syrinx by a fibrinonecrotic plug that was composed of an *A. fumigatus* mycelium with necrotic debris and inflammatory cells; hyphae had invaded the submucosa (Figure 20.4) (Stroud and Duncan 1982). Aspiration of food material such as grain can be the nidus of localized tracheal *Aspergillus* spp. infection.

The characteristic branching, septate hyphal structure of *Aspergillus* spp. is often visible in hematoxylin and eosin (H&E) stain. The fungi in tissue sections will stain with periodic acid-Schiff (PAS) and Grocott's methenamine silver (GMS) stains (Figure 20.5).

Lesions of aspergillosis are seen most frequently in the respiratory tract but also may occur in the esophagus, small intestine, liver, spleen (Adrian et al. 1978), kidney (Tham et al. 1974), eye, bone, brain (Chute and Richard 1997), skin, heart (Atkinson and Brojer 1998), and other internal organs. Lesions can be present at many sites in one bird. In addition to aspergillosis plaques in the liver, air sacs, and lungs of semi-wild Common Eider (*Somateria mollissima*) ducklings, large necrotic areas of meningoencephalitis in the

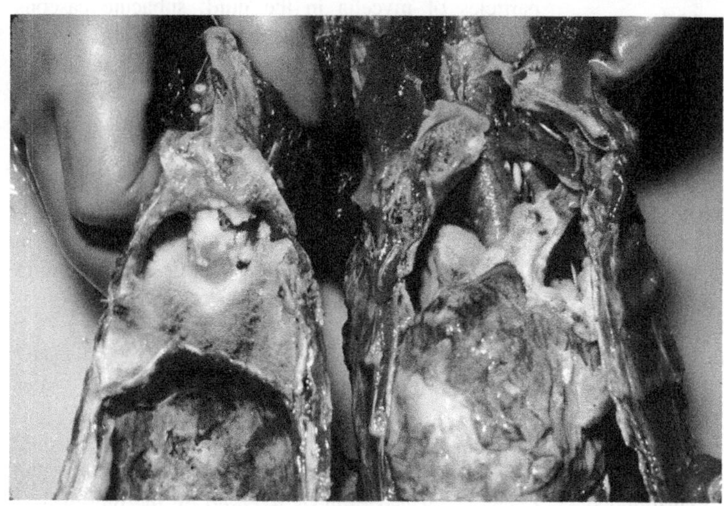

Figure 20.2. Severe chronic aspergillosis in an immature White-naped Crane (*Grus vipio*). The sternum has been reflected and placed on the left to view cervical and clavicular air sacs lined by a confluent white fungal plague with powdery spore production near the heart and surrounding the trachea.

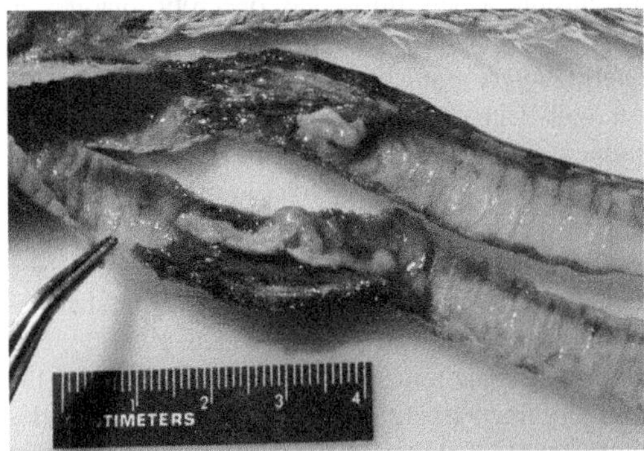

Figure 20.3. Tracheal aspergillosis in an adult Whooping Crane (*Grus americana*). A 3 cm length of the tracheal lumen was occluded by fungal mycelium, caseous material, and mucus.

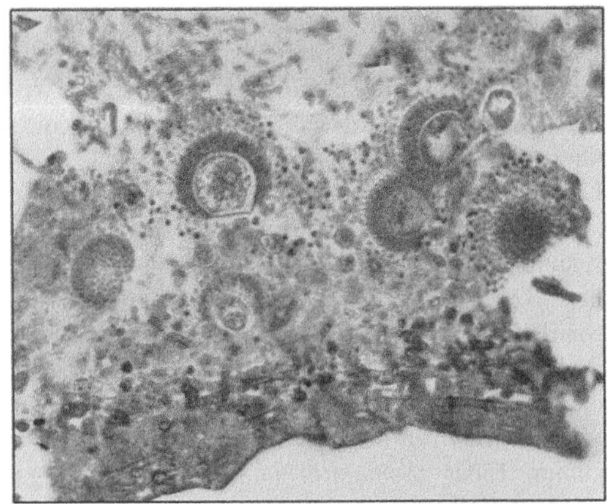

Figure 20.4. Exudate in the trachea of an Aleutian Canada Goose with obstructive tracheal aspergillosis. Fungal hyphae and fruiting bodies with radiating chains of condiospores are present among tracheal debris. (H&E stain; 400X)

cerebrum included perivascular cuffing, vessel thrombosis, and groups of monocytes clustered loosely around mycelia (Hubben 1958).

The progression of microscopic lesions of aspergillosis has been described from experimental infections in turkey poults (Chute and Richard 1997). In the earliest stages (one to seven days), lung lesions consisted of accumulations of lymphocytes and macrophages with few multinucleated giant cells scattered throughout the lungs. In the next stage (one to eight weeks), granulomas were formed around a necrotic center and consisted of heterophils surrounded

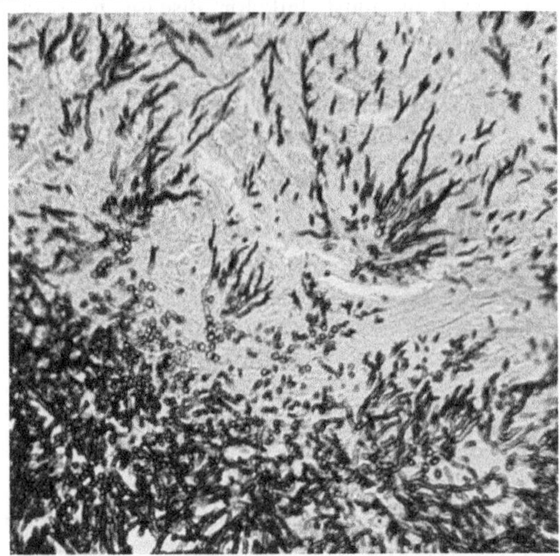

Figure 20.5. Fungal hyphae of *Aspergillus* sp. in the lung of a Golden Eagle (*Aquila chrysaetos*). (Grocott's methenamine-silver stain; 100X)

by macrophages, multinucleated giant cells, lymphocytes, and fibrous tissue. Poults that survived the first eight weeks had granulomas surrounded by giant cells and a thick layer of fibrous tissue with few heterophils. Fungal hyphae were present in necrotic areas and *A. fumigatus* was sporulating in well-oxygenated bronchi, bronchioles, and air sacs (Chute and Richard 1997).

Variation in lesions among individual birds in epizootics suggests differences in the progression of the disease, and, presumably, varied durations of exposure to *Aspergillus* spp. spores. Canada geese collected during an epizootic in Missouri had three distinct types of pneumonia: acute hemorrhage and edema with few particles of mycelia in the fluid; subacute caseous inflammation and necrosis with few multinucleated giant cells and hyphae growing outward into air spaces; and numerous chronic caseous granulomas containing cellular debris and mycelia, surrounded by heterophils and multinucleated giant cells with fibroplasia between adjacent lesions (McDougle and Vaught 1968). Similar variations in levels of acute, subacute, and chronic cellular reactions in lung parenchyma were reported in Mallards collected during an aspergillosis epizootic in Colorado (Adrian et al. 1978).

DIAGNOSIS

A post mortem diagnosis of aspergillosis can be supported by several factors: the animal's history and clinical signs, positive serologic tests, and grossly visible fungal plaques on tissues at necropsy. The confirmed diagnosis of aspergillosis is based on the presence of compatible lesions at necropsy and identification of one or more *Aspergillus* spp. in tissues by isolation or identification of characteristic fungal hyphae in tissue examined microscopically. A wide variety of tests is used to confirm the presence of *Aspergillus* spp. and identify the species. Isolation is accomplished by any of three methods: smearing tissues on plates of blood, Sabouraud's dextrose, or potato dextrose agar; plating ground tissue mixed with saline; or centrifuging fluid samples to obtain sediment for culture and microscopic examination (Kunkle and Richard 1998). Samples are incubated two to three days at 37°C until growth starts and then are kept at room temperature (25–30°C) for up to one month. After an isolate is obtained, hyphae and conidia can be collected using cellophane tape and stained with lactophenyl blue to enhance structures for microscopic examination and identification (USGS-NWHC).[1] For direct microscopy, small samples of scrapings, sediment, or tissue can be added to 10% KOH supplemented with ink dye to improve visualization of the short, branching, septate hyphae (Kunkle and Richard 1998). The complete and frequently used classification, morphology, and key for identification of the *Aspergillus* spp. are provided by Raper and Fennell (1965).

An immunohistochemical (IHC) label using monoclonal and polyclonal antibodies can be used to detect *Aspergillus* spp. in formalin fixed tissues (Carrasco et al.1993). This test can be used to identify the fungus retrospectively, as well as to differentiate aspergillosis from concurrent yeast infections or other zygomycosis.

Antemortem diagnosis of aspergillosis is based on clinical signs, positive serologic tests, culture of tracheal washes, endoscopy, and radiographs. The chronic nature of aspergillosis and the difficulty of antemortem diagnosis of this disease in wild birds during rehabilitation led to refinement of techniques for serologic diagnosis of aspergillosis. An indirect enzyme-linked immunosorbent assay (ELISA) was developed to detect *Aspergillus* spp. infections and can be used in captive birds to chart the progress of the disease and determine the prognosis in specific birds (Brown and Redig 1994). The test is based on a correlation between an optical density reading (OD) and the magnitude of antibody response. Given a range of negative, low, medium, and high thresholds, an immune response can be estimated. An initial diagnosis of aspergillosis infection would be indicated if the OD indicates an increasing antibody level. Success of treatment for aspergillosis is monitored by a subsequent decline in the OD; no decrease in the OD after treatment may mean uncontained spread of the disease. The success of this indirect antibody test is contingent on the ability of the host species to generate antibodies and adequate antibody production at the time the bird is tested (Brown and Redig 1994).

Under anesthesia, deep tracheal washes for culture can be obtained from live sick birds, or endoscopic examination of the respiratory tract and abdominal cavity can allow visualization of granulomas and collection of culture specimens (Redig 1998). Radiographs may help support a diagnosis of aspergillosis but only in later stages of the disease (Redig 1998).

If their eggs are tested to detect antibodies, adult free-ranging birds can be indirectly tested without the necessity of capturing them for blood sampling. Embryonated eggs from captive reared Cape (Jackass) Penguins (*Spheniscus demersus*), removed from a penguin colony during population reduction efforts, contained maternal IgG against *Aspergillus* spp., and these titers were significantly correlated with the specific antibody levels of their mothers (Graczyk and Cranfield 1996).

Gene sequences for human isolates of *A. fumigatus* were used to develop a polymerase chain reaction (PCR) method for detection as little of as 1 pg of *A. fumigatus* DNA in Ostriches (*Struthio camelus*) (Katz et al. 1996). Use of this very sensitive technique would allow early treatment to be initiated.

IMMUNITY

Adult birds are more resistant than chicks to aspergillosis, indicating that mechanisms for innate resistance exist, but little definitive data has been developed on birds' immunity to *Aspergillus* spp. Birds can produce specific antibodies to *Aspergillus* spp., but the presence of antibodies does not guarantee their protection from disease; birds with clinical disease can have positive antibody titers (Brown and Redig 1994). The humoral response of Rock Pigeons (*Columba livia*) was studied during development of an immunological model of avian aspergillosis. Weekly injections of *A. fumigatus* extracts produced an *Aspergillus*-specific humoral immune response in six to nine weeks that decreased over time. A booster after 10 months induced a rapid IgM and IgG response (Martinez-Quesada et al. 1993).

Maternal antibody may provide transient protection from infection in very young birds. Embryonated eggs from captive-reared Jackass Penguins contained maternal IgG against *Aspergillus* spp. and aspergillosis was not observed in any penguin chicks during the first four weeks after hatching, suggesting that maternal antibodies provided protection (Graczyk and Cranfield 1995).

During development of an *Aspergillus* spp. ELISA, it was demonstrated that antibody titers increased during the course of disease and decreased as disease was successfully resolved by treatment. However, the role of antibodies in protection from infection or in recovery from disease was not investigated (Brown and Redig 1994).

PUBLIC HEALTH CONCERNS

Aspergillus fumigatus is responsible for more than 90% of the pulmonary mycoses in humans, and an increase in these infections in the past 10 to 20 years has corresponded with an increase in immunosuppressed humans and use of immunosuppressive therapies (Latgé 2001). Aspergillosis is not a contagious disease, but exposure of humans to the same environmental source of *Aspergillus* spp. as wild birds could lead to development of acute respiratory infection and the potential for spread to other organs (Friend 1999). The risk of development of aspergillosis in humans is higher in individuals who have organ transplants, are leucopenic, have allergies, or have other respiratory illnesses such as tuberculosis or cancer (Coleman and Kaufman 1972; Ruchel and Reichard 1999). Because *A. fumigatus* is usually not pathogenic to immunocompetent humans, the virulence is poorly understood. DNA fingerprinting (southern blot) did not discriminate between isolates from immunosupressed humans and environmental isolates, therefore essentially any environmental strain of *A. fumigatus* is potentially pathogenic (Debeaupuis et al. 1997). A face mask is recommended when cleaning cages or buildings where there is an accumulation of moldy feed and litter, when working in dense bird colonies where mold has grown on the accumulations of fecal material, and when conducting field or necropsy investigations of aspergillosis mortality or cleaning up suspected environmental sources of *Aspergillus* spp.

DOMESTIC ANIMAL HEALTH CONCERNS

Aspergillosis is not transmissible to domestic animals directly from wild birds but could be present in birds sharing the same habitats as domestic animals. House Sparrows (*Passer domesticus*) were the most common species shot and cultured during sampling of avian populations on university farms in India and they had the highest number of *A. fumigatus* in "throat" cultures. (Monga 1972). This high prevalence could indicate either recent infections or high levels of the fungus in that environment. An outbreak of aspergillosis in wild birds that use the same environment as domestic animals may provide an indicator of the prevalence of the organism, presence of a contaminated source of the fungus, or a greater susceptibility to *Aspergillus* spp. in that wild avian species.

WILDLIFE POPULATION IMPACTS

Aspergillosis epizootics have resulted in losses of hundreds of free-living birds (Adrian et al. 1978; Bair et al. 1988; Bowes 1990). Aspergillosis can also be a serious problem in wild birds that are placed in permanent captivity (Fix et al. 1988), or housed in captivity during research studies (Friend and Trainer 1969) or relocation programs (Kocan and Perry 1976; Cork et al. 1999).). Marine birds placed in rehabilitation appear to be particularly prone to aspergillosis (Advisory Committee on Oil Pollution of the Sea 1974; Jauniaux and Coignoul 1994); *Aspergillus* spp. infections were present in 23/38 (61%) wild-caught Magellanic Penguins (*Spheniscus magellanicus*) that died within one year of transfer to a zoo (Fix et al. 1988). *Aspergillus fumigatus* detected in Wild Turkeys (*Meleagris gallopavo*) was teratogenic in chick embryos; because it is ubiquitous in the forest floor, it could contribute to mortality of poults and, if present in eggs, lower the hatching rate (Hopkins et al. 1990).

TREATMENT AND CONTROL

After a bird contracts an aspergillosis infection, there are few effective treatments. Treatments for birds in temporary or permanent captivity include the antifungal agent amphotericin B (usually in combination with other drugs such as 5-fluorocystocine, itraconazole, fluconazole, or clotrimazole) and, in some cases, surgical removal of lesions (Redig 1998). Discussion of current diagnostic methods and treatment for aspergillosis in captive wild birds is provided by Redig (1998).

Aspergillus spp. are so widely distributed in the environment that eliminating exposure in free-living wild birds is not practical (Cork et al. 1999). Mortality events have been attributed to the availability of discarded moldy grain, rice, or corn in agricultural areas. Therefore, at the onset of an aspergillosis mortality event a thorough search of the surrounding geographic area used by the affected avian species may reveal a source of moldy feed that can be plowed under, buried, or covered. Often grains that are deemed unfit for human or domestic animal use are discarded in large piles that are easily accessible to birds. If sources of moldy grains or silage are found and cannot be removed, then covering the source or hazing birds away can remove or reduce the risk. Some waste grains, such as corn, may be left on the ground after harvest and become moldy after periods of rain or snow. If aspergillosis occurs in these areas, the risk can be lowered by plowing fields prior to winter use by birds.

The use of moldy feed (especially corn) in supplemental feeding programs is potentially dangerous. Any grains used for baiting or trapping wild birds should be stored under temperature and humidity conditions that are not conducive to mold growth. Wildlife managers and landowners can avoid contributing to aspergillosis by keeping bird feeders free of moldy grain and nest boxes free of damp and molding nesting materials. Food plots grown and left standing for use by wildlife can be inspected to detect excessive mold growth and, if present, the crops can be cut down or plowed under. If mold on food plots becomes an annual problem, then a change in the type of crop or crop management may be indicated.

Guidelines for prevention and control of aspergillosis in domestic poultry apply to captive wild birds (Chute and Richard 1997). If wild birds will be trapped and transported, protocols to minimize stress, provide adequate food and water, and prevent exposure to extremes of heat and moisture should be carefully followed. Boxes, cages, and pens used for transporting and holding birds should be cleaned and disinfected between uses. Natural plant bedding such as hay or corn cobs may be particularly hazardous to species that are prone to aspergillosis (Pokras 1996). Frequent cleaning of, and around, food and water utensils used in pens will help prevent fungal growth. Game-farm incubators need to be thoroughly cleaned between hatches to remove fungi. Eggs being incubated should be periodically candled and infertile eggs and dead embryos removed to reduce sites for fungus growth (O'Meara and Witter 1971; Olsen et al. 1990). Aspergillosis caused mortality for two consecutive years in captive eider ducklings raised in a greenhouse that was hotter and more humid than their natural northern habitats. On the third year, ducklings were raised outside on a pond and acute aspergillosis infection did not occur (Hubben 1958).

UNPUBLISHED DATA

1. Diagnostic Microbiology Laboratory Protocol Manual, U.S. Geological Survey, National Wildlife Health Center, Madison, Wisconsin, U.S.A.

LITERATURE CITED

Adrian, W.J., T.R. Spraker, and R.B. Davies. 1978. Epornitics of aspergillosis in mallards (*Anas platyrhynchos*) in north central Colorado. *Journal of Wildlife Diseases* 14:212–217.

Advisory Committee on Oil Pollution in the Sea. 1974. *Research unit on the rehabilitation of oiled seabirds. Fifth Annual Report.* Department of Zoology, University of Newcastle upon Tyne, 24 pp.

Ainsworth, G.C., and R.E. Rewell. 1949. The incidence of aspergillosis in captive wild birds. *Journal of Comparative Pathology and Theraputics* 59:213–224.

Al-Doory, Y. 1985. The mycology of the Aspergilli. In *Aspergillosis,* Al-Doory, Y., and G.E. Wagner (eds.). Charles C. Thomas, Springfield, MA, U.S.A., pp. 274.

Alley, M.R.I. Castro, and J.E.B. Hunter. 1999. Aspergillosis in hihi (*Notiomystis cincta*) on Mokoia Island. *New Zealand Veterinary Journal* 47:88–91.

Atasever, A. and K.S. Gumussoy. 2004. Pathological, clinical and mycological findings in experimental aspergillosis infections in starlings. *Journal of Veterinary Medicine* 51:19–22.

Atkinson, R., and C. Brojer. 1998. Unusual presentations of aspergillosis in wild birds. In *Proceedings of the Annual Conference of the Association of Avian Veterinarians 1998,* pp.177–181.

Austwick, P.K.C. 1968. Mycotic Infections. *Symposium of the Zoological Society of London* 24:249–271.

Bair, W.C., S.G. Simpson, and R.M. Windingstad. 1988. Acute aspergillosis in mallards at Oahe Seep near Pierre, South Dakota. *Prairie Naturalist* 20:153–156.

Bellrose, F.C. 1945. Aspergillosis in wood ducks. *Journal of Wildlife Management.* 9:325–326.

Bowes, V.A. 1990. An outbreak of aspergillosis in wild waterfowl. *Canadian Veterinary Journal* 31:303–304.

Brand, C.J., R.M. Windingstad, L.M. Siegfried, R.M. Duncan, and R.M. Cook. 1988. Avian mortality from botulism, aspergillosis, and Salmonellosis at Jamaica Bay Wildlife Refuge, New York, U.S.A. *Colonial Waterbirds* 11:284–292.

Brown, M.J., E. Linton, and E.C. Rees. 1992. Causes of mortality among wild swans in Britain. *Wildfowl* 43:70–79.

Brown. P.A., and P.T. Redig. 1994. *Aspergillus* ELISA: A tool for detection and management. In *Proceedings of the Annual Conference of the Association of Avian Veterinarians,* Reno, NV, U.S.A., pp. 295–300.

CABI Bioscience Databases. 2004. *Index of fungal hierarchy.* CABI Bioscience, Egham, United Kingdom. [Online.] Retrieved from the World Wide Web: www.cabi-bioscience.org.

Carrasco, L., M.J. Bautista, J.M. de las Mulas, and H.E. Jensen. 1993. Application of enzyme-immunohistochemistry for the diagnosis of aspergillosis, candidiasis and zygomycosis in three lovebirds. *Avian Diseases* 37:923–927.

Chute, H.L., and D.C. O'Meara. 1958. Experimental fungous infections in chickens. *Avian Diseases* 2:154–166.

Chute, H.L., and J.L. Richard. 1997. Fungal infections. In *Diseases of Poultry,* 10th Ed., B.W. Calnek, H.J. Barnes, C.W. Beard. L.R. McDougle, and Y.M. Saif (eds.). Iowa State University Press, Ames, IA, U.S.A., pp. 351–360.

Chute, H.L., S.L. Hollander, E.S. Barden, and D.C. O'Meara. 1965. The pathology of mycotoxicosis of certain fungi in chickens. *Avian Diseases* 9:57–66.

Clark, G.M. 1960. Aspergillosis in naturally infected cowbirds and grackles. *Avian Diseases* 4:94–96.

Clark, F.D., A.D. Chinnah, and S.A. Garner. 1987. Aspergillosis in a great horned owl (*Bubo virginianus*). *Companion Animal Practice* 1:56.

Coleman R.M., and L. Kaufman. 1972. Use of the immunodiffusion test in the serodiagnosis of aspergillosis. *Applied Microbiology* 23:301–308

Coon, N.C., and L.N. Locke. 1968. Aspergillosis in a bald eagle (*Haliaeetus leucocephalus*). *Bulletin of the Wildlife Disease Association* 4:51.

Cooper, J. 1973. Post-mortem findings in East African birds of prey. *Journal of Wildlife Diseases* 9:368–375.

Cork, S.C., M.R. Alley, A.C. Johnstone, and P.H.G. Stockdale. 1999. Aspergillosis and other causes of mortality in the stitchbird in New Zealand. *Journal of Wildlife Diseases* 35:481–486.

Cowan, I. McT. 1945. Aspergillosis in a Thayer gull. *Murrelet* 24:29.

Dane, D.S. 1948. A disease of manx shearwaters (Puffinus puffinus). *Journal of Animal Ecology* 17:158–164.

Davidson, W.R., V.F. Nettles, C.E. Couvillion, and E.W. Howerth. 1985. Diseases diagnosed in wild turkeys (*Meleagris gallopavo*) of the southeastern United States. *Journal of Wildlife Diseases* 21:386–390.

Davis, W.A., and L.S. McClung.1940.Aspergillosis in wild herring gulls. *Journal of Bacteriology* 40:321–323.

Daoust, P-Y., G. Conboy, S. McBurney, and N. Burgess. 1998. Interactive mortality factors in common loons from maritime Canada. *Journal of Wildlife Diseases.* 34:524–531.

Debeaupuis, J.P, J. Sarfati, V. Chazalet and J.P. Latgé. 1997. Genetic diversity among clinical and environmental isolates of *Aspergillus fumigatus. Infection and Immunity* 65:3080–3085

Falandysz, J., and P. Szefer. 1983. Metals and organochlorines in a specimen of white-tailed eagle. *Environmental Conservation* 10:256–258.

Fix, A.S., C. Waterhouse, E.C. Greiner, and M.K. Stoskopf. 1988. *Plasmodium relictum* as a cause of avian malaria in wild-caught Magellanic penguins (*Spheniscus magellanicus*). *Journal of Wildlife Diseases* 24:610–619.

Forrester, D.J., W.R. Davidson, R.E. Lange Jr., R.K. Stroud, L.L. Alexander, J.C. Franson, S.D. Haseltine, R.C. Littell, and S.A. Nesbitt.1997. Winter mortality of common loons in Florida coastal waters. *Journal of Wildlife Diseases* 33:833–847.

Franson, J.C., N.J. Thomas, M.R. Smith, A.H. Robbins, S. Newman, and P.C. McCartin. 1996. A retrospective study of postmortem findings in red-tailed hawks. *Journal of Raptor Research* 30:7–14.

Friend, M. 1999. Aspergillosis. In *Field Manual of Wildlife Diseases,* M. Friend, and J.C. Franson (eds.), U.S. Geological Survey, *Biological Resources Division Information and Technology Report* 1999–001. pp. 129–133.

Friend, M., and D.O. Trainer. 1969. Aspergillosis in captive herring gulls. *Bulletin of the Wildlife Disease Association* 5:271–275.

Graczyk, T.K., and M.R. Cranfield. 1995. Maternal transfer of anti-*Aspergillus* spp. immunoglobulins in African black-footed penguins (*Spheniscus demersus*). *Journal of Wildlife Diseases* 31:545–549.

———1996. A model for the prediction of relative titres of avian malaria and *Aspergillus* spp. IgG in jackass penguin (*Spheniscus demersus*) females based on maternal IgG in egg-yolk. *International Journal for Parasitology* 26:749–754.

Gross, A.O. 1925. Diseases of the ruffed grouse. *Science* LXII:55–57.

Gullion, G.W. 1952. Some diseases and parasites of American coots. *California Fish and game* 38:421–423.

———1957. Gambel quail disease and parasite investigation in Nevada. *American Midland Naturalist* 40:414.

Gumussoy, K.S., F. Uyanik, A. Atasever, and Y. Cam. 2004. Experimental *Aspergillus fumigatus* infection in quails and results of treatment with itraconazole. *Journal of Veterinary Medicine* 51:34–38.

Hasegawa, I., S. Shoya, and T. Horiuchi. 1971. Brain lesions in chicken aspergillosis. National Institute of Animal Health Quarterly (Tokyo) 11:122–123.

Herman, C.M. 1943. An outbreak of mycotic pneumonia in mallards. *California Fish and Game* 29:204.

Herman, C.M., and G. Bolander. 1943. Fungus disease in a glaucous-winged gull. *Condor* 45:160–161.

Hillgarth, N., and J. Kear. 1979. Diseases of sea ducks in captivity. *Wildfowl Trust* 30:135–141.

Honess, R.F. and K.B. Winter. 1956. Diseases of wildlife in Wyoming. *Wyoming Game and Fish Commission Bulletin* 9:34–35.

Hopkins, B.A., J.K. Skeeles, G.E. Houghten, D. Stagle, and K. Gardner. 1990. A survey of infectious diseases in wild turkeys (*Meleagris gallopavo silvestris*) from Arkansas. *Journal of Wildlife Diseases* 26:468–472.

Hubben, K. 1958. *Aspergillus* meningoencephalitis in turkeys and ducks. *Avian Diseases* 2:110–116.

Hülphers, G., K. Lilleengen, and T. Henricson. 1941. Aspergillosis in hares, ducks, capercaillie, and blackcock. *Svensk Jaaroverz* 6:250.

Jacobson, E.R., B.L. Raphael, H.T. Nguyen, E.C. Greiner, and T. Gross. 1980. Avian pox infection, aspergillosis and renal trematodiasis in a royal tern. *Journal of Wildlife Diseases* 16:627–631.

Jauniaux, T., and F. Coignoul. 1994. Aspergillose chez les oiseaux marins echoues sur la cote belge. *Annules de Medecine Veterinaire* 138:277–281.

Katz, M.E., S.C.J. Love, H.S. Gill, and B.F. Cheetham. 1996. Development of a method for the identification, using the polymerase chain reaction, of *Aspergillus fumigatus* isolated from ostriches. *Australian Veterinary Journal* 74:50–54.

Kocan, R.M., and M.C. Perry. 1976. Infection and mortality in captive wild-trapped canvasback ducks. *Journal of Wildlife Diseases* 12:30–33.

Kunkle, R.A., and J.L. Richard. 1998. Mycoses and mycotoxicoses. In *A Laboratory Manual for the Isolation and Identification of Avian Pathogens,* 4th Ed., D.E. Swayne, J.R. Glisson, M.W. Jackwood, J.E. Pearson, and W. M. Reed (eds.). American Association of Avian Pathologists, University of Pennsylvania, Kennett Square, PA, U.S.A., 311 pp.

Latgé, J.P. 2001. The pathobiology of *Aspergillus fumigatus. Trends in Microbiology* 9:362–389.

Leotta, G.A., J.A. Pare, L. Sigler, D. Montalti, G. Vigo, M. Petruccelli, and E.H. Reinoso. 2002. *Thelebolus microsporus* mycelial mats in the trachea of wild brown skua *(Catharacta antarctica lonnbergi)* and south polar skua (*C. maccormicki*) carcasses. 2002. *Journal of Wildlife Diseases* 28:443–447.

Locke, L.N. 1965. Additional records of aspergillosis among passerine birds in Maryland and the Washington, D.C. metropolitan area. *Chesapeake Science* 6:120.

Locke, L.N., G.E. Bagley, D.N. Frickie, and L.T. Young. 1969. Lead poisoning and aspergillosis in an Andean condor. *Journal of the American Veterinary Medical Association* 155:1052–1056.

Machin, K. 1993. Aspergillosis outbreak in Stellar's jays (*Cyanocitta stelleri*) from central Vancouver Island. *Canadian Veterinary Journal* 34:247–248.

Manwell, R.D. 1954. A case of aspergillosis in a song sparrow. *Journal of Parasitology* 40:231.

Martinez-Quesada, J, A. Nieto-Cadenazzi, and J.M. Torres-Rodriguez. 1993. Humoral immunoresponse of pigeons to *Aspergillus fumigatus* antigens. *Mycopathologia* 124:131–137.

McDiarmid A. 1955. Aspergillosis in free living wild birds. *Journal of Comparative Pathology and Therapeutics* 65:246–249.

McDougle, H.C., and R.W. Vaught. 1968. An epizootic of aspergillosis in Canada geese. *Journal of Wildlife Management* 32:415–417.

Meade, G.M., and D. Stoner. 1942. Aspergillosis in a snowy owl. *The Auk* 50:577–578.

Mikaelian, I., F. Gauthier, G. Fitzgerald, R. Higgins, R. Claveau, and D. Martineau. 1997. Causes primaires de deces des oiseaux de la faune au Quebec. *Le Medecin Veterinaire du Quebec* 27:94–102.

Monga, D.P. 1972. Prevalence of pathogenic fungi in wild birds. *Indian Journal of Medical Research* 60:517–519.

Neff, J.A. 1955. Outbreak of aspergillosis in mallards. *Journal of Wildlife Management* 19:415–416.

Obendorf, D.L., and K. McColl. 1980. Mortality in little penguins (*Eudyptula minor*) along the coast of Victoria, Australia. *Journal of Wildlife Diseases* 16: 251–259.

Olsen, G.H., J.M. Nicolich, and D.J. Hoffman. 1990. A review of some causes of death in avian embryos. In *Proceedings of the Association of Avian Veterinarians,* Phoenix, AZ, U.S.A., pp. 106–111.

Olson, L.D. 1969. Aspergillosis in Japanese quail. *Avian Diseases* 13:225–227.

O'Meara D.C., and H.L. Chute. 1959. Aspergillosis experimentally produced in hatching chicks. *Avian Diseases* 3:404–406.

O'Meara D.C., and J.F. Witter. 1971. Aspergillosis. In *Infectious and Parasitic Diseases of Wild Birds,* Davis, J.N., R.C. Anderson, L. Karstad, and D.O. Trainer, (eds.). Iowa State University Press, Ames, IA, U.S.A., pp. 153–162.

Onofri, S., M. Fenice, A.R. Cicalini, S. Tosi, A. Magrino, S. Pagano, L. Selbmann, L. Zucconi, H.S. Vishniac, R. Ocampo-Friedmann, and E.I. Friedman. 2000. Ecology and biology of microfungi from Antartica rocks and soils. 2000. *Italian Journal of Zoology* 67:163–167.

Pennycott, T.W. 1999. Causes of mortality in mute swans (*Cygnus olor*) in Scotland 1995–1996. *Wildfowl* 50: 11–20.

Pokras, M.A.1996. Biomedicine of seabirds. In *Diseases of Cage and Aviary Birds,* 3rd Ed., Rosskopf, W., and R. Woerpel (eds.). Williams and Wilkins, Baltimore, MD, U.S.A., pp. 981–1001.

Quortrup, E.R., and J.E. Shillinger. 1941. 3,000 Wild bird autopsies on western lake areas. *Journal of the American Veterinary Medical Association* 99:382–387.

Raper, K.B., and D.I. Fennell. 1965. *The Genus Aspergillus.* The Williams and Wilkins Company, Baltimore, MD, U.S.A., pp. 686.

Reavill, D. 1996. Fungal diseases. In *Diseases of Cage and Aviary birds,* 3rd Ed., Rosskopf, W., and R. Woerpel (eds.). Williams and Wilkins, Baltimore, MD, U.S.A., pp. 989–591.

Redig, P.T., M.R. Fuller, and D.L. Evans. 1980. Prevalence of *Aspergillus fumigatus* in free-living goshawks (*Accipiter gentilis atricapillus*). *Journal of Wildlife Diseases* 16:169–174.

Redig, P.T.: 1998. Aspergillosis in avians, an update. In *Proceedings of the 19th Annual Conference on Avian Medicine and Surgery,* Mid-Atlantic States Association of Avian Veterinarians, Lancaster, PA, U.S.A., pp. 172–177.

Richard, J.L., and J.R. Thurston. 1983. Rapid hematogenous dissemination of *Aspergillus fumigatus* and *A. flavus* spores in turkey poults following aerosol exposure. *Avian Diseases* 27:1025–1033.

Rosen, M.N. 1964. Aspergillosis in wild and domestic fowl. *Avian Diseases* 8:1–6.

Ruchel, R., and U. Reichard. 1999. Pathogenesis and clinical representation of aspergillosis. In *Aspergillus fumigatus, Biology, Clinical Aspects and Molecular Approaches to Pathogenicity,* A.A.A. Brakhage, J.B. Schmidt, and A. Jahn (eds.). Karger, New York, NY, U.S.A., pp. 21–43.

Schneemann and Schaffner. 1999. Host defense mechanism in *Aspergillus fumigatus* infections. *In Aspergillus fumigatus, Biology, Clinical Aspects and Molecular Approaches to Pathogenicity,* A.A.A. Brakhage, J.B. Schmidt, and A. Jahn (eds.). Karger, New York, NY, U.S.A., pp. 57–68.

Smeenk, J. 1972. Aspergillose bij zilvermeeuwen (Larus argentatus) in Drenthe. *Netherlands Journal of Veterinary Science* 97:408–411.

Souza, M.J., and L.A. Degernes. 2005. Mortality due to aspergillosis in wild swans in northeast Washington state, 2000–2002. *Journal of Avian Medicine and Surgery* 19:98–106.

Stone, W.B., and J.C. Okoniewski. 2001. Necropsy findings and environmental contaminants in common loons from New York. *Journal of Wildlife Diseases* 37:178–184.

Stroud, R.K., and R.M. Duncan. 1982. Occlusion of the syrinx as a manifestation of aspergillosis in Canada geese. *Journal of the American Veterinary Medical Association* 181:1389–1390.

Tham, V.L., D.A. Purcell, and D.J. Schultz. 1974. Fungal nephritis in a grey-headed albatross. *Journal of Wildlife Diseases* 10:306–309.

Thom, C., and K.B. Raper. 1945. *A Manual of the Aspergilli.* Williams and Wilkins, Baltimore, MD, U.S.A., pp. 373.

Ulloa, J., V. Cubillos, M.I. Montecinos, and A. Alberdi. 1987. Aspergilosis en ganso silvestre (*Chloephaga poliocephala Scl.,* 1857) en Chile. *Journal of Veterinary Medicine* 34:30–35.

Wobeser, G. 1997. Aspergillosis. In *Diseases of Wild Waterfowl,* 2nd Ed. Plenum Press, New York, NY, U.S.A., pp. 95–101.

Wobeser, G., and J.R. Saunders. 1975. Pulmonary oxalosis in association with *Aspergillus niger* infection in a Great Horned owl (*Bubo virginianus*). *Avian Diseases* 19:388–92.

Work, T.M., and J. Hale. 1996. Causes of owl mortality in Hawaii, 1992–1994. *Journal of Wildlife Diseases* 32:266–273.

Young, E.A., T.E. Cornish, and S.E. Little. 1998. Concomitant mycotic and verminous pneumonia in a blue jay from Georgia. *Journal of Wildlife Diseases* 34:625–628.

Zinkl, J.G., J. M. Hyland, and J.J. Hurt. 1977. Aspergillosis in common crows in Nebraska, 1974. *Journal of Wildlife Diseases* 13:191–193.

Section 3: Biotoxins

21
Avian Botulism

Tonie E. Rocke and Trent K. Bollinger

INTRODUCTION

On a worldwide basis, avian botulism is the most significant disease of migratory birds, especially waterfowl and shorebirds. More than a million deaths from type C avian botulism have been reported in localized outbreaks in some wetlands in North America and elsewhere in a single year. Outbreaks with losses of 50,000 birds or more are relatively common. However, botulism losses vary a great deal from year to year and from species to species. Only a few hundred birds may die in a wetland one year, whereas tens of thousands or more may die the following year at the same location. The epizootiology of botulism in birds is very complex and also quite diverse, depending on the type of bacteria present, local environmental factors, and the primary species of birds involved.

Botulism in both animals and humans is caused by neurotoxins that are produced by a heterogeneous group of bacteria known as *Clostridium botulinum*. The disease is typically a "food poisoning" resulting from ingestion of toxin-laden food items, but it can also be caused by "toxico-infections," when botulinum toxin-producing bacteria colonize the intestinal tract of an individual or secondarily infect a wound. At least seven different neurotoxins are produced by strains of *C. botulinum*. These have been designated types A, B, C_1, D, E, F, and G (Smith and Sugiyama 1988). Most botulism outbreaks in birds are caused by type C_1 toxin, but sporadic die-offs among fish-eating birds, such as Common Loons (*Gavia immer*) and gulls (*Larus* spp.), have been caused by type E toxin. Type A toxin occasionally causes botulism in domestic chickens (Dohms 1987). Types B, D, F, and G toxin are not known to be causes of avian botulism in North America, but type D has been reported to have killed Pink-backed Pelicans (*Pelicanus rufescens*) in Senegal (Doutre 1979). Human botulism is rare but is typically caused by types A, B, or E toxin.

SYNONYMS

Limberneck, western duck sickness, duck disease, alkali poisoning.

HISTORY

Type C Botulism

Large outbreaks of a "duck sickness" later thought to be type C avian botulism have occurred in the western United States and Canada since the beginning of the twentieth century and possibly even as early as 1890 in California (Hobmaier 1932). Biologists first took notice of a "mysterious malady" causing disastrous losses among waterfowl in western states in the period between 1909–1913 (Kalmbach 1968). Heavy losses of waterfowl, estimated in the millions, occurred in three widely separated regions of North America: on the river deltas of the Great Salt Lake in Utah; on lakes in the southern part of the San Joaquin Valley in California; and in the Elfros region of Saskatchewan, 180 miles north of the U.S. border. Over the next several decades, similar outbreaks of what became known as "western duck sickness" were reported in the U.S. in Montana, southeastern Oregon, Nevada, and the Dakotas (Table 21.1). In Canada, outbreaks were reported at Lake Johnstone in Saskatchewan, Lake Newell in Alberta, and Whitewater Lake in Manitoba (Kalmbach 1968). Outside North America, Wetmore reported a waterfowl disease in Uruguay in 1921 that was similar to duck sickness in the U.S. (Kalmbach 1968).

Early attempts (1911–1918) to determine the cause of "duck sickness" resulted in several theories that later were not substantiated, including intestinal coccidiosis, alkaline poisoning (Wetmore 1915), and salt toxicity (Wetmore 1918). At that time, type C botulism was unknown; only types A and B botulism had been described, and neither was considered a threat to wild birds. Finally, in 1923, Dr. Ida A. Bengston isolated a toxin-producing anaerobe from fly larvae (Bengston 1923) and identified the organism as *C. botulinum* type C. This bacterium was quickly associated with limberneck in poultry (Graham and Boughton 1923), but it was seven years later, in 1930, before its connection with duck sickness was established by Kalmbach (1930) and Giltner and Couch (1930), when

Table 21.1. Major type C botulism outbreaks in waterfowl.

Location	Year	Estimated Loss
Utah and California, U.S.A.	1910	"Millions"
Lake Malheur, Oregon, U.S.A.	1925	100,000
Great Salt Lake, Utah, U.S.A.	1929	100,000–300,000
Tulare Basin, California, U.S.A.	1941	250,000
Tule Lake, California, U.S.A.	1948	65,000–150,000
California, U.S.A.	1969	140,000
Montana, U.S.A.	1979	100,000
Great Salt Lake, Utah, U.S.A.	1980	110,000
Caspian Sea, USSR	1982	600,000–1 million
Alberta, Canada	1995	100,000
Manitoba, Canada	1996	117,000
Saskatchewan, Canada	1997	1 million
Great Salt Lake, Utah, U.S.A.	1997	514,000

inadequately refrigerated liver tissue reproduced the disease upon feeding to gulls. Hobmaier (1930) first demonstrated the presence of type C botulinum toxin in the bloodstream of sick wild birds. Shortly afterward, the presence of the bacteria, as well as toxin, was demonstrated in a variety of invertebrates that birds prey upon in shallow water or on mud flats (Kalmbach 1932). Type C botulism was soon confirmed to be the cause of waterfowl disease in lakes in Alberta, Canada (Shaw and Simpson 1936) and similar die-offs of waterbirds in Australia (Pullar 1934; Rose 1935).

After the disease was correctly identified, outbreaks of type C botulism were detected and confirmed on numerous wetlands in the U.S. and Canada, with some locations experiencing outbreaks nearly every year, for example, marshes around the Great Salt Lake in Utah, the Tulare Basin in central California, Klamath Falls in northern California, and Whitewater Lake, Manitoba. In 1941, an estimated 250,000 birds died from botulism in the Tulare Basin (McLean 1946), and in 1952, 4–5 million mortalities from botulism were estimated in western states (Rosen 1971), although independent confirmation of this figure could not be found in the literature.

During the 1930s and '40s, investigators attempted to determine the environmental substrate for toxin production and the source of botulinum toxin for waterbirds (Kalmbach and Gunderson 1934; Quortrup and Holt 1941). Bell et al. (1955) assembled the available data and formulated two alternative theories to explain the occurrence of botulism outbreaks. The first, called the "sludge-bed hypothesis," suggested that large quantities of decaying organic matter leads to a depletion of oxygen, which allows germination of botulinum spores and toxin production; temperature, pH, and dissolved salts in the water were considered important corollary factors. The second hypothesis, which Bell et al. favored, proposed that *C. botulinum* type C germinates and produces toxin in small, discrete, particulate substances (invertebrate carcasses) that are independent of the ambient environment. Environmental conditions that kill invertebrates, such as anoxic conditions and the flooding of mud flats or drainage of wetlands during warm summer months, were thought to precipitate outbreaks (Hunter 1970). For many years this concept prevailed over other hypotheses and became the paradigm used to explain the occurrence of botulism in waterbirds.

Meanwhile, the first outbreaks of type C botulism in wild birds outside North America were recorded (Figure 21.1) in Russia in 1957 (Kuznetzov 1992) and in Europe in 1963 (Jensen and Price 1987), first in Sweden and shortly after in Denmark (1965), Great Britain (1969), and the Netherlands (1970). During this period, the disease was also first recognized in South Africa (1965), New Zealand (1971) and Japan (1973) and later in Argentina (1979) and Brazil (1981), although none of the outbreaks described were as large as those reported in North America at the same time.

For the next several decades, research on botulism focused on the agent itself and its mechanism of action. In the early 1970s, Eklund and others (1987) conducted laboratory experiments that suggested that the gene for type C_1 neurotoxin was carried by a bacteriophage; this was later confirmed by DNA hybridization analysis (Fuji et al. 1988). Molecular studies conducted from 1990–1993 revealed the complete DNA sequences of the botulinum neurotoxins (Minton 1995), and by 1993 the enzymatic action of each toxin and its specific substrates in nerve cells were determined (Schiavo et al.

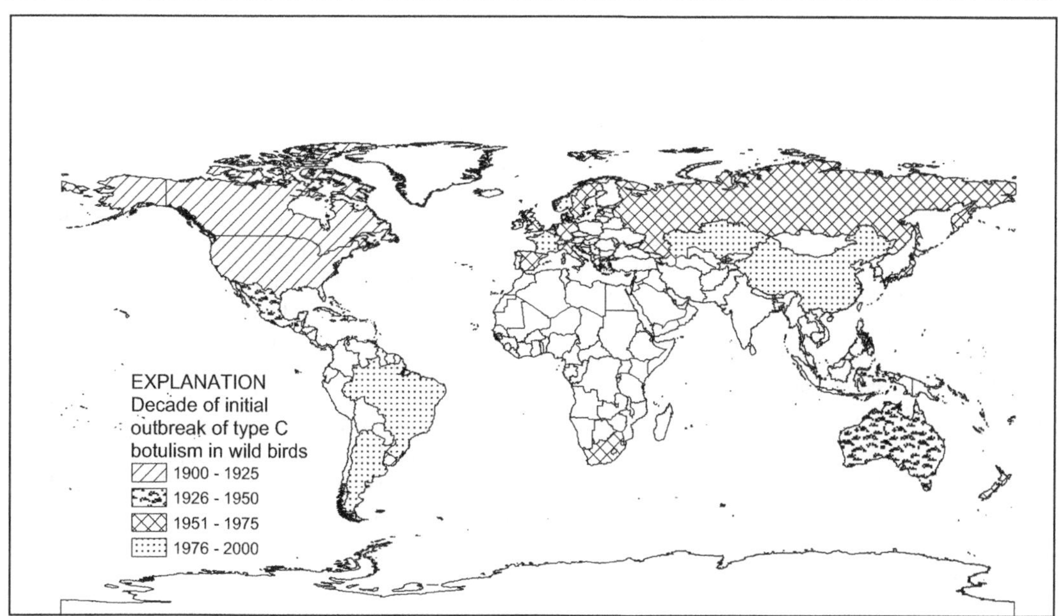

Figure 21.1. Countries with confirmed type C botulism outbreaks in wild waterbirds and the decade the first outbreak occurred.

1992a; Blasi et al. 1993). Understanding how the toxin is produced and how it causes disease in animals has furthered our basic knowledge regarding botulism and also led to the application of new technologies in the study of the disease. The importance of botulism in wild waterfowl has not abated, as the 1980s and '90s brought some of the worst recorded die-offs, with losses of nearly 1 million birds in Russia in 1982 and 1.5 million or more birds in North America in 1997.

Type E Botulism

Botulism in humans associated with the consumption of fish, likely caused by *C. botulinum* type E, has been reported in the Russian literature since 1818 (Hobbs 1976). Gunnison et al. (1935) were the first to propose that an isolate of *C. botulinum* from fish be designated as type E, recognizing that it was different from the types A, B, C, and D strains previously isolated. The disease continues to be a small but important cause of botulism in humans eating fish or marine mammals that were improperly cooked or processed.

Type E botulism in birds has a more recent history, with the first reported die-off occurring in late 1963 on the shores of Lake Michigan's Lower Peninsula, U.S.A. Another outbreak was reported along the north shore of Lake Michigan in 1964. At least 12,600 birds were estimated to have died over the two years, primarily Common Loons and gulls (Fay et al. 1965). In 1965, bird mortalities were reported again in northern Lake Michigan and also from the southeast shores of Lake Superior and the shores of Saginaw Bay in Lake Huron (Graikoski et al. 1968; Fay 1966). Dead fish and gulls were observed in Saginaw Bay from June to early fall, with peak gull mortality occurring in July. Type E toxin was demonstrated in cultured tissues from dead fish and gulls, and type E toxin was demonstrated in the blood of dying waterfowl in one case. Type E botulism die-offs continued to be reported on Lake Michigan every few years thereafter through 1983. Mortality tended to occur in October and November, frequently involving hundreds of birds. Gulls, loons, grebes, mergansers, and other fish-eating birds were primarily involved (Brand et al. 1983, 1988a).

Beginning in 1998 and annually through 2001, type E botulism was again confirmed as a cause of die-offs in the Great Lakes involving hundreds to thousands of fish-eating birds in southern Lake Huron and western Lake Erie (NWHC, CCWHC, unpublished data)[1,2]. Mortality occurred primarily in late fall, but type E botulism was confirmed as early as late July in some years. Common Loons, Ring-billed Gulls (*Larus delawarensis*), Herring Gulls (*L. argentatus*), and Bonaparte's Gulls (*L. philadelphia*), diving ducks, Horned Grebes (*Podiceps auritus*), Red-throated Loons (*Gavia stellata*), and mergansers all have been involved. In one location, 90% of the affected birds were

Red-breasted Mergansers (*Mergus serrator*). Small, undetected avian mortalities due to type E botulism likely occur annually. Type E botulism potentially can occur in birds wherever the bacterium has been identified in fish or in the environment, but few cases have been reported outside the Great Lakes.

The only other site where significant bird mortality from type E botulism has been documented is the Canche Estuary, Pas-de-Calais, France (Gourreau et al. 1998). In February 1996, 5,000 to 10,000 birds, mainly Black-headed Gulls (*L. ridibundus*) and Herring Gulls, died in the estuary, and diagnostic testing confirmed type E botulism as the cause of death. In November of that same year, the disease recurred, killing 4,000 to 6,000 individuals of the same species. Contaminated fish waste in a nearby dump where the birds were known to feed was the suspected source of toxin.

DISTRIBUTION

Type C Botulism

Type C botulism outbreaks have been reported in wild birds from every continent, except the Antarctic (Figure 21.1), and from at least 28 countries or territories (Jensen and Price 1987 for references, except where noted): Argentina (Polero et al. 1980), Australia, Brazil (Schonhofen and Ferreira 1981), Canada, China (Li 1990), Czechoslovakia, Denmark, England, France (Jubilo and LaMarque 1998), Germany, Hungary (Mikuska et al. 1986), Israel (Gophen et al. 1991), Italy, Japan, Mexico, The Netherlands, New Zealand, Norway (Skulberg and Holt 1987), Russia (Kuznetzov 1992), Scotland, South Africa, Spain, Sweden, the U.S.A., Uruguay, Yugoslavia (Mikuska et al. 1986), Venezuela (Leon et al. 1989), and the Virgin Islands (Norton 1986). Most of the largest die-offs (losses of 100,000 birds or more) have occurred in North America (Table 21.1), with the exception of an outbreak reported on the Caspian Sea in Russia in 1982, where an estimated 600,000 to 1 million birds died (Kuznetzov 1992). Both type C and E botulism outbreaks also occur with greatest frequency in the U.S. and Canada compared to other countries, with confirmed die-offs of type C botulism reported every year. In the United States, most type C botulism outbreaks occur west of the Mississippi River; however, their distribution appears to have expanded greatly since 1934, with outbreaks now reported in nearly every state (Figure 21.2).

In Canada, large outbreaks occur almost exclusively in the prairie regions of Alberta, Saskatchewan, and Manitoba (Figure 21.2). More recently, outbreaks have been detected in parkland and boreal regions of central and northwestern Alberta, although anecdotal reports exist of die-offs in this region prior to this time (CCWHC, unpublished data).[2] The highest reported losses on the Canadian prairies occurred in the middle to late 1990s.

Type E Botulism

Type E botulism outbreaks in birds are much less frequent than type C outbreaks and, within North America, have been confined to the Great Lakes Region, with the exception of a few isolated cases from Alaska and the Salton Sea in California. The location of the more recent type E outbreaks on the Great Lakes is different than those reported in the 1960s and 1980s (Figure 21.3) (Fay et al. 1965; Fay 1966; Brand et al. 1983; Brand et al. 1988a; Ian Barker, pers. comm.).[3] Outside North America, outbreaks of type E botulism have, to our knowledge, been reported only in the Canche Estuary area of France, although small isolated cases may have occurred elsewhere.

HOST RANGE

All birds are probably susceptible to botulinum toxin, with the exception of vultures and other scavenging birds, which may be resistant to the disease. In 1934, Kalmbach and Gunderson (1934) reported 74 species of birds believed to have been afflicted with type C botulism. Rosen (1971) added three more species to this list, and in 1987, Jensen and Price (1987) added another 117 species not recorded by the previous authors. A review of the literature since 1987 and more than 2,000 diagnostic records with confirmed diagnoses of type C botulism (NWHC, unpublished data),[1] revealed many additional species not previously recorded (Table 21.2), bringing the total thought to have died from type C botulism to at least 263 avian species in 39 families. However, the frequency of occurrence of the disease varies considerably among species, as does the epizootiology. Noticeably absent from this list are certain scavengers, such as crows, ravens, and vultures. It is possible that these species die in upland habitats not typically searched during botulism outbreaks, although available evidence suggests they may have some innate resistance (Ohishi et al. 1979). Scavenging raptors, such as harriers and bald eagles, have been found dead in association with botulism outbreaks (NWHC, CCWHC, unpublished data).[1,2] For type E botulism, the number of species thought to have been afflicted is much smaller: 31 species in 10 families of birds (Table 21.3).

Foraging behavior appears to be the most significant risk factor for botulism. Filter feeding and dabbling waterfowl, such as Mallards (*Anas platyrhynchos*), teal, and shovelers, are among the species at greatest risk for contracting type C botulism, as well as probing shorebirds, such as avocets and stilts (Rocke and Friend

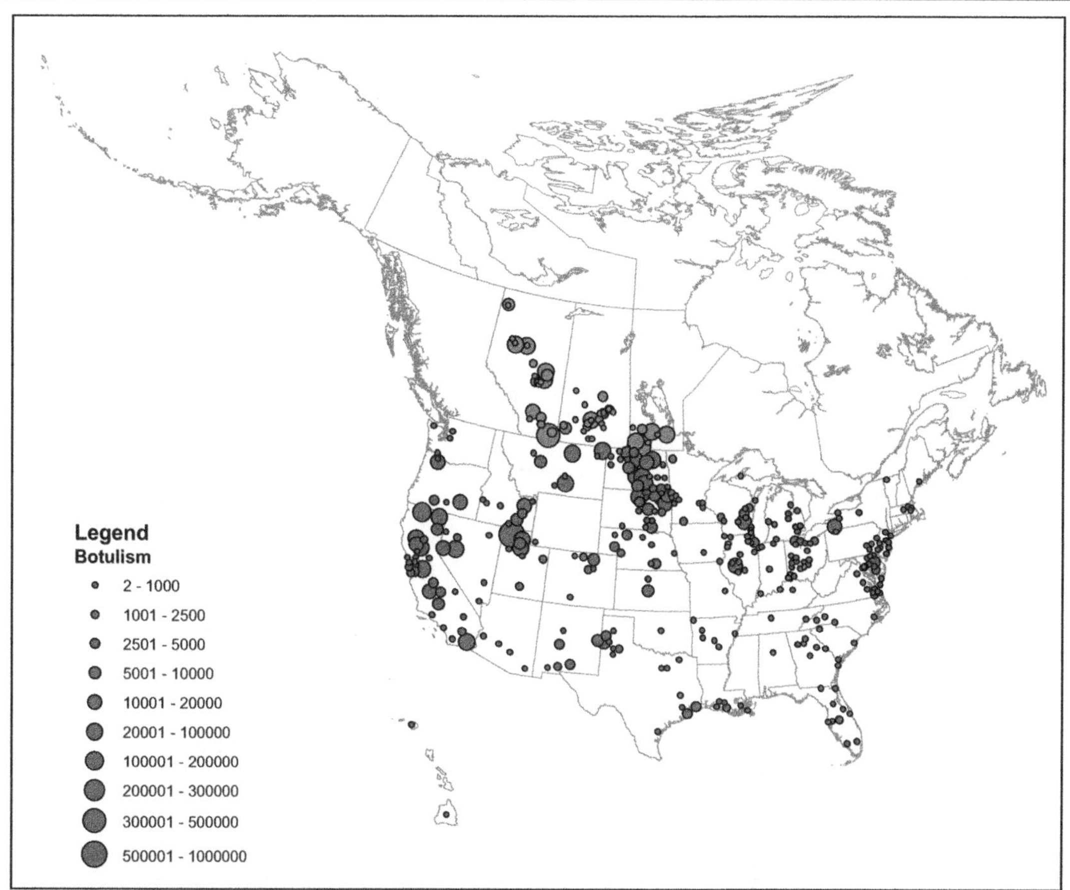

Figure 21.2. Location and cumulative magnitude of type C botulism outbreaks in North America.

1999). Shorebird species that feed near the surface of wetland soils and sediments, such as small *Calidris spp.* sandpipers, appear to be at greater risk of contracting botulism than shorebirds that probe deeply into the substrate for food (Adams et al. 2003). Diving ducks may also die in large numbers. In 1998, at Utikima Lake, Alberta, Canada, diving ducks comprised approximately 50% of the species collected and an estimated 100,000–250,000 Buffleheads (*Bucephela albeola*) died (CCWHC, unpublished data).[2] Fish-eating birds, such as Common Loons and gulls, are at greatest risk for contracting type E botulism in the Great Lakes, although fish-eating birds at the Salton Sea, a large inland water body in southern California, are more likely to die from type C botulism (NWHC, unpublished data).[1] Mortality of wild raptors from botulism in North America has been associated with improper disposal of poultry carcasses (NWHC, unpublished data),[1] and in England and elsewhere, botulism in gulls has been associated with landfills (Ortiz and Smith 1994).

Threatened or endangered bird species in the U.S. that have contracted botulism and are at risk for further exposure include the Bald Eagle *(Haliaeetus leucocephalus),* California Condor (*Gymnogyps californianus*), Hawaiian Coot (*Fulica alai*), Hawaiian Duck (*Anas wyvilliana*), Hawaiian Goose (*Branta sandvicensis*), Hawaiian Stilt (*Himantopus knudseni*) and the Brown Pelican (*Pelicanus occidentalis*) (NWHC, unpublished data).[1]

ETIOLOGY

The organisms that comprise the group of bacteria known as *C. botulinum* are Gram-positive rods, with oval subterminal spores. In culture, the cells vary considerably in size, from 2 to 22 µm in length and 0.5 to 2 µm in width (Cato et al. 1986), depending on the growth medium and other factors. The vegetative bacteria are motile by means of peritrichous flagella and may occur individually or in short chains. The seven serotypes of *C. botulinum* (A, B, C_1, D, E, F,

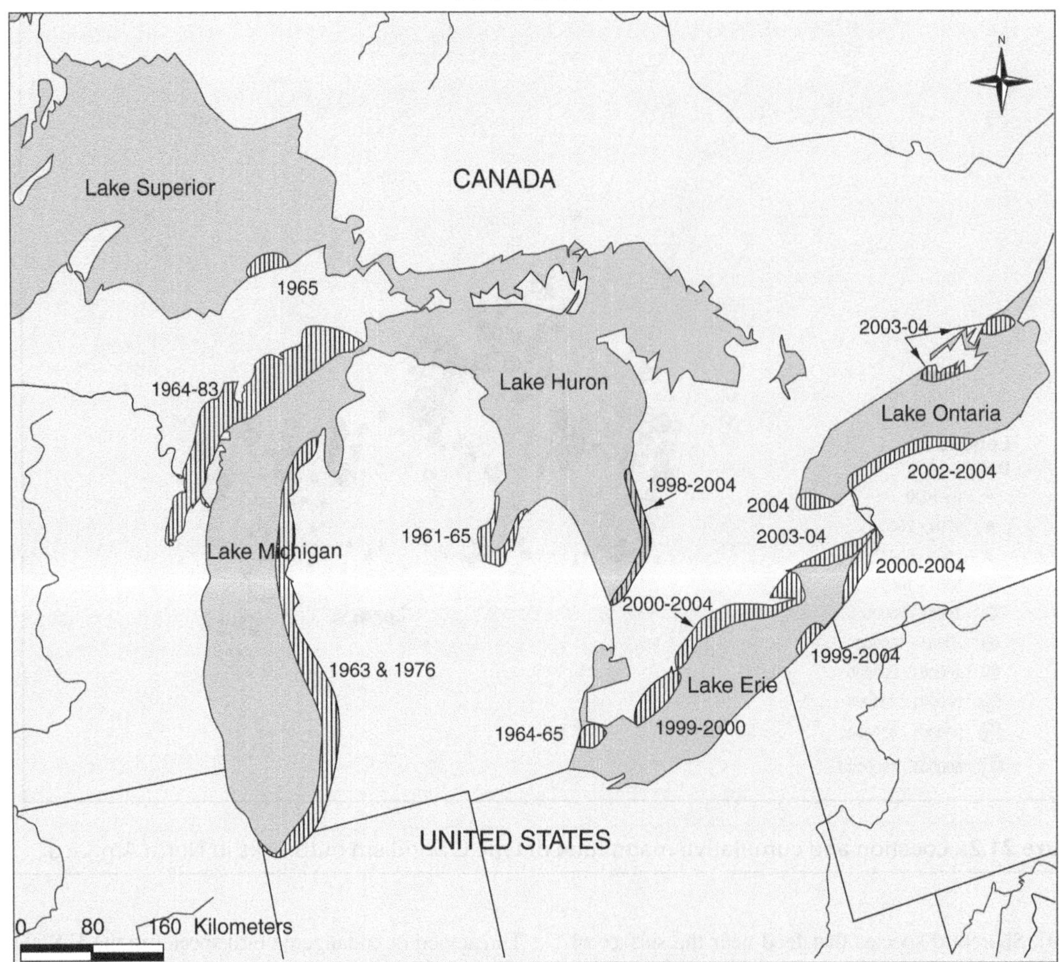

Figure 21.3. Change in distribution of type E botulism outbreaks (vertically banded areas) in birds in the Great Lakes region of North America. Outbreaks moved from Lake Michigan in the 1960s and 1980s to the eastern Great Lakes in the late 1990s and early 2000s.

and G) cannot be distinguished based on morphological characteristics; however, the neurotoxins they produce are serologically distinct. Bergey's Manual of Systematic Bacteriology (Cato et al. 1986) categorizes *C. botulinum* strains into four groups (I–IV), based on their cultural and physiological characteristics (Table 21.4) and later confirmed by DNA comparison (Lee and Riemann 1970) and phylogenetic analysis of 16S RNA sequences (Lawson et al. 1993).

Vegetative growth and toxin production of *C. botulinum* is affected by many factors including temperature (Smith and Turner 1987), pH, oxygen tension/redox potential (Smith and Pierson 1979), water vapor pressure (Emodi and Lechowich 1969), and the presence of a suitable growth medium containing appropriate amino acids (Leyer and Johnson 1990). The rate of growth under various environmental conditions is also dependent on the strain of bacteria (Segner et al. 1971; Leyer and Johnson 1990; Emodi and Lechowich 1969). Most type C and E strains are nonproteolytic or weakly proteolytic and do not digest complex protein substrates such as cooked meat, coagulated egg-white, coagulated serum, or iron and milk, as do strains of other toxin types. Glucose or another carbohydrate is required for an energy source. Ammonia can be used as a nitrogen source, although growth is markedly enhanced by organic nitrogenous compounds (Whitmer and Johnson 1988).

As are other clostridia, *C. botulinum* strains are strict anaerobes that can survive extreme environmental conditions by producing dormant spores. The spores are resistant to heating and drying and can remain viable for years (Hofer and Davis 1972). *Clostridium botulinum* spores are widely, but unevenly, distributed in soils and wetland sediments throughout the world (Smith and Sugiyama 1988). Type C spores are primarily found in freshwater habitats and occasionally marine environments; they are rarely found in soil. Type E is also primarily associated with mud or sediments in or near freshwater. Type C and E spores can also be found in invertebrates (Jensen and Allen 1960; Eklund and Poysky 1970), vertebrate tissues (Bott et al. 1966; Reed and Rocke 1992), and the feces of some animals. Matveev and Konstantinova (1974) cultured 171 soil samples contaminated with the feces of wild birds (guillemots, loons, puffins, sandpipers, phalaropes, kittiwakes, eiders, and others) inhabiting islands in the Barents Sea and isolated *C. botulinum* type A, B, C, D, E, or F from 58 (34%) of the samples.

Clostridium botulinum is harmless in the dormant spore state; neurotoxin is produced only after the spores germinate and the cells begin dividing. The toxin is released when the bacterial cells undergo autolysis (Niemann 1991). In culture media, toxin titer is low during the logarithmic phase of growth but increases when cell growth ceases and cell membranes rupture. Interestingly, the toxin has no known role in the growth and physiology of the bacterium, and many naturally occurring isolates of *C. botulinum* do not produce toxin.

Type C strains of *C. botulinum* tend to have a higher temperature range than other types. The optimal temperature for type C growth is 40°C, but most strains grow well at temperatures as high as 45°C. Type C strains do not grow well at temperatures lower than 15°C (Segner et al. 1971). Type E spores germinate over a wide temperature range, from 2 to 50°C, and optimum germination occurs at 9°C (Grecz and Arway 1982). At all temperatures, except 50°C, germination is a two-stage process with a slow rate of germination through 18 to 26 hours of incubation and a sudden fourfold increase in germination after that. Vegetative growth of type E cells occurs from 6 to 41°C, but optimal growth occurs at 32.5°C. Only marginal growth occurs from 6 to 14°C, although certain strains can produce toxin at a slow rate at temperatures as low as 3.3°C.

Type C and D strains of *C. botulinum* are different from other botulinum types in that the production of neurotoxin depends on the presence of specific bacteriophages that infect the bacteria (Eklund et al. 1987). When type C and D strains are cured of bacteriophage infections by UV radiation or treatment with acridine orange, they lose the ability to produce C_1 or D neurotoxins. The cured strains resume production of neurotoxin only after they are re-infected with certain phages (TOX^+) derived from the toxigenic parent stock. Furthermore, TOX^+ phages isolated from type D strains can infect nontoxigenic type C strains and induce them to produce type D toxin, and vice versa (Eklund et al. 1987). Hybridization analysis has shown that the structural gene for neurotoxin is located on the genome of TOX^+ bacteriophages (Fujii et al. 1988). Because the relationship with type C and D host strains is unstable, TOX^+ phages have been described as pseudolysogenic (Eklund et al. 1987). The DNA of pseudolysogenic phages is not incorporated into the bacterial genome; however, as with lysogenic phages, they can suppress the lysis of cells through several generations (Eklund et al. 1989). Replication of bacteria that contain pseudolysogenic phages can result in uninfected cells and cells that lyse and liberate phages, as well as intact cells that contain the phage. The stability of the host-phage relationship depends on the bacterial strain, environmental conditions such as temperature, and the growth phase of the bacteria (Eklund et. al. 1989).

A similar mechanism for toxin production in types A, B, E, and F has not been discovered (Eklund et al. 1989). Toxin production in these types is much more stable than in types C and D, which are prone to lose toxigenicity after several passages. Bacteriophages have been detected in *C. botulinum* types A, B, E, and F; however, even after curing these bacteria of their phage infection with mitomycin C or acradine orange, they continue to produce neurotoxin. Also, no phages have been isolated that can induce toxigenicity in nontoxigenic, phage-sensitive bacteria. Although the gene responsible for type E toxin production is located on the bacterial chromosome, under some conditions gene transfer can occur, possibly via defective and helper phages (Zhou et al. 1993) or on plasmids. For instance, a couple of human cases of type E botulism resulted from infection with a strain of a different bacteria, *C. butyricum,* that was found to produce type E toxin (McCroskey et al. 1986). Hauser et al. (1992) located the type E toxin gene in this bacterial strain on a plasmid.

Despite differences in location of the toxin gene, all seven *C. botulinum* neurotoxin types possess a similar structure, and consequently, a similar pharmacologic action. Toxin is initially produced by bacteria as an inactive, single-chain protein with a molecular weight of 140 to 170 kDa. After lysis of the bacterial cell or secretion of toxin from the cell, this single-chain protein is "nicked" by proteases (or trypsin) that are either endogenous or exogenous to the bacteria. Unlike the

Table 21.2. Species of birds believed to have contracted type C botulism.

Common Name	Family	Scientific Name	Reference
	Accipitridae		
Bald Eagle		*Haliaeetus leucocephalus*	Jensen and Price 1987; NWHC[a]
Western Marsh-Harrier		*Circus aeruginosus*	Jensen and Price 1987; Horvath et al. 1994
Northern Harrier		*C. cyaneus*	Kalmbach and Gunderson 1934
Northern Goshawk		*Accipiter gentilis*	Horvath et al. 1994
Cooper's Hawk		*A. cooperii*	NWHC
Red-shouldered Hawk		*Buteo lineatus*	NWHC
Red-tailed Hawk		*B. jamaicensis*	NWHC
Whistling Kite		*Haliastur sphenurus*	Woodall 1982
	Alcidae		
Common Murre		*Uria aalge*	Jensen and Price 1987
	Alaudidae		
Horned Lark		*Eremophila alpestris*	Kalmbach and Gunderson 1934
	Anatidae		
Black Swan		*Cygnus atratus*	Jensen and Price 1987
Mute Swan		*C. olor*	Calsow et al. 1995; NWHC
Tundra Swan		*C. columbianus*	NWHC
Coscoroba Swan		*Coscoroba coscoroba*	Mereb et al. 1999
Greylag Goose		*Anser anser*	Jensen and Price 1987; Portugal et al. 1995
Greater White-fronted Goose		*A. albifrons*	Kalmbach and Gunderson 1934
Bar-headed Goose		*A. indicus*	Portugal et al. 1995
Swan Goose		*A. cygnoides*	Portugal et al. 1995
Pink-footed Goose		*A. brachyrhynchus*	Jensen and Price 1987
Egyptian Goose		*Alopochen aegyptiacus*	Hay et al. 1973
Ross's Goose		*Chen rossii*	NWHC
Snow Goose		*C. caerulescens*	NWHC
Canada goose		*Branta canadensis*	Kalmbach and Gunderson 1934; NWHC
Brant		*B. bernicla*	NWHC
Hawaiian Goose		*B. sandvicensis*	NWHC
Spur-winged Goose		*Plectropterus gambensis*	Hay et al. 1973
Australian Shelduck		*T. tadornoides*	Jensen and Price 1987
Cape Shelduck		*T. cana*	Jensen and Price 1987
Ruddy Shelduck		*T. ferruginea*	Jensen and Price 1987
Wood Duck		*Aix sponsa*	NWHC
Marbled Teal		*Marmaronetta angustirostris*	Jensen and Price 1987
Northern Pintail		*Anas acuta*	Kalmbach and Gunderson 1934; Jensen and Price 1987; NWHC
Yellow-billed Pintail		*A. georgica*	Mereb et al. 1999
Green-winged Teal		*A. crecca*	Kalmbach and Gunderson 1934; Jensen and Price 1987; Calsow et al. 1995; NWHC
Blue-winged Teal		*A. discors*	Kalmbach and Gunderson 1934; NWHC
Gray Teal		*A. gibberifrons*	Jensen and Price 1987
Cinnamon Teal		*A. cyanoptera*	Kalmbach and Gunderson 1934; NWHC
Garganey		*A. querquedula*	Trnovak and Nemeth 1983; Jensen and Price 1987

Table 21.2. (Continued)

Common Name	Family	Scientific Name	Reference
Mallard		*A. platyrhynchos*	Kalmbach and Gunderson 1934 Jensen and Price 1987; Portugal et al. 1995; Calsow et al. 1995; NWHC
Spot-billed Duck		*A. poecilorhyncha*	Jensen and Price 1987
Northern Shoveler		*A. clypeata*	Kalmbach and Gunderson 1934; Calsow et al. 1995; NWHC
Australian Shoveler		*A. rhynchotis*	Jensen and Price 1987
Red Shoveler		*A. patalea*	Mereb et al. 1999
Cape Shoveler		*A. smithii*	Jensen and Price 1987
Gadwall		*A. strepera*	Kalmbach and Gunderson 1934; Jensen and Price 1987; Calsow et al. 1995; NWHC
Australian Black Duck		*A. superciliosa*	Jensen and Price 1987
Yellowbill Duck		*A. undulate*	Jensen and Price 1987
Cape Wigeon		*A. capensis*	Jensen and Price 1987
Eurasian Wigeon		*A. penelope*	Jensen and Price 1987; Calsow et al. 1995; NWHC
American Wigeon		*A. americana*	Kalmbach and Gunderson 1934; NWHC
American Black Duck		*A. rubripes*	Kalmbach and Gunderson 1934; NWHC
Mottled Duck		*A. fulvigula*	NWHC
Hawaiian Duck		*A. wyvilliana*	NWHC
White-cheeked Pintail		*A. bahamensis*	Mereb et al. 1999
White-eyed duck		*Aythya australis*	Jensen and Price 1987
Canvasback		*A. valisineria*	Kalmbach and Gunderson 1934; NWHC
Common Pochard		*A. ferina*	Calsow et al. 1995
Redhead		*A. americana*	Kalmbach and Gunderson 1934; NWHC
Tufted Duck		*A. fuligula*	Jensen and Price 1987; Horvath et al. 1994; Calsow et al. 1995; NWHC
Ferruginous Duck		*A. nyroca*	Horvath et al. 1994
Ring-necked Duck		*A. collaris*	Kalmbach and Gunderson 1934; NWHC
Lesser Scaup		*A. affinis*	Kalmbach and Gunderson 1934; NWHC
Greater Scaup		*A. marila*	NWHC
Common Goldeneye		*Bucephela clangula*	Kalmbach and Gunderson 1934; NWHC
Bufflehead		*B. albeola*	Kalmbach and Gunderson 1934; NWHC
Plumed Tree-Duck		*Dendrocygna eytoni*	Jensen and Price 1987
Fulvous Tree-Duck		*D. bicolor*	Kalmbach and Gunderson 1934
White-faced Tree-Duck		*D. viduata*	Jensen and Price 1987; Portugal et al. 1995
Southern Pochard		*Netta erythrophthalma*	Jensen and Price 1987
Red-crested Pochard		*N. rufina*	Jensen and Price 1987
Blue-billed Duck		*Oxyura australis*	Jensen and Price 1987
White-headed Duck		*O. leucocephala*	Jensen and Price 1987

(Continued)

Table 21.2. (Continued)

Common Name	Family	Scientific Name	Reference
Maccoa Duck		*O. maccoa*	Jensen and Price 1987
Ruddy Duck		*O. jamaicensis*	Kalmbach and Gunderson 1934; NWHC
Common Merganser		*Mergus merganser*[b]	Smith 1977
Red-breasted Merganser		*M. serrator*	Kalmbach and Gunderson 1934
Hooded Merganser		*Lophodytes cucullatus*	NWHC
Pink-eared Duck		*Malacorhynchus membranaceus*	Woodall 1982
Common Eider		*Somateria mollisima*	Jensen and Price 1987
Black Scoter		*Melanitta nigra*	Jensen and Price 1987
White-winged Scoter		*M. fusca*	NWHC
Muscovy Duck		*Cairina moschata*	Portugal et al. 1995; NWHC
Brazilian Duck		*Amazonetta brasiliensis*	Portugal et al. 1995
Australian Wood Duck		*Chenonetta jubata*	Woodall 1982
	Ardeidae		
Great Blue Heron		*Ardea herodias*	Kalmbach and Gunderson 1934; NWHC
Gray Heron		*A. cinerea*	Jensen and Price 1987; Horvath et al. 1994
White-faced Heron		*A. novaehollandiae*	Woodall 1982
Black-crowned Night-heron		*Nycticorax nycticorax*	Kalmbach and Gunderson 1934
American Bittern		*Botaurus lentiginosus*	Kalmbach and Gunderson 1934
Least Bittern		*Ixobrychus exilis*	NWHC
Purple Heron		*Ardea purpurea*	Jensen and Price 1987
Little Egret		*Egretta garzetta*	Jensen and Price 1987
Snowy Egret		*E. thula*	Kalmbach and Gunderson 1934; NWHC
White-faced Heron		*E. novaehollandiae*	Jensen and Price 1987
Great Egret		*Ardea alba*	NWHC
Cattle Egret		*Bubulcus ibis*	NWHC
	Cathartidae		
California Condor		*Gymnogyps californianus*	NWHC
	Charadriidae		
Snowy Plover		*Charadrius alexandrinus*	Jensen and Price 1987
Common Ringed Plover		*C. hiaticula*	Jensen and Price 1987
Kittlitz's Plover		*C. pecuarius*	Jensen and Price 1987
Semipalmated Plover		*C. semipalmatus*	Jensen and Price 1987
Three-banded Plover		*C. tricollaris*	Jensen and Price 1987
Red-capped Plover		*C. ruficapillus*	Jensen and Price 1987
Little ringed Plover		*C. dubius*	Horvath et al. 1994
Killdeer		*C. vociferus*	Kalmbach and Gunderson 1934; NWHC
Northern Lapwing		*Vanellus vanellus*	Jensen and Price 1987
Blacksmith Plover		*V. armatus*	Jensen and Price 1987
Spur-winged Plover		*V. spinosus*[b]	Smith 1977
Southern Lapwing		*V. chilensis*	Mereb et al. 1999
Black-bellied Plover		*Pluvialis squatarola*	Kalmbach and Gunderson 1934; Jensen and Price 1987
American Golden Plover		*P. dominica*	Kalmbach and Gunderson 1934
Pacific Golden Plover		*P. fulva*	NWHC

Table 21.2. (Continued)

Common Name	Family	Scientific Name	Reference
	Ciconiidae		
White Stork		*Ciconia ciconia*	Jensen and Price 1987
	Cisticolidae		
Zitting Cisticola		*Cisticola juncidis*	Jensen and Price 1987
	Columbidae		
Common Wood Pigeon		*Columba palumbus*	Jensen and Price 1987
Mourning Dove		*Zenaida macroura*	NWHC
	Corvidae		
Black-billed Magpie		*Pica hudsonia*	Kalmbach and Gunderson 1934
	Diomedeidae		
Laysan Albatross		*Phoebastria immutabilis*	NWHC
	Emberizidae		
Savannah Sparrow		*Passerculus sandwichensis*	NWHC
	Falconidae		
Peregrine Falcon		*Falco peregrinus*	Kalmbach and Gunderson 1934
Prairie Falcon		*F. mexicanus*	Kalmbach and Gunderson 1934
	Gaviidae		
Common Loon		*Gavia immer*	NWHC
	Gruidae		
Sandhill Crane		*Grus canadensis*	NWHC
Brolga		*G. rubicunda*[b]	Smith 1977
Sarus Crane		*G. antigone*	NWHC
	Haematopodidae		
Eurasian Oystercatcher		*Haematopus ostralegus*	Jensen and Price 1987
African Oystercatcher		*H. moquini*	Blaker 1967
	Hirundinidae		
Cliff Swallow		*Petrochelidon pyrrhonota*	Kalmbach and Gunderson 1934
Purple Martin		*Progne subis*	NWHC
	Icteridae		
Western Meadowlark		*Sturnella neglecta*	Kalmbach and Gunderson 1934; NWHC
Yellow-headed Blackbird		*Xanthocephalus xanthocephalus*	Kalmbach and Gunderson 1934; NWHC
Red-winged Blackbird		*Agelaius phoeniceus*	Kalmbach and Gunderson 1934; NWHC
Rusty Blackbird		*Euphagus carolinus*	Kalmbach and Gunderson 1934
Brewer's Blackbird		*E. cyanocephalus*	Kalmbach and Gunderson 1934
	Laridae		
Common Black-headed Gull		*Larus ridibundus*	Calsow et al. 1995
Bonaparte's Gull		*L. philadelphia*	Kalmbach and Gunderson 1934; NWHC
California Gull		*L. californicus*	Kalmbach and Gunderson 1934
Franklin's Gull		*L. pipixcan*	Kalmbach and Gunderson 1934; NWHC
Laughing Gull		*L. atricilla*	NWHC
Ring-billed Gull		*l. delawarensis*	Kalmbach and Gunderson 1934; NWHC
Mew Gull		*L. canus*	Jensen and Price 1987
Gray-hooded Gull		*L. cirrocephalus*	Jensen and Price 1987
Kelp Gull		*L. dominicanus*	Jensen and Price 1987

(Continued)

Table 21.2. (Continued)

Common Name	Family	Scientific Name	Reference
Great Black-backed Gull		*L. marinus*	Jensen and Price 1987
Lesser Black-backed Gull		*L. fuscus*	Jensen and Price 1987
Iceland Gull		*L. glaucoides*	Jensen and Price 1987
Hartlaub's Gull		*L. hartlaubii*	Jensen and Price 1987
Little Gull		*L. minutus*	Jensen and Price 1987
Silver Gull		*L. novaehollandiae*	Jensen and Price 1987
Herring Gull		*L. argentatus*	Horvath et al. 1994; NWHC
Western Gull		*L. occidentalis*	NWHC
Black-legged Kittiwake		*Rissa tridactylus*	Jensen and Price 1987
	Motacillidae		
Cape Wagtail		*Motacilla capensis*	Jensen and Price 1987
Yellow Wagtail		*M. flava*	Jensen and Price 1987
American Pipit		*Anthus rubescens*	Kalmbach and Gunderson 1934
	Pelecanidae		
Australian Pelican		*Pelicanus conspicillatus*	Jensen and Price 1987
Brown Pelican		*P. occidentalis*	Jensen and Price 1987; NWHC
American White Pelican		*P. erythrorhynchos*	Kalmbach and Gunderson 1934; Jensen and Price 1987; NWHC
Great White Pelican		*P. onocrotalus*	Blaker 1967
	Phalacrocoracidae		
Great Cormorant		*Phalacrocorax carbo*	Jensen and Price 1987
Double-crested Cormorant		*P. auritus*	Kalmbach and Gunderson 1934; NWHC
	Phasianidae		
Northern Bobwhite		*Colinus virginianus*	NWHC
Ring-necked Pheasant		*Phasianus colchicus*	Kalmbach and Gunderson 1934
Helmeted Guineafowl		*Numidia meleagris*	Jensen and Price 1987
	Phoenicopteridae		
Greater Flamingo		*Phoenicopterus ruber*	Jensen and Price 1987; NWHC
	Podicipedidae		
Great Crested Grebe		*Podiceps cristatus*	Jensen and Price 1987
Eared Grebe		*P. nigricollis*	Kalmbach and Gunderson 1934; Jensen and Price 1987; NWHC
Horned Grebe		*P. auritus*[b]	Smith 1977
Red-necked Grebe		*P. grisegena*[b]	Smith 1977
Little Grebe		*Tachybaptus ruficollis*	Jensen and Price 1987
Pied-billed Grebe		*Podilymbus podiceps*[b]	Smith 1977
Western Grebe		*Aechmophorus occidentalis*	Kalmbach and Gunderson 1934; NWHC
Clark's Grebe		*A. clarkia*	NWHC
White-tufted Grebe		*Rollandia rolland*	Mereb et al. 1999
	Procellariidae		
Northern Fulmar		*Fulmarus glacialis*	Jensen and Price 1987
	Rallidae		
Water Rail		*Rallus aquaticus*	Jensen and Price 1987
Virginia Rail		*R. limicola*	NWHC
Spotted Crake		*Porzana porzana*	Jensen and Price 1987
Sora		*P. carolina*	NWHC
Eurasian Coot		*Fulica atra*	Jensen and Price 1987; Calsow et al. 1995
Red-knobbed Coot		*F. cristata*	Jensen and Price 1987

Table 21.2. (Continued)

Common Name	Family	Scientific Name	Reference
American Coot		*F. americana*	Kalmbach and Gunderson 1934; NWHC
White-winged Coot		*F. leucoptera*	Mereb et al. 1999
Hawaian Coot		*F. alai*	NWHC
Common Moorhen		*Gallinula chloropus*	Jensen and Price 1987; Mikuska et al. 1986
Purple Swamphen		*Porphyrio porphyrio*	Jensen and Price 1987
	Recurvirostridae		
Black-winged Stilt		*Himantopus himantopus*	Jensen and Price 1987
White-headed Stilt		*H. leucocephalus*	Jensen and Price 1987
Black-necked Stilt		*H. mexicanus*	Kalmbach and Gunderson 1934; NWHC
Black-necked Stilt (Hawaiian)		*H. m. knudseni*	NWHC
White-backed Stilt		*H. melanurus*	Mereb et al. 1999
Pied Avocet		*Recurvirostra avosetta*	Jensen and Price 1987; Mikuska et al. 1986
Red-necked Avocet		*R. novaehollandiae*	Jensen and Price 1987
American Avocet		*R. americana*	Kalmbach and Gunderson 1934; NWHC
	Scolopacidae		
Sharp-tailed Sandpiper		*Calidris acuminata*	Jensen and Price 1987
Dunlin		*C. alpine*	Kalmbach and Gunderson 1934; Jensen and Price 1987; Calsow et al. 1995
Curlew Sandpiper		*C. ferruginea*	Kalmbach and Gunderson 1934; Jensen and Price 1987; Mikuska et al. 1986
Little Stint		*C. minuta*	Jensen and Price 1987
Red-necked Stint		*C. ruficollis*	Jensen and Price 1987
Great Knot		*C. tenuirostris*	Jensen and Price 1987
Red Knot		*C. canutus*	Kalmbach and Gunderson 1934; NWHC
Least Sandpiper		*C. minutilla*	Kalmbach and Gunderson 1934; NWHC
Semipalmated Sandpiper		*C. pusilla*	NWHC
Temminck's Stint		*C. temminckii*	Calsow et al. 1995
Pectoral Sandpiper		*C. melanotos*	Kalmbach and Gunderson 1934; NWHC
Baird's Sandpiper		*C. bairdii*	Kalmbach and Gunderson 1934
Stilt Sandpiper		*C. himantopus*	Kalmbach and Gunderson 1934
Western Sandpiper		*C. mauri*	Kalmbach and Gunderson 1934; NWHC
Sanderling		*C. alba*	Kalmbach and Gunderson 1934; NWHC
Spotted Redshank		*Tringa erythropus*	Jensen and Price 1987
Wood Sandpiper		*T. glareola*	Jensen and Price 1987
Common Greenshank		*T. nebularia*	Jensen and Price 1987
Green Sandpiper		*T. ocrophus*	Jensen and Price 1987;
Solitary Sandpiper		*T. solitaria*	Kalmbach and Gunderson 1934; Jensen and Price 1987; NWHC

(Continued)

Table 21.2. (Continued)

Common Name	Family	Scientific Name	Reference
Marsh Sandpiper		*T. stagnatilis*	Blaker 1967
Common Redshank		*T. tetanus*	Jensen and Price 1987; Calsow et al. 1995
Greater Yellowlegs		*T. melanoleuca*	Jensen and Price 1987; NWHC
Lesser Yellowlegs		*T. flavipes*	Kalmbach and Gunderson 1934; NWHC
Common Snipe		*Gallinago gallinago*	Jensen and Price 1987; NWHC
African Snipe		*G. nigripennis*	Jensen and Price 1987
Eurasian Curlew		*Numenius arquata*	Jensen and Price 1987
Ruff		*Philomachus pugnax*	Jensen and Price 1987
Spotted Sandpiper		*Actitis macularia*	Jensen and Price 1987; NWHC
Common Sandpiper		*A. hypoleucos*	Horvath et al. 1994
Ruddy Turnstone		*Arenaria interpres*	Kalmbach and Gunderson 1934; NWHC
Long-billed Dowitcher		*Limnodromus scolopaceus*	Kalmbach and Gunderson 1934; NWHC
Short-billed Dowitcher		*L. griseus*	NWHC
Marbled Godwit		*Limosa fedoa*	Kalmbach and Gunderson 1934; NWHC
Black-tailed Godwit		*L. limosa*	Mikuska et al. 1986
Willet		*Catoptrophorus semipalmatus*	Kalmbach and Gunderson 1934
Wilson's Phalarope		*Phalaropus tricolor*	Kalmbach and Gunderson 1934
Red-necked Phalarope		*P. lobatus*	Kalmbach and Gunderson 1934; NWHC
	Stercorariidae		
Parasitic Jaeger		*Stercorarius parasiticus*	Kalmbach and Gunderson 1934
	Sternidae		
Black Tern		*Chlidonias niger*	Kalmbach and Gunderson 1934
White-winged Tern		*C. leucopterus*	Jensen and Price 1987
Whiskered Tern		*C. hybrida*	Horvath et al. 1994
Caspian Tern		*Sterna caspia*	Jensen and Price 1987; Mikuska et al. 1986
Least Tern		*S. antillarum*	Smith 1977
Great Crested Tern		*S. bergii*	Jensen and Price 1987
Common Tern		*S. hirundo*	Jensen and Price 1987; Mikuska et al. 1986
Fairy Tern		*S. nereis*	Jensen and Price 1987
Arctic Tern		*S. paradisaea*	Jensen and Price 1987
Sandwich Tern		*S. sandvicensis*	Jensen and Price 1987
Forster's Tern		*S. forsteri*	NWHC
Snowy-crowned Tern		*S. trudeaui*	Mereb et al. 1999
	Strigidae		
Great Horned Owl		*Bubo virginianus*[b]	Smith 1977
Snowy Owl		*B. scandiacus*[b]	Smith 1977
Short-eared Owl		*Asio flammeus*[b]	Smith 1977
	Struthionidae		
Ostrich		*Struthio camelus*	Allwright et al. 1994
	Sulidae		
Northern Gannet		*Morus bassanus*	Jensen and Price 1987
Masked Booby		*Sula dactylatra*	NWHC

Table 21.2. (Continued)

Common Name	Family	Scientific Name	Reference
	Sylviidae		
Eurasian Reed-warbler		*Acrocephalus scirpaceus*	Jensen and Price 1987
	Threskiornithidae		
Sacred Ibis		*Threskiornis aethiopicus*	Jensen and Price 1987
White-faced Ibis		*Plegadis chihi*	Kalmbach and Gunderson 1934; NWHC
Glossy Ibis		*P. falcinellus*	NWHC
Yellow-billed Spoonbill		*Platalea flavipes*	Jensen and Price 1987; Woodall 1982
Eurasian Spoonbill		*P. leucorodia*	Jensen and Price 1987
Royal Spoonbill		*P. regia*	Jensen and Price 1987
Black-faced Spoonbill		*P. minor*	BirdLife International 2004
	Turdidae		
American Robin		*Turdus migratorius*	NWHC
Eurasian Blackbird		*T. merula*	Jensen and Price 1987
Song Thrush		*T. philomelos*[b]	Smith 1977

a: Unpublished data, U. S. Geological Survey, National Wildlife Health Center, Madison, WI, U.S.A.
b: Presumed, species names not provided.

other types, type E strains do not produce any proteases; thus exogenous enzymes are required for activation (DasGupta and Sugiyama 1972). Pure cultures of type E botulinum typically require the addition of trypsin to activate the toxin, but in decomposing tissue where proteases are plentiful, the addition of trypsin is not required to enhance toxicity (Smith et al. 1988).

The nicked protein is a dichain molecule, composed of a heavy (H) chain (85 to 100 kDa) and a light (L) chain (50 to 59 kDa) joined by a disulfide bond. This interchain disulfide bond plays an important role in cell penetration, and its cleavage by reduction abolishes toxicity (dePaiva et al. 1993). The dichain molecule is folded into three functional domains, which play different roles in the intoxication of nerve cells that leads to paralysis. The carboxy-terminal half of the H chain is primarily responsible for binding specifically to receptors on nerve cells, and the amino-terminal half governs cell penetration. The L chain has enzymatic activity and acts intracellularly to disrupt the release of the neurotransmitter, acetylcholine.

A unique aspect of type C and D strains of *C. botulinum* is that many strains produce another toxin, designated C_2, that does not act on the nervous system. Strains of type C may produce both C_1 and C_2 or only one of them. C_2 is a binary toxin with ADP-ribosylating activity, and it is highly lethal when injected into laboratory animals (Simpson 1989), causing an increase in vascular permeability that induces pulmonary hemorrhage and edema. Unlike the neurotoxin, the gene for C_2 toxin is located on the bacterial genome and not a bacteriophage. Although C_2 toxin has been implicated in the pathogenesis of botulism in some animals, such as horses, its role in avian botulism, if any, remains unknown.

EPIZOOTIOLOGY

Type C Botulism

Much of the collective knowledge about avian botulism derives from observations of the massive outbreaks in waterfowl in wetlands in western North America. However, it is becoming increasingly clear that the epizootiology of botulism in birds is more complex than previously believed and also quite diverse, depending on a number of factors, that include local environmental conditions and climatic events, as well as the foraging behavior of the bird species involved. Still, some common generalities exist. *Clostridium botulinum* requires an environment devoid of oxygen, as well as other appropriate environmental conditions, in order for spore germination, cell replication, and thus toxin production to occur. As with most other bacteria, temperature plays a critical role in the multiplication of *C. botulinum,* with optimal growth between 25 and 40°C for type C strains.

Table 21.3. Species of birds believed to have contracted type E botulism.

Common Name	Family	Scientific Name	Reference[a]
	Anatidae		
Long-tailed Duck		*Clangula hyemalis*	R,C
Common Goldeneye		*Bucephela clangula*	R,N
Bufflehead		*B. albeola*	R
Ring-necked Duck		*Aythya collaris*	R
Greater Scaup		*A. marila*	R,C
Common Merganser		*Mergus merganser*	R,C
Red-breasted Merganser		*M. serrator*	R,C
Hooded Merganser		*Lophodytes cucullatus*	R
White-winged Scoter		*Melanitta fusca*	R
Surf Scoter		*M. perspicillata*	C
Canada Goose		*Branta canadensis*	R
Snow Goose		*Chen caerulescens*	R
Trumpeter Swan		*Cygnus buccinator*	N
	Ardeidae		
Great Blue Heron		*Ardea herodias*	C
	Columbidae		
Mourning Dove		*Zenaida macroura*	R
	Gaviidae		
Common Loon		*Gavia immer*	R,C,N
Red-throated Loon		*G. stellata*	C
	Laridae		
Herring Gull		*Larus argentatus*	R,C,N
Ring-billed Gull		*L. delawarensis*	R,C,N
Bonaparte's Gull		*L. philadelphia*	R,C,N
Great Black-backed Gull		*L. marinus*	C,N
	Pelecanidae		
Brown Pelican		*Pelicanus occidentalis*	N
American White Pelican		*P. erythrorhynchos*	N
	Podicipedidae		
Pied-billed Grebe		*Podilymbus podiceps*	R
Horned Grebe		*Podiceps auritus*	R,C
Red-necked Grebe		*P. grisegena*	R,C
	Scolopacidae		
Sanderling		*Calidris alba*	C
Semipalmated Sandpiper		*C. pusilla*	N
Spotted Sandpiper		*Actitis macularia*	C
	Sternidae		
Caspian Tern		*Sterna caspia*	N
	Strigidae		
Short-eared Owl		*Asio flammeus*	R

a: N = Unpublished data, U.S. Geological Survey, National Wildlife Health Center, Madison, WI, U.S.A.; R = Rosen 1971; C = Carpentier 2000

Table 21.4. Characteristics of bacteria that produce botulinum neurotoxin. (Modified from Hatheway, 1995.)

	Clostridium botulinum group I	II	III	IV
Toxin type	A,B,F	B,E,F	C,D	G
Lipase	+	+	+	–
Lecithinase	–	–	–	–
Milk digestion	+	–	±	+
Gelatin	+	+	+	+
Glucose	+	+	+	–
Lactose	–	–	–	–
Mannose	–	+	+	–
Growth temperature (°C)				
Optimum	5–40	18–25	40	37
Minimum	12	3.3	15	
Spore heat resistance temperature (°C)	112	80	104	104
Toxin gene locale	C	C	P	C

Most type C botulism outbreaks in birds take place during the summer and fall, when ambient temperatures are higher and the bacteria are multiplying, although in some wetlands, evidence suggests that preformed toxin may persist in some form over winter and cause outbreaks in winter or spring. In addition to permissive environmental conditions, *C. botulinum* also requires an energy source for growth and multiplication. Because it lacks the ability to synthesize certain essential amino acids, the bacterium requires a high protein substrate for replication. Decomposing tissue is an ideal medium, but the organism will grow readily in media containing protein in solution.

Botulism in Waterbirds Associated with Wetlands

Type C botulinum spores or cells are widely distributed in wetlands that birds frequent (Smith et al. 1978). High prevalence of the bacteria has been reported in wetland sediments in California, U.S.A. (Sandler et al. 1993), Saskatchewan, Canada (Wobeser et al. 1987), and elsewhere (Borland et al. 1977; Azuma and Itoh 1987). Wobeser et al. (1987) sampled sediments from wetlands throughout the province of Saskatchewan, Canada, and found a strong association between the prior occurrence of avian botulism in a marsh and the presence of the bacteria as demonstrated by toxin production from sediments cultured in growth medium. Nearly 60% of samples from marshes with a prior history of botulism outbreaks contained botulinum spores compared to 6% from lakes with no prior history. These results indicated that lakes with a history of outbreaks remain contaminated with spores, and the authors hypothesized that these lakes are likely at a higher risk of subsequently developing botulism than lakes without a history of botulism. During the past 15 years (CCWHC, unpublished data)[2] since the survey, 13 of 19 lakes that contained botulinum spores in at least one soil sample have had one or more botulism outbreaks, including three lakes without a prior history of the disease at the time of the survey, whereas only one of the nine lakes without spores had a subsequent outbreak (Yate's Corrected Chi-squared 5.89; P= 0.015).

Using similar sampling methods, Sandler et al. (1993) tested the hypothesis that botulinum spore prevalence was directly associated with the likelihood of outbreaks in 10 marshes within a 40 km^2 wetland complex in California, U.S.A., but found no such relationship. The prevalence of botulinum spores did not differ between marshes with and without outbreaks. The authors concluded that in wetlands where the disease has occurred in the past, the prevalence of the bacteria is probably not an important limiting factor in the occurrence of outbreaks in waterbirds. In fact, available evidence suggests that some level of replication of the bacteria can occur year round in certain environments (Sandler et al. 1993; Rocke, unpublished data).[4]

Although some wetlands can be identified as botulism-prone based on their history, outbreaks can occur and have certainly been documented in recent years in wetlands without a known history of the disease (NWHC, CCWHC, unpublished data).[1,2] Spores can be carried in the tissues of birds (Reed and Rocke 1992) and can be distributed to new environments in their feces (Matveev and Konstantinova 1974), but must compete with other soil bacteria that may inhibit their growth (Smith 1976; Graham 1978;

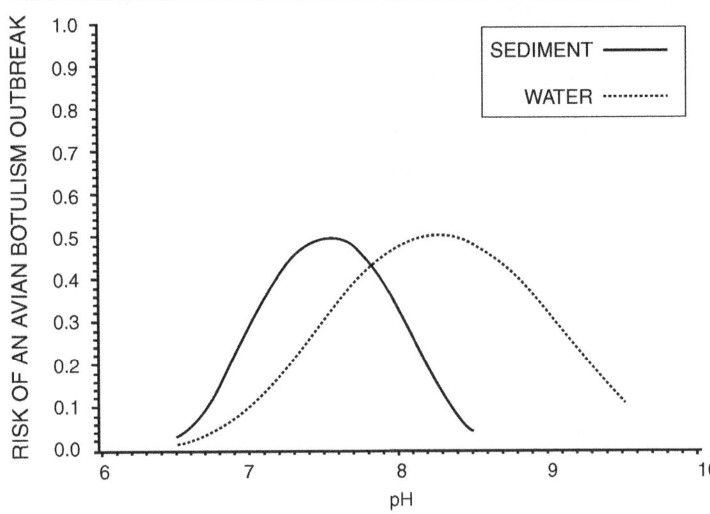

Figure 21.4. Predictive model depicting the relationship between sediment and water pH and the relative risk of botulism outbreaks in U.S. wetlands. (Reprinted from Rocke and Samuel 1999, courtesy of the Journal of Wildlife Management.)

Sandler et al. 1998). Factors that determine whether or not *C. botulinum* becomes established on a wetland are not known, largely because suitable methods to identify, quantify, and distinguish botulinum cells and spores were lacking. New molecular techniques recently developed for the selective isolation (Williamson et al. 1999; Nol et al. 2004) and quantification (Miyamoto 2002) of type C botulinum cells are currently being used in microbial ecology studies to address this question.

Outbreaks of avian botulism in wetlands are unpredictable, sometimes occurring annually in certain wetlands but not in adjacent ones. For many years, freshwater or alkali wetlands with large mud flats, fluctuating water levels, and feather edges were typically thought to be the most likely locations for type C botulism outbreaks to occur (Hunter 1970), and certainly, massive die-offs from botulism have been documented in wetlands with these physical characteristics (Barras and Kadlec 2000). However, these conditions do not characterize the timing and location of many outbreaks; the disease also occurs in deep, well-oxygenated wetlands with stable water levels (Kalmbach and Gunderson 1934; NWHC, unpublished data),[1] and even in river systems (NWHC, unpublished data).[1]

Decomposing vertebrate carcasses (see Carcass Maggot Cycle below) have been shown to support high levels of toxin production by *C. botulinum* type C (Bell et al. 1955; Hunter 1970; Reed and Rocke 1992) and can readily propagate an outbreak under some conditions. However, it has been demonstrated that botulism outbreaks in waterbirds have occurred in the absence of vertebrate carcasses (Rocke and Brand 1994), and in some outbreaks, the patterns of mortality are not consistent with a carcass source. Any decaying organic matter, insect remains, or other protein particulates can serve as a growth medium for *C. botulinum* (Kalmbach and Gunderson 1934; Bell et al. 1955; Rocke, unpublished data).[4] Decaying vegetation is frequently cited as a poor substrate for vegetative growth of *C. botulinum* (Coburn and Quortrup 1938; Bell et al. 1955; Wobeser 1997), yet the data is contradictory. Quortrup reversed his initial conclusions and subsequently stated that "common aquatic and emergent vegetation . . . may serve as an excellent medium for growth and toxin production of *C. botulinum* type C." (Quortrup and Holt 1941). He later showed that inoculation of water containing vegetation with *Pseudomonas aeruginosa* created anaerobic and alkaline conditions allowing *C. botulinum* to grow and produce toxin (Quortrup and Sudheimer 1943b). Supernatant from these cultures given orally to ducks readily produced signs of botulism and death, but confirmation of type C botulism was not attempted. Bell et al. (1955) could not demonstrate toxin production in decaying vegetation placed on mud in open-ended tubes on the Bear River Refuge, Utah, U.S.A., but showed that decaying duck livers and invertebrates could produce type C toxin. Because several species of bacteria in mud have been shown to inhibit *C. botulinum* type C growth (Graham 1978) and other aerobic bacteria rapidly destroy toxin (Quortrup and Holt 1941), further research is required to clearly demonstrate that decaying vegetation is not a suitable substrate for *C. botulinum* growth or that stagnant water cannot contain toxin before the "sludge-bed hypothesis" (Bell et al. 1955) is rejected.

In addition to natural processes of death and decomposition in wetlands, human activity can increase the available substrate for toxin production. For example, flooding and draining, pesticides, and other chemical inputs into wetlands from agricultural activities may kill aquatic life, thereby providing more substrate for toxin production. Rotting vegetation and raw sewage are other potential sources of energy; a number of botulism outbreaks in recent years have been associated with sewage oxidation ponds (NWHC, unpublished data).[1]

Until recently, the prevailing theory used to explain the occurrence of botulism outbreaks in wetlands was the "microenvironment concept" put forth by Bell et al. (1955). This hypothesis suggested that invertebrate carcasses or other decaying matter provided suitable substrate for toxin production independent of ambient environmental conditions. Jensen and Allen (1960) reported that botulism outbreaks in Utah coincided with a marked decline in invertebrate populations, following a population high, suggesting a relationship between dead invertebrates and the occurrence of botulism. However, as the authors conceded, conclusive data to support this hypothesis was lacking. At least one attempt to initiate botulism outbreaks by killing invertebrates in experimental ponds seeded with type C botulinum spores failed (Moulton et al. 1976). The investigators concluded that other factors must play a role in the occurrence of botulism outbreaks, and the microenvironment concept, as originally defined, was called into question.

A recent study of 32 wetlands with botulism outbreaks and paired control wetlands in nine states in the U.S. (Rocke and Samuel 1999) demonstrated that the risk of botulism outbreaks was associated with several measurable wetland characteristics. These relationships could be modeled but they were complex, involving both nonlinear and multivariate associations. The risk of outbreaks in wetlands was most strongly associated with water pH (Figure 21.4), but the effect of pH was strongly influenced by water temperature and redox potential (Figure 21.5). In general, the risk of botulism outbreaks was increased when water pH was between 7.5 and 9.0, redox potential was negative, and water temperature was > 20 C. Risk declined in wetlands with a pH < 7.5 or > 9.0, when redox potential was positive (> +100 mv), and water temperature was lower (10–15° C). All of these variables have been shown to influence spore germination and bacterial replication in the laboratory, but the underlying mechanism for their association with the risk of botulism outbreaks in wetlands was not determined. The authors cautioned that although their models identified potentially important wetland conditions associated with the risk of botulism outbreaks, they should not be used to predict the probability of an outbreak in a specific wetland, but to assess relative or potential risk (high, medium, or low). Even when wetland conditions are permissive and indicative of high risk for an outbreak, other factors, such as invertebrate density, bird abundance, and other sediment and water characteristics, probably interact to determine whether botulism actually occurs in a specific wetland and may also influence its severity. For example, in a multi-wetland refuge complex in northern California, U.S.A., botulism outbreaks in high-risk wetlands were temporally associated with increasing invertebrate abundance and increasing temperature (Rocke et al. 1999).

Currently, the mechanisms for the complex associations among environmental conditions and risk of avian botulism outbreaks is unclear. Presumably, wetland conditions enable bacterial growth and toxin production, resulting in a high-risk situation, but in order for an outbreak to actually occur, toxic food items must be encountered and ingested by birds. In some instances, decaying organic matter that contains toxin may be directly ingested by birds. Although this mechanism of transfer has not been clearly demonstrated in natural outbreaks, empirical evidence is compelling. Toxin has been produced readily in the laboratory in high-protein organic matter and decaying invertebrate tissues (Hobmaier 1932; Kalmbach and Gunderson 1934; Bell et al. 1955; Rocke, unpublished data).[4] Birds that sift through the mud to feed, such as Mallards and other dabbling ducks, and filter feeders, such as shovelers, are likely to encounter a wide variety of decaying organic matter or dead invertebrates that may contain sufficient levels of toxin to cause botulism. Unfortunately, it is not possible to pinpoint likely sources of toxin by examination of food remains in botulism-intoxicated birds because toxin is adsorbed through the small intestine; thus, the toxin-laden food is digested long before the bird becomes ill or dies from the disease. Furthermore, quantification and toxin analysis of dead invertebrates and other decaying matter in wetlands is quite difficult.

In other instances, waterbirds may be secondarily poisoned upon consumption of zooplankton or wetland invertebrates that inadvertently consumed toxic material. The carcass-maggot cycle, described in more detail later, is a classic example of secondary poisoning through consumption of toxin-laden invertebrates, but other aquatic animals may serve in this role as well. Wetlands are home to numerous invertebrates and zooplankton that consume organic debris, particularly in the benthos, and type C botulinum toxin has been demonstrated in free-living aquatic invertebrates (Kalmbach and Gunderson 1934), crustacea (Rocke, unpublished data),[4] and zooplankton (Neubauer et al. 1988), although most of these have been incidental findings, and toxin concentrations in

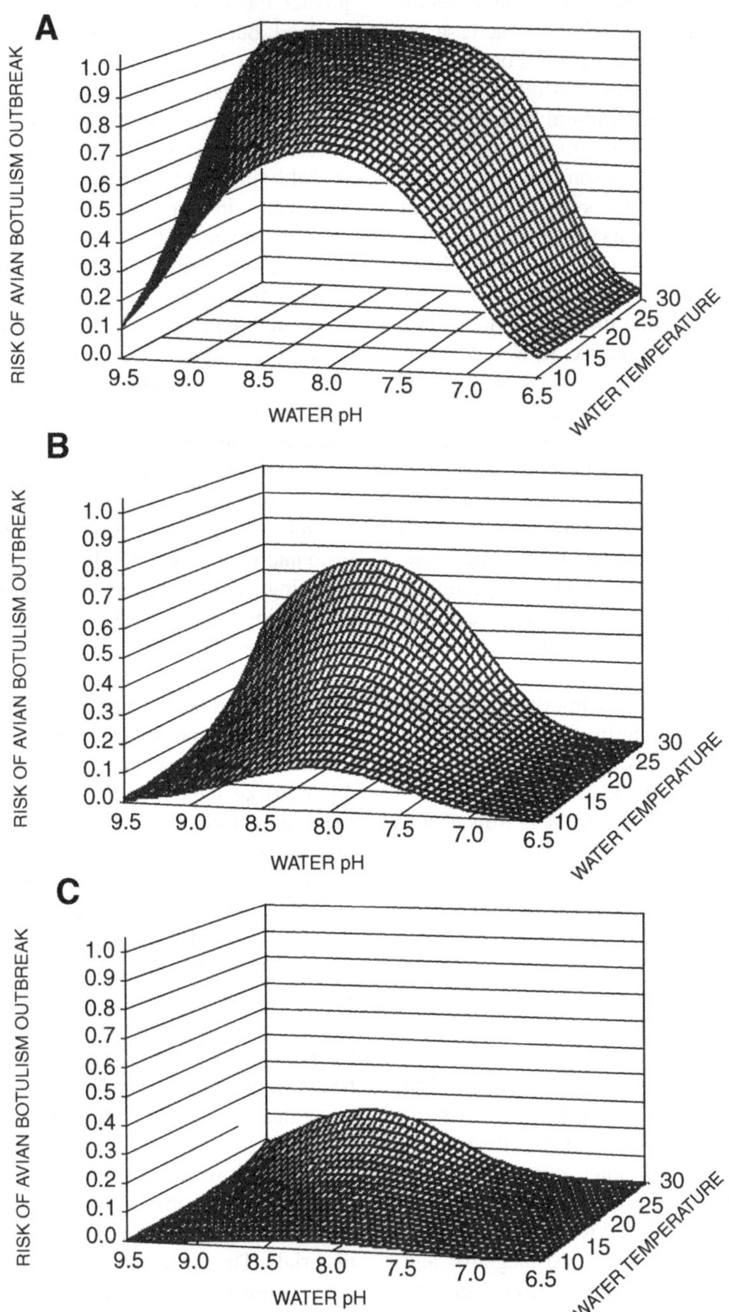

Figure 21.5. Predictive models showing the relationship between water pH and temperature and the relative risk of botulism outbreaks in U.S. wetlands with water redox potentials of: A = – 200 mv, B = +100 mv, and C = +300 mv. (Reprinted from Rocke and Samuel 1999, courtesy of the Journal of Wildlife Management.)

a limited sampling of insects appeared to be low compared to fly larvae (Bollinger, unpublished data).[5] Recently, a significant association was found between the occurrence of botulism outbreaks in birds and increasing invertebrate abundance and biomass within a California wetland complex (Rocke et al. 1999). However, direct and conclusive evidence that clarifies the role of aquatic invertebrates in initiating botulism outbreaks is lacking. Systematic studies designed to evaluate the availability of toxin in potential waterbird food items have not been undertaken, mainly because of the large scope of the problem and difficulties in sampling invertebrates on a large scale in wetlands that are often thousands of acres in size. Instead, most research has focused on the role of sarcophagous larvae on carcasses and the carcass maggot-cycle of botulism.

Carcass-Maggot Cycle of Botulism

Laboratory studies demonstrated long ago that decomposing flesh seeded with botulinum cells or spores can support the production of high levels of botulinum toxin (Kalmbach and Gunderson 1934; Bell et al. 1955). Waterbirds and other vertebrates inadvertently ingest botulinum spores while feeding and carry them for some period of time in their tissues. In one study in California, type C botulinum spores were detected in the liver or intestines of about 50% of healthy Mallards sampled in one botulism-prone wetland (Reed and Rocke 1992). Upon death, the resulting anaerobic environment and rich protein source of carcasses is optimal for germination of spores, vegetative cell growth, and toxin production. Decomposing carcasses also generate high internal temperatures suitable for toxin production, which can be independent of ambient temperatures, allowing for continued toxin production during cool weather (Wobeser and Galmut 1984).

Ingestion of fly larvae from decaying bird carcasses was suspected to cause "limberneck" in poultry, even before the disease was recognized as botulism (Bishopp 1923). Fly larvae and other invertebrates appear to be unaffected by the toxin, and as they feed on decaying matter, they effectively concentrate toxin. During an outbreak of botulism in waterfowl in Utah, U.S.A., Duncan and Jensen (1976) reported toxin levels as high as 409,600 mouse minimum lethal doses of toxin per gram in blow fly larvae collected from carcasses of a variety of waterbirds. Although most waterfowl will not directly consume a vertebrate carcass, they will readily ingest any maggots that fall off. In this way, botulism outbreaks in waterbirds often become self-perpetuating. This has become known as the carcass-maggot cycle of avian botulism, and it is thought that toxic maggots have the greatest potential to cause massive die-offs of birds (Wobeser 1997). Wobeser (1997) proposed that the dynamics of the carcass-maggot cycle of botulism are very similar to an infectious disease.

Waterbirds that have fed in environments contaminated with botulinum spores and that die from any cause are as likely to carry spores and initiate outbreaks through the carcass-maggot cycle of botulism as those that ingested preformed toxin and died from the disease (Hunter et al. 1970; Reed and Rocke 1992). Bird collisions with power transmissions lines have been implicated as the initiating factor in botulism outbreaks in Montana, U.S.A. (Malcolm 1982) and elsewhere (NWHC, unpublished data).[1] Other sources of mortality, such as hailstorms, algal poisoning, and other disease agents (Brand et al. 1988b; Soos 2004), may also precipitate type C botulism outbreaks in waterbirds through the carcass-maggot cycle.

Many factors likely play a role in the carcass-maggot cycle of botulism, including fly density and environmental conditions, such as temperature and wind speed, that facilitate fly egg-laying, maggot development, and maggot dispersal from carcasses (Reed and Rocke 1992; Wobeser 1997). The most critical factor is the density of carcasses that are "toxigenic", that is, contain type *C. botulinum* spores that will germinate and produce toxin. In some studies, 85–90% of maggot-infested carcasses were found to contain toxic maggots (Duncan and Jensen 1976; Bollinger, unpublished data)[5], and in another this rate varied from 29–69% (Reed and Rocke 1992). Although not every carcass in a wetland will become maggot infested or produce toxic maggots, factors that reduce the availability of decomposing carcasses, such as the presence of scavenging predators and carcass pick-up, may lower the risk of waterbird exposure to botulinum toxin (Reed and Rocke 1992).

Winter-Spring Outbreaks of Botulism in Waterbirds

Occasionally, outbreaks of type C botulism in waterbirds have been documented in late winter or early spring (Rosen and Cowan 1953; Parrish and Hunter 1969; Haagsma 1973; Graham et al. 1978; Wobeser et al.1983; Hubalek and Halouzka 1991). Typically these outbreaks are preceded by a die-off in the same location the previous fall. The epizootiology of winter-spring outbreaks has not been well studied, although several observations are pertinent. Wobeser et al. (1983) found that most of the affected ducks in a spring outbreak in Saskatchewan were diving ducks, although primarily dabblers had died the previous fall, and both types of ducks were present in both fall and spring. It was suggested that the spring die-off in divers resulted from toxin-bearing maggots that had fallen to the bottom of the wetland the previous fall and were accessible in the spring only to diving ducks. This hypothesis was supported by laboratory experiments on the thermal resistance of type C botulinum toxin (Hubalek and Halouzka 1988), in which sterile suspensions of toxin were held at various temperatures and their toxicity was measured in mice. At 5° C, the time required for 100-fold reduction of toxicity was six months, suggesting that in temperate climates, the toxin could persist through the winter season and cause intoxication in early spring. In further experiments with toxin-bearing maggots placed in perforated bottles that were then buried in wetland sediments overwinter, Hubalek and Halouzka (1991) demonstrated that toxin was still present 131 days later at levels that could potentially cause disease in waterbirds, although toxin titers dropped 25- to 40-fold.

Type C Botulism in Fish-Eating Birds at Salton Sea

Fish-eating birds are usually associated with type E botulism, but in 1996, more than 15,000 pelicans, herons, and other fish-eating birds became sick or died from type C botulism at the Salton Sea, a large inland sea in southern California, U.S.A. (Rocke et al. 2004). The majority of affected birds (> 8000) were American White Pelicans (*Pelecanus erythrorhynchos*), and the loss represented nearly 15% of the western American White Pelican population. In addition, more than 1500 endangered Brown Pelicans were afflicted, although a number of the sick birds were ultimately rehabilitated and released. Since 1996, type C botulism has recurred in fish-eating birds at the Sea every year, but the numbers of dead birds have been lower (1,000 to 3,000). In these die-offs at Salton Sea, fish (tilapia) are thought to be the primary source of toxin for birds. In 1996, type C botulinum toxin was found in a large percentage (35–50%) of fish found sick or dead in fresh postmortem condition, and toxin was also found in undigested fish remains regurgitated by sick pelicans. Although studies are still ongoing, available data and empirical evidence suggests that botulinum spores germinate in the gut of stressed or morbid fish, and the high summer water temperatures (often > 37°C) promote toxin production. The epizootiology of the disease at Salton Sea appears to be fairly unique, although type C botulism has been documented previously in pelicans at other locations (NWHC, unpublished data).[1]

Botulism in Gulls Associated with Landfills

Several outbreaks of type C botulism in gulls have been associated with landfills and refuse disposal sites in Britain (Lloyd et al. 1976), Scotland (MacDonald and Standring 1978), Ireland (Quinn and Crinion 1984), the Virgin Islands (Norton 1986), and most recently Israel (Gophen et al. 1991). Ortiz and Smith (1994) surveyed landfill sites in the United Kingdom and found spores of *C. botulinum* type B, C, and D at > 60% of the 19 sites sampled; type E was detected at one site, and the other toxin types (A, F, and G) were not detected. The authors speculated that the refuse was not the source of the bacteria; rather, the spores were probably transferred by birds attracted to the sites. The presence of the spores, coupled with rotting organic matter, and the concomitant rise in environmental temperatures, promoted bacterial replication and toxigenesis and ultimately resulted in botulism in the gulls that were scavenging on the site. In the case of the die-off in Israel, waste products from a chicken slaughterhouse were found to be improperly buried and likely contributed to the die-off.

Botulism in Raptors Associated with Poultry Farms

Botulism in raptors is fairly rare compared with other species and most often involves a single individual; however, at least one documented outbreak involved improperly discarded chicken carcasses (NWHC, unpublished data).[1] In Arkansas, in 1992, approximately 30 Red-tailed Hawks (*Buteo jamaicensis*) were found sick or dead in the vicinity of a "chicken dump." Presumably, the hawks were feeding on decaying flesh of carcasses, although there were reports of live chickens in the dump as well.

Botulism in Passerines

Botulism in songbirds occurs infrequently, although at least 16 species (Table 21.2) have been confirmed with the disease. In 1995, an unusual type C botulism outbreak occurred in Purple Martins (*Progne subis*) on a farm in Indiana (NWHC, unpublished data),[1] killing approximately 90% (112) of the adults in a large nesting colony; consequently, numerous nestlings starved to death, and unhatched eggs also died (Chambers 1995). Although the precise source of toxin was not identified, the die-off presumably originated in a small, stagnant pond where the birds frequently drank and fed on emerging insects.

Botulism in Captive-Reared Birds

Game farm pheasants and Ostriches (*Struthio camelus*) frequently develop botulism from direct contact with "toxic" carcasses. Ostriches are known to pick at carrion and bones, and carcass-associated type C botulism has been documented in captive Ostriches in South Africa (Allwright et al. 1994). In game-farm pheasants, the carcass-maggot cycle of botulism is probably the most significant source of the disease (Lee et al. 1962). In zoological collections, botulism has been associated with decaying food and organic material that accumulates in the bottom of artificial ponds or lagoons.

Botulism As a Result of Gut Toxigenesis

Although most botulism cases in birds are probably the result of ingestion of toxin through food items, another possible route, gut toxigenesis or "toxico-infection," deserves mention. Gut toxigenesis is the formation of toxin upon proliferative growth of *C. botulinum* in the gastrointestinal (GI) tract and is the primary means by which human infants acquire botulism. It occurs when an animal is debilitated or when GI function or normal GI flora is disrupted for some reason, and an anaerobic environment in the gut becomes established.

In chickens, gut toxigenesis, most likely in the ceca, combined with fecal contamination is a unique mode of botulism intoxication (Miyazaki and Sakaguchi 1978; Dohms 1987). Chickens inoculated intracecally with spores of *C. botulinum* type C or that were fed botulism spores did not develop botulism (Sakaguchi and Kaji 1980; Hyun and Sakaguchi 1989), even though the spores germinated and toxin was detected in their fecal droppings for as long as three days. However, chickens fed type C spores that subsequently fed on contaminated fecal droppings developed botulism and died (Hyun and Sakaguchi 1989). Presumably, the amount of toxin produced in the gut and absorbed there was not sufficient to intoxicate the host chicken, but ingestion and absorption of cell-bound toxin in fecal droppings was sufficient to cause intoxication.

Empirical evidence suggests that gut toxigenesis may also occur occasionally in wild birds, although it is difficult to distinguish from ingestion of preformed toxin. Several cases of type C botulism have been confirmed in moribund waterfowl that were simultaneously diagnosed with severe cases of lead poisoning and vitamin A deficiency (Rocke, unpublished data)[4] while other birds in the vicinity remained healthy. The sick birds were severely emaciated and were clearly not ingesting food. Because the wetlands they inhabited were heavily seeded with botulinum spores, it was postulated that these debilitated birds developed botulism secondarily through gut toxigenesis. This route of exposure to the toxin is probably not significant in most populations of free-ranging birds, but it should be a consideration in the care and management of captive-reared birds.

Type E Botulism

The preferred habitat of *C. botulinum* type E appears to be temperate, fresh, and brackish water sediments (Sugiyama et al. 1970; Huss 1980), although cases of type E avian botulism have occurred infrequently at the Salton Sea in southern California (NWHC, unpublished data),[1] a hot, marine environment. Occurrences of disease and systematic surveys for the bacterium indicate that the organism has a wide geographic distribution, primarily in northern temperate zones. The ability of type E spores to germinate at cold temperatures and cold tolerance of vegetative cells likely gives *C. botulinum* type E an ecological advantage over other anaerobic bacteria in cold water environments.

Surveys on the distribution of type E botulinum spores have been reviewed previously (Hobbs 1976; Smith and Sugiyama 1988). In most locations, the prevalence of type E spores is low; however, in some locations, such as the Great Lakes of North America and the Baltic Sea, high concentrations of *C. botulinum* type E were found in aquatic sediments in areas where type E botulism was diagnosed in fish, birds, and/or humans. Sugiyama, et al. (1970) found *C. botulinum* type E in more than 90% of wet sediment samples and in 56% of fish in Lake Michigan near Green Bay, Wisconsin, U.S.A. In contrast, only 5% of the soil samples from terrestrial environments surrounding Green Bay contained the organism. Johannsen (1963) found that 100% of bottom samples from the Baltic Sea and its tributaries contained *C. botulinum* type E, and, depending on the location, between 33 and 84% of shore samples contained the bacterium. He also found the bacterium in terrestrial samples and suggested that the organism was of terrestrial origin and accumulated in waterways due to runoff, but this is now thought not to be the case. *Clostridium botulinum* type E appears to be a true aquatic organism and fish or a rich aquatic fauna appear to contribute to its high prevalence in some locations (Huss 1980).

Type E spores and possibly bacteria are ingested routinely by healthy fish and cause no harm as germination and/or growth of *C. botulinum* type E does not appear to take place in or on living fish (Sugiyama et al. 1970; Eklund et al. 1984). Ingested spores pass through the digestive tract in a matter of days and, under experimental conditions, most fish fed approximately 1,000 type E spores were no longer carrying spores after two days (Sugiyama et. al. 1970). However, in dead fish, the bacterium can replicate in the decomposing anaerobic carcass and produce type E toxin. Vertebrate carcasses are a highly suitable substrate for growth of *C. botulinum* type E (Smith et al. 1988), and carrion is a common source of toxin for animals (Smith and Turner 1989), including other fish. In hatchery-reared fish, type E botulism appears to be a cyclic process, driven by post-mortem toxin formation in carcasses. Initially only a few fish are involved in the outbreak, but as concentrations of bacteria and toxin increase and numbers of carcasses increase, the mortality rate can rise rapidly (Eklund et al. 1984).

Apparently, fish are very sensitive to type E toxin. The toxic oral dose in coho salmon (*Oncorhynchus kisutch*) was reported at approximately six mouse lethal doses per g of fish at 20°C (Eklund et al. 1984), and by intraperitoneal inoculation, fish are even more sensitive than mice. In addition, it appears that fish are much more sensitive to type E toxin than type C. Carp orally administered type E toxin died from doses as low as 0.24 mouse lethal doses per g of fish, but survived oral dosing with type C up to 427 mouse lethal doses/g of fish (Haagsma 1975).

The source of toxin in outbreaks of type E botulism in birds is not known with certainty, although fish are strongly implicated in most cases. In outbreaks of the early 1960s on Lake Michigan, avian mortality occurred in association with die-offs of alewife (*Alosa pseudoharengus*). Alewife were the predominant species of fish found in the digestive tract of most of the dead birds examined, and dead alewife fed to gulls produced botulism under experimental conditions (Fay 1966). Alewife are small (average length 6 inches), anadromous fish of eastern North America that invaded the upper Great Lakes through the Welland and Erie Barge Canals, which were completed in the mid 1820s. These canals bypassed Niagara Falls, which had previously prevented the movement of fish from Lake Ontario into the upper Great Lakes. Alewife were first reported in Lake Michigan in 1949 but by the 1960s were the most predominant fish. Very large die-offs of Alewife occurred annually throughout most of the Great Lakes in spring and early summer (Scott and Crossman 1973). Alewives are thought to be the source of toxin for many of the scavenging birds throughout the 1960s (Fay 1966; Monheimer 1968); however, spores and toxin have been reported in other fish species.

The sources of type E toxin in the most recent die-offs in Lake Huron and Lake Erie are less clear. Gobies (*Proterorhinus marmoratus* and *Neogobius melanostomus*) were the most common food item in dead birds from some of the die-offs, and investigators reported gobies with signs of partial paralysis suggestive of botulism (Campbell, pers. comm.).[6] Similar to alewives, gobies are an introduced species. Native to the Black and Caspian seas, gobies were first detected in the St. Clair River, between Lake Erie and Lake Huron, in 1990, and were most likely transported to the Great Lakes in bilge water (Jude 1992). These fish are now widespread throughout most of the Great Lakes and are the predominant fish in some areas of Lake Erie and elsewhere (Domske and Obert 2001). Fish die-offs, involving various species, occur commonly on the Great Lakes, and where they overlap with areas of high spore densities in the environment and high concentrations of birds, type E avian botulism may occur. In most cases, the causes of fish die-offs are not clearly established. Fish die-offs, of any cause, have the potential to be amplified by fish botulism if other fish feed on the decomposing carcasses (Eklund et al. 1984). Although perhaps only coincidental, the association of type E botulism with the introduction of non-native species to the Great Lakes and the alteration of fish community structure warrants further study. Die-offs of mudpuppies (*Necturus maculosus*) also have been tentatively linked to type E avian botulism at some sites on the Great Lakes (Domske and Obert 2001; D. Campbell, pers. comm.).[6]

The role of sarcophagous invertebrates in type E botulism has not been investigated. Blow fly larvae may be a source of type E toxin in some situations but do not appear to play a similar role to the carcass-maggot cycle of type C botulism in ducks. Involvement of shore birds in some type E botulism die-offs indicates that invertebrates or sources of toxin other than fish are available.

Conditions unsuitable for vegetative growth of *C. botulinum* type E result in production of a resistant resting stage or spore form that can persist in sediments for years. The location of spores in sediments has been investigated only on fish farms, where they occur in highest densities (28,000 to 150,000 spores/gram) in the top 1.5 cm of the sediment. This top sediment contains waste feed, fecal material, and dead fish, and when suitable environmental conditions occur, vegetative growth probably occurs, resulting in the accumulation of more spores (Eklund et al. 1984). Growth of *C. botulinum* type E in sediments is thought to account for the high concentration of spores in Green Bay of Lake Michigan (Bott et al. 1968); however in other locations, bacteria within the substrate produce exotoxins that inhibit growth of *C. botulinum* type E (Dautter et al. 1996). Currents and inflow from rivers and creeks may redistribute spores.

CLINICAL SIGNS

Botulinum toxins interfere with transmission in the peripheral nervous system, specifically in cholinergic nerves of the motor and autonomic nervous system; clinical signs reflect this mechanism of action. The rate at which clinical signs develop, severity and duration of clinical signs, and time to death or recovery depend on several factors, including the quantity and type of toxin consumed and species affected. The rapidity of onset and severity of clinical signs is proportional to the amount of toxin consumed (Kalmbach 1930).

In general, affected birds show signs of progressive weakness, paresis, and flaccid paralysis of skeletal muscles. The earliest sign of botulism in birds is weak flight (Haagsma et al. 1972). Birds are reluctant to fly when disturbed, have difficulty taking off and landing, have a weak wing-beat, and fly for only short distances before stopping. Eventually birds may completely lose the ability to fly and will propel themselves across the water and land using their wings as "oars." Paresis of the legs results in a stumbling gait and eventually an inability to stand. In early stages of the disease, even with significant paralysis, birds remain mentally alert. The disease can progress to involve skeletal muscles of the neck, a condition occasionally referred to as "limber-neck," and birds on water can drown because they are unable to keep their head above water. Waterbirds, such as ducks, will frequently drag themselves out of the water onto shorelines, muskrat houses, or matted vegetation. Wind, excessive heat, and inclement weather can exacerbate clinical signs. Recumbent birds exposed to sun and heat rapidly dehydrate. Paralysis of skeletal muscles involved in respiration leads to death by asphyxiation. Hunter et al. (1970) divided affected birds into three categories: Class I birds were bright and alert, walking but flightless; Class II birds had difficulty walking and problems in holding their heads erect; Class III birds were prostate and almost totally paralyzed. These classes have been used by researchers and managers to evaluate treatment options and the probability of survival.

Botulism-weakened and recumbent waterfowl may become heavily infected with leeches in oral and nasal cavities, resulting in severe anemia. The nictitating membrane touch reflex gradually disappears (Blaker 1967), and debilitated birds frequently have partially or completely closed eyelids. Lacrimal fluid may accumulate behind the eyelids and spill out at the margins. Anorexia (Smith et al. 1975) and green diarrhea (Kalmbach 1930) are occasionally reported. Mildly affected birds may recover and other birds may show intermittent clinical signs. Chronic botulism or persistent clinical signs have not been described in birds but have been in other species (Kriek and Odendaal 1994). In humans, muscle weakness may persist for weeks in recovered individuals (Koenig et al. 1964), and given the common mechanism of action of botulinum toxin, similar residual effects may occur in wild birds with potential impacts on survival of what appear to be recovered birds.

Given that botulinum toxin also affects acetylcholine release of the autonomic nervous system, it is doubtful that the full range of physiological effects and clinical signs of botulism in birds has been described, and some of these effects may have implications for survival. Cooch (1964) proposed that botulism toxin impaired avian salt gland function by inhibiting acetylcholine release by parasympathetic nerve fibers of cranial nerve VII, which innervates this gland. In Mallards and Northern Pintails (*Anas acuta*), he was able to demonstrate a significant decrease in LD_{50} when a high oral dose of NaCl was given in conjunction with type C toxin either via oral or intraperitoneal inoculations. However, exposure of Mallard ducklings to saline water from lakes with a known history of botulism prior to challenge with type C toxin did not consistently increase the occurrence or severity of clinical signs (Wobeser 1988). In humans, in whom the full range of clinical signs can be more readily assessed and monitored over time, a wider range of physiological alterations are observed and effects are normally of long duration (Rogers et al. 1964; Jenzer et al. 1975). These include blurred vision, dysphagia, dry mouth, dizziness, and general weakness. The biological activity of different types of botulinum toxins are not identical (Bittner et al. 1989; Montecucco and Schiavo 1994), and species vary in susceptibility to different types of botulinum toxin; therefore, extrapolations among species and types should be made only with caution. In humans, significant neuromuscular blockade occurs for two to three months after intramuscular inoculation of type A and type C toxin (Eleopra et al. 1997), whereas with type E toxin, the effects are reversed far more rapidly (Eleopra et al. 1998). Research is needed on the range and duration of physiological impairment in birds poisoned with botulinum type C and E.

PATHOGENESIS

Botulinum neurotoxins are the most toxic substances known, with mouse LD_{50}'s between 0.1 and 1.0 ng/kg of body weight. In birds, the oral LD_{50} of type C toxin appears to be quite variable, with reports as low as 500 mouse intraperitoneal (IP) LD_{50} units for American Coots (*Fulica americana*)(Hunter et al. 1970) to 2,500,000 mouse lethal doses for gulls and crows (Haagsma 1987). Waterfowl, the family of birds most commonly afflicted with botulism, appear to be only moderately susceptible to type C toxin, with oral toxicities reported in the range of 14,000–80,000 mouse IP LD_{50} units/bird (Table 21.5). On a body weight basis, the sensitivity to type *C botulinum* toxin is similar among the few species tested experimentally (36,000–43,000 mouse IP LD_{50} units)(Rocke et al. 2000). A few reported values for Mallards are considerably higher than this at 190,000 (Itoh et al. 1978) and 320,000 mouse IP LD_{50} units/bird (Haagsma 1987); however, these authors did not describe the medium that was used to deliver the toxin. Oral toxicities determined in different experimental trials are difficult to compare because the results are dependent on the protein substrate in which the toxin is delivered; much lower toxicity has been observed in birds fed toxin prepared in culture media versus suspensions of fly larvae that contain the same level of toxin (Rocke, unpublished data).[4]

Table 21.5. Toxic oral dose of *Clostridium botulinum* type C toxin for several species in mouse intraperitoneal (IP) 50% lethal dose units. (Modified from Wobeser 1981.)

Mallard	45,000–80,000	Hunter et al. 1970
	20,000–80,000	Duncan and Jensen 1976
	45,000	Martinez and Wobeser 1999
Northern Pintail	16,000–76,000	Hunter et al. 1970
	22,500	Martinez and Wobeser 1999
Cinnamon Teal	30,000	Hunter et al. 1970
Green-winged Teal	17,000	Hunter et al. 1970
	14,000	Rocke et al. 2000
American Coot	500	Hunter et al. 1970

Botulinum neurotoxin in both natural substrates and in vitro cultures is generally found associated with one or more nontoxin proteins (Sugiyama 1980). The toxin complexes are usually either bimolecular or trimolecular and vary in molecular weight from 230–900 kDa. Some of the nontoxin proteins have hemagglutinin activity, but their function is unknown. The complex of neurotoxin and nontoxin proteins appears to protect these proteins during exposure to acid and proteolytic enzymes in the gastrointestinal tract (Chen et al. 1998). When administered perorally, toxin complexes are considerably more toxic than purified neurotoxin, and trimolecular complexes are more toxic than bimolecular complexes (Ohishi 1984). One or more of these proteins may also be involved in transport of the toxin across the gut membrane to the circulatory system via receptor binding to epithelial cells. Some evidence suggests the ligand binding property is found on the hemagglutinin antigen (Fujinaga et al. 1997), although other work supports the hypothesis that the binding site is on the botulinum toxin molecule itself (Maksymowych et al. 1999). Recent studies implicate glycoproteins, such as mucin, as receptor and transporter of botulinum toxin in intestinal epithelium (Nishikawa et al. 2004).

Once in the general circulation, the toxin is delivered to its target organs, which are cholinergic nerve cells. The neurotoxin exerts its paralytic effects by blocking the release of the neurotransmitter, acetylcholine. The toxin acts on the peripheral nervous system, including cholinergic neuromuscular junctions, autonomic ganglia, postganglionic parasympathetic sites, postganglionic sympathetic nerves that release acetylcholine, and the adrenal glands (Simpson 1981). The extreme toxicity of botulinum neurotoxins is due to their high affinity to presynapatic membranes and their persistent and specific inhibition of the release of neurotransmitter. Neurotoxin does not kill neurons but disrupts their most essential function of synaptic transmission. Botulinum toxin does not cross the blood-brain barrier.

The toxin's interference with neuromuscular transmission occurs in a three-step process: (1) specific binding to receptors on nerve cells; (2) internalization of the toxin by endocytosis and translocation of the L chain across the endosomal membrane; and (3) enzymatic cleavage of target proteins in the cytosol that disrupts the cell's ability to release neurotransmitter (for recent reviews, see Pellizzari et al. 1999; Herreros et al. 1999; Humeau et al. 2000; Simpson 2004).

Neurospecific Binding

Binding of botulinum neurotoxin to nerve cell membranes is the first critical step toward paralysis. After diffusion through body fluids from the site of toxin production or absorption, botulinum toxin binds rapidly and irreversibly to the presynaptic membrane of cholinergic nerve terminals (Simpson 1989). Available evidence suggests that the region of the neurotoxin molecule that contains the binding site (binding domain) probably resides on the carboxy terminus of the H chain (Bandyopadhyay et al. 1987). Isolated preparations of the H and L chains of neurotoxin are not paralytic when applied to tissues singly; both are required for neuromuscular blockage. In addition, the H chain must be applied before the L chain in order for paralysis to occur.

Although identification of the presynaptic receptor(s) of botulinum neurotoxin has been attempted by several investigators, the data supporting a specific receptor is equivocal. Polysialogangliosides are involved (Halpern and Neale 1995) but are not the sole receptors. Recent evidence suggests that binding of neurotoxin to the nerve cell may involve multiple interactions with both glycoprotein and glycolipid binding sites (Herreros et al. 1999). However, it is clear from competition experiments that different neurotoxin types do not share the same receptor (with the exception of types C and D, which are closely related).

Internalization

Botulinum neurotoxins do not enter the cell directly via the plasma membrane; rather, they are internalized into an endosome through receptor-mediated endocytosis. Electron microscope studies have shown that after binding, neurotoxin enters the lumen of vesicular structures by a temperature- and energy-dependent process (Black and Dolly 1986 a, 1986b). After the toxins are internalized, the amino terminus of the H chain is believed to mediate the translocation of the L chain across the endosomal membrane into the cytoplasm. The low pH environment of the endosome may trigger a conformational change in the translocation domain, thus forming a channel for the L chain to enter the nerve cell cytosol (Simpson 1989), although there are numerous hypotheses as to how this process might occur (Pellizzari et al. 1999).

Intracellular Action

The final step in the intoxication of nerve cells involves catalytic hydrolysis of key proteins in acetylcholine-containing vesicles. The L chains of botulinum neurotoxins are zinc-dependent endoproteases (Schiavo et al. 1992b) that inactivate essential proteins involved in the docking and fusion of synaptic vesicles to the plasma membrane. This inactivation prevents release of the neurotransmitter by the cell, resulting in neuromuscular paralysis. Three synaptic proteins, the so-called SNARE (soluble N-ethylmaleimide-sensitive-factor attachment protein receptor) proteins, have been identified as targets of botulinum neurotoxins (Pelizzarri 1999; Herreros 2000). Types B, D, F, and G have been demonstrated to cleave VAMP (synaptic vesicle-associated membrane protein), each at a single, distinct peptide bond; types A, C_1, and E cleave a protein called SNAP-25 (synaptosomal-associated protein of 25kDa), each at a single, distinct peptide bond. Type C_1 is unique in that it is the only neurotoxin that has been demonstrated to cleave syntaxin, as well as SNAP-25 (Blasi et al. 1993). Recently, numerous isoforms of the SNARE proteins have been identified in different species and tissues, but only some of them are susceptible to the proteolytic activity of botulinum neurotoxins, which may account for species insensitivity to certain types of toxin (Humeau et al. 2000). Toxin resistance may also be caused by the absence of specific membrane receptors.

Tetanus, another clostridial neurotoxin produced by *C. tetani*, has a similar molecular mechanism of action as botulinum toxin; however, tetanus toxin affects central nervous system synapses of the spinal cord (Wellhoner 1992) rather than peripheral nerves. Interestingly, studies have shown that tetanus cleaves VAMP at the exact same peptide bond as botulinum neurotoxin B (Schiavo 1992a), but because of their different sites of action, when injected into an animal they cause the opposite syndromes of tetanus (spastic paralysis) and botulism (flaccid paralysis). Another important distinction is that tetanus toxin is not complexed with other proteins as are the seven botulinum neurotoxins; therefore, it does not survive oral administration but rather enters the body solely through wounds.

C_2 Toxin

C_2 toxin, the other protein toxin associated with *C. botulinum* types C and D strains, is not a neurotoxin and does not block neurotransmitter release or neuromuscular function (Simpson 1982). Instead, effects in laboratory animals are characterized by increased movement of fluids across membranes, including increased vascular permeability, effusive secretions into the airway, pulmonary edema and bleeding, collection of fluids in the thoracic cavity, and extreme hypotension. C_2 is a binary toxin consisting of two separate and independent polypeptides, an H and an L chain, that require activation with trypsin. The H chain mediates binding of the toxin to cell membranes (Ohishi 1983), and the L chain has been shown to possess ADP-ribosylating activity similar to toxins produced by *C. perfringens* and *C. spiriforme* (Simpson 1989).

Jensen and Duncan (1980) evaluated the potential hazard of C_2 toxin for waterbirds with experimental studies in Mallards. By intravenous (IV) inoculation, C_2 toxin was found to have an LD_{50} for Mallards of 2.4 mouse IP LD_{50}'s compared to 3,000 mouse IP LD_{50}'s for C_1 (Table 21.6); C_2 toxin was greater than 1,000-fold more toxic than C_1. In peracute cases in which Mallards received > 32 mouse IP LD_{50}'s of C_2 toxin, birds died within two hours after inoculation, with respiratory distress and convulsions. Upon necropsy, massive pulmonary edema and congestion were observed; lungs were saturated with serous fluid, sometimes quite bloody. However, oral administration of C_2 toxin did not produce the same result; most birds showed no signs at doses as high as 6,000 mouse IP LD_{50}'s. These results are similar to those obtained by Ohishi and Das-Gupta (1987) in mice and geese, where lethality by IV administration was nearly equivalent in the two species despite their great difference in size, and much greater than the lethality of C_1 toxin by IV administration (Table 21.6). The significance of these findings are unknown. The presence of C_2 toxin in wild birds has never been demonstrated; however, organisms that produce C_2 toxin are quite prevalent in wetland sediments that waterbirds frequent and in which botulism outbreaks are common (Sandler et al. 1993).

Adjuvant Effect of Type C and E Toxin

On occasion, both type C and type E toxin have been found in different birds during a botulism die-off or even in the same carcass (Brand et al. 1983). Jensen and Gritman (1966) reported a synergistic effect on

Table 21.6. Lethality of C_1 and C_2 toxins in mice, geese, and mallards in mouse intraperitoneal (IP) 50% lethal dose units. (Modified from Ohishi and DasGupta 1987, and Jensen and Duncan 1980.)

		Lethality in		
Toxin	Route	Mice	Geese	Mallards
C_1	IV	4.8	100,000	3,000
	Oral	120,000	10,000,000	>50,000
C_2	IV	0.11	0.5	2.4
	Oral	6,000	5,000	

toxicity in birds that was not simply additive when the two toxin types were administered together. The mechanism for this synergism is unknown, as is its importance in outbreaks in wild birds.

PATHOLOGY

Animals dead of botulism typically have no obvious lesions. Congestion and/or hyperemia of various organs has been described but is a nonspecific finding. The crop, proventriculus, and gizzard are frequently empty, except for grit and, occasionally, small quantities of food material. Dilation of the colon with fluid and urates has been described (Hobmaier 1932). Infrequently, ingesta containing botulinum toxin is present in the digestive tract. Maggots are occasionally detected in the upper digestive tract, especially in ducklings, and if present, is highly suggestive of type C intoxication. Fish in the digestive tract may be the source of type E toxin. Maggots and other invertebrates are broken down within hours of ingestion, often prior to the animal's death, and may still be the source of toxin even when they are not detected in the upper digestive tract (Wobeser and Galmut 1984). Carcasses may be dehydrated and leeches may be present in the nasal and oral cavity. Marked pulmonary edema and congestion, and, occasionally, hemorrhage have been reported in ducks experimentally challenged with C_2 toxin (Jensen and Duncan 1980).

DIAGNOSIS

A presumptive diagnosis of botulism is often based on a combination of clinical signs observed in sick birds (bilateral paralysis of wings and legs, paralysis of the nictitating membrane, and limberneck) and the absence of obvious lesions of disease upon necropsy of sick and dead birds. However, this assumption must be confirmed by laboratory tests that demonstrate the presence of botulinum toxin in blood or tissue in order to separate avian botulism from algal toxicoses, castor-bean poisoning, and other toxic processes. During a group die-off, when botulism is suspected, it is important to collect blood for botulism testing from moribund birds or very freshly dead birds, because post-mortem formation of botulinum toxin may occur in older carcasses, making interpretation of the results subject to question. Individual birds afflicted with botulism may have low quantities of toxin in their blood, not detectable by current methods. Therefore, in a die-off event, it is advisable to test a number of birds with varying degrees of morbidity.

The most widely used test for the diagnosis of avian botulism is the mouseprotection test (Quortrup and Sudheimer 1943a). Blood samples are collected from sick birds by venipuncture or from the hearts of freshly dead birds and centrifuged. The serum fraction is inoculated into two groups of laboratory mice, one of which has been previously protected with type-specific antitoxin. The sample is considered positive for botulinum toxin if the protected mouse survives and the unprotected mouse either dies or is observed sick with characteristic signs (hind limb paralysis, contracted abdomen typically called wasp waist, and labored breathing). Although the mouse test is still considered the most sensitive test for all botulinum types, false negatives are possible (Thomas 1991; Rocke et al. 2004). Cattle and horses (Galey et al. 2000), and possibly some birds, may be more sensitive to botulinum toxin than the bioassay mouse. Nonspecific mortality in test mice from bacteria or other contaminants can obscure the results.

Various enzyme-linked immunosorbent assays (ELISA) have been described and used with varying success for the detection of botulinum neurotoxin, including type C toxin (Thomas 1991). The advantages of ELISA over traditional mouse neutralization tests are that it is significantly cheaper and does not use live animals. Most of these tests are performed using microplates, which require a plate reader and other specialized equipment. Unfortunately, blood and tissue samples from dead animals are not always suitable for testing on microplates, because they often result in high background staining and nonspecific reactions. Rocke et al. (1998) recently described a very simple, antigen-capture ELISA, utilizing immunosticks as the solid substrate, for diagnosis of type C botulism in wild birds using whole blood or serum. The advantage of this ELISA is that large volumes of blood can be tested, effectively concentrating toxin in the sample. This test has been used successfully for confirming type C botulism in birds as well as mammals (Galey et al. 2000; Swift et al. 2000).

Some investigators have used molecular techniques for detection of *C. botulinum* type C bacteria in animal tissues and environmental samples. Both Franciosa et al. (1996) and Fach et al. (1996) described polymerase chain reaction (PCR) assays that were used to detect C_1 toxin gene after enrichment of tissues or intestinal contents in culture media. However, these assays are not valid for diagnosis of botulism in waterfowl and other animals because dormant spores of *C. botulinum* that would germinate in culture media can be found in the tissues of healthy animals (Reed and Rocke 1992). Nol et al. (2004) described a more appropriate PCR assay, whereby only the DNA from vegetative cells (not spores) is extracted directly from environmental samples or tissues without an initial enrichment step. Because this PCR assay detects the C_1 toxin gene only in vegetative cells, it might be useful for diagnosing toxico-infections, although it would be difficult to conclude with any certainty that botulinum cells were replicating *in vivo* and not just recently ingested along with toxin.

IMMUNITY

In most animals, natural host immune defenses probably do not play a significant role in either the pathogenesis of botulism or in prevention of the disease. The toxin is so poisonous that the amount required to immunize an animal is much higher than the lethal dose. However, in one study (Ohishi et al. 1979), naturally occurring antibodies to botulinum neurotoxins (types A–F) were found in several carrion-eating species, including 18/20 Turkey Vultures (*Cathartes aura*), 5/12 American Crows (*Corvus brachyrhynchos*), and 25/110 coyotes (*Canis latrans*) tested with a passive hemagglutination assay (PHA). It is unknown whether these antibodies were protective for the host, because none of the animals were challenged; however, neutralization tests in mice confirmed the PHA results. The highest antibody titer was found in a vulture; antibody titers against type C toxin were 1:8192, and measurable antibody titers were found in descending order against types D, F, E, A, and B toxins. Botulism has never been reported in any of these species, and it is possible that they are innately more resistant to the paralytic effects of neurotoxin. Turkey vultures are highly resistant to both orally administered and injected type C toxin, as well as injected type A and B toxins (Kalmbach 1939). This may be explained by failure of toxin to bind at presynaptic nerve endings (Cohen 1970).

Another possibility is that the sero-positive animals developed antibody to toxin in response to a nonlethal toxico-infection in the gut (Ohishi et al. 1979) or through repeated ingestion of sublethal doses of toxin. Ring-billed Gulls administered low doses of type E toxin over a period of three weeks were more resistant to challenge (80% survival) with lethal doses of the toxin compared to nonimmunized control gulls (17% survival; Kaufmann and Crecelius 1967). Interestingly, in 1999, type C botulism was confirmed in a captive-bred California Condor (*Gymnogyps californianus*) with signs of acute progressive paralysis (NWHC, unpublished data).[1] This bird was fed dead calves and road-killed rabbits. It was speculated that the absence of exposure to botulinum toxin early in life may have resulted in a lack of resistance to the toxin upon ingestion of natural carrion.

Botulinum toxin can be inactivated with formaldehyde to produce a toxoid that is immunogenic upon administration to animals. These toxoids have been used to prevent botulism in domestic and captive-reared animals. Type C toxoids have been used to vaccinate game-farm pheasants (Kurazono et al. 1985), captive ducks (Schwartz and Smart 1963), and waterbirds in a zoological collection (Cambre and Kenny 1993). Although none of these animals were challenged experimentally with botulinum toxin, higher survival rates of vaccinated birds compared to unvaccinated birds in the face of natural botulism die-offs provide some empirical evidence that immunization was successful in these cases. Further experimental studies in captive birds by Martinez and Wobeser (1999) and Rocke et al. (2000) demonstrated that a single dose of type C botulinum toxoid administered by subcutaneous injection could improve the survival of Mallards and Green-winged Teal (*Anas crecca*) during botulism epizootics; however, the level of protection afforded was limited and decreased with increasing amounts of toxin in the challenge dose. A second immunization significantly enhanced immunity in one study (Schwartz and Smart 1963), and the addition of adjuvant also improved vaccine efficacy (Boroff and Reilly 1959). More recently, a vaccine derived from recombinant whole heavy chain fragments of type C toxin has been used to successfully immunize ducks (Arimitsu et al. 2004).

In captive birds, where boosters can be administered at regular intervals, vaccination against botulism is probably useful. Vaccination might also be considered a potential option for protecting small populations of endangered species that can be safely captured. However, current methods of immunization that require inoculation of individual animals are impractical for protecting most free-ranging populations of birds.

PUBLIC HEALTH CONCERNS

Humans contract botulism through food poisoning, gut toxigenesis, or infected wounds, but in no case has botulism in wild birds been associated with the disease in humans. Type A and B botulism occur most commonly in humans, but type E also occurs with some regularity and is typically associated with consumption of contaminated fish or other marine products (McLaughlin et al. 2004). In 1963 the occurrence of type E botulism in birds in the Great Lakes coincided with increased cases in humans (Hobbs 1976) and potentially could have been used as a warning system for spore contamination of fish products from these areas.

Type C botulism has been confirmed in only one case, an infant with gut toxigenesis (Oguma et al. 1990), and humans are not thought to be very susceptible to this serotype. However, type C botulism has been confirmed in several primate species (Smart et al. 1980; Smith et al. 1985) that consumed contaminated meat, and *in vitro* studies have demonstrated that type C toxin can paralyze human neuromuscular transmission (Coffield et al. 1997).

DOMESTIC ANIMAL HEALTH CONCERNS

Type C and E botulism occur in a number of domestic animals, but the disease is very rarely the result of association with wild birds. Type C is the most common form of botulism in dogs, but the disease occurs infrequently. Most reports have been in the hound breeds and have been linked to feeding on carrion or improperly processed or raw meat (Darke et al. 1976; Barsanti et al. 1978). In one report, young dogs became sick with type C botulism after feeding on a rotten duck carcass (Farrow et al. 1983). *Clostridium botulinum* type C was isolated from other duck carcasses and soil from the pond where the original carcass was eaten.

Type C botulism has been reported in poultry, pheasants, horses, and cattle (Rocke 1993). Outbreaks are often associated with the consumption of decaying carcasses in feed, consumption of maggots from carcasses, and contaminated poultry litter. Recently, cattle contracted type C botulism after grazing immediately adjacent to a lake with a large botulism outbreak in waterfowl. Although the source of toxin was not determined, duck carcasses and/or maggots were likely involved, as both were abundant on shore and in the water where the cattle drank (Wobeser et al. 1997). This was the first report of type C botulism in livestock associated with botulism in wild waterfowl.

Type E botulism is a frequent cause of mortality in fish-rearing operations, and accumulation of carcasses on fish farms can result in heavy contamination of the environment with spores (Eklund et al. 1984).

WILDLIFE POPULATION IMPACTS

Avian botulism is arguably the most significant disease of ducks and various other aquatic birds, yet its effect on populations is poorly understood. Samuel (1992) attempted to evaluate the effects of botulism on mid-continent Mallards and determined that more reliable estimates of daily probability of mortality are needed before conclusions can be drawn. Information on annual and spatial variation in botulism occurrence, as well as estimates of the proportion of birds at risk, are required. Furthermore, research has shown that estimates of total mortality based on carcass retrieval alone underestimates mortality by three (Cliplef 1993) to as much as 10 times (Stutzenbaker et al. 1986; Bollinger, unpublished data)[5]; therefore, current estimates of known outbreaks significantly underestimate losses. Numerous outbreaks are thought to go undetected, because scavenging animals can consume fairly large numbers of carcasses (Stutzenbaker et al. 1986). Survival rate estimates of radio-marked, molting Mallards have shown that severe botulism on lakes can reduce 30-day survival rates to as low as 5% (Evelsizer 2002); however, there is significant variability among lakes and years.

Botulism outbreaks often involve several species; some may be able to withstand high losses, whereas populations of other species may not be as resilient. Mallards, which are numerous, geographically widespread, and have a high reproductive potential, may be able to withstand sporadic heavy losses from botulism. Other less common species, whose populations are disproportionately exposed to botulism, may be more severely impacted by the disease. During the 1990s, Northern Pintail populations remained low, whereas populations of other dabbling ducks increased in response to improving water conditions on the prairies. During the same period, numerous Northern Pintail carcasses were being found during botulism outbreaks. For example, at Old Wives Lake, Saskatchewan; Whitewater Lake, Manitoba; and Pakowki Lake, Alberta, Canada; an estimated 350,000 Northern Pintails died of botulism in 1997 (Bollinger, unpublished data).[5] In the same year, botulism killed an estimated 100,000 Northern Pintails on the Bear River Refuge, Utah, U.S.A. (Miller and Duncan 1999). Botulism may be one of several factors contributing to low Northern Pintail numbers. Virtually nothing is known of the impact of avian botulism on populations of shorebirds, which are frequently involved in type C outbreaks, or fish-eating birds involved in type E outbreaks.

Although the emphasis in migratory birds is often placed on continental or total breeding populations, the effects of botulism on local or regional populations can also be important, because many waterfowl species demonstrate breeding, molting, and wintering-site philopatry (Anderson et al. 1992). Botulism mortality on individual wetlands frequently can reach thousands and occasionally up to a million birds. Outbreaks affecting a large proportion of birds with strong philopatry to these areas can result in local declines. Similarly, if botulism-prone lakes consistently attract birds from a larger geographic area for critical life stages, such as molt and migration, population effects could be regional in scale. One outbreak at Salton Sea in 1996 killed nearly 15% of the western American White Pelican population (Anderson, pers. comm.).[7] Miller and Duncan (1999) suggested that botulism mortality in prairie Northern Pintails could disproportionately affect Pacific Flyway wintering populations.

Losses from avian botulism are best documented for waterfowl. This group of birds is intensively managed for sport hunting, and large sums of money are invested in enhancing habitat for waterfowl production. In some years, losses from avian botulism can reduce production gains. For example, waterfowl mortality in the mid-1990s on a large lake in southeastern Alberta, Canada, exceeded estimated production on North American Waterfowl Management Plan wetlands in prairie Alberta (Neraasen, pers. comm.).[8] The value of a single Mallard has been estimated at U.S. $50 (Cowardin et al. 1995), and although these types of estimates are highly subjective, they can provide an approximation of the cost of botulism outbreaks.

TREATMENT AND CONTROL

Treatment of botulinum-intoxicated ducks (type C) is generally highly successful; survival rates range from 75–90% (Rocke and Friend 1999), although rates may be lower in immature ducks (Hammond 1950) and other waterbird species. Mildly affected birds can be treated by providing easy access to water, food, and shade, and protection from inclement weather and predators. Birds with more severe clinical signs, such as difficulty in walking or complete recumbency, should be orally dosed with water. Injection with type C antitoxin improves survival rates of ducks with moderate to severe clinical signs (Rocke and Friend 1999) and, if given to birds in early stages of the disease, may prevent disease progression. Despite good recovery rates with type C antitoxin, treatment of botulism-intoxicated birds is uncommon due to cost and logistics, especially during large outbreaks. Recovered birds remain susceptible to botulinum toxin and therefore must be moved to botulism-free locations to ensure that they are not re-exposed. Although type E antitoxin is available, it has not been commonly used to treat large numbers of birds during outbreaks, and nothing is known about its effectiveness in treating birds.

Vaccination, either single or with a booster, may be a beneficial adjunct to treatment. A single immunization of intoxicated ducks with botulinum toxoid can protect against subsequent toxin exposure as early as 10 days post-vaccination; it does not interfere with antitoxin treatment and recovery (Martinez and Wobeser 1999).

Although numerous strategies for controlling type C avian botulism have been proposed and implemented, few have been evaluated as to their effectiveness. Virtually nothing is known regarding the control of type E botulism in birds. The most common method of managing type C botulism outbreaks in waterfowl is by removal of carcasses prior to development of maggots in an attempt to prevent transmission of toxin to other birds. This is a logical response, given that research has repeatedly demonstrated the importance of carcasses in propagating outbreaks. Reed and Rocke (1992) found that daily survival rates of sentinel Mallards in field enclosures containing carcasses at densities of 12.5 carcasses per hectare were 4.5 times lower than Mallards in similar pens with no carcasses. In a related study (Rocke, unpublished data),[4] penned Mallards were maintained at a density of 25 to 29 birds/hectare in two adjacent 1.7 ha enclosures and monitored over a three-month period during the summer. When mortality in sentinels from lead poisoning or other causes occurred in both enclosures, carcasses were removed from one (8.8 carcasses/ha removed) but not the other (10.6 carcasses/ha remained). No botulism morbidity or mortality occurred in the enclosure with carcass removal, but 22% of the sentinels contracted botulism in the enclosure without carcass removal.

Unfortunately, carcass removal is quite difficult in some wetlands because of their large acreage and the poor visibility of dead birds in heavily vegetated areas. Cliplef and Wobeser (1993) found that only 1/3 of marked carcasses were detected during clean up operations of a botulism outbreak. In a similar study of seven lakes in Canada, only 7% to 42% of marked carcasses were detected (Bollinger, unpublished data).[5] In several heavily vegetated wetlands, carcass densities of 30–50 per ha were found immediately after cleanup (Bollinger, unpublished data).[5] In these same wetlands, toxic maggots were found on more than 90% of carcasses tested (Bollinger, unpublished data),[5] so the potential for disease spread through the carcass-maggot cycle was very high in this case. However, this number of toxigenic carcasses may not be present during all outbreaks at all locations. In another study, the percentage of carcasses that produced toxic maggots was much lower (29–69%) and not all carcasses became maggot-infested (Rocke and Reed 1992).

Because maggots can develop on carcasses within three to five days (Rocke and Reed 1992; Cliplef and Wobeser 1993), wetlands must be searched frequently to reduce maggot availability for birds. The logistics and costs of this level of carcass cleanup can be very high. For example, the annual cost of carcass removal on Canadian wetlands during the mid 1990s was several hundred thousand dollars Canadian (Cd), peaking at approximately $1 million Cd in 1998 (Kehoe, pers. comm.).[9] A recent study of large wetlands (ranging in size from 400–6,680 ha) found that the survival rate of radio-marked, adult, molting

Mallards was not significantly different between several sites with and without cleanup during botulism outbreaks (Evelsizer, 2002), seriously questioning the cost effectiveness of carcass cleanup for botulism control. However, where wetlands are considerably smaller (< 400 ha) and monitoring for carcasses for early outbreak detection occurs on a regular basis during the summer and fall, carcass pick-up is thought to be effective in reducing losses but has not been formally tested.

Water manipulation has been used, where feasible, to drain known "hot spots" or problem wetlands prior to the warm weather season to prevent outbreaks and also in an attempt to "flush" toxin or dilute toxic material through a wetland complex after an outbreak has started. Again, these strategies have not been formally tested for their effectiveness. Attempts have also been made to control outbreaks by dispersing birds with aircraft (Parrish and Hunter 1969) and with the use of auditory deterrents (Butterworth and Calverley 1997), but neither were very successful.

MANAGEMENT IMPLICATIONS

Prevention of the disease would be a more effective strategy than controlling an outbreak after it begins. However, a better understanding of the ecology of type C botulism is needed to identify host, agent, or environmental factors associated with botulism outbreaks that are amenable to manipulation or management. Because the agent in this case produces dormant spores that are viable for years and widely distributed in the environment, little can be done to reduce botulinum spore prevalence.

Immunization of birds against botulism via vaccine injection is possible for captive-reared or zoo animals, but is not currently feasible for free-ranging waterfowl. Vaccination of endangered species is an option for species at high risk of exposure to botulinum toxin if capture and handling are feasible.

Management or manipulation of wetland factors related to germination of botulinum spores, vegetative cell growth, and toxin availability for birds would appear to be the most feasible alternative for managing the disease in wild waterfowl. One strategy is to reduce available substrate for the growth of the bacteria. Because any vertebrate carcass on a botulism-prone wetland may contain botulinum spores, efforts to reduce vertebrate mortality would likely be beneficial. Power transmission lines are a significant source of avian mortality, and if they cross wetlands heavily utilized by birds, may initiate, or at least exacerbate, botulism outbreaks (Malcolm 1982). On some lakes, high mortality of juvenile colonial aquatic birds, such as Franklin's Gulls and grebes, coincides with botulism outbreaks in ducks. Because these carcasses support toxin production and may be involved in the initiation of botulism outbreaks (Soos 2004; Bollinger, unpublished data),[5] habitat management to reduce densities of birds in these colonies and reduce mortality may be beneficial.

Other forms of organic input into wetlands should be minimized where possible. Flooding and drawdowns of wetlands during the summer are thought to result in die-offs of invertebrates that could provide substrate for toxin production. Toxin has been demonstrated in invertebrate carcasses, but their role in initiating outbreaks has not been clearly established. In zoos and in other urban pond settings where waterfowl congregate, feeding by humans should be discouraged or steps should be taken to reduce or clean up feed that accumulates in the sediments.

Another potential strategy to consider is manipulation of wetland conditions previously shown to be associated with a high risk of botulism outbreaks. The risk-assessment models previously discussed (Figures 21.4, 21.5) could be useful in identifying high-risk wetlands and evaluating appropriate actions for preventing botulism outbreaks when they are most likely to occur (Rocke and Samuel 1999). For example, these risk-assessment models suggest that in alkaline wetlands, management actions that increase water temperature or decrease redox potential could further increase the risk of an outbreak, whereas actions that reduce temperature (that is, flushing with cold water) may help reduce risk. Research to evaluate management practices (for example, timing, level, and duration of flooding, and vegetation management) for their effects on the risk of botulism outbreaks, using the risk-assessment models for guidance, is needed in order to identify those strategies that reduce risk or avoid increasing risk on problem wetlands.

Many botulism-prone wetlands are terminal basins or wetlands created for waterfowl habitat and water retention in otherwise arid environments. In some cases these wetlands may be a net drain on local waterfowl production due to frequent and large botulism outbreaks. Without a better understanding of environmental factors that influence botulism outbreaks, wetland management practices may, in fact, enhance occurrence of the disease in some locations, negating any benefits. Although we have made progress in understanding the ecology of avian botulism in waterbirds, unfortunately our ability to prevent and control catastrophic outbreaks has not improved since the disease was first recognized a century ago.

UNPUBLISHED DATA

1. U. S. Geological Survey, National Wildlife Health Center (NWHC), Madison, WI, U.S.A. NWHC unpublished data is derived from computerized databases that

include information collected by federal, state, territorial, and nongovernment wildlife agencies in the United States; see www.nwhc.usgs.gov/.

2. Canadian Cooperative Wildlife Health Centre (CCWHC), Western College of Veterinary Medicine, University of Saskatchewan, Saskatoon, Saskatchewan, Canada. CCWHC unpublished data is derived from a computerized database that includes information collected by federal, provincial, territorial, and nongovernment wildlife agencies in Canada; see //wildlife.usask.ca.
3. Ian K. Barker, CCWHC, Department of Pathology, Ontario Veeterinary College, University of Guelph, Guelph, Ontario, Canada.
4. Tonie E. Rocke, NWHC.
5. Trent K. Bollinger, CCWHC, Western College of Veterinary Medicine, University of Saskatchewan, Saskatoon, Saskatchewan, Canada.
6. Douglas G. Campbell, CCWHC, Department of Pathology, Ontario Veterinary College, University of Guelph, Guelph, Ontario, Canada.
7. Daniel W. Anderson, Department of Wildlife, Fish, and Conservation Biology, University of California, Davis, CA, U.S.A.
8. Terry Neraasen, Ducks Unlimited Canada, Stonewall, Manitoba, Canada.
9. Pat Kehoe, Ducks Unlimited Canada, Edmonton, Alberta, Canada.

LITERATURE CITED

Adams, S.G., F.M. Conly, C.L. Gratto-Trevor, K.J. Cash, and T. Bollinger. 2003. Shorebird use and mortality at a large Canadian prairie lake impacted by botulism. *Waterbirds* 26:13–125.

Allwright, D.M., M. Wilson, and W.J.J. Van Rensurg. 1994. Botulism in ostriches (Struthio camelus). *Avian Pathology* 23:183–186.

Anderson, M.G., J.M. Rhymer, and F.C. Rohwer. 1992. Philopatry, dispersal, and the genetic structure of waterfowl populations. In *Ecology and Management of Breeding Waterfowl,* B.D.J. Batt, A.D. Afton, M.G. Anderson, C.D. Ankney, D.H. Johnson, J.A. Kadlec, and G.L. Krapu (eds.), University of Minnesota Press, Minneapolis, MN, U.S.A., pp. 365–395.

Arimitsu, H., J-E. Lee, Y. Sakaguchi, Y. Hayakawa, M. Hayashi, M. Nakaura, H. Takai, S-N. Lin, M. Mukamoto, T. Murphy, K. Oguma. 2004. Vaccination with recombinant whole heavy chain fragments of *Clostridium botulinum* type C and D neurotoxins. *Clinical and Diagnostic Immunology* 11:496–502.

Azuma, R. and T. Itoh. 1987. Botulism in waterfowl and distribution of *C. botulinum* type C in Japan. In *Avian Botulism: An International Perspective,* M. W. Eklund and V. R. Dowell Jr. (eds.). Charles C Thomas, Springfield, IL, U.S.A., pp. 167–190.

Bandyopadhyay, S., A.W. Clark, B.R. DasGupta, and V. Sathyamoorthy. 1987. Role of the heavy and light chains of botulinum neurotoxin in neuromuscular paralysis. *Journal of Biological Chemistry* 262:2260–2263.

Barras, S.C., and J.A. Kadlec. 2000. Abiotic predictors of avian botulism outbreaks in Utah. *Wildlife Society Bulletin* 28:724–729.

Barsanti, J.A., M. Walser, C.L. Hatheway, J.M. Bowen, and W. Crowell. 1978. Type C botulism in American foxhounds. *Journal of the American Veterinary Association* 172:809–813.

Bell, J.F., G.W. Sciple, and A.A. Hubert. 1955. A microenvironment concept of the epizoology of avian botulism. *Journal of Wildlife Management* 19:352–357.

Bengston, I.A. 1923. A toxin-producing anaerobe isolated principally from fly larvae. *Public Health Reports* 38:340–344.

BirdLife International 2004. *State of World's Birds 2004: Indicators for Our Changing World.* Cambridge, U.K., p. 45.

Bishopp, F.C. 1923. Limberneck of fowls produced by fly larvae. *Journal of Parasitology* 9:170–173.

Bittner, M.A., B.R. DasGupta, and R.W. Holz. 1989. Isolated light chains of botulinum neurotoxins inhibit exocytosis. *The Journal of Biological Chemistry* 264:10354–10360.

Black, J.D., and J.O. Dolly. 1986a. Interaction of ^{125}I-labeled botulinum neurotoxins with nerve terminals. I. Ultrastructural autoradiographic localization and quantitation of distinct membrane acceptors for types A and B on motor nerves. *Journal of Cell Biology* 103:521–534.

Black, J.D., and J.O. Dolly. 1986b. Interaction of ^{125}I-labeled botulinum neurotoxins with nerve terminals. II. Autoradiographic evidence for its uptake into motor nerves by acceptor-mediated endocytosis. *Journal of Cell Biology* 103:535–544.

Blaker, D. 1967. An outbreak of botulism among waterbirds. *Ostrich* 32:144–147.

Blasi, J.E., R. Chapman, S. Yamasaki, T. Binz, H. Niemann and R. Jahn. 1993. Botulinum neurotoxin C1 blocks neurotransmitter release by means of cleaving HPC-1/syntaxin. *The EMBO Journal* 12:4821–4828.

Borland, E.D., C.J. Moryson, and G.R. Smith. 1977. Avian botulism and the high prevalence of *Clostridium botulinum* in the Norfolk Broads. *The Veterinary Record* 100:106–109.

Boroff, D.A., and J.R. Reilly. 1959. Studies of the toxin of *Clostridium botulinum* V. Prophylactic immunization of pheasants and ducks against avian botulism. *Journal of Bacteriology* 77:142–146.

Bott, T.L., J.S. Deffner, E. McCoy, and E.M. Foster. 1966. *Clostridium botulinum* type E in fish from the Great Lakes. *Journal of Bacteriology* 91(3):919–924.

Bott, T.L., J. Johnson Jr., E.M. Foster, and H. Sugiyama. 1968. Possible origin of the high incidence of *Clostridium botulinum* type E in an inland bay (Green Bay of Lake Michigan). *Journal of Bacteriology* 95:1542–1547.

Brand, C.J., R.M. Duncan, S.P. Garrow, D. Olson, and L.E. Schumann. 1983. Waterbird mortality from botulism type E in lake Michigan: An update. *Wilson Bulletin* 95: 269–275.

Brand, C.J., S.M. Schmitt, R.M. Duncan, and T. M. Cooley. 1988a. An outbreak of type E botulism among common loons (*Gavia immer*) in Michigan's Upper Peninsula. *Journal of Wildlife Diseases* 24:471–476.

Brand, C.J., R.M. Windingstad, L.M. Siegfried, R.M. Duncan, and R. M. Cook. 1988b. Avian morbidity and mortality from botulism, aspergillosis, and salmonellosis at Jamaica Bay Wildlife Refuge, New York, U.S.A. *Colonial Waterbirds* 11:284–292.

Butterworth, E.W., and B.K. Calverley. 1997. Efficacy of the Phoenix Wailer Mark III, an auditory avian deterrent, to reduce bird populations near focal points of botulism mortality on Pakowki lake. Ducks Unlimited Canada, Edmonton, Alberta, CA, 39 pp.

Calsow, P., H. Helbing, C. Ludwig, and R. Schlegelmilch. 1995. An epidemic of botulism in waterfowl on a reservoir. *Tierarztliche Umschau* 50:477–480.

Cambre, R.C., and D. Kenny. 1993. Vaccination of zoo birds against avian botulism with mink botulism vaccine. *Proceedings of the American Association of Zoo Veterinarians* 1993:383–385.

Carpentier, G. 2000. Avian botulism outbreak along the lower Great Lakes. *Ontario Birds* 18:84–81.

Cato, E.P., W.L. George, and S.M. Finegold. 1986. Genus *Clostridium*. In *Bergey's Manual of Systematic Bacteriology,* Vol. 2, P.H.A. Sneath, N.S. Mair, M.E. Sharpe, and J.G. Holt (eds.). Williams and Wilkins, Baltimore, U.S.A., pp. 1141–1200.

Chambers, L. 1995. Purple martin die-offs during the summer of 1995. *Purple Martin Update* 6:24–25.

Chen, F., G.M. Kuziemko, and R.C. Stevens. 1998. Biophysical characterization of the stability of the 150-kilodalton botulinum toxin, the nontoxic component, and the 900-kilodalton botulinum toxin complex species. *Infection and Immunity* 66:2420–2425.

Cliplef, D.J., and G. Wobeser. 1993. Observations on waterfowl carcasses during a botulism epizootic. *Journal of Wildlife Diseases* 29:8–14.

Coburn, D.R., and E.R. Quortrup. 1938. The distribution of botulinus toxin in duck sickness areas. *Transactions of the North American Wildlife Conference* 3:869–876.

Coffield, J.A., N. Bakry, R. Zhang, J. Carlson, L.G. Gomella, and L.L. Simpson. 1997. In vitro characterization of botulinum toxin types A, C and D action on human tissues: combined electrophysiologic, pharmacologic and molecular biologic approaches. *Journal of Pharmacology and Experimental Therapeutics* 280:1489–1498.

Cohen, G.M. 1970. Studies on the resistance of roosters and vultures to type A botulinal toxin. Ph.D. thesis. Florida State University, Tallahassee, FL, U.S.A., 94 pp.

Cooch, F.G. 1964. A preliminary study of the survival value of a functional salt gland in prairie anatidae. *The Auk* 81:380–393.

Cowardin, L.M., T.L. Shaffer, and K.M. Kraft. 1995. How much habitat management is needed to meet mallard production objectives? *Wildlife Society Bulletin* 23:48–55.

Darke, P.G.G., T.A. Roberts, J.L. Smart, and P.R. Bradshaw. 1976. Suspected botulism in foxhounds. *Veterinary Record* 99:98–99.

DasGupta, B.R., and H. Sugiyama. 1972. Role of protease in natural activation of *Clostridium botulinum* neurotoxin. *Infection and Immunity* 6:587–590.

Dautter, D.A., S.M. Harmon Jr. R.K. Lynt, and T. Lilly Jr. 1996. Antagonistic effect on *Clostridium botulinum* type E by organisms resembling it. *Applied Microbiology* 14:616–622.

de Paiva, A., B. Poulain, G.W. Lawrence, C.C. Shone, L. Tauc and J.O. Dolly. 1993. A role for the interchain disulfide or its participating thiols in the internalization of botulinum neurotoxin A revealed by a toxin derivative that binds to ecto-acceptors and inhibits transmitter release intracellularly. *Journal of Biological Chemistry* 268:20838–20844.

Dohms, J.E. 1987. Laboratory investigation of botulism in poultry. In *Avian Botulism: An International Perspective,* M.W. Eklund and V.R. Dowell Jr. (eds.). Charles C Thomas, Springfield, IL, U.S.A., pp. 295–314.

Domske, H.M., and E.C. Obert. 2001. *Avian Botulism in Lake Erie: Workshop Proceedings.* New York Sea Grant and Pennsylvania Sea Grant, Pennsylvania State University, Erie, PA, U.S.A. [Online.] Retrieved from the World Wide Web: www.pserie.psu.edu/seagrant/extension/extension.html

Doutre, M.P. 1979. Un foyer de botulisme de type D, lie a des modifications du mileu naturel, observe chez des pelicans (*Pelicanus rufescens*) du Senegal (Petite Cote). *Revue D'Elevage et de Médecine Vétérinaire des Pays Tropicaux* 32:131–134.

Duncan, R.M., and W.I. Jensen. 1976. A relationship between avian carcasses and living invertebrates in the epizootiology of avian botulism. *Journal of Wildlife Diseases* 12:116–126.

Eklund, M.W., and F.T. Poysky. 1970. Distribution of *Clostridium botulinum* on the Pacific Coast of the United States. In *Toxic Microorganisms,* M. Herzberg (ed.),

U.S. Department of the Interior, Washington, D.C., U.S.A., pp. 304–308.

Eklund, M.W., F.T. Poysky, M.E. Peterson, L.W. Peck, and W.D. Brunson. 1984. Type E botulism in salmonids and conditions contributing to outbreaks. *Aquaculture* 41:293–309.

Eklund, M.W., F.T. Poysky, E. Oguma, H. Iida, and K. Inoue. 1987. Relationship of bacteriophages to toxin and hemagglutinin production by *Clostridium botulinum* types C and D and its significance in avian botulism outbreaks. In *Avian Botulism: An International Perspective,* M.W. Eklund and V.R. Dowell Jr. (eds.). Charles C Thomas, Springfield, IL, U.S.A., pp. 191–222.

Eklund, M.W., F.T. Poysky, and W.H. Habig. 1989. Bacteriophages and plasmids in *Clostridium botulinum* and *Clostridium tetani* and their relationship to production of toxins. In *Botulinum Neurotoxin and Tetanus Toxin,* L.L. Simpson (ed.). Academic Press, Inc., San Diego, CA, U.S.A., pp. 25–51.

Eleopra, R., V. Tugnoli, O. Rossetto, C. Montecucco, and D. De Grandis. 1997. Botulinum neurotoxin serotype C: a novel effective botulinum toxin therapy in human. *Neuroscience Letters* 224:91–94.

Eleopra, R., V. Tugnoli, O. Rossetto, D. De Grandis, and C. Montecucco. 1998. Different time courses of recovery after poisoning with botulinum neurotoxin serotypes A and E in humans. *Neuroscience Letters* 256:135–138.

Emodi, A.S., and R.V. Lechowich. 1969. Low temperature growth of type E Clostridium botulinum spores. (2) Effects of solutes and incubation temperature. *Journal of Food Science* 34:82–87.

Evelsizer, D.D. 2002. Management of avian botulism and survival of molting mallards. MSc thesis. University of Saskatchewan, Saskatoon, Sask, CA, 59 leaves.

Fach, P., M. Gibert, R. Griffais, and M.R. Popoff. 1996. Investigation of animal botulism outbreaks by PCR and standard methods. *FEMS Immunology and Medical Microbiology* 13:279–285.

Farrow, B.R.H., W.G. Murrell, M.L. Revington, B.J. Stewart, and R. M. Zuber. 1983. Type C botulism in young dogs. *Australian Veterinary Journal* 60:374–377.

Fay, L.D., O. W. Kaufmann, and L.A. Ryel. 1965. Mass mortality of water-birds in Lake Michigan 1963-64. In *Proceedings: Eighth Conference on Great Lakes Research 1965.* Great Lakes Research Division Publication, University of Michigan, Anne Arbor, MI, U.S.A., pp. 36–46.

Franciosa, G., L. Fenicia, C. Caldiani, and P. Aureli. 1996. PCR for detection of *Clostridium botulinum* type C in avian and environmental samples. *Journal of Clinical Microbiology* 34:882–885.

Fujii, N., K. Oguma, N. Yukosawa, K. Kimura, and K. Tsuzuki. 1988. Characterization of bacteriophage nucleic acids obtained from *Clostridium botulinum* types c and d. *Applied Environmental Microbiology* 54:69–73.

Fujinaga Y., K. Inoue, S. Watanabe, K. Yokota, Y. Hirai, E. Nagamachi, and K. Oguma. 1997. The haemagglutinin of *Clostridium botulinum* type C progenitor toxin plays an essential role in binding of toxin to the epithelial cells of guinea pig small intestine, leading to the efficient absorption of the toxin. *Microbiology* 143:3481–3487.

Galey, F.D., R. Terra, R. Walker, J. Adaska, M.A. Etchebarne, B. Puschner, R. H. Whitlock, T.E. Rocke, D. Willoughby, E. Tor. 2000. Type C botulism in dairy cattle from feed contaminated with a dead cat. *Journal of Veterinary Diagnostic Investigation* 12:204–209.

Giltner, I.T., and J.F. Couch. 1930. Western duck sickness and botulism. *Science* 72:660.

Gophen, M., A. Cohen, K. Grinberg, S. Pokamunski, E. Nili, D. Wynne, A. Yawetz, A. Dotan, A. Zook-Rimon, M. Ben-Shlomo, and Z. Ortenberg. 1991. Implications of botulism outbreaks in gulls (*Larus ridibundus*) on the watershed management of Lake Kinneret (Israel). *Environmental Toxicology and Water Quality: An International Journal* 6:77–84.

Gorreau, J.M., O. Debaere, P. Raevel, F. Lamarque, P. Fardel, H. Knockaert, J. Catel, F. Moutou and M. Popoff. 1998. Study of a type E botulism outbreak in gulls (*Larus ridibundus* and *L. argentatus*) in the Bay of Canche (Pas-de-Calais, France). *Gibier Faune Sauvage* 15:357–363.

Graham, J.M. 1978. Inhibition of *Clostridium botulinum* type C by bacteria isolated from mud. *Journal of Applied Microbiology* 45:205–211.

Graham, J.M., G.R. Smith, E.D. Borland, and J.W. MacDonald. 1978. Botulism in winter and spring and the stability of *Clostridium botulinum* type C toxin. *Veterinary Record* 102:40–41.

Graham, R. and I.B. Boughton. 1923. *Clostridium botulinum* type C, a pathogenic anaerobe associated with limberneck-like disease in chickens and ducks. *Illinois Agricultural Experiment Station, Bulletin 246,* 34 pp.

Graikoski, J.T., E.W. Bowman, R.A. Robohm, and R.A. Koch. 1968. Distribution of *Clostridium botulinum* in the ecosystem of the Great Lakes. In *Proceedings of the First U.S.-Japan Conference on Toxic Microorganisms. Mycotoxins, Botulism.,* M. Herzberg (ed.), U.S. Government Printing Office, Washington, D.C., U.S.A., pp. 271–277.

Grecz, N., and L.H. Arvay. 1982. Effect of temperature on spore gemination and vegetative cell growth of *Clostridium botulinum. Applied and Environmental Microbiology* 43:331–337.

Gunnison, J.B., J.R. Cummings, and K.F. Meyer. 1935. *Clostridium botulinum* type E. *Proceedings of the Society for Experimental Biology and Medicine* 35:278–280.

Haagsma, J. 1973. Etiology and epidemiology of botulism in waterfowl in the Netherlands. *Hydrobiological Bulletin* 7:96–105.

Haagsma, J. 1975. Sensitivity of eels (*Anguilla anguilla*) and carp (*Cyprinus carpio*) to type C and Type E botlinum toxin. *Zentralblatt fur Bakteriologie, Parasitenkiunde, Infecktionshkrankheiten und Hygiene, Abeilung I Originale* A 230:59–66.

Haagsma, J. 1987. Laboratory investigation of botulism in wild birds. In *Avian Botulism: An International Perspective,* M.W. Eklund, and V.R. Dowell Jr. (eds.). Charles C Thomas, Springfield, IL, U.S.A., pp. 283–293.

Haagsma, J., H.J. Over, Th. Smit, and J. Hoekstra. 1972. Botulism in waterfowl in the Netherlands in 1970. *Netherland Journal of Veterinary Science* 5:12–33.

Halpern, J.L., and E. A. Neale. 1995. Neurospecific binding, internalization, and retrograde axonal transport. *Current Topics in Microbiology and Immunology* 195:221–241.

Hammond, M.C. 1950. Some observations on sex ratio of ducks contracting botulism in North Dakota. *Journal of Wildlife Management* 14:209–214.

Hatheway, C.L. 1995. Botulism: the present status of the disease. *Current Topics in Microbiology and Immunology* 195:55–75.

Hauser, D., M. Gibert, P. Boquet, and M.R. Popoff. 1992. Plasmid localization of a type E botulinal neurotoxin gene homologue in toxigenic *Clostridium butyricum* strains, and absence of this gene in non-toxigenic *C. butyricum* strains. *FEMS Microbiological Letters* 99:251–256.

Hay, C.M., H.N. van der Made, and P.C. Knoetze. 1973. Isolation of *Clostridium botulinum* type C from an outbreak of botulism in geese. *Journal of the South African Veterinary Medical Association* 44:53–56.

Herreros, J.G. Lalli, C. Montecucco, and G. Schiavo. 1999. Pathophysiological properties of clostridial neurotoxins. In *The Comprehensive Sourcebook of Bacterial Protein Toxins,* J.E. Alouf and J.H. Freer (eds.). Academic Press, London, U.K., pp. 292–228.

Hobbs, G. 1976. *Clostridium botulinum* in fishery products. *Advances in Food Research* 22:135–185.

Hobmaier, M. 1930. Duck disease caused by the toxin of *Clostridium botulinum* type C. *Proceedings of the Society of Experimental Biology and Medicine* 28: 339–340.

Hobmaier, M. 1932. Conditions and control of botulism (duck disease) in waterfowl. *California Fish and Game* 18:5–21.

Hofer, J.W., and J. Davis. 1972. Survival and dormancy. *Texas Medicine* 68:80–81.

Horvath, J., A. Lelkes, E. Futo, and J. Lakatos. 1994. Botulism at Kis-Balaton in 1988 and 1993. *Aquila* 101:225–226.

Hubalek, Z., and J. Halouzka. 1988. Thermal sensitivity of *Clostridium botulinum* type C toxin. *Epidemiology and Infection* 101:321–325.

Hubalek, Z., and J. Halouzka. 1991. Persistence of *Clostridium botulinum* type C toxin in blow fly (Calliphoridae) larvae as a possible cause of avian botulism in spring. *Journal of Wildlife Diseases* 27:81–85.

Humeau, Y., F. Doussau, N.J. Grant, and B. Poulain. 2000. How botulinum and tetanus neurotoxins block neurotransmitter release. *Biochimie* 82:427–446.

Hunter, B. F. 1970. Ecology of waterfowl botulism toxin production. *Transactions of the Thirty-fifth North American Wildlife and Natural Resources Conference* 35:64–72.

Hunter, B.F., W. E. Clark, P.J. Perkins, and P.R. Coleman. 1970. *Applied Botulism Research including Management Recommendations—A Progress Report.* California Department of Fish and Game, Sacramento, CA, U.S.A., 87 pp.

Huss, H.H. 1980. Distribution of *Clostridium botulinum. Applied and Environmental Microbiology* 39:764–769.

Hyun, S., and G. Sakaguchi. 1989. Implication of coprophagy in pathogenesis of chicken botulism. *Japanese Journal of Veterinary Science* 51:582–586.

Itoh, T.S., and T. Kiyoshi. 1978. Experimental botulism in wild ducks and toxin production of *Clostridium botulinum* type C. *Bulletin of Azabu Veterinary College* 3:75–81.

Jensen, W.I., and J.P. Allen. 1960. A possible relationship between aquatic invertebrates and avian botulism. *Transactions of the North American Wildlife and Natural Resources Conference* 25:171–180.

Jensen, W.I., and R.M. Duncan. 1980. The susceptibility of the mallard duck (*Anas platyrhynchos*) to *Clostridium botulinum* C_2 toxin. *Japanese Journal of Medical Science and Biology* 33:81–86.

Jensen, W.I., and R.B. Gritman. 1966. An adjuvant effect between *Clostridium botulinum* type C and E toxins in the mallard duck (*Anas platyrhynchos*). In *Botulism,* M. Ingram and T. A. Roberts (eds.). Chapman and Hall Limited, London, U.K., pp. 407–413.

Jensen, W.I., and J.I. Price. 1987. The global importance of type C botulism in wild birds. In *Avian Botulism: An International Perspective,* M. W. Eklund and V. R. Dowell Jr. (eds.). Charles C Thomas, Springfield, IL, U.S.A., pp. 33–54.

Jenzer, G., M. Mumenthaler, H.P. Ludin, and F. Robert. 1975. Autonomic dysfunction in botulism B: A clinical report. *Neurology* 25:150–153.

Johannsen, A. 1963. *Clostridium botulinum* in Sweden and the adjacent waters. *Journal of Applied Bacteriology* 26:43–47.

Jubilo, K. and F. Lamarque. 1998. Botulism in waterfowl: situation in France in 1996. *Gibier Faune Sauvage* 15:507–512.

Jude, D.J. 1992. Establishment of Gobiidae in the Great Lakes Basin. *Canadian Journal of Fish and Aquatic Science* 49:416–421.

Kalmbach, E.R. 1930. Western duck sickness produced experimentally. *Science* 72:658–659.

Kalmbach, E.R. 1932. Progress in western duck sickness studies. *Science* 75:57–58.

Kalmbach, E.R. 1939. American vultures and the toxin of *Clostridium botulinum. Journal of American Veterinary Medical Association* 47:187–191.

Kalmbach, E.R. 1968. Type C botulism among wild birds—A historical sketch. *Bureau of Sport Fisheries and Wildlife Special Scientific Report* No. 110, 8 pp.

Kalmbach, E.R., and M.F. Gunderson. 1934. Western duck sickness: a form of botulism. *U.S. Department of Agriculture Technical Bulletin 411,* 82 pp.

Kaufmann, O.W. and E.M. Crecelius. 1967. Experimentally induced immunity in gulls to type E botulism. *American Journal of Veterinary Research* 28: 1857–1862.

Koenig, M.G., A. Spickard, M.A. Cardella, and D. E. Rogers. 1964. Clinical and laboratory observations on type E botulism in man. *Medicine* 43:517–545.

Kriek, N.P.J,. and M.W. Odendaal. 1994. Botulism. In *Infectious Diseases of Livestock with Special Reference to Southern Africa,* J.W.W. Coetzer, G.R. Thomson, and R.C. Tustin (eds.). Oxford University Press, Oxford, U.K., pp. 1354–1368.

Kurazono, H.K. Shimozawa, G. Sakaguchi, M. Takahashi, T. Shimizu, and H. Kondo. 1985. Botulism among penned pheasants and protection by vaccination with C1 toxoid. *Research in Veterinary Science* 38:104–108.

Kuznetzov, E.A. 1992. Botulism in wild waterfowl in the USSR. In *Diseases and Parasites of Wild Animals.* Ministry of Ecology and Natural Resources of Russia, Moscow, Russia, pp. 112–122. (In Russian.)

Lawson, P.A. P. Llop-Perez, R. A. Hutson, H. Hippe, M.D. Collins. 1993. Towards a phylogeny of the clostridia based on 16S rRNA sequences. *FEMS Microbiology Letters* 113:87–92.

Lee, V.H., V. Srikrishnan, and R.P. Hanson. 1962. Blow fly larvae as a source of botulinum toxin for game farm pheasants. *Journal of Wildlife Management* 26:411–413.

Lee, W.H., and H. Riemann. 1970. Correlation of toxic and nontoxic strains of Clostridium botulinum by DNA composition and homology. *Journal of Genetics and Microbiology* 60:117–123.

Leon, A.J., D.M. Infante, C. de Noguera, E. Pulgar, G.C. Quiroz, A. J. Herrera, and P. Valdillo. 1989. Brotes de botulismo tipo C en Aves. *Veterinaria Tropical* 14:37–42.

Leyer, G.J., and E.A. Johnson. 1990. Repression of toxin production by tryptophan in Clostridium botulinum type E. *Archives of Microbiology* 154:443–447.

Li, Z.J. 1990. Study on animal botulism in Anxi-Dunhuang grasslands of China. *Journal of Toxicology* 9:113.

Lloyd, C.S., G.J. Thomas, J.W. MacDonald, E.D. Borland, K. Standring, J.L. Smith. 1976. Wild bird mortality caused by botulism in Britain 1975. *Biological Conservation* 10:119–129.

MacDonald, J.W., and K.T. Standring. 1978. An outbreak of botulism in gulls on the Firth of Forth, Scotland. *Biological Conservation* 14:149–155.

Maksymowych, A.B., M. Reinhard, C.J. Malizio, M.C. Goodnough, and E.A. Johnson. 1999. Pure botulinum neurotoxin is absorbed from the stomach and small intestine and produces peripheral neuromuscular blockade. *Infection and Immunity* 67:4708–4712.

Malcolm, J.M. 1982. Bird collisions with a power transmission line and their relation to botulism at a Montana wetland. *Wildlife Society Bulletin* 10:297–304.

Martinez, R. and G. Wobeser. 1999. Immunization of ducks for type C botulism. *Journal of Wildlife Diseases* 35:710–715.

Matveev, K.I., and N.D. Konstantinova. 1974. The role played by migrating birds in the distribution of the botulism agent. *Hygiene and Sanitation* 12:91–92.

McCroskey, L.M., C.L. Hatheway, L. Fenicia, B. Pasolini, and P. Aureli. 1986. Charcterization of an organism that produces type E botulinal toxin but which resembles *Clostridium butyricum* from the feces of an infant with type E botulism. *Journal of Clinical Microbiology* 23:201–202.

McLaughlin, J.B., J. Sobel, T. Lynn, E. Funk, J.P. Middaugh. 2004. Botulism type E associated with eating a beached whale, Alaska. *Emerging Infectious Diseases* 10:1685–1687.

McLean, D.D. 1946. Duck disease at Tulare Lake. *California Fish and Game* 32:71–80.

Mereb, G., F. Rosetti, E. Castelli, R. Ganuza, L. Ottavioni, D. Cavallero, and A. Calderon. 1999. Description of a botulism type C outbreak among waterbirds in the province of La Pampa Argentina. *Anaerobe* 5:191–193.

Mikuska, J., T. Mikuska, I. Pelle, and Z. Pelle. 1986. The dying of birds at Slano Kopovo near Novi Becej in the summer of 1982. *Larus* 36–37:311–315.

Miller, M.R., and D.C. Duncan. 1999. The northern pintail in North America: status and conservation needs of a struggling population. *Wildlife Society Bulletin* 27:788–800.

Minton, N.P. 1995. Molecular genetics of clostridial neurotoxins. *Current Topics in Microbiology and Immunology* 195:161–194.

Miyamoto, A. 2002. Risk assessment of type C botulism in freshwater wetlands surrounding the Salton Sea of southern California. M.S. thesis. University of California, Riverside, CA, U.S.A., 65 pp.

Miyazaki, S., and G. Sakaguchi. 1978. Experimental botulism in chickens: the cecum as the site of production and absorption of botulinum toxin. *Japanese Journal of Medical Science and Biology* 31:1–15.

Monheimer, R.H. 1968. The relationship of Lake Michigan waterbird mortalities to naturally occurring Clostridium botulinum type E toxin. *Bulletin of the Wildlife Disease Association* 4:81–85.

Montecucco, C., and G. Schiavo. 1994. Mechanism of action of tetanus and botulinum neurotoxins. *Molecular Microbiology* 13:1–8.

Moulton, D.W., W.I. Jensen, and J.B. Low. 1976. Avian botulism epizootiology on sewage oxidation ponds in Utah. *Journal of Wildlife Management* 40:735–742.

Neubauer, M., K. Hudec, and J. Pellantova. 1988. The occurrence of *Clostridium botulinum* type C bacterium and botulotoxin in an aquatic environment in southern Moravia. *Folia Zoologica* 37:255–262.

Niemann, H. 1991. Molecular biology of clostridial neurotoxins. In *A Sourcebook of Bacterial Protein Toxins,* J.E. Alouf and J.H. Freer (eds.). Academic Press, London, U.K., pp. 303–348.

Nishikawa, A., N. Uotsu, H. Arimitsu, J-C. Lee, Y. Miura, Y. Fujinaga, H. Nakada, T. Watanabe, T. Ohyama, Y. Saskana, and K. Oguma. 2004. The receptor and transporter for internalization of *Clostridium botulinum* type C progenitor toxin into HT-29 cells. *Biochemical and Biophysical Research Communications* 319:327–333.

Nol, P., J.L. Williamson, T.E. Rocke, and T.M. Yuill. 2004. Detection of *Clostridium botulinum* type C cells in the gastrointestinal tracts of Mozambique tilapia (*Oreochromis mossambicus*) by polymerase chain reaction. *Journal of Wildlife Diseases* 40:749–753.

Norton, R.L. 1986. Case of botulism in laughing gulls at a landfill in the Virgin Islands, Greater Antilles. *Florida Field Naturalist* 14:97–98.

Oguma, K., K. Yokota, S. Hayashi, K. Takeshi, M. Kumagai, N. Itoh, N. Tachi, and S. Chiba. 1990. Infant botulism due to *Clostridium botulinum* type C toxin. *The Lancet* 336:1449–1450.

Ohishi, I. 1983. Lethal and vascular permeability activities of botulinum C_2 toxin induced by separate injections of the two toxin components. *Infection and Immunity* 40:336–339.

Ohishi, I.G. 1984. Oral toxicities of *Clostridium botulinum* type A and B toxins from different strains. *Infection and Immunity* 43:487–490.

Ohishi, I.G.G., and B.R. DasGupta. 1987. Molecular structure and biological activities of *Clostridium botulinum* C_2 toxin. In *Avian Botulism: An International Perspective,* M.W. Eklund and V.R. Dowell Jr. (eds.). Charles C. Thomas, Springfield, IL, U.S.A., pp. 222–247.

Ohishi, I.G., G. Sakaguchi, H. Riemann, D. Behymer and B. Hurvell. 1979. Antibodies to *Clostridium botulinum* toxins in free-living birds and mammals. *Journal of Wildlife Diseases* 15:3–9.

Ortiz, N.E., and G.R. Smith. 1994. Landfill sites, botulism and gulls. *Epidemiology and Infection* 112:385–391.

Parrish, J.M., and B.F. Hunter. 1969. Waterfowl botulism in the southern San Joaquin Valley, 1967–1968. *California Fish and Game* 55:265–272.

Pellizzari, R., O. Rossetto, G. Schiavo, and C. Montecucco. 1999. Tetanus and botulinum neurotoxins: mechanism of action and therapeutic uses. *Philosophical Transactions of the Royal Society of London* B 354:259–268.

Polero, B.J., T.E. Smitsaart, J. Beaudoin, J. Carreira. 1980. Botulismo en aves acuaticas en semi-cautiverio. *Revista Investigaciones Agropecuarias* 14:667–72.

Portugal, M.A.S.C., L. Baldassi, and E.M.B. Calil. 1995. An outbreak of fowl botulism in a commercial pen in Valinhos County, state of Sao Paulo. *Arquivos do Instituto Biológico* 62:45–52.

Pullar, E.M. 1934. Enzootic botulism amongst wild birds. *Australian Veterinary Journal* 10:128–135.

Quinn, P.J., and R.A.P. Crinion. 1984. A two year study of botulism in gulls in the vicinity of Dublin Bay. *Irish Veterinary Journal* 38:214–219.

Quortrup, E.R., and A.L. Holt. 1941. Detection of botulinus-toxin producing areas in western duck marshes, with suggestions for control. *Journal of Bacteriology* 41:363–372.

Quortrup, E.R., and R.L. Sudheimer. 1943a. Detection of botulinus toxin in the blood stream of wild ducks. *Journal of the American Veterinary Medical Association* 102:264–266.

Quortrup, E.R., and R.L. Sudheimer. 1943b. Some ecological relations of *Pseudomonas aeruginosa* to *Clostridium botulinum* type C. *Canadian Journal of Bacteriology* 45:551–554.

Reed, T.M., and T.E. Rocke. 1992. The role of avian carcasses in botulism epizootics. *Wildlife Society Bulletin* 20:175–182.

Rocke, T. E. 1993. Clostridium botulinum. In *Pathogenesis of Bacterial Infections in Animals,* Second Edition, C. L. Gyles and C. O. Thoen (eds.). Iowa State University Press, Ames, IA, U.S.A., pp. 86–96.

Rocke, T.E., and C.J. Brand. 1994. Use of sentinel mallards for epizootiologic studies of avian botulism. *Journal of Wildlife Diseases* 30:514–522.

Rocke, T.E., and M. Friend. 1999. Avian Botulism. In *Field Manual of Wildlife Diseases: General Field Procedures and Diseases of Birds,* M. Friend and J.C. Franson (eds.). Biological Resources Division Information and Technology Report 1999-001, U.S. Geological Survey, Washington, D.C., U.S.A., pp. 271–281.

Rocke, T.E., and M.D. Samuel. 1999. Water and sediment characteristics associated with avian botulism outbreaks in wetlands. *Journal of Wildlife Management* 63:1249–1260.

Rocke, T.E., S.R. Smith, and S.N. Nashold. 1998. A preliminary evaluation of an in vitro test for the diagnosis of botulism in waterfowl. *Journal of Wildlife Diseases* 34:744–751.

Rocke, T.E., N. Euliss, and M.D. Samuel. 1999. Environmental characteristics associated with the occurrence of avian botulism in wetlands on a northern California wetland. *Journal of Wildlife Management* 63:358–368.

Rocke, T.E., M.D. Samuel, P.K. Swift, and G.S. Yarris. 2000. Efficacy of a type C botulism vaccine in green-winged teal. *Journal of Wildlife Diseases* 36:489–493.

Rocke, T.E., P. Nol, C. Pelliza, and K. Sturm. 2004. Type C botulism in pelicans and other fish-eating birds at the Salton Sea. *Studies in Avian Biology* 27:136–140.

Rogers, D.E., M.G. Koenig, and A. Spickard. 1964. Clinical and laboratory manifestations of type E botulism in man. *Transactions of the Association of American Physicians* 77:135–144.

Rose, A.L. 1935. Enzootic botulism amongst wild birds. *Australian Veterinary Journal* 10:175–177.

Rosen, M.N. 1971. Botulism. In *Infectious and Parasitic Diseases of Wild Birds,* J.W. Davis, R.C. Anderson, L. Karstad, and D.O. Trainer (eds.). Iowa State University Press, Ames, IA, U.S.A., pp. 100–117.

Rosen, M.N., and J.B. Cowan. 1953. Winter botulism: A sequel to a severe summer outbreak. *Conference of the Western Association of State Game and Fish Commission Annual Proceedings* 33:189–193.

Sakaguchi, G. and R. Kaji. 1980. Avian botulism. *Journal of Japanese Society of Poultry Diseases* 16:37–49.

Samuel, M.D. 1992. Influence of disease on a population model of mid-continent mallards. *Transactions of the 57th North American Wildlife and Natural Resource Conference,* pp. 486–498.

Sandler, R.J., Rocke, T.E., Samuel, M.D., and T. M. Yuill. 1993. Seasonal prevalence of *Clostridium botulinum* type C in sediments of a northern California wetland. *Journal of Wildlife Diseases* 29:533–539.

Sandler, R.J., T.E. Rocke, and T.M. Yuill. 1998. Inhibition of *Clostridium botulinum* type C by other bacteria in wetland sediments. *Journal of Wildlife Diseases* 34:803–833.

Schiavo, G., F. Benfenati, B. Poulain, O. Rossetto, P. Polverino, de Laureto, B. R. DasGupta, and C. Montecucco. 1992a. Tetanus and botulinum-B neurotoxins block neurotransmitter release by proteolytic cleavage of synaptobrevin. *Nature* 39:832–835.

Schiavo, G., O. Rosetto, A. Santucci, B.R. DasGupta and C. Montecucco. 1992b. Botulinum neurotoxins are zinc proteins. *Journal of Biology and Chemistry* 267:23479–23483.

Schonhofen, C.A., and R.G. Ferreira. 1981. First outbreaks of botulism in wild ducks in Curitiba. *Brazilian Archives of Biology and Technology* 24:433–435.

Schwartz, L.K., and G. Smart. 1963. Control of botulism in wild fowl. *Journal of the American Veterinary Medical Association* 143:163.

Scott, W.B., and E.J. Crossman. 1973. *Freshwater Fishes of Canada.* Bulletin 966, Fisheries Research Board of Canada, Ottawa, ON, Canada, 184 pp.

Segner, W.P., C.F. Schmidt, and J.K. Boltz. 1971. Enrichment, isolation, and cultural characteristics of marine strains of *Clostridium botulinum* type C. *Applied Microbiology* 22:1017–1024.

Shaw, R.M., and G.S. Simpson. 1936. *Clostridium botulinum,* type C, in relation to duck sickness in Alberta. *Journal of Bacteriology* 32:79–88.

Simpson, L.L. 1981. The origin, structure, and pharmacological activity of botulinum toxin. *Pharmacological Reviews* 33:155–188.

Simpson, L.L. 1982. A comparison of the pharmacological properties of *Clostridium botulinum* type C_1 and type C_2 toxins. *Journal of Pharmacology and Experimental Therapeutics* 223:695–701.

Simpson, L.L. 1986. Molecular pharmacology of botulinum toxin and tetanus toxin. In *Annual Review of Pharmacology and Toxicology,* R. George, R. Okun, and A.K. Cho (eds.). Annual Reviews, Inc., Palo Alto, CA, U.S.A., pp.427–453.

Simpson, L.L. 1989. Peripheral actions of the botulinum toxins. In *Botulinum Neurotoxin and Tetanus Toxin,* L. L. Simpson (ed.). Academic Press, New York, NY, U.S.A., pp. 153–178.

Simpson, L.L. 2004. Identification of the major steps in botulinum toxin action. *Annual Review of Pharmacology and Toxicology* 44:167–193.

Skulberg, A., and F. Holt. 1987. Avian botulism in Scandinavia. In *Avian Botulism: An International Perspective,* M.W. Eklund and V.R. Dowell Jr. (eds.). Charles C Thomas, Springfield, IL, U.S.A., pp. 107–110.

Smart, J.L., T.A. Roberts, K.G. McCullagh, V.M. Lucke, and H. Pearson. 1980. An outbreak of type C botulism in captive monkeys. *Veterinary Record* 126:216.

Smith, G.R. 1976. Botulism in waterfowl. *Wildfowl* 27:129–138.

Smith, G.R., and A. Turner. 1987. Factors affecting the toxicity of rotting carcasses containing *Clostridium botulinum* type C. *Epidemiology and Infection* 98:345–351.

Smith, G.R., and A. Turner. 1989. The production of *Clostridium botulinum* toxin in mammalian, avian and piscine carrion. *Epidemiology and Infection* 102: 467–471.

Smith, G.R., J.M. Hime, I.F. Keymer, J.M. Graham, P.J.S. Olney, and M.R. Brambell. 1975. Botulism in captive birds fed commercially-bred maggots. *The Veterinary Record* 97:204–205.

Smith, G.R., R.A. Milligan, and C.J. Moryson. 1978. *Clostridium botulinum* in aquatic environments in Great Britain and Ireland. *Journal of Hygiene* 80:431–438.

Smith, G.R., M.R. Brambell, W.T. Gaynor, G.R. Gree, and W. De Meurichy. 1985. Botulism in zoological collections. *Veterinary Record* 117:534.

Smith, G.R., A. Turner, and D. Till. 1988. Factors affecting the toxicity of rotting carcasses containing *Clostridium botulinum* type E. *Epidemiology and Infection* 100:399–405.

Smith, L. DS. 1977. *Botulism: The Organism, Its Toxins, the Disease.* Charles C Thomas, Springfield, IL, U.S.A., 236 pp.

Smith, L. DS., and H. Sugiyama. 1988. *Botulism: The Organism, Its Toxins, the Disease,* Second Edition. Charles C Thomas, Springfield, IL, U.S.A., 171 pp.

Smith, M.V. and M.D. Pierson. 1979. Effect of reducing agents on oxidation-reduction potential and the outgrowth of *Clostridium botulinum* type E spores. *Applied and Environmental Microbiology* 37:978–984.

Soos, C. 2004. Links between avian botulism outbreaks in waterfowl, hatching asynchrony, and life history trade-offs of prefledgling Franklin's gulls. Ph.D. thesis. University of Saskatchewan, Saskatoon, Sask, Ca., 144 pp.

Stutzenbaker, C.D., K. Brown, and D. Lobpries. 1986. Special report: an assessment of the accuracy of documenting waterfowl die-offs in a Texas coastal marsh. In *Lead Poisoning in Wild Waterfowl,* J.S. Feierabend and A.B. Russel (eds.). National Wildlife Federation, Washington, D.C., U.S.A., pp. 88–95.

Sugiyama, H. 1980. *Clostridium botulinum* neurotoxin. *Microbiology Reviews* 44:419–448.

Sugiyama, H., T.L. Bott, and E.M. Foster. 1970. *Clostridium botulinum* type E in an inland bay (Green Bay of Lake Michigan). In *Proceedings of the First U.S.-Japan Conference on Toxic Micro-organisms. Mycotoxins, Botulism.* M. Herzberg (ed.). U.S. Government Printing Office, Washington, D.C., U.S.A., pp. 287–291.

Swift. P.K., J. D. Wehausen, H.B. Ernest, R.S. Singer, A.M. Pauli, H. Kinde, T.E. Rocke and V.C. Bleich. 2000. Desert bighorn sheep mortality due to presumptive type C botulism in California. *Journal of Wildlife Diseases* 36:184–189.

Thomas, R.J. 1991. Detection of *Clostridium botulinum* type C and D toxin by ELISA. *Australian Veterinary Journal* 68:111–113.

Wellhoner, H.H. 1992. Tetanus and botulinum neurotoxins. In *Handbook of Experimental Pharmacology,* Vol. 102, H. Hechen and F. Hucho (eds.). Springer-Verlag, New York, NY, U.S.A., pp.357–417.

Wetmore, A. 1915. Mortality among waterfowl around Great Salt Lake, Utah. U.S. Department of Agriculture, Bulletin 217, 10 pp.

Wetmore, A. 1918. The duck sickness in Utah. U.S. Department of Agriculture, Bulletin 672, 26 pp.

Whitmer, M.E., and E.A. Johnson. 1988. Development of improved defined media for Clostridium botulinum serotypes A, B, and E. *Applied and Environmental Microbiology* 54:753–759.

Williamson, J.L., T.E. Rocke, and J.M. Aiken. 1999. In situ detection of the Clostridium botulinum type C_1 toxin gene in wetland sediments with a nested PCR assay. *Applied and Environmental Microbiology* 65:3240–3243.

Wobeser, G.A. 1981. *Diseases of Wild Waterfowl.* Plenum Press, New York, NY, U.S.A., 300 pp.

Wobeser, G. 1988. Effects of botulism on ducks drinking saline water. *Journal of Wildlife Diseases* 24:240–245.

Wobeser, G.A. 1997. Avian botulism—another perspective. *Journal of Wildlife Diseases* 33:181–186.

Wobeser, G., and E.A. Galmut. 1984. Rate of digestion of blowfly maggots by ducks. *Journal of Wildlife Diseases* 20:154–155.

Wobeser, G.A., D.J. Rainnie, T.B. Smith-Windsor, and G. Bogdan. 1983. Avian botulism during late autumn and early spring in Saskatchewan. *Journal of Wildlife Diseases* 19:90–94.

Wobeser, G.A., S. Marsden, and R.J. MacFarlane. 1987. Occurrence of toxigenic *Clostridium botulinum* type C in the soil of wetlands in Saskatchewan. *Journal of Wildlife Diseases* 23:67–76.

Wobeser, G., K. Baptiste, E.G. Clark, and A.W. Deyo. 1997. Type C botulism in cattle in association with a botulism die-off in waterfowl in Saskatchewan. *Canadian Veterinary Journal* 38:782.

Woodall, P.F. 1982. Botulism outbreak in waterbirds at Seven-Mile Lagoon in south-east Queensland. *Australian Wildlife Research* 9:533–539.

Zhou, Y., H. Sugiyama, and E.A. Johnson. 1993. Transfer of neurotoxigenicity from *Clostridium butyricum* to a nontoxigenic *Clostridium botulinum* type E-like strain. *Applied and Environmental Microbiology* 59:3825–3831.

22
Mycotoxicosis

Charlotte F. Quist, Todd Cornish, Roger D. Wyatt

INTRODUCTION

"Mycotoxin" is a general term applied to a class of potent toxins that affect birds and other animals primarily via food contamination. The primary commonality among mycotoxins is that they are all produced by fungi; the chemical structures of the mycotoxins vary widely. The many genera of fungi capable of producing mycotoxins, including *Acremonium, Alternaria, Aspergillus, Claviceps, Fusarium,* and *Penicillium,* account for the marked structural heterogeneity among the compounds (Bennett and Klich 2003). Animals become affected accidentally upon ingestion of contaminated foodstuffs. The illnesses produced by the toxins are as different as the species of birds, mammals, and fish that have been shown to be affected. These toxins are metabolic by-products of the fungi; thus, the illnesses caused in animals and birds by mycotoxins are intoxications, not actual infections with fungal agents.

Production of mycotoxins in foodstuffs contaminated with fungi can occur both in the field and in storage, and varies from year to year, depending on climatic conditions such as temperature and humidity. Other factors, including insect damage, agronomic conditions, and harvesting practices, also may affect production of toxins by the specific fungi. Although some of the mycotoxins have been shown to be plant pathogens (Joffe 1986), the raison d'être for others remains unclear.

Although ingestion is the primary route of exposure to mycotoxins, disease due to inhalation and direct contact has also been reported in mammals including domestic livestock (Pang et al. 1988; Wu et al. 1997). The effects of these diverse toxins range from low-level chronic effects, including poor weight gains and/or failure to grow, immunosuppression, and reproductive problems, to overt clinical disease including liver dysfunction or failure, carcinogenesis, and death. In general, the diversity of effects is dose related. Lower doses of mycotoxins encountered over longer time frames tend to cause subclinical disease or growth effects. Progressively higher doses cause more severe effects, which ultimately can lead to organ failure, cancer, or death, depending on the dosage level and duration of exposure.

Mycotoxins initially were recognized in the mid-1950s (Forgacs and Carll 1955; Forgacs et al. 1958) when an association was made between illness in poultry and ingestion of moldy feed. Since that time, the number of mycotoxins identified has expanded markedly, with the majority of research on mycotoxins being concentrated on human and domestic animal health. Research studies indicate that differing species' susceptibilities to various mycotoxins are due to differing ability of animals to metabolize the toxins. Despite reports of morbidity and mortality caused by mycotoxins in wildlife, only limited research has been conducted on the effects of these toxins on wildlife species.

Large-scale die-offs of wild birds have been documented on a few occasions. Generally, these scenarios involve large flocks of birds gathering during the colder months to feed on some type of grain-stuffs lying in fields. Granivorous birds are particularly at risk because grain is the primary source of many of the more common mycotoxins. Unfortunately, smaller mortality events due to mycotoxins might easily be overlooked unless an obvious source of mycotoxins was present and mortality was detected. Finally, morbidity due to low-level mycotoxin exposure is, in all likelihood, severely under-recognized and therefore underestimated. Mycotoxin testing is not usually part of a routine post-mortem or diagnostic evaluation, so isolated exposures of unknown source may go undetected.

Aflatoxins were the first of the mycotoxins whose effects were recognized, and they remain the most studied and best classified in all species. Since that first discovery of aflatoxin, other mycotoxins, including the trichothecenes, fumonisins, zearalenone, and many others have been identified and their effects characterized. However, most of the research that has been performed on wild birds has been in relation to aflatoxins. Wild bird mortality due to other mycotoxins has been documented, but the range of effects of many of the other mycotoxins in wildlife is poorly researched and may provide an emerging area of interest.

Aflatoxins

ETIOLOGY

Aflatoxins are a class of mycotoxins predominantly produced by species of *Aspergillus,* most notably *Aspergillus flavus* and *Aspergillus parasiticus.* The general term "aflatoxin" (AF) refers to a group of closely related compounds that includes AFB_1, AFB_2, AFG_1 AFG_2, AFM_1, and AFM_2, which can be separated chromatographically (Uraguchi 1971). Structurally, aflatoxins are ringed compounds consisting of a coumarin nucleus fused to a bifuran and, depending on the metabolite, a pentanone (AFB_1 and AFB_2) or six-membered lactone (AFG_1 and AFG_2) ring (Palmgren and Hayes 1987). The varied structures of the many metabolites of the parent compound are factors in their relative toxicity (Uraguchi 1971). Of these metabolites, AFB_1 is by far the most prevalent and the most toxic, and thus is the most common cause of toxicosis. Metabolites AFM_1 and AFM_2 are secreted in milk via the mammary gland, so are not of importance in avian species.

HISTORY

In 1960, approximately 100,000 domestic turkeys (*Meleagris gallopavo*) and fewer pheasants and ducklings died in England from what was termed "turkey X disease" (Blount 1961). Eventually, the link between the turkey feed, a Brazilian groundnut (peanut) meal, and turkey X disease was identified, with the causative agent being discovered and two years later named "aflatoxin" (Hendrickse 1997). Subsequently, aflatoxins were shown to cause liver tumors in rainbow trout (Halver 1965). Since the association between aflatoxins and disease was recognized, extensive research has been conducted to determine the effects of aflatoxin on domestic animals, fish, and humans.

DISTRIBUTION

Aflatoxin production on grain substrates can occur in any part of the world that has a combination of moderate temperatures and relatively high humidity. Official estimates indicate that as much as 25% of the world's annual food supply is contaminated with mycotoxins (Coulombe 1993). Based on reports of human disease caused by aflatoxins, which are better documented than exposure of domestic or wild animals, aflatoxin exposure is highest in developing countries in Asia and Africa (Williams et al. 2004; Wogan et al. 2004). In the United States, aflatoxin contamination is most common in grain in the southeastern states, due to climatic conditions, but it is not restricted to that portion of the country.

HOST RANGE

Morbidity and mortality due to acute aflatoxicosis has occurred in field cases involving Snow Geese (*Chen caerulescens*), Ross's Geese (*Chen rossi*), Greater White-fronted Geese (*Anser albifrons*), Mallards (*Anas platyrhynchos*), and Northern Pintails (*Anas acuta*) (Robinson et al. 1982) (NWHC, SCWDS unpublished data).[1, 2]

Numerous species, including fish, birds, and mammals, are susceptible to aflatoxins. Although some species are more resistant than others, no species has been shown to be completely resistant to the toxic effects (Hendrickse 1997), though the degree of host susceptibility to aflatoxins varies tremendously even among closely related species (Gumbmann et al. 1970; Arafa et al. 1981). Young animals are more susceptible than older animals, presumably due to the lack of the well-developed hepatic enzymatic systems that are required to degrade the toxins (Cheeke and Shull 1985). Species such as rats, rabbits, and white Pekin ducks that metabolize the parent aflatoxin compounds more rapidly suffer greater effects from the toxic metabolites than do species that metabolize aflatoxins more slowly (Coulombe 1993; Cheeke and Shul 1985). Ruminants, in general, are more resistant to the effects of aflatoxins, possibly due to dilution and slower metabolism within the rumen.

Experimental studies are the best means of determining toxic concentrations of aflatoxins in various species. Only a limited amount of research, mostly using game bird species, has been conducted with wild birds, but some studies have shown parallels between wildlife species and their domestic counterparts. Among the avian species tested, domestic ducklings appear the most susceptible to aflatoxins. Domestic turkey poults and Wild Turkey poults (*Meleagris gallopavo*) show a similar susceptibility to aflatoxins after a relatively short-term exposure of two to three weeks, with effects being marginal at 100 ppb and significant at 200 and 400 ppb (Arafa et al. 1981; Quist et al. 2000). Of game birds, Ring-necked Pheasants (*Phasianus colchicus*) are the most susceptible, followed by Northern Bobwhite (*Colinus virginianus*), and Chukar (*Alectoris chukar*). Japanese Quail (*Coturnix japonica*) are more resistant (Table 22.1) (Stewart 1985; Ruff et al. 1990; Ruff et al. 1992).

Table 22.1. Experimentally determined effects of aflatoxin in the feed of wild bird species.

Species	Age	Aflatoxin Concentration	Duration	Decreased Weight Gain	Decreased Feed Consumption	Hepatic Lesions	Immune Function Effects	Deaths	Literature Citation
Duck, domestic	1 day	500 ppb	3 wk	yes	yes	yes		30%	Muller et al. 1970
Mallard (*Anas platyrhynchos*)	6 wks	33 ppb	9 day	no				no	Neiger et al. 1994
Goose, domestic	1 day	500 ppb	2 wk	yes	yes	yes		40%	Muller et al. 1970
Chukar (*Alectoris chukar*)	1 day	500 ppb	3 wk	yes		no		no	Ruff et al. 1990
	1–2 days	800 ppb		yes		yes		no	Gumbmann et al. 1970
Guineafowl	1–2 days	800 ppb	4–6 wk	no		yes		no	Gumbmann et al. 1970
Ring-necked Pheasant (*Phasianus colchicus*)	1 day	500 ppb	2 wk	yes		yes		10%	Muller et al. 1970
	1 day	1250 ppb	2 wk	yes				10%	Huff et al. 1992
	1 day	2500 ppb	2 wk	yes				30%	Huff et al. 1992
Northern Bobwhite (*Colinus virginianus*)	1 day	125 ppb	2 wk	yes				10%	Ruff et al. 1992
	16 wks	250 ppb	4 wk	no		yes		no	Stewart 1985
	1–2 days	800 ppb	4–6 wk	yes		yes			Gumbmann et al. 1970
Japanese Quail (*Coturnix japonica*)	1 day	500 ppb	3 wks	yes				no	Ruff et al. 1992
	1–2 days	800 ppb	4–6 wk	no		yes		no	Gumbmann et al. 1970
Turkey, domestic	12 wks	62.5 ppb	12 wk	yes				21%	Hamilton et al. 1972
	12 wks	125 ppb	3 wk	yes				8%	Hamilton et al. 1972

(Continued)

Table 22.1. *(Continued)*

Species	Age	Aflatoxin Concentration	Duration	Decreased Weight Gain	Decreased Feed Consumption	Hepatic Lesions	Immune Function Effects	Deaths	Literature Citation
	4 wks	250 ppb	3 wk[a]	yes		yes	yes[a]	20%	Pier and Heddleston 1970
	4 wks	500 ppb	3 wk[a]	yes		yes	yes[b]	82%	Pier and Heddleston 1970
	1–2 days	800 ppb	2–3 wk	yes		yes		20–50%	Gumbmann et al. 1970
Wild Turkey (*Meleagris gallopavo*)	4 mo	100 ppb	2 wk	slight		no	no[b]	no	Quist et al. 2000
	4 mo	200 ppb	2 wk	yes	yes	yes	no[b]	no	Quist et al. 2000
	4 mo	400 ppb	2 wk	yes	yes	yes	yes[b]	10–15%	Quist et al. 2000

a = Immune challenge occurred three weeks after aflatoxin exposure.
b = Immune challenge occurred during aflatoxin exposure.

EPIZOOTIOLOGY

Fungi that produce aflatoxins grow on a wide variety of cereal grains and oil seeds, particularly corn, cottonseed, and peanuts (Coulombe 1993). Fungal contamination of these crops generally occurs prior to harvest. In contrast to corn, peanuts, and cotton, contamination of soybeans and other grains usually occurs during storage (Cheeke and Shull 1985). Aflatoxins are produced when the appropriate species of fungi are subjected to environmental stress from a combination of relatively high ambient temperature and humidity. Generally, a mean temperature of 27°C and relative humidity of approximately 80–90% maximize aflatoxin production by the *Aspergillus* spp. (Hendrickse 1997). Drought stress is recognized as one the key factors in weakening corn plants, allowing the fungi to invade and subsequently begin producing aflatoxins (Bingham et al. 2003). However, even pristine corn can become contaminated with aflatoxins if handled and stored improperly after harvest (Bingham et al. 2003), particularly if the humidity remains high during storage.

Two significant epizootics of aflatoxicosis have been described in free-ranging waterfowl in the United States. In the winter of 1977–1978, approximately 7,500 ducks and geese died in two areas of Texas (Harris and Comanche/Eastland counties), with mortality attributed to ingestion of aflatoxin-contaminated feeds (corn, rice, and peanuts). Corn and rice from upper gastrointestinal tracts of dead birds at the first site contained 500 ppb aflatoxin B_1, and peanuts from a field at the second site contained 110 ppb aflatoxin B_1 (Robinson et al. 1982). A similar epizootic of aflatoxicosis occurred in the Tensas and Concordia parishes of Louisiana in the winter of 1998–1999. More than 10,000 birds, predominantly Snow Geese with fewer Ross's Geese, Greater White-fronted Geese, and Mallards, died during that outbreak. Aflatoxin B_1 was detected in corn found in the upper gastrointestinal contents from geese and also was detected at very high concentrations (up to 8200 ppb) in corn from fields where geese were found dead or dying. Testing of corn samples from throughout Louisiana demonstrated that much of the corn that had survived a drought in 1998 was contaminated with moderate to high concentrations of aflatoxin (approximately 56% of all samples originating from farms) (NWHC unpublished data).[1]

The United States Food and Drug Administration (FDA) regulates concentrations of AFB_1 allowed in food stuffs (FDA, 1989): <20 ppb in corn intended for immature animals including immature poultry, and <100 ppb in corn intended for mature poultry. The threat to wildlife of aflatoxicosis through contaminated feed, both harvested and unharvested, has been documented in several studies. Unharvested grain that is determined to be highly contaminated with aflatoxins and thus unmarketable is often left standing in the fields where it is available to a variety of wildlife species. Aflatoxin concentrations were tested in standing corn on the Mississippi Sandhill Crane National Wildlife Refuge, Gautier, Mississippi, U.S.A., and from corn that was either on the ground or left standing in nearby fields (Couvillion et al. 1991). Overall, >200 ppb aflatoxin B_1 were found in 32% of the corn sampled. Aflatoxin B_1 concentrations were highest (≤5,000 ppb) in waste corn on the ground. In southern Georgia/northern Florida, corn left standing in fields on a pine plantation to provide food for Northern Bobwhite and other wildlife species was found to contain 42 to 1210 ppb total aflatoxin, depending on the year and site of sampling (Stewart 1985). Crop and gizzard contents of quail in those areas contained up to approximately 500 ppb aflatoxin (Stewart 1985). Corn in legal deer bait piles in North and South Carolina contained up to 750 ppb aflatoxin (Fischer et al. 1995). Though this grain was intended to feed white-tailed deer, a species more resistant to the effects of aflatoxins (Quist et al. 1997), contaminated feed would likely be consumed by sympatric species, including birds. Aflatoxins also have been found in corn sold for use as wildlife feed in Georgia (Schweitzer et al. 2001), in corn and sorghum sampled from supplemental feeders in Texas and Oklahoma (Oberheu and Dabbert 2001), and in commercially sold birdseed in Texas (Henke et al. 2001). Thus, ample potential exists for avian species to consume aflatoxin-contaminated grain.

CLINICAL SIGNS

Clinical signs in acute aflatoxicosis include apparent blindness, lack of response to environmental stimuli, weakness, inability to fly, repeated flapping of wings, assuming sitting positions, and, terminally, unconsciousness (Robinson et al. 1982).

Chronic aflatoxicosis in domestic mammals most commonly is manifest by reduced growth rates, and similarly, birds have been shown to have reduced growth rates in experimental studies. Both domestic (Arafa et al. 1981) and Wild Turkey poults (Quist et al. 2000) fed aflatoxin-contaminated feed at 100 to 400 ppb had decreased feed consumption and decreased weight gains compared to control birds. Neoplasia attributable to aflatoxins has not been documented in wild birds, but hepatomas have been reported in domestic ducklings fed low levels of peanut meal (Carnaghan 1965).

PATHOGENESIS

After ingestion, the parent aflatoxin compound is transported via the blood to various organs, where it is converted into toxic metabolites by cytochrome P_{450}

mixed-function oxidases within microsomes. The liver is the main target for toxicity and pathological changes because it contains more of the microsomal mixed-function oxidase systems required to metabolize the compounds (Cheeke and Shull 1985). However, the lungs and kidneys also contain mixed-function oxidases and can be affected. The ultimate effect of aflatoxins on the liver is dependent on the level of aflatoxin exposure over time.

The reactive and electrophilic aflatoxin metabolites have an affinity for cellular nucleophiles such as RNA and DNA, resulting in the toxic and carcinogenic effects of the toxins. Aflatoxins interfere with RNA translation by binding to DNA, causing altered protein synthesis through inhibition of nucleic acid transcription (Yu et al. 1988). This disruption of protein synthesis disrupts basic metabolic pathways of the cell by affecting key enzyme processes including carbohydrate and lipid metabolism (Cheeke and Shull 1985). The Krebs cycle and phosphorylation of substrates also are inhibited via alterations in mitochondrial function (Cheeke and Shull 1985). Clotting factor synthesis is depressed or eliminated, and steroid binding sites in tissues are blocked (Hendrickse 1997). Host immunity is diminished through both hepatic (altered globulin synthesis) and nonhepatic mechanisms (Hendrickse 1997).

Interaction of aflatoxin metabolites with DNA produces alkylation (resulting in loss of a DNA base) or DNA adducts (wherein an amino acid is substituted for a second, inappropriate amino acid) (Coulombe 1993). Though cellular mechanisms are in place to recognize and enzymatically repair these DNA defects, occasional permanent DNA alterations can occur, potentially leading to carcinogenesis. Liver cancer, mainly hepatomas and hepatocellular carcinomas, is well documented in humans exposed to aflatoxins (Bennett 2003; Williams et al. 2004; Wogan et al. 2004), and hepatomas have been reported in domestic ducklings (Carhaghan 1965). By virtue of the multiplicity of actions aflatoxins have on the liver and other systems, the effects of aflatoxins on animals are profound and far reaching.

Experimentally, domestic and Wild Turkeys exposed to aflatoxins suffer hepatocellular damage resulting in hypoalbuminemia, hypoproteinemia, and increased aspartate aminotransferase activity (Arafa et al. 1981; Quist et al. 2000). Alterations in serum protein levels are considered the most sensitive indicators of aflatoxin intoxication (Gumbmann et al. 1970). Reductions in serum triglycerides also have been reported in Wild Turkey poults (Quist et al. 2000) and chickens (Huff et al. 1986) exposed to high concentrations of aflatoxin. Aflatoxins interfere with lipid metabolism, resulting in altered carotenoid levels in Wild Turkeys and domestic poultry (Quist et al. 2000). Release of triglycerides by the liver is also thought to be impaired (Cheeke and Shull 1985).

Less well-documented effects of aflatoxins may be significant in wild birds. Reduced hepatic synthesis of clotting factors by liver damage from aflatoxins can result in delayed blood clotting. Prolonged clotting times have been shown experimentally in chickens (Doerr et al. 1976) and domestic turkey poults (Witlock and Wyatt 1981), and evidence of delayed clotting was seen in Wild Turkey poults exposed to aflatoxins (Quist et al. 2000). Because trauma can be a significant mortality factor for wild birds, increased hemorrhage from impaired hemostasis and increased capillary and vascular fragility might become important in chronic aflatoxicosis. Tissue trauma and a hemorrhagic syndrome were attributed to aflatoxicosis in an early study using domestic poultry (Tung et al. 1970).

Aflatoxin exposure may increase morbidity and mortality in wild birds that have been exposed to pesticides. An interesting study in chickens showed that white leghorn chickens exposed to aflatoxins had significantly more inhibition of brain and serum acetyl cholinesterase levels after malathion exposure than did birds given malathion alone (Ehrich et al. 1985). Significant morbidity and mortality of wild birds is due to pesticides (Fleischli et al. 2004), but no documented studies have examined birds killed by pesticides for aflatoxin exposure.

PATHOLOGY

The pathologic effects of aflatoxins vary depending on whether the exposure is short term, causing acute morbidity or mortality, or long term, resulting in signs of chronic aflatoxicosis. Exposure of even resistant species, such as white-tailed deer, to high levels of aflatoxin in a single dose can cause fatalities due to acute massive hepatic necrosis (V.F. Nettles, unpublished data)[3]; whereas many species can tolerate short-term exposure to low levels of aflatoxin.

Gross pathology in wild birds dying from acute aflatoxicosis ranges from none to discoloration and enlargement of the liver, hemorrhage in the liver, shrinkage and fibrosis of the liver, swelling and pallor of the kidneys, and pallor or mottling of the spleen and pancreas. Most birds examined in two reports from Texas (Robinson et al. 1982) were in fair to good nutritional condition; however, some birds found dead during an epizootic in Louisiana were in poor nutritional condition with atrophy of subcutaneous and internal adipose stores and some atrophy of pectoral skeletal muscles (NWHC, SCWDS unpublished data).[1,2] Whether the poor body condition seen in these birds was an effect of the aflatoxin exposure is unknown.

Microscopic lesions observed in waterfowl dying from acute aflatoxicosis are most prominent in the liver, consisting of varying degrees of hepatocellular degeneration, fatty change, and necrosis, together with mild to severe biliary hyperplasia and portal tract inflammation (predominantly mononuclear cells). Portal fibrosis may be present in livers of some birds, particularly those birds in poorer nutritional condition, suggesting a more prolonged course of disease. Less commonly, hepatocytes with enlarged nuclei (karyomegaly) or multi-lobed nuclei may be seen. Renal, splenic, and pancreatic lesions including patchy tubular degeneration and necrosis in kidneys, congestion and mild necrosis in spleens, and necrosis and hemorrhage in pancreases can be seen (Robinson et al. 1982) (NWHC, SCWDS unpublished data).[1,2]

Chronic aflatoxicosis in both birds and mammals causes decreased body weights (or failure to grow in young animals), hepatic dysfunction, immunosuppression, and ultimately death. The chronic effects of aflatoxin exposure that have been documented in birds through experimental studies are summarized in Table 22.1. No confirmed cases of neoplasia have been reported in wild birds, though hepatic tumors have been reported in domestic ducklings fed diets containing aflatoxin (Carnaghan 1965).

Unfortunately, the sublethal effects of low concentrations of aflatoxins (<100 ppb) over prolonged time periods (over three weeks) have been poorly documented in both mammalian and avian species.

DIAGNOSIS

Diagnosis of aflatoxicosis is most easily made on the basis of appropriate history, clinical signs, and postmortem lesions referable to hepatic failure, with confirmation of the presence of aflatoxins in the feed or in stomach contents. As little as 0.1 ng/ml of mycotoxin can be detected in feed by available tests, including enzyme linked immunosorbent assays (ELISA) and radioimmunoassays. Several commercial kits are available that can be used in the field, and most veterinary diagnostic laboratories conduct these tests. Measurement of aflatoxins in tissues is much more difficult due to the rapid degradation of the compounds by liver enzymes. Therefore, tissue analyses may not be a sensitive measure of aflatoxin exposure. Assay for the presence of aflatoxins in tissues requires high-performance liquid chromatography (Helferich et al. 1986), which is conducted by relatively few laboratories.

Unfortunately, the most common form of intoxication may be low-level chronic exposures that produce significant, but nonspecific, clinical effects (Pier 1992). These types of exposures would be difficult to recognize and may go undiagnosed. Conditions suggestive of this type of chronic aflatoxicosis would include weight loss, immune suppression, and hepatic dysfunction. Long-term focused studies that include feed and/or tissue analysis may be required to diagnose these exposures.

IMMUNITY

There is no evidence that animals develop specific immunity to aflatoxins. In contrast, exposure to aflatoxins causes a reduction in the immune response to other infectious agents, primarily through a deficiency in cell-mediated immunity, but also through decreased phagocytosis (Pier 1992). Mycotoxin poisoning in livestock is often manifest by increased losses due to infectious organisms (Sharma, 1993). Similarly, immune compromise to pathogens may be one of the most important effects aflatoxins have on birds. Aflatoxicosis has been speculated to be a predisposing factor for avian cholera outbreaks in the Rainwater Basin of Nebraska (Smith et al. 1990). Pier and Heddleston (1970) demonstrated immunosuppression in response to *Pasteurella multocida* in domestic turkey poults fed aflatoxins. This impaired acquired resistance, which included a reduction in plasma proteins other than gamma globulins, was seen when poults were vaccinated during or prior to aflatoxin exposure, but the immune response returned to normal three weeks post-exposure. Decreased humoral immunity evidenced by altered antibody responses (IgA and IgG, not IgM) is generally seen only at very high levels of aflatoxin (Pier 1992). However, domestic chicks that had been fed aflatoxin but were apparently recovered remained less resistant to coccidiosis than control chicks, suggesting continued interference with hepatic synthesis of immunoglobulins (Edds and Simpson 1976). Cell-mediated immunity is inhibited by aflatoxins in many species (Cheeke and Shull 1985; Williams et al. 2004), including domestic and Wild Turkey poults (Giambrone et al. 1985a; Giambrone et al. 1985b; Quist et al. 2000), probably through suppression of T-helper or cytotoxic T-cell activity (Sharma 1993).

Trichothecenes

ETIOLOGY

The trichothecenes are a complex group of more than 60 related mycotoxins produced by several genera of fungi. The most significant of the trichothecene-producing fungi are in the genus *Fusarium,* with *Fusarium sporotrichioides* and *Fusarium graminearum* being among the most common toxin producers. Chemically, the trichothecene mycotoxins are structurally related sesquiterpenes, with the various metabolites having hydroxyl and acetoxy substitutions at different ring carbons (Savard and Blackwell 1994).

These compounds are divided into groups based on these functional structural similarities (Bennett and Klich 2003). Examples of trichothecenes include T-2 toxin, nivalenol, and deoxynivalenol (DON or vomitoxin). Of these, T-2 toxin has been the most widely studied and appears to be the most toxic (Bennett and Klich 2003).

DISTRIBUTION

Trichothecenes are widely distributed throughout the world in cereal crops including wheat, barley, and corn. However, the trichothecenes that are most prominent in North America are of lesser toxicity or tend to be present in lower concentrations that do not present as great a threat to humans or animals (Prelusky 1994). Different trichothecenes may be more prevalent in certain areas depending on environmental conditions and which fungi are present.

HOST RANGE

Epizootics involving trichothecenes have been documented only in Sandhill Cranes (*Grus canadensis*), Whooping Cranes (*Grus americana*), unidentified geese, and domestic ducks. However, studies have shown that most mammalian and avian species can be affected by trichothecenes; differences in both susceptibility of different species to the toxins and the manifestations of the toxic effects exist (Bondy and Pestka 2000). Perceived limitations on host range may stem more from lack of detection of toxic effects than from the lack of effects.

EPIZOOTIOLOGY

In contrast to the aflatoxins, where toxin is produced at warmer temperatures, cool temperatures enhance production of trichothecenes, although high humidity remains a necessary component (Coulombe 1993). As with the aflatoxins, trichothecenes can be produced on a variety of grain substrates including corn, wheat, barley, and peanuts. In wildlife species, outbreaks of fusariotoxicosis have typically occurred in the winter months, when weather conditions (cool temperatures and high humidity) are most conducive to toxin production.

Morbidity and mortality attributable to trichothecenes has occurred intermittently since the mid-1980s in Texas during winter months in Sandhill Cranes feeding on peanuts left in the field after harvest. A variety of *Fusarium* fungi and associated mycotoxins were identified in initial outbreaks (Windingstad et al. 1989).

Morbidity and mortality occurred in Sandhill Cranes and Whooping Cranes at the Patuxent Wildlife Research Center in Laurel, Maryland, U.S.A., in September 1987 (Olsen et al. 1995). Illness was reported in 80% of 300 captive cranes at the facility, with 15 deaths.

Field outbreaks of fusariotoxicosis occurred in winter in British Columbia when geese (species unidentified) feeding in barley fields were poisoned by grain that had become contaminated with *Fusarium* sp. (Greenway and Puls 1976; Puls and Greenway 1976). Domestic ducks, horses, and swine were also affected, but mortality occurred only among the geese (Greenway and Puls 1976). The fusariotoxin, T-2, was identified as the likely agent (Puls and Greenway 1976).

CLINICAL SIGNS, PATHOGENESIS, AND PATHOLOGY

In mammals, the mechanism of action of the trichothecenes is marked inhibition of protein synthesis through inhibition of both RNA and DNA synthesis (Osweiler 2000). Similar effects are thought to occur in birds.

As might be expected with such a large group of toxins, the effects of trichothecenes are varied, but are often characterized by gastrointestinal disturbances such as feed refusal, oral ulceration, vomiting, and diarrhea. Dermal irritation, anemia, leukopenia, and coagulopathies also are reported, and abortion can occur in mammals (Coloumbe 1993; Osweiler 2000). Many animals refuse trichothecene-contaminated feed (Osweiler 2000), which may be due to either the unpalatability of the feed or discomfort associated with toxin-induced oral lesions, or a combination of both.

Clinical signs in intoxicated Sandhill Cranes from Texas consisted of paresis, frequently of the muscles of the head and neck, resulting in a drooped neck posture while standing and during flight. Wing and leg weakness also were reported, resulting in the birds' inability or reduced ability to fly. Gross lesions seen in affected birds included subcutaneous edema of the head and multifocal hemorrhages throughout skeletal muscles, with the dorsal neck, cranial tibial, and pectoralis muscles being the most often affected. Histologically, vascular thrombosis and subsequent ischemia were observed in damaged skeletal muscles (Roffe et al. 1989).

The lesions seen in sick and dead cranes from the epizootic at Patuxent were not consistent with the clinical signs and lesions seen in Texas cranes. The lesions seen in Patuxent cranes were compatible with debilitation plus other lesions attributed to secondary complications (Olsen et al. 1995). It may be that the combination and concentration of trichothecenes found in each event may have played a role in the differing signs and lesions seen.

Gross lesions seen in geese (species unidentified) in a natural outbreak of fusariotoxicosis (T2 toxin) in Canada included necrosis of the lining of the esophagus, proventriculus, and gizzard, and degeneration and complete necrosis of mucous membranes was confirmed histologically (Greenway and Puls 1976).

Mallards and several species of upland game birds had weight loss and oral and upper gastrointestinal ulceration after ingestion of experimental diets containing T-2 toxin. After the mortality in British Columbia, young Mallards fed diets containing 20–30 ppm of T-2 toxin for two or three weeks had reduced weight gains and delayed development of adult plumage (Hayes and Wobeser 1983). At necropsy, caseonecrotic plaques were present throughout the upper gastrointestinal tract, particularly the oropharynx and ventriculus. In another study (Neiger et al. 1994), six-week-old Mallard ducklings fed 2 ppm of T-2 toxin-contaminated feed for nine days had decreased feed consumption, weight loss, and decreased thymic, bursal, and splenic weights. At necropsy, birds had erosive lesions of the upper gastrointestinal tract extending from the oral cavity throughout the length of the esophagus. Ducklings were considered more susceptible to the effects of T-2 toxin than turkey poults or chickens (Neiger et al. 1994).

Experimentally, the effects of T-2 toxin have been examined in Ring-necked Pheasants (Huff et al. 1992), Northern Bobwhites, Japanese Quail, (Ruff et al. 1992), and Chukar (Ruff et al. 1990). As in other species, oral lesions, increasing in severity with toxin dosage, were seen in pheasants, Chukar, and Northern Bobwhite, but were less severe in Japanese Quail. Ingested T-2 toxin fed at levels from 8 to 16 ppm resulted in decreased body weights in Chukar, Japanese Quail, and Ring-necked Pheasants, but mortality was seen only in Ring-necked Pheasants, Chukar, and Northern Bobwhites, not Japanese Quail.

Reproductive effects have been associated with T-2 toxin. In domestic geese, egg yield and hatchability are reduced by exposure to T-2 toxin (Vanyi et al. 1994a). Lesions in the reproductive tracts of affected geese included ovarian follicle degeneration, oviduct involution, and peritonitis. Spermatogenesis was not affected (Vanyi et al. 1994b).

DIAGNOSIS

As with the aflatoxins, diagnosis of trichothecenes can be difficult. Detection of fungal growth or the presence of fungal spores alone does not support a diagnosis of mycotoxicosis. Accurate diagnosis must be based on laboratory confirmation of the presence of the mycotoxin combined with the presence of compatible lesions. Many trichothecenes are readily detected in feed using thin-layer chromatography and enzyme-linked immunosorbent assay (ELISA) techniques (Osweiler 2000). Because concentrations of toxins can vary within a given sample, it is recommended that multiple samples be taken from feed storage facilities or suspected grain fields (Osweiler 2000). Many *Fusarium*-produced mycotoxins are rapidly metabolized and eliminated from tissues; thus, confirming a diagnosis of mycotoxicosis months after an outbreak can be difficult or impossible if appropriate feed samples have not been collected during the event (Osweiler 2000). Diagnosis can further be complicated by the presence of multiple mycotoxins, as was thought to be occurring in the crane mortalities (Windingstad et al. 1989; Olsen et al. 1995).

IMMUNITY

Specific immunity to effects of the *Fusarium*-produced mycotoxins has not been reported. The T-2 toxin has been shown to cause altered immune responses in a variety of domestic species (Sharma 1993). Although the immunotoxic effects of these mycotoxins have not been evaluated in wildlife species, altered immune responses are likely in these species as well.

Other Fusarium-Produced Mycotoxins

ETIOLOGY

Other *Fusarium*-produced mycotoxins include the fumonisins, B_1 and B_2, and zearalenone. The fumonisins, which form the most recently discovered family of *Fusarium* toxins, have a structure similar to that of sphingosine, a component of sphingolipid, and have been shown to inhibit sphingolipid synthesis (Savard and Blackwell 1994). Of these, fumonisin B_1 (FB_1), produced by *Fusarium verticillioides* (formerly *moniliforme*), is thought to be the most toxic (Coloumbe 1993). Unlike most mycotoxins, the fumonisins are hydrophilic, which makes them more difficult to study (Bennett and Klich 2003).

Zearalenone, which is produced by *Fusarium graminearum* and a few less common *Fusarium* species, is a phenolic resorcyclic acid lactone that is unique in having estrogenic properties. It may be better classified as mycoestrogen than a mycotoxin (Newberne 1987; Bennett and Klich 2003).

DISTRIBUTION

Fusarium verticillioides commonly contaminates corn, and its presence does not necessarily indicate contamination by fumonisins. In actuality, most fungal strains do not produce toxins (Bennett and Klich 2003). The fumonisins are produced only under specific conditions including dry conditions and insect damage (Miller 1994).

The *Fusarium* species that produce zearalenone are common on cereal crops, primarily corn and wheat, and are found worldwide.

HOST RANGE

No disease outbreaks in wildlife have been attributed to either the fumonisins or zearalenone, though disease events have been reported in domestic birds and mammals.

PATHOLOGY AND PATHOGENESIS

The fumonisins can affect different species in different ways. Fumonisin B1 causes leukoencephalomalacia in horses and rabbits, yet pulmonary edema is seen in swine (Bondy and Pestka 2000; Bennett and Klich 2003). Hepatotoxic and carcinogenic effects are seen in rats, and there is a link with esophageal cancers in humans (Bennett and Klich 2003). The effects of fumonisin exposure on wild species have not been evaluated, but there has been extensive work with fumonisins in domestic poultry. Poultry appear more resistant to the effects of the fumonisins (Bondy and Pestka 2000), but numerous changes have been reported in domestic poultry, turkeys, and ducks including decreased body weight, increased liver weights, and biliary hyperplasia (Ledoux et al. 1992; Weibking et al. 1993; Weibking et al. 1994).

Zearalenone is unique among the mycotoxins in its effects on the reproductive system of animals. Though not a steroid compound, zearalenone binds to the cytoplasmic estrogen receptor (Coulombe 1993), and through this receptor interaction, specific RNA synthesis is initiated, leading to signs of estrogenism (Osweiler 2000). Among mammals, swine are particularly sensitive (Cheeke and Shull 1985). Male pigs fed the compound undergo signs of femininization including mammary enlargement and testicular atrophy. In females, the secretion and release of follicle-stimulating hormone is inhibited, resulting in inhibition of ovarian follicle maturation in sows and clitoral enlargement in gilts. Zearalenone also binds to estrogenic receptors in chickens (Fitzpatrick et al. 1989) and Japanese Quail (Robinson and Gibbins 1984), and testicular atrophy and infertility were seen in farmed pheasants (Willemart and Schricke 1981). These data suggest that the potential exists for hyperestrogenism in birds, though no such problems have been documented in wild species.

IMMUNITY

Specific immunity to effects of the *Fusarium*-produced mycotoxins has not been reported. However, experimental studies using various fumonisins (FB_1, FB_2) have demonstrated reduced immune function involving humoral, cellular, and innate immunity in a number of species including domestic poultry, pigs, calves, and rodents (Bondy and Pestka 2000).

DIAGNOSIS

The primary analytic method used for fumonisins is high-performance liquid chromatography with fluorescent detection. The hydrophilic nature of the fumonisins makes detection of these compounds particularly difficult because they are lost in the common water-based methods for preparing samples (Bennett and Klich 2003). Gas and thin-layer chromatographic methods are used for detection of zearalenone (Joffe 1986).

Ochratoxins

ETIOLOGY AND DISTRIBUTION

The mycotoxin ochratoxin A, produced by a number of common molds including *Aspergillus ochraceus* and *Penicillium verrucosum* (Bennett and Klich 2003), is a food contaminant that is found worldwide. Ochratoxin A is found in a wide variety of foodstuffs including barley, oats, rye, wheat, coffee beans, and other plant products, but barley is more often implicated as the source of the toxin (Bennett and Klich 2003).

EPIZOOTIOLOGY

Natural occurrences of ochratoxicoses have not been reported in wildlife, but have been reported in domestic turkeys and chickens.

CLINICAL SIGNS, PATHOLOGY, AND PATHOGENESIS

Ochratoxins are potent nephrotoxins for all species studied to date, with nephrotoxic, hepatotoxic and immunosuppressive effects being documented in humans, swine, rats, ducklings, and chickens. Abortion has been documented in cattle (Munro et al. 1973), and immunosuppressive effects have been reported (Bondy and Pestka 2000). It is deemed a potential human carcinogen (Bennett and Klich 2003). This toxin acts by inhibition of macromolecule syntheses primarily through enzymes involved in phenylalanine metabolism, increasing lipid peroxidation, and inhibiting mitochrondrial function (Bondy and Pestka 2000; Bennett and Klich 2003).

Clinical signs and lesions seen in natural occurrences of ochratoxicoses in domestic turkeys and chickens include necrosis of renal tubules, decreased egg production by layers, and reduced growth rates in broilers (Hamilton et al. 1982). Experimentally, Chukars, Japanese Quail, Northern Bobwhite, and Ring-necked Pheasants appeared more resistant to the effects of ochratoxin (1–4 ppm) than were chickens (Ruff et al. 1990; Huff et al. 1992; Ruff et al. 1992).

Mycotoxicosis

HUMAN HEALTH AND DOMESTIC ANIMAL CONCERNS

The human and domestic animal health concerns from primary exposure to mycotoxins are considerable and have been mentioned under the specific sections above. Secondary exposure to aflatoxins through ingestion of contaminated wildlife has been explored, but birds fed aflatoxins present a limited threat to hunters or other individuals or animals such as dogs that consume affected carcasses. Domestic turkey poults fed 500 ppb aflatoxin for 18 days had low levels (0.01–0.19 ppb) of detectable aflatoxin in the liver with lesser amounts in other tissues such as breast and thigh muscles (Gregory et al. 1983). Unless affected bird organs (liver, kidney, or gizzard) were consumed in high levels over a prolonged period of time, this low concentration of toxin would probably not present a human health concern. Additionally, any delay between the bird's ingestion of aflatoxin and hunter harvest reduces tissue burdens of aflatoxins because aflatoxins are cleared rapidly from tissues. After turkey poults were withdrawn from affected feeds, tissue concentrations of aflatoxins diminished within two to three days (Gregory et al. 1983). Only one of 18 domestic turkey poults fed 50 to 150 ppb aflatoxins and then placed on a control diet for one or two weeks had detectable aflatoxin (0.01 ppb) in the kidney and none detectable in the liver (Richard et al. 1986).

WILDLIFE POPULATION IMPACTS

The impact of acute or chronic mycotoxicosis on wildlife populations is not well documented despite reported epizootics in wild birds. Although major epizootics involving mycotoxins are rare, the effects of low-dose chronic exposures may be more significant than the few epizootics involving bird mortality indicate. For example, chickens fed aflatoxins have reduced egg production (Huff et al. 1975). After a one-week exposure to aflatoxins, Northern Bobwhite fed 200- and 400-ppb aflatoxin halted egg production (Stewart 1985), while control birds and birds fed 100 ppb aflatoxin had steady egg production. If aflatoxins have a similar effect on egg production in wild birds, population impacts of low-level chronic aflatoxicosis could be significant.

TREATMENT AND CONTROL

The best treatment and control for any of the mycotoxicosis is prevention. Nonetheless, there is a continued threat of exposure of wild birds to mycotoxins, particularly during winter months, because birds (especially waterfowl) commonly use harvested grain fields as feeding sites (Smith et al. 1990). Studies in domestic poultry and livestock indicate that tricothecene-contaminated feed is unpalatable, suggesting that birds might avoid consumption of contaminated feed if alternate foods are available. Should a food source be documented as being contaminated with trichothecenes or other mycotoxins, hazing of birds, plowing under of contaminated grains, and provision of alternate food sources should be considered to reduce morbidity and mortality.

The only practical treatment remains supportive care of affected birds.

MANAGEMENT IMPLICATIONS

Wildlife professionals should consider testing feeds, whether purchased or grown, for mycotoxins such as aflatoxins if those mycotoxins are a problem in their area. Local university extension agents should be able to provide guidance on the necessity of such testing. When sampling either standing crops or purchased feeds, efforts should be made to take samples from several areas or multiple bags of feed to ensure adequate testing.

Regarding aflatoxins, the best management recommendation, based on currently available literature and given the wide variability in susceptibility of avian species, is to avoid feeds contaminated with more than 100 ppb total aflatoxin, though complete avoidance of the toxins is, obviously, preferable. However, because this recommendation is based on the response of birds experimentally exposed to aflatoxins, the effects of aflatoxins on wild birds under field conditions could vary. Experimental birds are maintained under optimal conditions with regard to feed quality and availability, yet wild birds under field conditions are exposed to environmental stressors, differential rates of ingestion, and different durations of exposures to aflatoxin-contaminated feed.

Many attempts have been made to reduce aflatoxin-contamination of feed by dilution of contaminated feed with uncontaminated feed or inclusion of aflatoxin-binding agents such as clay compounds (Phillips 1999). Few of these methods work when the contaminated feed remains in the field, and few wildlife agencies have the financial resources to attempt these sometimes costly procedures.

Specific recommendations for limits of exposure of the other mycotoxins have not been established.

UNPUBLISHED DATA

1. U.S. Geological Survey, National Wildlife Health Center (NWHC), Madison, Wisconsin, U.S.A.
2. Southeastern Cooperative Wildlife Disease Study (SCWDS), College of Veterinary Medicine, University of Georgia, Athens, Georgia, U.S.A.
3. V.P. Nettles, Southeastern Cooperative Wildlife Disease Study, College of Veterinary Medicine, University of Georgia, Athens, Georgia, U.S.A.

LITERATURE CITED

Arafa, A.S., R.J. Bloomer, H.R. Wilson, C.F. Simpson, and R.H. Harms. 1981. Susceptibility of various poultry species to dietary aflatoxins. *British Poultry Science* 22:431–436.

Bennett, J.W., and M. Klich. 2003. Mycotoxins. *Clinical Microbiology Reviews* 16:497–516.

Bingham, A.K., T.D. Phillips, and J.E. Bauer. 2003. Potential for dietary protection against the effects of aflatoxins in animals. *Journal of the American Veterinary Medical Association* 222:591–596.

Blount, W.P. 1961. Turkey "X" disease. *Journal of the British Turkey Federation* 1:52,55,61.

Bondy, G.S., and J.J. Pestka. 2000. Immunomodulation by fungal toxins. *Journal of Toxicology and Environmental Health* B 3:109–143

Carnaghan, R.B.A. 1965. Hepatic tumors in ducks fed a low level of toxic ground nut meal. *Nature* 208:308.

Cheeke, P.R., and L.R. Shull. 1985. *Natural Toxicants in Feeds and Poisonous Plants.* AVI Publishing Company, Inc., Westport, CT, U.S.A., pp. 402–471.

Coulombe, Roger A. 1993. Symposium: Biological action of mycotoxins. *Journal of Dairy Science* 76:880–891.

Couvillion, C.E., J.R. Jackson, R.P. Ingram, L.W. Bennett, and C.P. McCoy. 1991. Potential natural exposure of Mississippi sandhill cranes to aflatoxin B_1. *Journal of Wildlife Diseases* 27:650–656.

Doerr, J.A., R.D. Wyatt, and P.B. Hamilton. 1976. Impairment of coagulation function during aflatoxicosis in young chickens. *Toxicology and Applied Pharmacology* 35:437–446.

Edds G.T., and C.F. Simpson. 1976. Cecal coccidiosis in poultry as affected by prior exposure to aflatoxin B_1. *American Journal of Veterinary Research* 37:65–68.

Ehrich M., C. Driscoll, and W.B. Gross. 1985. Effect of dietary exposure to aflatoxin B_1 on resistance of young chickens to organophosphate pesticide challenge. *Avian Diseases* 29:715–720.

Fitzpatrick, D.W., C.A. Picken, L.C. Murphy, and M.M. Buhr. 1989. Measurement of the relative binding affinity of zearalenone, alpha-zearalenol and beta-zearalenol for uterine and oviduct estrogen receptors in swine, rats and chickens: an indicator of estrogenic potencies. *Comparative Biochemical Physiology* C 94:691–694.

Fischer, J.R., A.V. Jain, D.A. Shipes, and J.S. Osborne. 1995. Aflatoxin contamination of corn used as bait for deer in the southeastern United States. *Journal of Wildlife Diseases* 31:570–572.

Fleischli, M.A., J.C. Franson, N.J. Thomas, D.L. Finley, and W. Wiley Jr. 2004. Avian mortality events in the United States caused by anticholinesterase pesticides: a retrospective summary of National Wildlife Health Center Records from 1980 to 2000. *Archives of Environmental Contamination and Toxicology* 46: 542–550.

Food and Drug Administration. 1989. Corn shipped in interstate commerce for use in animal feeds; action levels for aflatoxins in animal feeds. Revised compliance policy guide; availability; FDA's policy on blending of aflatoxin-contaminated corn from the 1988 harvest with noncontaminated corn for use in animal feeds. *Federal Register 54,* Vol. 100. U.S. Government Printing Office, Washington, D.C., U.S.A., pp. 22622–22624.

Forgacs, J., and W.T. Carll. 1955. Preliminary mycotoxic studies on hemorrhagic disease in poultry. *Veterinary Medicine* 50:172.

Forgacs, J., H. Koch, W.T. Carll, and R.H. White-Stevens. 1958. Additional studies on the relationship of mycotoxicosis to the poultry hemorrhagic syndrome. *American Journal of Veterinary Research* 19:744–753.

Giambrone, J.J., U.L. Deiner, N.D. Davis, A.S. Panagala, and F. J. Hoerr. 1985a. Effect of purified aflatoxin on turkeys. *Poultry Science* 64:859–865.

———1985b. Effect of purified aflatoxin on turkeys and broiler chickens. *Poultry Science* 64:1678–1684.

Gregory, J.F., S.L. Goldstein, and G.T. Edds. 1983. Metabolite distribution and rate of residue clearance in turkeys fed a diet containing aflatoxin B_1. *Food and Chemical Toxicology* 21:463–467.

Greenway, J.A., and R. Puls. 1976. Fusariotoxicosis from barley in British Columbia. I. Natural occurrence and diagnosis. *Canadian Journal of Comparative Medicine* 40:12–15.

Gumbmann, M.R., S.N. Williams, A.N. Booth, P. Vohra, R.A. Ernst, and M. Bethard. 1970. Aflatoxin susceptibility in various breeds of poultry. In *Proceedings of the Society of Experimental Biological Medicine* 134:683–688.

Halver, J.E. 1965. Aflatoxicosis and rainbow trout hepatoma. In *Mycotoxins in Foodstuffs,* G.N. Wogan (ed.). MIT Press, Cambridge, MA, U.S.A., pp. 209–234.

Hamilton, P.B., H.T. Tung, J.R. Harris, J.H. Gainer, and W.E. Donaldson. 1972. The effect of dietary fat on aflatoxicosis in turkeys. *Poultry Science* 51:165–170.

Hamilton, R.D., W.E. Huff, J.R. Harris, and R.D. Wyatt. 1982. Natural occurrences of ochratoxicosis in poultry. *Poultry Science* 61:1832–1841.

Hayes, M.A., and G.A. Wobeser. 1983. Subacute toxic effects of dietary T-2 toxin in young mallard ducks. *Canadian Journal of Comparative Medicine* 47: 180–187.

Helferich, W.G., W.N. Garrett, D.P.H. Hsieh, and R.L. Baldwin. 1986. Feedlot performance and tissue residues of cattle consuming diets contain aflatoxins. *Journal of Animal Science* 62:691–696.

Hendrickse, R.G. 1997. Of sick turkeys, kwashiorkor, malaria, perinatal mortality, heroin addicts and food poisoning: research on the influence of aflatoxins on child health in the tropics. *Annals of Tropical Medicine and Parasitology* 91:787–793.

Henke, S.E., V.C. Gallardo, B.Matinez, and R.Bailey. 2001. Survey of aflatoxin concentrations in wild bird seed purchased in Texas. *Journal of Wildlife Diseases* 37:831–835.

Huff, W.E., R.D. Wyatt, P.B. Hamilton. 1975. Effects of dietary aflatoxin on certain egg yolk parameters. *Poultry Science* 54:2014–2018.

Huff, W.E., L.F. Kubena, R.B. Harvey, D.E. Corrier, and H.H. Mollenhauer. 1986. Progression of aflatoxicosis in broiler chickens. *Poultry Science* 65:1891–1899.

Huff, W.E., M.D. Ruff, and M.B. Chute. 1992. Characterization of the toxicity of the mycotoxins aflatoxin, ochratoxin, and T-2 toxin in game birds. II Ringneck pheasant. *Avian Diseases* 36:30–33.

Joffe, A.Z. 1986. *Fusarium Species: Their Biology and Toxicology.* John Wiley and Sons, New York, NY, U.S.A., pp. 588.

Ledoux, D.R., T.P. Brown, T.S. Weibking, and G.E. Rottinghaus. 1992. Fumonisin toxicity in broiler chicks. *Journal of Veterinary Diagnostic Investigation* 4:330–333.

Miller, J.D. 1994. Epidemiology of *Fusarium* ear diseases of corn.. In *Mycotoxins in Grain: Compounds Other Than Aflatoxin.* J.D. Miller and H.L. Trenholm (eds.). American Association of Cereal Chemists, Inc. St. Paul, MN, U.S.A., pp. 19–36.

Muller, R.D., C.W. Carlson, G. Semeniuk, and G.S. Harshfield. 1970. The response of chicks, ducklings, goslings, pheasants, and poults to graded levels of aflatoxin. *Poultry Science* 49:1346–1350.

Munro, I.C., P.M. Scott, C.A. Moodie, and R.F. Willes. 1973. Ochratoxin A—occurrence and toxicity. *Journal of the American Veterinary Medical Association* 163:1269–73.

Neiger, R.D., T.J.Johnson, D.J. Hurley, K.F. Higgins, G.E. Rottinghaus, and H. Stahr. 1994. The short-term effect of low concentrations of dietary aflatoxin and T-2 toxin on Mallard ducklings. *Avian Diseases* 38:738–743.

Newberne, P.M. 1987. Interaction of nutrients and other factors with mycotoxins. In *Mycotoxins in Food.* P. Krogh (ed.). Academic Press, New York, NY, U.S.A., pp. 177–216.

Oberheu, D.G., and C.B. Dabbert. 2001. Aflatoxin production in supplemental feeders provided for Northern Bobwhite in Texas and Oklahoma. *Journal of Wildlife Diseases* 37:475–480.

Olsen, G.H., J.W. Carpenter, G. F. Gee, N.J. Thomas, and F.J. Dein. 1995. Mycotoxin-induced disease in captive Whooping Cranes (*Grus americana*) and Sandhill Cranes (*Grus canadensis*). *Journal of Zoo and Wildlife Medicine* 26:569–576.

Osweiler, G.D. 2000. Mycotoxins: contemporary issues of food animal health and productivity. *Veterinary Clinics of North America Food Animal Practice* 16:511–531.

Palmgren, M.S., and A.W. Hayes. 1987. Aflatoxins in food. In *Mycotoxins in Food.* P. Krogh (ed.). Academic Press, New York, NY, U.S.A., pp 65–95.

Pang, V.F., R.J. Lambert, P.J. Felsburg, V.R. Beasley, W.B. Buck, and W.M. Haschek. 1988. Experimental T-2 toxicosis in swine following inhalation exposure: clinical signs and effects on hematology, serum biochemistry, and immune response. *Fundamentals of Applied Toxicology* 11:100–109.

Phillips, T.D. 1999. Dietary clay in the chemoprevention of aflatoxin-induced disease. *Toxicological Sciences* 52 (Supplement):118–126.

Pier, A.C. 1992. Major biological consequences of aflatoxicosis in animal production. *Journal of Animal Science* 70:3964–3967.

Pier, A.C., and K.L. Heddleston. 1970. The effect of aflatoxin on immunity in turkeys. I. Impairment of actively acquired resistance to bacterial challenge. *Avian Diseases* 14:797–809.

Preluskey, D.B. 1994. Residues in food products of animal origin. In *Mycotoxins in Grain: Compounds Other Than Aflatoxin.* J. D. Miller and H. L. Trenholm (ed.). American Association of Cereal Chemists, Inc. St. Paul, MN, U.S.A., pp. 405–420.

Puls, R. and J.A Greenway. 1976. Fusariotoxicosis from barley in British Columbia. II. Analysis and toxicity of suspected barley. *Canadian Journal of Comparative Medicine* 40:16–19.

Quist, C.F., E.W. Howerth, J.R. Fischer, R.D. Wyatt, D.M. Miller, and V.F. Nettles. 1997. Evaluation of low-level aflatoxin in the diet of white-tailed deer. *Journal of Wildlife Diseases* 33:112–121.

Quist, C.F., D.I. Bounous, J.V. Kilburn, V.F. Nettles, and R.D.Wyatt. 2000. The effect of dietary aflatoxin on wild turkey poults. *Journal of Wildlife Diseases* 36:436–444.

Richard, J.L., R.D. Stubblefield, R.L. Lyon, W.M. Peden, J.R. Thurston, and R.B. Rimler. 1986. Distribution and clearance of aflatoxins B_1 and M_1 in turkeys fed diets containing 50 or 150 ppb aflatoxin from naturally contaminated corn. *Avian Diseases* 30:788–793.

Robinson, G.A. and A.M. Gibbins. 1984. Induction of vitellogenesis in Japanese quail as a sensitive indicator of the estrogen-mimetic effects of a variety of environmental contaminants. *Poultry Science* 63:1529–1536.

Robinson, R.M., A.C. Ray, J.C. Reagor, and L.A. Holland. 1982. Waterfowl mortality caused by aflatoxicosis in Texas. *Journal of Wildlife Diseases* 18:311–313.

Roffe, T.J., R.K. Stroud, and R.M. Windingstad. 1989. Suspected fusariomycotoxicosis in sandhill cranes (*Grus canadensis*): clinical and pathological findings. *Avian Diseases* 33:451–457.

Ruff, M.D., W.E. Huff, and G.C. Wilkins. 1990. Characterization of the toxicity of the mycotoxins aflatoxin, ochratoxin, and T-2 toxin in game birds. I. Chukar partridge. *Avian Diseases* 34:717–720.

Ruff, M.D., W.E. Huff, and G.C. Wilkins. 1992. Characterization of the toxicity of the mycotoxins aflatoxin, ochratoxin, and T-2 toxin in game birds. III. Bobwhite and Japanese quail. *Avian Diseases* 36:34–39.

Savard, M.E. and B.A. Blackwell. 1994. Spectral characteristic of secondary metabolites from *Fusarium* fungi. In *Mycotoxins in Grain: Compounds Other Than Aflatoxin.* J.D. Miller and H.L. Trenholm (eds.). American Association of Cereal Chemists, Inc. St. Paul, MN, U.S.A., pp. 59–69.

Schweitzer, S.H., C.F. Quist, G.L. Grimes, and D.L. Forster. 2001. Aflatoxin levels in corn available as wild turkey feed in Georgia. *Journal of Wildlife Diseases* 37:657–659.

Sharma, R.P. 1993. Immunotoxicity of mycotoxins. *Journal of Dairy Science* 76:892–897.

Smith, B.J., K.F. Higgins, and W.L. Tucker. 1990. Precipitation, waterfowl densities, and mycotoxins: their potential; effect on avian cholera epizootics in the Nebraska rainwater basin area. *Transactions of the North American Wildlife and Natural Resources Conference* 55:269–282.

Stewart, R.G. 1985. Natural exposure of bobwhite quail to aflatoxin. PhD Dissertation, University of Georgia, Athens, GA, U.S.A., 65 pp.

Tung, H-T., J.W. Smith, and P.B. Hamilton. 1970. Aflatoxicosis and bruising in the chicken. *Poultry Science* 50:795–800.

Uraguchi, K. 1971. Hepatotoxic mycotoxins of *A. flavus.* In *Pharmacology and Toxicology of Naturally-Occurring Toxins,* Vol. II. G. Peters (ed.). Pergamon Press, Elmsford, NY, U.S.A., pp. 217–246.

Vanyi, A., A. Bata, and F. Kovacs. 1994a. Effects of T-2 toxin treatment on the egg yield and hatchability in geese. *Acta Veterinaria Hungarica* 42:79–85.

Vanyi, A., R. Glavits, A. Bata, V.A., and F. Kovacs. 1994b. Pathological changes caused by T-2 trichothecene fusariotoxin in geese. *Acta Veterinaria Hungarica* 2: 447–457.

Weibking, T.S., D.R. Ledoux, T.P. Brown, and G.E. Rottinghaus. 1993. Fumonisin toxicity in turkeys. *Journal of Veterinary Diagnostic Investigation* 5:75–83.

Weibking, T.S., D.R. Ledoux, A.J. Bermudez, and G.E. Rottinghaus. 1994. Individual and combined effects of feeding *Fusarium moniliforme* culture material, containing known levels of fumonisin B1, and aflatoxin B1 in the young turkey poult. *Poultry Science* 73:1517–1525.

Willemart, J.P., and E. Schricke. 1981. Un cas d'infecondite chez les faisans description—reproduction—etiology. *Avian Pathology* 10:489–498.

Williams, J.H., T.D. Phillips, P.E. Jolly, J.K. Stiles, C.M. Jolly, and D. Aggarwal. 2004. Human aflatoxicosis in developing countries: a review of toxicology, exposure, potential health consequences, and interventions. *American Journal of Clinical Nutrition* 80: 106–1122.

Windingstad, R.M., R.J. Cole, P.E. Nelson, T.J. Roffe, R.R. George, and J.W. Dorner. 1989. *Fusarium* mycotoxins from peanuts suspected as a cause of sandhill crane mortality. *Journal of Wildlife Diseases* 25: 38–46.

Witlock, D.R. and R.D. Wyatt. 1981. Effect of dietary aflatoxin on hemostasis of young turkey poults. *Poultry Science* 60:528–531.

Wogan, G.N., S.S. Hecht, J.S. Felton, A.H. Conney, and L.A. Loeb. 2004. Environmental and chemical carcinogenesis. *Seminars in Cancer Biology* 14: 4732–486.

Wu, W., M.E. Cook, F.S. Chu, T. Buttles, J. Hunger, and P. Sutherland. 1997. Case study of bovine dermatitis caused by oat straw infected with *Fusarium sporotrichioides. The Veterinary Record* 140:399–400.

Yu, Fu-Li, I.H. Geronimo, W. Bender, and J. Permthansin. 1988. Correlation studies between the biding of aflatoxin B_1 to chromatin components and the inhibition of RNA synthesis. *Carcinogenesis* 9:527–532.

23
Algal Biotoxins

Jan H. Landsberg, Gabriel A. Vargo, Leanne J. Flewelling, Faith E. Wiley

INTRODUCTION

Over the last 20 years the number of microalgal species in marine and fresh water environments that are known to produce toxins (phycotoxins) and cause Harmful Algal Blooms (HABs) has increased. A variety of dinoflagellates and several diatom species are associated with HABs, many of which produce potent neurotoxins. There is a growing body of evidence that seabird mortalities accompany HABs worldwide (Shumway 2003), but with only a few exceptions, most avian mortalities associated with HAB events are anecdotal. For example, more than 1,000 deaths of Magellanic Penguins (*Spheniscus magellanicus*) in colonies at Chubut, Argentina (Quintana et al. 2001, cited in Shumway et al. 2003), co-occurred with HABs, although no direct cause and effect has yet been demonstrated. Black-browed Albatross (*Diomedea melanophris*) and Rockhopper Penguin (*Eudyptes crestatus*) mortalities in the Falkland Island region have also been associated with HAB events (BirdLife International 2004). In the last few years with persistent red tides along the west coast of Florida, the frequency of circumstantial bird mortalities has escalated. Rehabilitation centers are increasingly reporting admissions of sick birds or dead birds during red tide events, yet few studies have been done to characterize the chronic or differential effects of these toxins on bird communities and populations.

There is a convincing historical record that freshwater cyanobacteria have been responsible for avian deaths around lakes and rivers. Given the variety of neurotoxins and hepatotoxins produced by cyanobacteria, it is surprising that there are not more documented incidents of avian morbidity and mortality associated with such freshwater blooms.

In this chapter we summarize basic information on the most common HAB phycotoxins in marine and freshwater ecosystems. For each toxin group, we provide, where known, a description of the clinical signs and pathology associated with the toxin, levels that may elicit toxicity in humans, and circumstances and signs reported in wild bird mortalities.

SYNONYMS

Phycotoxicosis is an intoxication caused by an algal toxin. In humans, exposure to phycotoxins results in syndromes indicative of the effect of the toxins, for example, Paralytic Shellfish Poisoning (PSP) from saxitoxin, Neurotoxic Shellfish Poisoning (NSP) from brevetoxin, Amnesic Shellfish Poisoning (ASP) from domoic acid, and Diarrhetic Shellfish Poisoning (DSP) from okadaic acid. No systematic toxicoses syndromes are applied to wildlife impacted by HABs, probably because the symptoms may vary in different species or phyla. Brevetoxicosis is the syndrome traditionally ascribed to marine mammals lethally exposed to brevetoxins from *K. brevis* (Bossart et al. 1998) and can equally apply to birds.

HISTORY

In 1984, approximately 22 marine species and perhaps six fresh-water species of microalgae were known to produce toxins (Steidinger and Baden 1984; Hallegraeff 1993). Almost 80 toxic marine and 55 toxic freshwater species belonging to 10 classes of microalgae are now recognized (Table 23.1). This increase in HAB species can be partially attributed to a worldwide enhancement in trained scientists conducting shellfish monitoring programs for public health, to expanded toxicity testing of aquaculture products, and to major advances in detection methodologies for toxins.

The co-occurrence of HABs and bird deaths has been reported since the 1880s from Florida (Glazier 1882; Moore 1882; Walker 1884). Walker's (1884) account describes the effects of a red tide bloom: "At Tampa, ducks were dying. I saw dead vultures at Anna Maria Key, and at Passage Key, large flocks of cormorants were sick and dying. I also saw the carcasses of terns, gulls, and frigate birds. The cormorants sat on

Table 23.1. Estimates of the numbers of "red tide" species and the numbers of marine and freshwater species that are known to produce toxins among several classes of marine and fresh–water microalgae. Compiled from various sources and Landsberg 2002.

Common Name/Class	Total # of Species	Marine Red Tide Species	Marine & FW Toxic Species
Cyanobacteria			
Cyanophyceae	2000[a]	3–4	55
Diatoms			
Bacillariophyceae			
Centric	870–1000	30–65	1–2
Pennate	500–780	15–18	11
Dinoflagellates			
Dinophyceae	1500–1800	95–125	70–80
Golden–brown algae			
Chrysophyceae	95–125	6	0
Other monads and flagellates			
Cryptophyceae	55–75	5–6	1
Dictyochophyceae	1–3	1–2	0 (?)
Euglenophyceae	36–37	6–8	1
Prasinophyceae	100–135	5	1
Prymnesiophyceae	245–300	8–9	4–5
Raphidophyceae	11–12	7–9	4–6

a: depends upon nomenclature used.

the beach with their heads under their wings, and could be approached and handled." Other records of wild bird deaths associated with HABs are summarized in Table 23.2.

There is an interesting account in the fossil record that may be the first report of avian mortalities due to algal toxins. A late Pliocene death assemblage of marine birds and fish in Florida was hypothesized to be caused by blooms of saxitoxin-producing *Pyrodinium bahamense* (Emslie et al. 1996). Excavations of fossils revealed thousands of bones and partial skeletons of the extinct cormorant (*Phalacrocorax filyawi*), fewer bones from ten avian taxa, and numerous fish species. Parallel sediment cyst analyses revealed high densities of fossil dinocysts of *Polysphaeridium zoharyi* (nomenclature for fossil *Pyrodinium bahamense*). The two scenarios proposed were: (1) upwelling leading to a movement of fish, reduction in ideal prey, and ultimate starvation, or (2) a red tide event involving food chain transfer of toxins, likely saxitoxins originating from *P. bahamense.* It is unclear why this dinoflagellate species was proposed when unarmored *Karenia brevis* (for which there is no known fossilizable cyst [K. Steidinger, pers. comm.][1]) is known in this region to bloom annually and be associated with mass mortalities of birds. In our opinion, the role of saxitoxin in avian mortalities in the fossil record remains ambivalent, but nonetheless the record provides intriguing evidence of possible ancient phycotoxicosis.

EPIZOOTIOLOGY

The HABs about which most is known tend to be planktonic, visible, and quickly lead to acute shellfish poisonings or mass mortalities of aquatic organisms. Higher organisms are directly exposed to microalgal cells and their toxins by drinking them or ingesting them via various feeding modes (for example, filter feeding, predation), or, in cases in which toxins can be aerosolized (for example, brevetoxins), by inhalation (Landsberg 2002).

"Harmful algae" include all aquatic microalgal species that are known to produce toxins or to cause harm, directly or indirectly, to aquatic organisms or to terrestrial organisms associated with aquatic habitats or their products. The groups of microalgae considered to be harmful are shown in Table 23.1. In common usage, HABs are often called "red tides," so named for the discoloration caused by dense populations of cells in the water column. The term may be a misnomer because HABs are typically not red nor are they related to the tide. Typical water discolorations are red-brown to yellow-green due to both the primary pigment for photosynthesis, chlorophyll-a, and to accessory pigments such as chlorophyll-b, peridinin,

Table 23.2. Harmful algal bloom (HAB) species, toxins, and associated field mortalities or health impacts on wild and domestic birds (modified from Landsberg 2002).

Toxins[a]	HAB Species	Avian Species Affected	Year	Location	Reference
	Dinoflagellates				
Saxitoxins	*Alexandrium catenella*	Approximately 2,000 dead birds, Herring Gull *(Larus argentatus),* Western Gull *(L. occidentalis),* White-winged Scoter *(Melanitta fusca),* Common Murre *(Uria aalge californica),* Pacific Loon *(Gavia arctica pacifica),* Tufted Puffin *(Fratercula cirrhata),* Sooty Shearwater *(Puffinus griseus),* Black-footed Albatross *(Diomedea nigripes).* Several human PSP fatalities. Deaths of cats, chickens; vector: razor clams.	1942	Copalis and Grayland beaches, Washington coast, U.S.A.	McKernan and Scheffer 1942
		[b]More than 18 seabirds: Black Oystercatcher *(Haematopus moquini),* Kelp Gull *(Larus dominicanus),* Hartlaub's gull *(L. hartlaubii).*	1978	Lamberts Bay to False Bay, Marcus and other islands, Saldanha Bay, Ysterfontein shore, South Africa	Popkiss et al. 1979; Hockey and Cooper 1980
		Penguins, other marine bird species	1991–1992	Southern Chile and southern Argentina	Carreto and Benavides 1993
	Alexandrium tamarense	[b]636 bird mortalities: European Shag *(Phalacrocorax aristotelis),* Northern Fulmar *(Fulmarus glacialis),* Northern Gannet *(Morus bassanus),* Great Cormorant *(P. carbo),* Black Scoter *(Melanitta nigra),* Common Eider *(Somateria mollissima),* Great Black-backed Gull *(Larus marinus),* Lesser Black-backed Gull *(L. fuscus)* Herring Gull, Mew Gull *(L. canus),* Black-headed Gull *(L. ridibundus),* Black-legged Kittiwake *(Rissa tridactyla),* Common Tern *(Sterna hirundo),* Arctic tern *(S. paradisaea),*	1968	Sunderland to Holy Island, northeastern England	Adams et al. 1968; Coulson et al. 1968a, 1968b

(Continued)

Table 23.2. (Continued)

Toxins[a]	HAB Species	Avian Species Affected	Year	Location	Reference
		Roseate Tern *(S. dougallii),* Sandwich Tern *(S. sandvicensis),* Razorbill *(Alca toda),* Common Murre *(Uria aalge),* Atlantic Puffin *(Fratercula arctica);* suspected poisoning in Rock Pigeon (*Columba* sp.)			
		Gulls, shorebirds, 620 waterfowl, and 1600 Black Ducks *(Anas rubripes)*	1972	Northern coast of Massachusetts, U.S.A.	Bicknell and Walsh 1975; Sasner et al. 1975
		490 birds: European Shag, Northern Fulmar, Northern Gannet, Great Cormorant, Common Eider, Lesser Black- backed Gull, Herring Gull, Mew (Common) Gull, Black-legged Kittiwake, Common Tern, Arctic Tern, Sandwich Tern, Common Murre	1975	Northeastern England	Armstrong et al. 1978
	(as *A. excavata)*	[b] 73 Common Terns, 2 Arctic Tern, 1 Roseate Tern, 38 Herring Gull, 2 Laughing Gull *(Larus atricilla)*	1978	Monomoy National Wildlife Refuge, Massachusetts, U.S.A.	Nisbet 1983
		Black-legged Kittiwake	1984–1987	Northeastern England	Coulson and Strowger 1999
		Birds	1986	Bering Sea, northeast Kamchatka, Russia	Konovalova 1989, 1993
		Few dead eiders	1992	Trondheimsfjord, Norway	Tangen et al. 1992
		Herring gull	1996	St. Lawrence estuary, Quebec, Canada	Levasseur et al. 1996 in Shumway et al. 2003
		Black-legged Kittiwake	1997–1998	Northeastern England	Coulson and Strowger 1999
Brevetoxins	*Karenia brevis*	[b] Terns, gulls, frigatebirds, ducks, vultures, sick cormorants	1880	Tampa Bay to Key West, Florida, U.S.A.	Glazier 1882; Moore 1882; Walker 1884
		[b] Pelicans, seagulls	1946–1947	Dry Tortugas to Boca Grande, Florida, U.S.A.	Gunter et al. 1947, 1948

Table 23.2. (Continued)

		[b] Several thousand Lesser Scaup *(Aythya affinis)*, Double-crested Cormorant *(Phalacrocorax auritus)*, Red-breasted Merganser *(Mergus serrator)*	1973–1974	West coast, Florida, U.S.A.	Quick and Henderson 1974; Forrester et al. 1977
		[b]Double-crested Cormorant	1982	West coast Florida, U.S.A.	O'Shea et al. 1991
		Birds	1990	Southwestern Florida, U.S.A.	ICES 1991
		613 sick Double-crested Cormorant	1995–1999	Southwestern Florida, U.S.A.	Kreuder et al. 2002
Undescribed	*Prorocentrum micans*	Few dead cormorants	1956	Between Arica and Iquique, Chile	Manning 1957 in Avaria 1979
	Diatoms				
Domoic acid	*Pseudo-nitzschia australis*	43 Brown Pelicans *(Pelecanus occidentalis)*, 95 Brandt's Cormorants *(Phalacrocorax penicillatus)*, few Double-crested Cormorants, Western Gull, Pelagic Cormorant *(Phalacrocorax pelagicus)*	1991	Santa Cruz, California, U.S.A.	Work et al. 1992, 1993
	Pseudo-nitzschia sp.	More than 150 dead Brown Pelicans	1996	Baja California, Mexico	Sierra Beltran et al. 1996
	Prymnesiophytes				
?	*Prymnesium parvum*	Thirty species of water birds including young of the endangered Dalmatian Pelican *(Pelecanus crispus)*, White Spoonbill *(Platalea leucorodia)*, Great Egret *(Egretta alba)*	2004	Lake Koronia, Greece	Moustaka-Gouni et al. 2004
	Cyanobacteria				
Anatoxin–a, saxitoxins	*Anabaena circinalis*	24 Mallards *(Anas platyrhynchos)*, American Wigeon *(A. americana)*	1985	Steele Lake, Alberta, Canada	Pybus et al. 1986
Anatoxins, microcystins, saxitoxins	*Anabaena flos-aquae*, *Microcystis flos-aquae*, and *Aphanizomenon flos-aquae*	[b]47 turkey, 4 duck, 2 geese	1933	Lac Qui Parle, Milan, Minnesota, U.S.A.	Fitch et al. 1934

(*Continued*)

Table 23.2. (Continued)

Toxins[a]	HAB Species	Avian Species Affected	Year	Location	Reference
	Anabaena flos-aquae, Microcystis flos-aquae	[b]Pekin duck, wild birds, herons	1939	Fort Collins, Colorado, U.S.A.	Deem and Thorp 1939; Durrell and Deem 1939 in Schwimmer and Schwimmer 1968
Anatoxin-a, microcystins	*Anabaena flos-aquae*	[b]Chickens, turkeys, songbirds	1944–1945	East Okoboji, Lower Garn and Central Lakes, Iowa, U.S.A.	Rose 1953 in Schwimmer and Schwimmer 1968
		[b]7000 Franklin's Gulls *(Larus pipixcan)*, 560 ducks, 400 coots, 200 pheasants, 2 hawks, numerous songbirds	1952	Storm Lake, Iowa, U.S.A.	Rose 1953 and Firkins 1953 in Schwimmer and Schwimmer 1968
	Anabaena flos-aquae (with *Coelosphaerium kuetzingianum)*	Approx. 50 chickens	1918	Oaks Lake, Windom, Minnesota, U.S.A.	Fitch et al. 1934
Anatoxin-a(s)	*Anabaena lemmermanni*	Many ducks, chickens	1948	Fox Lake, Minnesota, U.S.A.	Olson 1951, 1952 in Schwimmer and Schwimmer 1968
		Birds	1993–1994	Lake Knud sø, Denmark	Henrickson et al. 1997; Onodera et al. 1997b
	Anabaena sp.	[b]Mergansers, Divers	1940–1942	Lake Ymsen, Mariestad, Skaraborg, Sweden	Berlin 1948 in Schwimmer and Schwimmer 1968
Microcystins, Anatoxin-a	*Arthrospira fusiformis*	Lesser Flamingos *(Phoenicopterus minor)*	2001	Lakes Bogoria, Nakuru, Kenya	Krienitz et al. 2003; Ballot et al. 2004
Microcystins	*Microcystis aeruginosa*	[b]Turkeys, ducks	1913–1943	Northeast Orange Free State and southeast Transvaal, South Africa	Steyn 1945; Stephens 1948
		[b]Water birds	1927	Amersfoort District, South Africa	Steyn 1945
		Pheasants, heron, snipe	1948	Round Lake, Minnesota, U.S.A.	Scott 1952 in Schwimmer and Schwimmer 1968
		Ducks, geese, waterfowl	1953	Lake Semekhovichi, Zhabchitskii District, Pinsk Province, Russia	Vinberg 1954 in Schwimmer and Schwimmer 1968

		7 Mallards	1989	Oklahoma, U.S.A.	Short and Edwards 1990
		20 Spot-billed Ducks *(Anas poecilorhyncha)*	1995	Nishinomiya, Hyogo Prefecture, Japan	Matsunaga et al. 1999
		Approx. 30 herons and ducks	1995	Jehay, Belgium	Wirsing et al. 1998
Microcystins	*M. aeruginosa* and *Anabaena flos-aquae*	579 Greater Flamingo, (*Phoenicopterus ruber*), Mallard, Eurasian Coot (*Fulica atra*), Purple Gallinule (*Porphyrio martinicus*), Common Moorhen (*Gallinula chloropus*)	2001	Doñana National Park, Spain	Alonso-Andicoberry et al. 2002
Microcystins	*M. flos-aquae* with *M. aeruginosa*	Numerous chickens	1933	Hall Lake, Fairmont, Minnesota, U.S.A.	Fitch et al. 1934
Microcystins	*M. botrys, M. viridis* and *M. wesenbergii*	Dead birds	2001	Lake Ontario, Lake Erie, Canada	Murphy et al. 2003
Microcystins	*Planktothrix agardhii*	[b] Waterfowl: 13 Mallards, 7 Common Terns, 6 Eurasian Coots, 4 Mew (Common) gulls, 4 Great Crested Grebe (*Podiceps cristatus*), 1 Common Goldeneye (*Bucephala clangula*), 12 unidentified birds	1984–1985	Lake Långsjon, Aland, Finland	Erikkson et al. 1986
Nodularins	*Nodularia spumigena*	400 duck	1963	Jasmunder Bodden, Germany	Kalbe and Tiess 1964
Unknown	*Nostoc rivulare*	Chickens, ducks, turkey	1956–1958	Waco, Texas, U.S.A.	Davidson 1959

a: Toxin known to be produced by these species—not necessarily confirmed to be present in the event.
b: Multispecies mortality event, birds only shown.

fucoxanthin, phycoerythrin, or phycocynanin. Dinoflagellate blooms produce red-brown discoloration due to the presence of fucoxanthin or peridinin, whereas blue-green algal (cyanobacteria) blooms may range from bright green due to chlorophyll-b to pink-red due to release of water-soluble phycoerythrin (Jeffrey et al. 1997; Mur et al. 1999). Because benign species can also cause water discolorations and hence be called red tides, the term HAB has been used to differentiate between blooms of benign and toxic species. However, not all HABs produce visibly obvious water discolorations. For example, blooms of *K. brevis* can cause fish kills at 100,000–250,000 cells/L but water discoloration does not occur until approximately one million cells/L is reached. Remote sensing technology can detect red tides, for example *K. brevis* can be visualized at a minimum of 100,000 cells/L (Tester et al. 1998), but because public health requirements for shellfish beds are often more stringent, traditional methods of routine water sampling are still required to determine cell concentrations.

Marine and freshwater HABs are worldwide phenomena. In general, their increased frequency, duration, and magnitude have been attributed to anthropogenic inputs of nutrients interacting with natural cycles (Smayda 1990; Hallegraeff 1993, 1995) and, in some cases, the global transport of species into areas where the lack of competition or predation may allow for extensive growth (Hallegraeff 1995). Changes in agriculture and aquaculture practices, over-fishing, and climate change may also be important factors in the global increase in HABs (HARRNESS 2005).

Negative impacts of HABs on fish and wildlife can result from several attributes: 1. toxin production; 2. the accumulation of biomass and concomitant oxygen depletion from the water column due to respiratory processes; and 3. physical damage based on the shape and composition of the microalgal species, for example, fish gill punctures from highly silicified diatom setae.

We are still in the early stages of understanding toxin production by HABs. Given the ubiquitous distribution and wide variety of toxic species, we might expect greater impacts on wildlife than are presently reported. However, the presence of a known toxic species alone does not necessarily mean that toxins are a significant risk factor. Toxin production, its availability and stability, and the degree of toxicity are dependent upon abiotic and biotic environmental conditions, such as temperature, the type and ratio of available macronutrients (for example, nitrogen and phosphorus) (Boyer et al. 1987; Anderson et al. 1990a, 1990b; Tomas and Baden 1993), clonal types present (Smith et al. 1990), and the presence of associated bacteria (Bates et al. 1995) that may produce toxin, for example, saxitoxin (Kodama et al. 1988; Doucette and Trick 1995).

Vertebrate mortalities may occur even in the absence of a visible HAB, because toxins can persist in the environment or food web for weeks or months after a bloom. For example, manatee (*Trichechus manatus latirostris*) deaths that occurred after a *K. brevis* red tide in Florida coastal waters were found to result from the accumulation of toxin on seagrass (*Thalassia testudinum*) blades (Flewelling et al. 2005) well after the red tide had dissipated.

There are three main types of algal toxins that are likely to be encountered by avian fauna: neurotoxins, hepatotoxins, and, minimally, dermatotoxins. Typically, marine dinoflagellates and diatoms largely produce the neurotoxic saxitoxins, brevetoxins, and domoic acid, while freshwater cyanobacteria produce neurotoxic saxitoxins and anatoxins, hepatotoxic microcystins, and the dermatotoxic lyngbyatoxins. Within each toxin group there are a number of derivatives, each having different levels of toxicity and hence being of varying risk to bird populations. In general, the microalgal species that produce these toxins are highly ubiquitous. For example, members of the genus *Alexandrium* that produce saxitoxins can be found in coastal regions of the northeast and northwest United States, Central and South American waters, European waters, the Mediterranean, and South African waters (Taylor et al. 2003). Toxin-producing cyanobacteria have the most ubiquitous distribution being found in lakes, rivers, and streams throughout the world (Carmichael 1992). Therefore, both aquatic and terrestrial birds that encounter water sources may be exposed to phycotoxins throughout their lives.

Bird deaths have been caused by the birds' consumption of contaminated fish or mollusks that have themselves consumed or otherwise bioaccumulated microalgal toxins. In other cases, birds have succumbed to toxins after drinking contaminated water, particularly after ingesting toxins from cyanobacterial blooms in freshwater systems (Landsberg 2002; Shumway et al. 2003). The toxins produced by HAB species and their documented involvement in bird mortalities are summarized in Table 23.2.

Harmful Algal Blooms can affect the foraging behavior of birds. It is possible that learned behavior and avoidance of saxitoxins by birds may depend on the differential familiarity of a species with red tide events, their choice of prey items, recognition of toxins, and their ability to switch to less ideal, nontoxic prey items. Kvitek and Bretz (2005) demonstrated that changes in the foraging behavior of shorebirds, particularly Black Oystercatchers *(Haematopus bachmani)* correlated with seasonal variation in toxicity of two major invertebrate prey species, sea mussels (*Mytilus californianus*) and sand crabs (*Emerita analoga*). They confirmed that shorebirds are able to detect and avoid consumption of lethal amounts of saxitoxins by opening and "testing" their molluskan prey to sense the presence of toxins in soft tissues and reject them if they are above a certain detectable threshold. These observations followed earlier studies by Kvitek (1991), which demonstrated that Glaucous-winged Gulls (*Larus glaucescens*) avoid saxitoxin exposure by conditioned aversions developed after regurgitation of contaminated bivalves. Kvitek suggested that avian predators generally are not at risk for paralytic shellfish poisoning via bivalve vectors because they can learn to avoid potentially toxic prey. Nonetheless, some mortality incidents associated with saxitoxins have involved toxic molluskan prey, so evidently some birds do not learn to avoid these items.

Most marine avian HAB-related mortality events appear to affect piscivorous species. This may in part reflect the inability of the predatory bird to discriminate toxic from nontoxic prey because fish are often ingested whole and toxins would not be released internally through digestion until well after feeding (Kvitek and Bretz 2005). Shags and cormorants appear in reports of intoxicated seabirds more often than most other avian families (Landsberg 2002; Shumway et al. 2003). This might be a function of their abundance, their piscivorous feeding habits, pelagic prey items, and their coastal habitat which, taken together, make them especially vulnerable to vectored phycotoxins, coastal HABs, and presence in locations where their mortalities are more likely to be noticed (Shumway et al. 2003). Double-crested Cormorants (*Phalocrocorax auritus*) are particularly susceptible to brevetoxin exposure by ingestion of fish in which toxin has been transferred up the food chain. Mollusks, crustacea, and other benthic infauna found along shore contaminated by brevetoxins during inshore red tides are also likely sources of ingestion exposure for many shorebirds, but this aspect has not been well studied.

The route of exposure, life history stage, immunocompetence, and risk of toxicosis may also determine a bird's susceptibility to toxins. For example, unlike manatees, which can be exposed to brevetoxins by inhalation and ingestion (Bossart et al. 1998; Flewelling et al. 2005), Double-crested Cormorants exhibited only mild evidence of pulmonary and tracheal lesions, indicating that inhalation was not a significant route of exposure (Kreuder et al. 2002). Immature Double-crested Cormorants were more likely to be admitted to rehabilitation clinics with brevetoxicosis than adults (Kreuder et al. 2002), suggesting that their lack of foraging experience made them more inclined to ingest dead or moribund brevetoxin-contaminated fish—a differential pattern that would not be explained if birds were exposed via inhalation, which should be nonselective by age class. Another possible explanation is that juveniles are more sensitive to brevetoxin than are adults.

ETIOLOGY, CLINICAL SIGNS, AND PATHOLOGY

Saxitoxins

Saxitoxins are a family of neurotoxins that occur worldwide in both marine and freshwater environments. They are produced by dinoflagellates (*Alexandrium* species, *Gymnodinium catenatum,* and *Pyrodinium bahamense*) and by cyanobacteria (*Anabaena circinalis, Aphanizomenon flos-aquae, Cylindrospermopsis raciborskii, Lyngbya wollei,* and *Planktothrix* sp.) (Landsberg 2002). *Alexandrium* and *Pyrodinium* are thecate dinoflagellates, 20–40 µm in diameter, with distinct plates composed of thickened cellulose. Most thecate dinoflagellates form resting stages called cysts that accumulate in the sediment, can resist harsh environmental conditions, and regenerate into vegetative cells when conditions are within limits for growth. *Gymnodinium catenatum* is an athecate (that is, does not have thickened cellulose plates) dinoflagellate but does produce a cyst (Steidinger and Tangen 1996). All of the cyanobacteria that produce saxitoxins are filamentous, and several (for example, *Amphanizomenon* and *Lyngbya*) also possess heterocysts for use in nitrogen fixation (Cronberg et al. 2003).

Saxitoxins are potent toxins with an intraperitoneal (i.p.) LD_{50} in mice of 10 µg/kg (as compared to an LD_{50} for sodium cyanide at 10 mg/kg) (Oshima et al. 1989). They are highly nitrogenous heterocyclic guanidines, and the guanidinium character is considered essential for their activity (Kao 1993). Saxitoxins restrict signal transmission between neurons by binding to site 1 on the voltage-dependent sodium channel, blocking the influx of sodium into excitable cells.

Oshima (1995) described more than 20 derivatives of saxitoxin, and that number continues to increase with new analogs recently identified from *Lyngbya wollei* (Onodera et al. 1997a) and *Gymnodinium catenatum* (Llewellyn et al. 2004). Derivatives include the most common and highly toxic carbamate toxins: saxitoxin, neosaxitoxin, and gonyautoxins (I-IV). The decarbamoyl analogues (dcSTX, dcNEO, dcGTX1-4) and the deoxydecarbamoyl analogues (doSTX, doGTX2, doGTX3) are of intermediate toxicity, whereas the least toxic derivatives are the N-sulfocarbamoyl toxins B1, B2, and C1-C4 (Oshima 1995).

No dinoflagellate or cyanobacteria population has been found to contain all naturally occurring saxitoxin derivatives, so the toxin profile is considered to be characteristic of the microalgal strain or species (Landsberg 2002). Toxin composition can also vary in relation to geographical range, environmental factors, and experimental conditions (Kodama 2000). Given this variation, the proportion of highly toxic saxitoxin derivatives, and therefore the overall toxicity, to which animals are exposed will differ from case to case.

In humans, consumption of bivalves that have accumulated saxitoxins results in Paralytic Shellfish Poisoning (PSP). Symptoms usually occur rapidly (5–30 minutes after consumption) and include headache, nausea and vomiting, dizziness, numbness and tingling of the face and neck, and muscle weakness. In more serious cases, a person may experience numbness and tingling of the arms and legs, incoherent speech, motor incoordination, drowsiness, light-headedness, paralysis, and difficulty breathing. Without emergency medical care, death can occur, typically within 1–12 hours after ingestion (Baden et al. 1995).

Similarly, birds can be affected by saxitoxins (Table 23.2). In May 1942, coincident with an *Alexandrium catenella* bloom, at least 2,000 dead seabirds were observed along the coastal beaches of Washington state, U.S.A. Concurrently, six human cases of fatal PSP had been reported; cats and chickens that had consumed razor clam (*Siliqua patula*) viscera were also dying. At least eight bird species (Table 23.2) were found dead with crustaceans and clams in their stomachs and with inflamed intestines. The peak of the mortality occurred about two weeks after the crest of the red tide, and the numbers of dead birds seen on the beaches began to decline two weeks after the disappearance of the bloom. McKernan and Scheffer (1942) suggested that the birds were killed by feeding on toxic fish and crustaceans that had ingested *A. catenella* cells.

In May 1968, dying sea birds and dead sand eels (*Ammodytes* sp.) were reported around the Farne Islands, northeast England. The first deaths of sand eels were recorded about one week after the peak of an *Alexandrium tamarense* bloom (Adams et al. 1968). Large numbers of the mollusks striped Venus (*Venus striatula*), edible cockles (*Cardium edule*), and Baltic macomas (*Macoma balthica*) were moribund along the shoreline. Blue mussels (*Mytilus edulis*) were found to be highly toxic. A total of 636 dead seabirds were found along 104 kilometers of the northeast coast. Many of the birds had been feeding on fish shortly before they died. Within a few days, 82% of the breeding European Shag (*Phalocrocorax aristotelis*) population had died. Dying European Shags found on the Farne Islands exhibited loss of equilibrium, lack of motor coordination, paralysis, constriction of pupils, excess vomiting, abnormal green-brown feces, intestinal hemorrhage, failure of the circulatory system, and congestion of organs, including the lungs. All these symptoms were remarkably similar to those observed in humans and domestic chicks affected by PSP. Seventy-eight human cases of PSP were caused from eating toxic blue mussels (Coulson et al. 1968a, 1968b). From May–June 1975, a similar mortality event in the same area affected an estimated 500 European Shags (Armstrong et al. 1978).

The first red tide bloom that led to a major PSP outbreak in the U.S.A. occurred in September 1972 from southern Maine to Cape Ann, Massachusetts. Hundreds of waterfowl and shorebirds died from saxitoxin exposure after feeding on contaminated bivalves (Bicknell and Walsh 1975). Blue mussels and soft-shell clams (*Mya arenaria*) were the bivalves most susceptible to saxitoxin accumulation and were the most toxic. Bird gastrointestinal contents contained small, filter-feeding bivalves including blue mussels and the Atlantic jacknife (*Ensis directus*). Many other birds apparently perished after feeding on toxic shellfish, but were not recovered (Bicknell and Walsh 1975; Sasner et al. 1975).

In 1978, following a red tide, at least 70 Common Terns (*Sterna hirundo*) were reported to have died in the Monomoy National Wildlife Refuge (NWR), Maine, U.S.A., and high concentrations of saxitoxins were confirmed in regurgitated fish, specifically sand lance (*Ammodytes americanus*). Dying birds fell forward, beat their wings ineffectually, stumbled across the sand, became paralyzed, and died within 5–10 minutes of their first signs of poisoning. In 13 birds the intestinal mucosa was thickened and the intestine contained pale mucoidal material, suggesting a tentative diagnosis of enteritis (Nisbet 1983). In 2005, an unprecedented and persistent *Alexandrium* red tide occurred along the New England states, U.S.A. On Monomoy NWR, at least 40 Common Terns died, with some showing clinical and postmortem lesions similar to the 1978 event. Several liver samples were positive for saxitoxin (SEANET 2005).

Brevetoxins

Brevetoxins (PbTxs) are potent marine neurotoxins produced by the dinoflagellate *Karenia brevis* (Baden 1983) and other *Karenia* species (Haywood et al. 2004). Brevetoxin production has also been documented in the raphidophytes *Chattonella* cf. *verruculosa* (Bourdelais et al. 2002) and *C. marina* (Ahmed et al. 1995), and has been reported, but not structurally confirmed, in the raphidophytes *C. antiqua* (Haque and Onoue 2002), *Heterosigma akashiwo* (Kahn et al. 1997), and *Fibrocapsa japonica* (Kahn et al. 1996). The overwhelming majority of documented brevetoxin-related impacts are the result of *K. brevis* blooms.

There are six described *Karenia* species (Haywood et al. 2004). All are athecate, motile dinoflagellates 30–50 μm in diameter. Typical water column background levels of the most abundant species, *K. brevis*, are 1,000 cells/L. Other *Karenia* species can be found mixed in with *K. brevis* blooms but are usually not as abundant. Although all are pigmented, photosynthetic cells, populations on the order of several million cells per liter are required before significant water discoloration occurs. *Karenia* species occur in the Gulf of Mexico from Mexico to Florida, on the east coast of Florida, Australia, Western Europe, and Japan (Steidinger and Tangen 1996; Haywood et al. 2004). *Karenia brevis* is principally distributed throughout the Gulf of Mexico, with occasional red tides along the mid and south Atlantic coast of the U.S.A. (Steidinger 1993). The raphidophyte species that produce brevetoxins range in size from 20–100 μm and are typically flattened dorsoventrally with two flagellae inserted apically. They are ubiquitous, found in discolored water blooms in neretic and brackish waters of the North and South Atlantic, Europe, Japan, Korea, and the west coast of the U.S.A. and Canada (Throndsen 1996).

Brevetoxins are a family of lipid-soluble polycyclic ether toxins. They are divided into two groups based on their backbone structure, with at least 12 derivatives identified that represent modifications of the two parent toxins, PbTx-1 and PbTx-2 (Baden et al. 2005). The most abundant brevetoxins are PbTx-2 and its derivatives, while the PbTx-1-type toxins are the most potent. Brevetoxins are neurotoxins that cause repetitive firing in nerves; they bind to site 5 on voltage-dependent sodium channels (Poli et al. 1986), with half-maximal binding in the nm concentration range. Binding results in opening of sodium channels at normal resting potential, which can lead to membrane depolarization (Poli et al. 1986; Baden et al. 1995). Mice administered brevetoxins i.p. show irritability immediately upon injection, followed by hind-quarter paralysis, dyspnea, salivation, lachrymation, urination, defecation, and death from respiratory paralysis. Whole LD_{50} for brevetoxins in mice ranges from 0.05 mg/kg body weight for intravenous (i.v.) administration to 0.5 mg/kg for oral and i.p. administration (Baden and Mende 1982; Baden 1989).

Brevetoxins have also been shown to inhibit cathepsins, key enzymes in the formation of antigenic determinants, which may result in suppression of antibodies (Sudaranam et al. 1992; Benson et al. 2005). Additionally, aerosolized brevetoxins are potent airway constrictors that induce effects at concentrations 1,000 times lower than has been found in neuronal studies, suggesting an additional pulmonary receptor (Abraham et al. 2005).

Brevetoxins are toxic to humans following ingestion of contaminated shellfish and can result in Neurotoxic Shellfish Poisoning (NSP). Toxicity is characterized by paresthesia, reversal of hot-cold temperature sensation, myalgia, vertigo, ataxia, abdominal pain, nausea, diarrhea, burning pain in the rectum, headache, bradycardia, and dilated pupils (Baden et al. 1995). People can also suffer from respiratory effects when brevetoxins become aerosolized through the disruption of *K. brevis* cells by breaking waves, surf, or on-shore winds (Pierce 1986). Until 1987, brevetoxin-induced human illnesses were limited to the Gulf of Mexico. Since then, NSP has been reported on the Atlantic coast of the U.S.A. at North Carolina (Fowler and Tester 1989) and in New Zealand (Bates et al. 1993).

Karenia brevis blooms, documented in Florida since the 1840s, are usually known to cause massive fish kills (Gunter et al. 1947, 1948; Galstoff 1948; Steidinger et al. 1973; Smith 1975), but bird die-offs also have been recorded (Table 23.2). During the *K. brevis* red tide of October 1973–May 1974 along the west coast of Florida, large numbers of Double-crested Cormorants, Red-breasted Mergansers (*Mergus serrator*), and Lesser Scaup (*Aythya affinis*) were found moribund or dead. During an eight-week period, several thousand Lesser Scaup died. All Lesser Scaup examined had abundant subcutaneous fat and normal pectoral muscle mass, indicating that the birds died quickly. Most of the ducks had recently fed, and the proventriculi contained several taxa of mollusks: turritellid, pyramidellid, and opisthobranch gastropods; and amethyst gemclams (*Gemma gemma*). Clinical signs included weakness, reluctance to fly, slumping of the head, clear nasal discharge, viscous oral discharge, oil gland dysfunction, excessive lacrimation, chalky yellow diarrhea, dyspnea, tachypnea, tachycardia, decreased blood pressure, depressed body temperature, diminished reflexes, and dehydration (Quick and Henderson 1974; Forrester et al. 1977).

To directly assess the effects of red tide toxins, white Pekin ducklings (*Anas platyrhynchos domesticus*) were force-fed toxic hard clams (*Mercenaria mercenaria*) (assayed at 48 MU/100 g tissue), or red tide water containing 2.2×10^4 *Karenia brevis* cells/ml. The ducklings showed signs of toxicity two days after exposure, appearing lethargic, and on day three developed ataxia, spastic movements of the head, and a tendency to droop the head to one side. Over the next few days some ducks died and others showed signs similar to those noted in field observations of moribund birds (Quick and Henderson 1974; Forrester et al. 1977).

Substantial numbers of sick and dying Double-crested Cormorants were found concurrently with six red tide events along the west Florida coast during 1995–1999 (Kreuder et al. 2002). Birds exhibited signs of severe cerebellar ataxia characterized by a broad-based stance, truncal incoordination, hypermetric gait, and intention tremors of the head similar to ataxia experimentally induced in ducklings with brevetoxin. Brevetoxin was found in the spleen and lung of four Double-crested Cormorants examined in 1997. In all, 360 birds were admitted to the rehabilitation clinics with neurologic signs, allowing the authors to demonstrate a significant ($p<0.05$) relationship with the presence of *K. brevis*.

In addition to neurotoxins, early characterization of *K. brevis* toxins also described hemolytic and anticoagulative components (Doig and Martin 1973; Baden 1983). This aspect of the pathogenesis of brevetoxins has not been well studied but may also impact avian health. There is evidence for hemolysis and excessive destruction of erythrocytes in fish (Quick and Henderson 1974) and marine mammals (Bossart et al. 1998, 2002) exposed to *K. brevis* red tides. In Double-crested Cormorants, histopathological findings demonstrated multi-organ hemosiderosis suggestive of chronic hemolysis (Kreuder et al. 2002), as well as acute neurotoxicity.

Domoic Acid

Domoic acid is a neurotoxin produced by marine diatoms. Originally isolated from the red macroalga (*Chondria armata*) (Takemoto and Daigo 1958), domoic acid was not known to be produced by microalgae prior to a human shellfish poisoning event in 1987 on Prince Edward Island, Canada, when the toxin was implicated for the first time in Amnesic Shellfish Poisoning (ASP). After the consumption of toxic blue mussels, three people died, 19 were hospitalized (12 remained in intensive care for a time), and more than 100 were taken ill with varying degrees of gastrointestinal and neurologic illness. Domoic acid toxicity in mussels was eventually linked to the diatom (*Pseudo-nitzschia multiseries*) (Subba Rao et al. 1988; Bates et al. 1989).

The production of domoic acid has been identified in 11 species of *Pseudo-nitzschia* and one species of *Nitzschia* (Bates 2000; Landsberg 2002; Cerino et al. 2005). *Pseudo-nitzschia* and *Nitzschia* are elongated, needle-like, pennate diatoms that form long chains of physiologically independent cells by overlapping valve ends. Cells range from 30–140 μm in length and 1–10 μm in width. These diatoms are ubiquitous, with one or more species found in Argentina, Chile, Tasmania, Brazil, both the Atlantic and Pacific coasts of the United States and Canada, the Gulf of Mexico, and European waters (Fryxell and Hasle 2003).

Domoic acid is a water-soluble, heat-stable low-molecular-weight amino acid. It is an analog of glutamate, an excitatory neurotransmitter that binds to both kainate and AMPA subtypes of glutamate receptors in nervous tissue (Hampson et al. 1992). These receptors are found in high densities on nerve cells in the hippocampus, an area of the brain associated with memory retention, hence the loss of memory associated in ASP cases. Domoic acid causes massive depolarization of the neurons, resulting in an increase in cellular Ca^{2+}, neuronal swelling, and cell death (Novelli et al. 1990; Bates et al. 1998).

Clinical symptoms of ASP include nausea, vomiting, abdominal cramps, diarrhea, a decreased level of consciousness, seizures, confusion, disorientation, and permanent short-term memory loss (Baden et al. 1995). The i.p. LD_{50} in rats is 3.6 mg/kg. Human illnesses occurred at oral dosages of 1–5 mg/kg; however, the oral potency in rats is much lower (35–70 mg/kg), demonstrating differences in sensitivities between susceptible humans and rats (Van Dolah 2000).

Although domoic acid–producing species are found worldwide, documented cases of ASP and domoic acid–related animal mortalities have thus far been restricted to North America. In September 1991 the first wildlife mortality event, and one that occurred in birds, was attributed to this toxin (Fritz et al. 1992; Work et al. 1992). In Santa Cruz, California, U.S.A., at least 43 Brown Pelicans (*Pelicanus occidentalis*) and 95 Brandt's Cormorants (*Phalacrocorax penicillatus*) died from ingesting Californian anchovies (*Engraulis mordax*) contaminated with domoic acid. The birds displayed a characteristic slow side-to-side head motion, held their wings partially extended, and were unable to fly for more than 10 minutes without having to land. Vomiting was common, and the birds would lose awareness of their surroundings, display torticollis, lose righting reflex, and lie either on their back or side with their feet paddling slowly prior to death. The only consistent gross and histopathologic lesions observed were hemorrhages and necrosis of the skeletal muscle. Serum blood urea nitrogen and creatinine phosphokinase were higher in affected birds than they were in controls. Domoic acid was detected in the stomach contents of the sick and dead birds, in the flesh and viscera of Californian anchovies, and in plankton samples dominated by *Pseudo-nitzschia* (Work et al. 1992, 1993). In this case, *P. australis* was demonstrated to produce domoic acid (Fritz et al. 1992; Garrison et al. 1992). As well as anchovies, planktivores such as krill (Bargu et al. 2002, 2003) are also key vector species for the transfer of domoic acid.

Sierra Beltran et al. (1997) reported another domoic acid event in Cabo San Lucas, Mexico, where Brown Pelicans were killed after feeding on domoic acid-contaminated chub mackerel (*Scomber japonicus*). At least 150 birds were found during a period of five days in January 1996. Live pelicans exhibited signs of intoxication including disorientation and agitation, difficulty in swimming, and inability to right themselves if they had turned upside-down during swimming, causing them to drown. At least 50% of the pelican colony died, and surviving birds still showed symptoms of weakness and disorientation two months after the event. *Pseudo-nitzschia* sp. frustules were found in the stomach contents of pelicans and mackerel; mouse bioassay of bird stomach contents and high performance liquid chromatography (HPLC) confirmed the presence of domoic acid.

Cyanotoxins

Blooms of cyanobacteria in freshwater and brackish systems have been responsible for a number of mass bird mortality events. Cyanotoxins are basically classified into two groups—hepatotoxins and neurotoxins—based on the symptoms they induce in animals. Neurotoxic cyanotoxins include saxitoxins and anatoxins. Hepatotoxic cyanotoxins are more common than the neurotoxins and include the microcystins, nodularin, and cylindrospermopsin.

Cyanobacteria are highly diverse, ranging from colonial filamentous forms such as *Anabaena* spp. to visible colonies (8 mm diameter) of 4–6 μm cells embedded in a gelatinous matrix (for example, *Microcystis aeruginosa, Nostoc* spp.). Most toxin-producing cyanobacteria are found worldwide in fresh water or, as with *Nodularia,* in brackish waters, but several *Lyngbya* species are marine. Many species produce gas vesicles that provide positive buoyancy and lead to dense surface accumulations and water discolorations (Cronberg et al. 2003).

Although documented primarily for their effects on poultry and waterfowl, cyanobacteria are significant emerging risk factors in wild bird mortalities. Primarily, anatoxins and microcystins have been associated with mass mortality events.

Anatoxin-a

Anatoxin-a was originally isolated from *Anabaena flos-aquae* and has also been reported from strains of *A. circinalis, A. planctonica, Aphanizomenon* sp., *Cylindrospermum* sp., and *Planktothrix* (= *Oscillatoria*)(Smith 2000).

Anatoxin-a is a low-molecular-weight secondary amine that is highly neurotoxic. It is a postsynaptic cholinergic nicotine agonist that causes death via a depolarizing blockage of neuromuscular transmission and subsequent respiratory paralysis. The i.p. LD_{50} in mice for purified toxin is about 200 μg/kg body weight, with a survival time of 4–7 minutes. Symptoms of anatoxin-a toxicity in mouse bioassays include muscle fasciculation, loss of coordination, gasping, convulsions, and death by respiratory arrest (Carmichael et al. 1990; Carmichael 1992).

Clinical signs of anatoxin-a in vertebrates are often difficult to distinguish from those of saxitoxin. Both result in all or some of the following symptoms: trembling, loss of coordination, staggering, and collapse and death by respiratory failure. Signs of poisoning in field reports for wild and domestic animals are similar and include staggering, muscle fasciculations, gasping, convulsions, and in birds, opisthotonus. Death occurs within minutes to a few hours depending on species, dosage, and prior food consumption. Animals need to ingest only a few milliliters to a few liters of the toxic surface bloom to receive a lethal bolus (Carmichael 1988).

Anatoxin-a from *Anabaena* blooms has been implicated in a few mortality events involving primarily waterfowl, domestic birds, and gulls (Table 23.2) but is usually reported in mixed cyanobacterial blooms with multiple toxins. Single bloom events and sole anatoxin-a responsibility for bird mortalities has not, to our knowledge, been reported.

Anatoxin-a(s)

Anatoxin-a(s) is a naturally occurring organophosphate produced by *Anabaena flos-aquae* and *A. lemmermannii,* first reported from a culture of *A. flos-aquae* isolated from Buffalo Pound Lake, Saskatchewan, Canada (Carmichael and Gorham 1978). As are synthetic organophosphates, anatoxin-a(s) is a potent acetylcholinesterase inhibitor. The i.p. LD_{50} in mice is 20–50 μg/kg, about 10 times more lethal than anatoxin-a. In mice or rat bioassays, anatoxin-a(s) induces marked viscous salivation (which is the basis for the [s] label for the toxin), lachrymation in mice, chromodacryorrhea (red-pigmented tears) in rats, urinary incontinence, muscular weakness, fasciculation, convulsion, and defecation prior to death due to respiratory failure (Carmichael et al. 1990; Smith 2000).

In July 1993 and June-July 1994 at lakes in Denmark, deaths of wild birds coincided with massive cyanobacterial blooms dominated by *A. lemmermannii* var. *minor.* Extracts of field samples were neurotoxic to mice and subsequently showed an anticholinesterase activity similar to anatoxin-a(s). Neither anatoxin-a nor saxitoxin or its derivatives were detected by HPLC, which together with the pharmacological evidence and unambiguous spectroscopic identification of anatoxin-a(s) confirmed for the first time that anatoxin-a(s) was the cause of avian mortalities (Henriksen et al. 1997; Onodera et al. 1997b).

Microcystins

Microcystins are the most common cause of water-based toxicosis caused by cyanobacteria. About

65 structural variants of microcystins are currently known, more than half of which have been isolated from species and strains of *Microcystis aeruginosa* and *M. viridis.* Other microcystins are produced by *Anabaena flos-aquae, Anabaena* spp., *Anabaenopsis milleri, Nostoc* spp., and *Planktothrix* (= *Oscillatoria*) *agardhii* (Sivonen and Jones 1999). As with other microalgal toxins, most information regarding the mechanism of action has been obtained from rodent bioassay models. The LD_{50} of microcystin-LR (i.p. or i.v.) in mice and rats is in the range of 36–122 µg/kg, and the inhalation toxicity in mice is similar: LCT_{50} 180mg/min/mm, LD_{50} = 43 µg/kg (Dawson 1998).

In mammals, symptoms of microcystin intoxication are diarrhea, vomiting, piloerection, weakness, and pallor (Bell and Codd 1994). Microcystin targets the liver, causing cytoskeletal damage, necrosis, and pooling of blood in the liver, with a consequent increase (up to 100%) in liver weight. At acutely toxic doses, microcystins cause rounding or shrinkage of the hepatocytes and loss of normal hepatocyte structure. This disorganization of the tissue leads to massive hepatic hemorrhage, often followed by the death of animals from hypovolemic shock or hepatic insufficiency. Death can occur within a few hours after a high dose (Bell and Codd 1994; Dawson 1998).

Microcystins are also potent tumor promoters in mammals, mediated through the inhibition of protein phosphatase type 1 and 2A activities. Their mode of action appears to be different from other protein phosphatase inhibitors such as okadaic acid (cause of Diarrheic Shellfish Poisoning) (Falconer 1993) and their effects are organ specific (liver) (Falconer 1991). Microcystins do not easily penetrate epithelial cells nor are they tumor promoters on mouse skin (Matsushima et al. 1990). The potential role of microcystins in the induction of hepatic neoplasia in birds has not been determined.

Bird mortalities associated with several microcystin-producing species have been documented (Table 23.2). The experimental effects of microcystins in birds such as the Northern Bobwhite (*Colinus virginianus*) suggested a possible organotropism for the spleen rather than the liver as in mammalian models (Takahashi and Kaya 1993), but a recent bird mortality event in Japan also indicated hepatotoxicity (Matsunaga et al. 1999). In the summer of 1995, approximately 20 Spot-billed Ducks (*Anas poecilorhyncha*) died during an *M. aeruginosa* bloom in a pond in Nishinomiya, Hyogo Prefecture, Japan. Lyophilized algal cell powder from the pond contained high concentrations of microcystins that were acutely toxic to mice. Algal samples from a neighboring pond (with no bird mortalities) were not acutely toxic. At necropsy, ducks had severely jaundiced, necrotic livers suggestive of microcystin toxicity. Apparently, there was a significant influx of untreated sewage into the pond following the Hanshinn earthquake in January 1995. Eutrophic conditions likely contributed to the development of the bloom (Matsunaga et al. 1999).

In the summer of 1995 in Jehay, Belgium, 30 duck and heron deaths coincided with a massive bloom of *M. aeruginosa.* Rat hepatocyte assays and HPLC confirmed microcystins in bloom material, but bird tissues were not examined (Wirsing et al. 1998).

Although *M. aeruginosa* blooms are more typically involved in microcystin mortality events, other bloom species have also been implicated. During 1984–1985, a bloom of *Planktothrix agardhii* (= *Oscillatoria agardhii*) in Lake Långsjon (southwest Finland) was associated with fish kills, mostly roach (*Rutilus rutilus*) and bream (*Abramis* brama), and bird deaths (Erikkson et al. 1986), including both herbivorous and piscivorous species. Toxins from bloom isolates were experimentally demonstrated to accumulate in swan mussels (*Anodonta cygnea*), which, together with liver lesions in dead fish, were considered to be strong circumstantial evidence of a role for hepatotoxic cyanotoxins in the mortality event. Although not characterized at the time, subsequent research demonstrated that the *Planktothrix* originally isolated from Lake Långsjon during 1984–1985 produce microcystins (Luukkainen et al. 1993).

Mixed Cyanobacteria Blooms

Generally, HABs are considered to be ephemeral acute events dominated by an increased biomass of planktonic forms suspended in the water column, but there is evidence for equivalent risks to birds from benthic (at the sea or lake bottom) cyanobacteria. In some cases during mixed cyanobacterial blooms, birds may be exposed to multiple toxins from both planktonic and/or benthic sources.

For decades, frequent mass mortalities of Lesser Flamingos (*Phoenicopterus minor*) have been observed in the alkaline-saline Rift Valley lakes in East Africa. Because flamingos normally feed on cyanobacteria, they may be at high risk for ingesting large doses of microcystins during persistent blooms. Since a 2001 mortality event in Lake Bogoria, Kenya, cyanobacterial mats at the inflow of hot springs along the shore are being investigated as a potential source of toxicity. Mats were dominated by *Phormidium terebriformis, Oscillatoria willei, Spirulina subsalsa,* and *Synechococcus bigranulatus.* Hepatotoxic microcystins-LR (221–845 µg eq/g dry weight of mat), -RR, -LF, and -YR, and the neurotoxin anatoxin-a (10–18 µg/g dry weight of mat) were present. Flamingos exhibited neurological signs of poisoning, and stomach and intestinal contents as well as fecal pellets showed high concentrations of microcystins and anatoxins, suggesting that cyanotoxins contributed to the mortality. Krienitz et al. (2003) proposed that intoxication from cyanotoxins could occur by uptake of detached cyanobacterial cells from the mats when flamingos drink inflowing fresh or brackish water, or bathe near the inflowing hot springs where salinity is lower than in the main water-body of the lake. A more expansive study investigated phytoplankton communities and cyanotoxins were in three Kenyan lakes (Ballot et al. 2004). *Arthrospira fusiformis*, generally considered nontoxic, was identified as one toxin source when an isolated strain from Lake Bogoria was found to produce both microcystin-YR and anatoxin-a. Because *A. fusiformis* blooms are characteristic of alkaline-saline lakes and Lesser Flamingo feed primarily on *Arthrospira*, it was proposed that further mortalities of this species from cyanotoxins might be anticipated (Ballot et al. 2004).

In July 2001, at least 579 Greater Flamingos (*Phoenicopterus ruber*) together with Mallards (*Anas platyrynchos*), Eurasian Coots (*Fulica atra*), Purple Gallinules (*Porphyrio martinica*), and Common Moorhens (*Gallinula chloropus*) died in the Doñana National Park, Spain, during the sudden appearance of a cyanobacterial bloom. *Microcystis aeruginosa* and *Anabaena flos-aquae* formed dense surface scum on the windward shores of the lagoon. Water, crop contents, and liver samples were positive for microcystins by mouse bioassay and rapid screening kits. Crop contents from six dead flamingo chicks contained high numbers of *M. aeruginosa* and *A. flos-aquae* with toxin concentrations of more than 600 μg microcystin-LR eq/ml, as compared to less than 10 μg microcystin-LR eq/ml in the water (Alonso-Andicoberry et al. 2002).

Nodularin

Nodularin is a hepatotoxin produced by *Nodularia spumigena*. Only *N. spumigena* has been found to produce nodularin, and not all strains of *Nodularia* are toxic. Several nodularins have been characterized. They are pentapeptides structurally related to microcystins, but they are much fewer in number. Both in experimental animals and based on observations in field reports, the toxicity and pathogenicity of nodularin is very similar to that of microcystin (Rinehart et al. 1994). Like microcystin, nodularin is a protein phosphatase 1 and 2A inhibitor, a tumor promoter (Yoshizawa et al. 1990), and a direct liver carcinogen (Ohta et al. 1994). In rodents, nodularin induces enlarged hemorrhagic livers, centrilobular necrosis, lysis of hepatocytes, and death within one to two hours (Runnegar et al. 1988).

Nodularia spumigena blooms associated with livestock, canine, and wildlife mortality events have principally occurred in brackish waters in Australia, New Zealand, and the Baltic Sea (Landsberg 2002). Nodularin may have impacts on bird populations, but evidence is scant.

Sipia et al. (2004) verified nodularin in blue mussels and fish, primarily flounder (*Platichthys flesus*), caught in the northern Baltic Sea from 1996–2002. Additionally, nodularin was confirmed by enzyme-linked immunosorbent assay (ELISA) and liquid chromatography-mass spectrometry in liver samples from Common Eiders (*Somateria mollissima*). Because Common Eiders feed extensively on blue mussels, they can be exposed to nodularin accumulated in contaminated shellfish. In August–September 2002, 15 eiders were shot and collected from three different sites in the western Gulf of Finland (northern Baltic Sea). Eider liver samples contained 3–180 μg nodularin/kg (dry weight) which, calculated by total liver weight, was equivalent to 0.1–5.8 μg nodularin/liver (dry wt). Although nodularin was found in one sick eider, the relationship between the lesions (that is, swollen organs) and the presence of the toxin was considered uncertain. This report was the first documentation of nodularin in seabirds and provides evidence for the trophic transfer of this toxin through the Baltic Sea food web (Sipia et al. 2004).

Suspected Cyanotoxin

Avian vacuolar myelinopathy (AVM) is a neurological disease primarily affecting Bald Eagles (*Haliaeetus leucocephalus*) and American coots (*Fulica americana*) in the southeastern U.S.A. The disease is characterized and diagnosed by spongy degeneration of the white matter of the central nervous system (CNS), particularly prominent in the optic tectum (Thomas et al. 1998). Birds with AVM may display clinical signs of neurological impairment, including difficulty in swimming, flying, and/or walking. Not all birds with AVM lesions display these signs, and clinical recovery has been documented despite the persistence of lesions (Larsen et al. 2002).

Avian vacuolar myelinopathy is site specific, can have a quick onset (as early as five days post-exposure), and is seasonal, with AVM events occurring during the late fall to early winter (Rocke et al. 2002). First observed during the winter of 1994–1995, the disease has been documented in five states and is responsible for the deaths of at least 100 Bald Eagles and estimates of more than a thousand American Coots (Wilde et al. 2005). Other species that have been diagnosed with AVM include the Mallard, Ring-necked Duck (*Aythya collari*), Bufflehead (*Buchephala albeola*), Canada Goose (*Branta canadensis*), Great Horned Owl (*Bubo virginianus*), and Killdeer (*Charadrius vociferous*)-(Fischer et al. 2002; Augspurger et al. 2003).

The cause of AVM has not yet been determined. Evidence gathered to date suggests a toxin of natural origin. The lack of inflammation in affected tissues, inability to detect infectious disease agents, and the character of the lesion suggest a toxic compound (Thomas et al. 1998). In addition, the disease has not been shown to be transmissible by direct contact with affected birds (Larsen et al. 2003). Extensive toxicological tests have been conducted on American Coot and Bald Eagle tissues and environmental samples, with no significant concentrations of known compounds detected (Thomas et al. 1998, Dodder et al. 2003).

Experimentally, coots and waterfowl developed AVM by ingestion of aquatic vegetation and associated materials (Birrenkott et al. 2004, Lewis-Weis et al. 2004). Bald Eagles likely become affected by feeding on affected prey species (Fischer et al. 2003). Vegetative material that induced AVM in laboratory studies contained large quantities of a novel cyanobacteria species of the Order Stigonematales (Birrenkott et al. 2004). Surveys of cyanobacterial epiphytes have revealed that this species is prevalent at all known AVM sites during epizootics, and is not present, or is present in very low numbers, at sites where AVM is not documented (Wilde et al. 2005). Scientists have postulated that this species may be producing a toxin responsible for AVM, and research is currently under way to explore this hypothesis.

DIAGNOSIS

In spite of historical and recent records of bird deaths associated with HAB occurrences, evidence for the role of HABs in causing bird mortalities remains sparse. The scientific literature contains few quantitative attempts to relate clinical signs and pathology with the presence of toxins in affected birds, and few measurements of toxin body burdens in wild birds have been done. Acute phycotoxicosis may result in death quickly and, though there may be defined clinical signs for specific toxins, there usually are few pathognomonic postmortem lesions. Because individual HAB species can produce multiple toxins that can have different mechanisms, and routes and degrees of exposure can vary, a complex suite of subtle pathological changes may confound diagnostic interpretation. Systematic documentation of such changes has not been done. To implicate HABs in bird mortality, extensive environmental and animal sampling is therefore a critical step toward developing a differential diagnosis. Knowledge would be greatly advanced if future investigations adopt a comprehensive approach that includes a thorough synthesis of environmental factors, provides for the collection of water or benthic samples for microalgal and phycotoxin testing, conducts routine screening for phycotoxins in tissues and gastrointestinal contents, and documents clinical, gross, and histopathological abnormalities in cases of suspected phycotoxicosis.

In recent years, improvements have been made in toxin detection methodologies that can be used to identify phycotoxin involvement in avian mortalities or disease. The availability of ELISAs for many toxins (for example, brevetoxins, saxitoxins, domoic acid, microcystins) and improvements in analytical techniques such as HPLC, have lowered limits of detection, reduced the time required for analyses, and can provide results that either sum or differentiate the multiple toxins and their derivatives. An immunohistochemical assay has been used to diagnose brevetoxin exposure in animals (Bossart et al. 1998), and could be developed for other toxins as well. However, as with ELISAs, the availability and appropriate specificity of antibodies present challenges. Many functional assays that detect the toxins' physiological activities or effects have also been developed and can be useful screening tools. For example, anticholinesterase assays and protein phosphatase inhibition assays can be used to screen for anatoxin-a(s) and microcystins respectively, and receptor-binding assays have been developed to detect many of the marine neurotoxins. However, few commercial laboratories perform such analyses, and they are in large part restricted to research laboratories and those that test water and food for the protection of public health. Many of these assays are highly susceptible to matrix effects from tissue extracts, or require the use of expensive equipment or radioisotope-linked toxins (many of which are not commercially available), and in all cases positive results require unambiguous structural confirmation. Although toxin detection methodologies are quickly being developed and continually improving, at present the best route to pursue testing (that is, development of in-house capabilities versus commercial laboratories or research partners) may be determined by the number of samples anticipated, the number and types of toxins suspected, existing capabilities, and available funds.

There is currently no systematic collection of specific prey species that might be associated with transfer of toxicity in HAB-related bird mortality events. Because of their risks to public health, shellfish have been well studied and used as an indicator of HAB occurrence (Shumway 1990). However, many bird HAB-associated mortality events do not correlate with shellfish toxin levels (Nisbet 1983; Scholin et al. 2000), demonstrating in part that different shellfish species retain variable concentrations of toxins and cannot always be used as a proxy for interpreting the trophic transfer of toxins. Knowledge of avian species ecology and feeding habits, as well as determination of toxic prey species in the wild, must be integrated to determine those higher trophic level species at risk.

The HABs or their phycotoxins may also be triggers or stressors for avian diseases, but definitive links are lacking. Murphy et al. (2000) speculated that toxic *Microcystis* and *Aphanizomenon* blooms could act as stressors during the winter when waterfowl molt. Unable to fly, already stressed birds that are further exposed to phycotoxins could be more susceptible to an outbreak of avian botulism. Such unknown but potential linkages must be resolved before the impacts of phycotoxins on avian fauna can be fully understood.

It is especially important to have a sound basis for linking cause and effect with HABs because there is always a high degree of uncertainty (Suter et al.1993). Koch (1891) developed a series of postulates that could be used to test the basis for cause and effect, but they applied to microbial related diseases. To establish causality between various chemicals and their impacts on organisms, ecotoxicologists modified Koch's original postulates (Adams 1963; Woodman and Cowling 1987). These reformulated postulates, as stated in Suter et al. 1993), are as follows:

1. The injury, dysfunction, or other putative effect of the toxicant must be regularly associated with exposure to the toxicant and any contributory causal factors.
2. Indicators of exposure to the toxicant must be found in the affected organisms.
3. The toxic effects must be seen when normal organisms or communities are exposed to the toxicant under controlled conditions, and any contributory factors should be manifested in the same way during controlled exposures.
4. The same indicators of exposure and effects must be identified in the controlled exposures as in the field.

A case can be made that finding a particular phycotoxin at high concentrations in avian species dying acutely in an area where an HAB was in progress and producing the same toxin would establish cause and effect. However, it is also possible that coincidental, unaccounted causal factors could be significant; positive confirmation of toxins does not necessarily prove direct effect.

At this time, lethal doses for phycotoxins and their metabolites are not known for individual bird species. Extrapolation of results obtained using experimental species as a substitute for the affected species could lead to uncertainties in data interpretation. Interpretive problems also arise because of differences in the temporal and spatial distributions of toxic blooms and affected organisms. Birds may be chronically, cumulatively, or sub-lethally exposed to toxins or move away from the implicated HAB area. Lag effects may occur.

There is a lack of knowledge about the body burden of toxins that can be carried by migratory birds that are exposed elsewhere to HABs, and about how sub-lethal toxin concentrations may affect avian health. Given the ubiquitous nature of phycotoxins, it is entirely possible that, as with environmental pollutants, most avian species carry background concentrations. For example, brevetoxins were detected in several species of dead seabirds found in southwest Florida when no *K. brevis* red tide blooms occurred (Vargo et al. 2006) (FWC, unpubl. data).[2] In order to firmly establish cause and effect, we urgently need to know the concentrations and characteristics of toxins that cause particular signs, lesions, or death. Until these questions are answered, and until diagnostic tests for phycotoxins become routine for cases of seemingly unexplained avian deaths, relationships between microalgal toxins and their avian impacts will largely remain anecdotal.

WILDLIFE POPULATION IMPACTS

The impact of HABs on wildlife populations is largely undocumented. It can be difficult to assess the magnitude of mortality associated with HABs. Unless mortality events occur acutely and in a small, localized area, accurate mortality estimates are difficult to obtain. Many HABs occur over hundreds of kilometers offshore or in inaccessible areas so that bird carcasses are unnoticed or become too badly decomposed for accurate diagnosis. Significant events may go unnoticed or are severely underestimated. Until a direct relationship is confirmed between HABs and wild bird mortality events, and the losses are evaluated in light of population trends, the role of HABs in declining bird populations will remain to be determined. For example, Rockhopper Penguin mortality events in the Falkland Islands frequently co-occur with toxic *Alexandrium* blooms. Based on recent population estimates, Rockhopper Penguins in the Falklands decreased 80% from 1932–1995, a reduction from 1.5 million to 263,000 breeding pairs (Pütz et al. 2003). Fishing pressure is considered a major factor (Bingham 2002), but to what extent HABs directly or indirectly contribute to this dramatic loss is uncertain.

Birrenkott (2003) examined the impact of AVM on South Carolina and Georgia's Bald Eagle population, concluding that AVM significantly affected local populations. Because Bald Eagles in these states are non-migratory and their breeding seasons coincide with AVM epizootics, AVM could pose a significant risk to statewide populations if it spread to other lakes. Impacts to coot and waterfowl populations are beginning to be explored. Although unsubstantiated, numbers of migrating American Coots appear to have declined over the past few years in South Carolina

(T. Murphy, pers. comm.)[3], and there is concern that AVM may be a contributing factor.

TREATMENT AND CONTROL

Phycotoxin exposures are usually lethal or sickened birds are not easily recovered from the wild. Records for successful rehabilitation and treatment are available from *K. brevis* and brevetoxin endemic areas in Florida.

Birds suffering from brevetoxicosis are usually dehydrated, weak, and unable to stand. At the Suncoast Seabird Sanctuary, over the last decade more than 200 Brown Pelicans have been admitted with brevetoxicosis (B. Suto, pers. comm.).[4] If birds are removed from the area of exposure and treated with supportive therapy, including plenty of fresh water to flush out brevetoxins, then birds can recover and are often released. Although birds recover when removed from the red tide area, birds that were banded and released were often readmitted within five days with recrudescence of clinical signs. Kreuder et al. (2002) suggested that birds were either becoming reexposed to brevetoxins or that they demonstrated signs of delayed effect from the initial exposure.

MANAGEMENT IMPLICATIONS

Reduction in the magnitude and duration of HAB events could significantly reduce the impact of phycotoxins on wildlife. Strategies to reduce the risk of bird mortalities would be to remove or reduce the magnitude and potency of the HAB, to prevent bird exposures by managing the affected habitat or toxic prey, or to treat birds after they are affected. However, on a large scale many of these strategies are impractical or economically prohibitive.

Recent studies on the management of HABs range from control of nutrient inputs in order to reduce biomass in both marine and freshwater environments, to research on the development of targeted probes for biological control of individual species, and to direct sedimentation of all water column particles, including cells, using fine clays (HARRNESS 2005). For many blooms, decreased eutrophication has dramatically reduced the impact of these events (Smayda 1990, 1992).

Control of cyanobacterial blooms by reduction of phosphorus inputs into freshwater ecosystems has been a proven management tool for decades (Vollenweider and Kerekes 1982; Cooke et al. 1993; Reynolds 1997), whereas the use of anti-algae chemicals such as copper sulfate typically leads to cell lysis and therefore the release of intracellular phycotoxins, which exacerbates the problem (Lam et al. 1995; references in Chorus and Bartram 1999). The pros and cons of a variety of management methods for control of freshwater cyanobacterial blooms can be found in the comprehensive review by Chorus and Bartram (1999).

Management of AVM epizootics will ultimately depend upon determination of the source of the disease. However, the knowledge that AVM is associated with aquatic vegetation, including certain invasive plants, has given researchers and managers an area of focus. Exotic aquatic weeds have been impacting the nation's waterways since the late 1800s, and management of these plants is still a major area of research today (Cofrancesco 1998). Researchers are currently studying grass carp (*Ctenopharyngodon idella*) as a potential control agent for aquatic weeds in AVM sites.

UNPUBLISHED DATA

1. Karen Steidinger, Fish and Wildlife Research Institute, Florida Fish and Wildlife Conservation Commission, St. Petersburg, FL, U.S.A.
2. Fish and Wildlife Research Institute, Florida Fish and Wildlife Conservation Commission, St. Petersburg, FL, U.S.A.
3. Tom Murphy, South Carolina Department of Natural Resources, Green Pond, SC, U.S.A.
4. Barbara Suto, Suncoast Seabird Sanctuary, Indian Shores, FL, U.S.A.

LITERATURE CITED

Abraham, W.M., A.J. Bourdelais, A. Ahmed, I. Serebriakov, and D.G. Baden. 2005. Effects of inhaled brevetoxins in allergic airways: toxin-allergen interactions and pharmacologic intervention. *Environmental Health Perspectives* 113:632–637.

Adams, D.F. 1963. Recognition of the effects of fluorides on vegetation. *Journal of Air Pollution Control Association* 13:360–362. Cited in G. W. Suter, III et al. 1993. *Ecological Risk Assessment.* Lewis Publishers, Boca Raton, FL, U.S.A., 438 pp.

Adams, J.A., D.D. Seaton, J. B. Buchanan, and M.R. Longbottom. 1968. Biological observations associated with the toxic phytoplankton bloom off the east coast. *Nature* 220:24–25.

Ahmed, M.S., O. Arakawa, and Y. Onoue. 1995. Toxicity of cultured *Chatonella marina.* In *Harmful Marine Algal Blooms,* C. Marcaillou (ed.). Lavoisier, Paris, France, pp. 499–504.

Alonso-Andicoberry, C., L. García-Villada, V. Lopez-Rodas, and E. Costas. 2002. Catastrophic mortality of flamingos in a Spanish national park caused by cyanobacteria. *The Veterinary Record* 151:706–707.

Anderson, D.M., D.M. Kulis, J.J. Sullivan, S. Hall, and C. Lee. 1990a. Dynamics and physiology of saxitoxin production by the dinoflagellates *Alexandrium* spp. *Marine Biology* 104:511–524.

Anderson, D.M., D.M. Kulis, J.J. Sullivan, and S. Hall. 1990b. Toxin composition variations in one isolate of the dinoflagellate *Alexandrium fundyense. Toxicon* 28:885–893.

Armstrong, I.H., J.C. Coulson, P. Hawkey, and M.J. Hudson. 1978. Further mass seabird deaths from paralytic shellfish poisoning. *British Birds* 71:58–68.

Augspurger, T.A., J.R. Fischer, N.J. Thomas, L. Sileo, R.E. Brannian, K.J.G. Miller, and T.E. Rocke. 2003. Vacuolar myelinopathy in waterfowl from a North Carolina impoundment. *Journal of Wildlife Diseases* 39:412–417.

Avaria, S. 1979. Red tides off the coast of Chile. In *Toxic Dinoflagellate Blooms,* D.L. Taylor and H.H. Seliger (eds.). Elsevier, New York, NY, U.S.A., pp. 161–164.

Baden, D.G. 1983. Marine food-borne dinoflagellate toxins. *International Review of Cytology* 82:99–149.

Baden, D.G. 1989. Brevetoxins: unique polyether dinoflagellate toxins. *Federation of American Societies for Experimental Biology Journal* 3:1807–1817.

Baden, D.G., and T.J. Mende. 1982. Toxicity of two toxins from the Florida red tide marine dinoflagellate, *Ptychodiscus brevis. Toxicon* 20:457–461.

Baden, D.G., L.E. Fleming, and J.A. Bean. 1995. Marine toxins. Handbook of Clinical Neurology 21(65): 141–175.

Baden, D.G., A. J. Bourdelais, H. Jacocks, S. Michelliza, and J. Naar. 2005. Natural and derivative brevetoxins: historical background, multiplicity, and effects. *Environmental Health Perspectives* 113:621–625.

Ballot, A., L. Krienitz, K. Kotut, C. Wiegand, J.S. Metcalf, G.A. Codd, and S. Pflugmacher. 2004. Cyanobacteria and cyanobacterial toxins in three alkaline Rift Valley lakes of Kenya–Lakes Bogoria, Nakuru and Elmenteita. *Journal of Plankton Research* 26: 925–935.

Bargu, S., C.L. Powell, S.L. Coale, M. Busman, G.J. Doucette, and M.W. Silver. 2002. Krill: a potential vector for domoic acid in marine food webs. *Marine Ecology Progress Series* 237:209–216.

Bargu, S., B. Barinovic, S. Mansergh, and M.W. Silver. 2003. Feeding responses of krill to the toxin-producing diatom *Pseudo-nitzschia. Journal of Experimental Marine Biology and Ecology* 284:87–104.

Bates, M., M. Baker, N. Wilson, L. Lane, and S. Handford. 1993. Epidemiologic overview of the New Zealand shellfish toxicity outbreak. In *Marine Toxins and New Zealand Shellfish,* J.A. Jasperse (ed.). SIR Publishing, Wellington, NZ, pp. 35–40.

Bates, S.S. 2000. Domoic-acid-producing diatoms: another genus added! *Journal of Phycology* 36:978–983.

Bates, S.S., C.J. Bird, A.S.W. de Freitas, R. Foxall, M. Gilgan, L.A. Hanic, G.R. Johnson, A.W. McCulloch, P. Odense, R. Pocklington, M.A. Quilliam, P.G. Sim, J.C. Smith, D.V. Subba Rao, E.C.D. Todd, J.A. Walter, and J.L.C. Wright. 1989. Pennate diatom *Nitzschia pungens* as the primary source of domoic acid, a toxin in shellfish from Eastern Prince Edward Island. *Canadian Journal of Fisheries and Aquatic Sciences* 46:1203–1215.

Bates, S.S., D.L. Garrison, and R.A. Horner. 1998. Bloom dynamics and physiology of domoic-acid-producing *Pseudo-nitzschia* species. In *Physiological Ecology of Harmful Algal Blooms,* D.M. Anderson, A.D. Cembella, and G.M. Hallegraeff (eds.). Springer-Verlag, Heidelberg, Germany, pp. 267–292.

Bell, S.G., and G.A. Codd. 1994. Cyanobacterial toxins and human health. *Reviews in Medical Microbiology* 5:256–264.

Benson, J., F.F. Hahn, T.H. March, J.D. McDonald, A.P. Gomez, M.J. Sopori, A.J. Bourdelais, J. Naar, J. Zaias, G.D. Bossart, and D.G. Baden. 2005. Inhalation toxicity of brevetoxin 3 in rats exposed for twenty-two days. *Environmental Health Perspectives* 113:626–631.

Bicknell, W.J., and D.C. Walsh. 1975. The first "red tide" in recorded Massachusetts history. In *Proceedings of the First International Conference on Toxic Dinoflagellate Blooms,* V.R. LoCicero (ed.). Massachusetts Science and Technology Foundation, Wakefield, Massachusetts, U.S.A., pp. 447–458.

Bingham, M. 2002. The decline of Falkland Islands penguins in the presence of a commercial fishing industry. *Revista Chilena de Historia Natural* 75:805–818.

Birdlife International. 2004. Dramatic declines on seabird island (16-02-2004). BirdLife International, Cambridge, United Kingdom. [Online.] Retrieved from the World Wide Web: www.birdlife.org/news/news/2004/02/falklands.html.

Birrenkott, A.H. 2003. Investigating the cause of avian vacuolar myelinopathy and the consequences to the South Carolina Bald Eagle (*Haliaeetus leucocephalus*) population. M.S. Thesis, Clemson University, Clemson, SC, U.S.A., 49 pp.

Birrenkott, A.H., S.B. Wilde, J.J. Hains, J.R. Fischer, T.M. Murphy, C.P. Hope, P.G. Parnell, and W.W. Bowerman. 2004. Establishing a food-chain link between aquatic plant material and avian vacuolar myelinopathy in mallards (*Anas platyrhynchos*). *Journal of Wildlife Diseases* 40:485–492.

Bossart, G.D., D.G. Baden, R.Y. Ewing, B. Roberts, and S.D. Wright. 1998. Brevetoxicosis in manatees (*Trichechus manatus latirostris*) from the 1996 epizootic: gross, histologic and immuno-histochemical features. *Toxicologic Pathology* 26:276–282.

Bossart, G.D., D.G. Baden, R.Y. Ewing, B. Roberts, and S.D. Wright. 2002. Manatees and brevetoxicosis. In *Molecular and Cell Biology of Marine Mammals,* C.J. Pfieffer (ed.). Krieger Publishing Company, Melbourne, FL, U.S.A., pp. 205–212.

Boyer, G.L., J.J. Sullivan, R.J. Andersen, P.J. Harrison, and F.J.R. Taylor. 1987. Effects of nutrient limitation on toxin production and composition in the marine dinoflagellate *Protogonyaulax tamarensis. Marine Biology* 96:123–128.

Bourdelais, A.J., C.R. Tomas, J. Naar, J. Kubanek, and D. G. Baden. 2002. New fish-killing alga in coastal Delaware produces neurotoxins. *Environmental Health Perspectives* 110:465–470.

Carmichael, W.W. 1992. Cyanobacteria secondary metabolites—the cyanotoxins. *Journal of Applied Bacteriology* 72:445–459.

Carmichael, W.W., and P.R. Gorham. 1978. Anatoxins from clones of *Anabaena flos-aquae* isolated from lakes of western Canada. *Mitteilungen Internationale Vereinigung für Theoretische und Angewandte Limnologie* 21:285–295.

Carmichael, W.W., N.A. Mahmood, and E.G. Hyde. 1990. Natural toxins from cyanobacteria (blue-green algae). In *Marine Toxins: Origin, Structure, and Molecular Pharmacology,* S. Hall and G. Strichartz (eds.). American Chemical Society, Washington, D.C., U.S.A., pp. 87–106.

Carreto, J.I., and H.R. Benavides. 1993. World record of PSP in southern Argentina. *Harmful Algae News* 5:2.

Castonguay, M., J.L. Levasseur, F.G. Beaulieu, S. Michaud, E. Bonneau, and S.S. Bates. 1997. Accumulation of PSP toxins in Atlantic mackerel: seasonal and ontogenic variations. *Journal of Fish Biology* 50:1203–1213.

Cerino, F, L. Orsini, D. Sarno, C. Dell'Aversano, L. Tartaglione, and A. Zingone. 2005. The alternation of different morphotypes in the seasonal cycle of the toxic diatom Pseudo-nitzschia galaxiae. *Harmful Algae* 4:33–48.

Chorus, I., and J. Bartram (eds.). 1999. *Toxic Cyanobacteria in Water: A Guide to Their Public Health Consequences, Monitoring, and Management.* E. and F. N. Spon, London, U.K., on behalf of WHO, 400 pp.

Cofrancesco, A. F. Jr. 1998. Overview and future direction of biological control technology. *Journal of Aquatic Plant Management* 36:49–53.

Cooke, G.D., E.B. Welch, S.A. Peterson, and P.R. Newroth (eds.). 1993. Restoration and Management of Lakes and Reservoirs, 2nd Ed. Lewis Publishers, CRC Press Inc., Boca Raton, FL, U.S.A., 548 pp.

Cronberg, G., E.J. Carpenter, and W.W. Carmichael. 2003. Taxonomy of harmful cyanobacteria. In *Manual of Harmful Marine Microalgae,* G. M. Hallegraeff, D. M. Anderson, and A.D. Cembella (eds.), UNESCO Publishing, Paris, FR, pp. 523–562.

Coulson, J.C., and J. Strowger. 1999. The annual mortality rate of black-legged kittiwakes in NE England from 1954 to 1998 and a recent exceptionally high mortality. *Waterbirds* 22:3–13.

Coulson, J.C., G.R. Potts, I. R Deans, and S.M. Fraser. 1968a. Mortality of shags and other seabirds caused by paralytic shellfish poison. *Nature* 220:23–24.

Coulson, J.C., G.R. Potts, I.R. Deans, and S. M. Fraser. 1968b. Exceptional mortality of shags and other seabirds caused by paralytic shellfish poison. *British Birds* 61:381–404.

Davidson, F.F. 1959. Poisoning of wild and domestic animals by a toxic waterbloom of *Nostoc rivulare* Kütz. *Journal of the American Water Works Association* 51:1277–1287.

Dawson, R.M. 1998. The toxicology of microcystins. *Toxicon* 36:953–962.

Deem, A.W., and F. Thorp. 1939. Toxic algae in Colorado. *Journal of the American Veterinary Medical Association* 95:542.

Dodder, N.G., B. Strandberg, T. Augspurger, and R.A. Hites. 2003. Lipophilic organic compounds in lake sediment and American coot (*Fulica americana*) tissues, both affected and unaffected by avian vacuolar myelinopathy. *The Science of the Total Environment* 311:81–89.

Doig, M.T., III, and D.F. Martin. 1973. Anticoagulant properties of a red tide toxin. *Toxicon* 11:351–355.

Doucette, G.J. and C.G. Trick. 1995. Characterization of bacteria associated with different isolates of *Alexandrium tamaraense.* In *Harmful Marine Algal Blooms,* P. Lassus, G. Arzul, E. Erard-Le Denn, P. Gentien, C. Marcaillou-Le Baut (eds.). Lavoisier Publishing, Paris, FR, pp. 33–38.

Emslie, S.D., W.D. Allmon, F.J. Rich, J.H. Wrenn, and S. D. de France. 1996. Integrated taphonomy of an avian death assemblage in marine sediments from the late Pliocene of Florida. *Palaeogeography, Palaeoclimatology and Palaeoecology* 124:107–136.

Eriksson, J.E., J.A.O. Meriluoto, and T. Lindholm. 1986. Can cyanobacterial peptide toxins accumulate in aquatic food chains? In *Perspectives in Microbial Ecology, Proceedings of the Fourth International Symposium on Microbial Ecology,* F. Megusar and M. Gantar (eds.). Slovene Society of Microbiology, Ljubljana, Slovenia, pp. 655–658.

Falconer, I.R. 1991. Tumor promotion and liver injury caused by oral consumption of cyanobacteria. *Environmental Toxicology and Water Quality.* 6:177–184.

Falconer, I.R. 1993. Mechanism of toxicity of cyclic peptide toxins from blue-green algae. In *Algal Toxins in Seafood and Drinking Water,* I. Falconer (ed.). Academic Press, London, U.K., pp. 177–186.

Fischer, J.R., L.A. Lewis, T.Augspurger, and T.E. Rocke. 2002. Avian vacuolar myelinopathy: a newly recognized fatal neurological disease of eagles, waterfowl, and other birds. *Transactions of the North American Wildlife and Natural Resources Conference* 67:51–61.

Fischer, J.R., L.A. Lewis, and C.M. Tate. 2003. Experimental vacuolar myelinopathy in red-tailed hawks. *Journal of Wildlife Diseases* 39:400–406.

Fitch, C.P., L.M. Bishop, and W.L. Boyd. 1934. "Waterbloom" as a cause of poisoning in domestic animals. *Cornell Veterinarian* 24:30–39.

Flewelling, L.J., J.P. Naar, J.P. Abbott, D.G. Baden, N. B. Barros, G.D. Bossart, M.-Y. D. Bottein, D.G. Hammond, E.M. Haubold, C.A. Heil, M.S. Henry, H.M. Jacocks, T.A. Leighfield, R.H. Pierce, T.D. Pitchford, S.A. Rommel, P.S. Scott, K.A. Steidinger, E.W. Truby, F.M.V. Dolah, and J.H. Landsberg. 2005. Brevetoxicosis: Red tides and marine mammal mortalities. *Nature* 435:755–756.

Forrester, D.J., J.M. Gaskin, F. H. White, N.P. Thompson, J.A. Quick, Jr., G. Henderson, and J.C. Woodard. 1977. An epizootic of waterfowl associated with a red tide episode in Florida. *Journal of Wildlife Diseases* 13:160–167.

Fowler, P.K., and P.A. Tester. 1989. Impacts of the 1997–88 North Carolina red tide. *Journal of Shellfish Research* 8:440.

Fritz, L., M.A. Quilliam, and J.L.C. Wright. 1992. An outbreak of domoic acid poisoning attributed to the pennate diatom *Pseudonitzschia australis. Journal of Phycology* 28:439–442.

Fryxell, G.A. and G.R. Hasle. 2003. Taxonomy of harmful diatoms. In *Manual on Harmful Marine Microalgae,* G.M. Hallegraeff, D.M. Anderson, and A.D. Cembella, United Nations Educational, Scientific and Cultural Organization (UNESCO) Publishers, Paris, FR, pp.465–509.

Galtsoff, P.S. 1948. Red tide. Progress report on the investigations of the cause of the mortality of fish along the west coast of Florida conducted by the U.S. Fish and Wildlife Service and cooperating organizations. *United States Fish and Wildlife Service Special Scientific Report* No. 46:1–44.

Garrison, D.L., S.M. Conrad, P.P. Eilers, and E.M. Waldron. 1992. Confirmation of domoic acid production by *Pseudonitzschia australis* (Bacillariophyceae) cultures. *Journal of Phycology* 28:604–607.

Glazier, W.C.W. 1882. On the destruction of fish by polluted water in the Gulf of Mexico. *Proceedings of the United States National Museum* 4:126–127.

Gunter, G., F.G.W. Smith, and R.H. Williams. 1947. Mass mortality of animals on the lower west coast of Florida, November 1946-January, 1947. *Science* 105: 256–257.

Gunter, G., R.H. Williams, C.C. Davis, and F.G.W. Smith. 1948. Catastrophic mass mortality of marine animals and coincident phytoplankton bloom on the west coast of Florida, November 1946 to August 1947. *Ecological Monographs* 18:309–324.

Hallegraeff, G.M. 1993. A review of harmful algal blooms and their apparent global increase. *Phycologia* 32:79–99.

Hallegraeff, G.M. 1995. Harmful algal blooms: a global overview. In *Manual on Harmful Marine Microalgae,* G.M. Hallegraeff, D.M. Anderson, and A. Cembella (eds.). United Nations Educational, Scientific and Cultural Organization, Paris, FR, pp. 1–22.

Hampson, D.R., X. Huang, J.W. Wells, J.A. Walter, and J.L.C. Wright. 1992. Interaction of domoic acid and several derivatives with kainic acid and AMPA binding sites in rat brain. *European Journal of Pharmacology* 218:1–8.

Haque, S.M., and Y. Onoue. 2002. Variation in toxin compositions of two harmful raphidophytes, *Chattonella antiqua* and *Chattonella marina,* at different salinities. *Environmental Toxicology* 17:113–118.

HARRNESS 2005. *Harmful Algal Research and Response: A National Environmental Science Strategy 2005–2015.* J.S. Ramsdell, D.M. Anderson, and P.M. Glibert (eds.). Ecological Society of America, Washington, D.C., U.S.A., 96 pp.

Haywood, A.J., K.A. Steidinger, E.W. Truby, P.R. Bergquist, and P.L. Bergquist. 2004. Comparative morphology and molecular phylogenetic analysis of three new species of the genus *Karenia* (Dinophyceae) from New Zealand. *Journal of Phycology* 40:165–179.

Henriksen, P., W.W. Carmichael, J. An, and Ø. Moestrup. 1997. Detection of an anatoxin-a(s)-like anticholinesterase in natural blooms and cultures of cyanobacteria/blue-green algae from Danish lakes and in the stomach contents of poisoned birds. *Toxicon* 35:901–913.

Hockey, P.A.R., and J. Cooper. 1980. Paralytic shellfish poisoning—a controlling factor in black oystercatcher populations? *Ostrich* 51:188–190.

ICES (International Council for the Exploration of the Sea) 1991. *Report on the Working Group on Phytoplankton and the Management of Their Effects,* Vigo, Spain, 18–21 March 1991. ICES, Copenhagen, Denmark, C.M.1991/Poll: 3:1–175.

Ingham, H.R., J. Mason, and P.C. Wood. 1968. Distribution of toxin in molluscan shellfish following the occurrence of mussel toxicity in north-east England. *Nature* 220:25–27.

Jeffrey, S.W., R.F. Mantoura, and S.W. Wright (eds.). 1997. *Phytoplankton Pigments in Oceanography.* United Nations Educational, Scientific and Cultural Organization, Paris, FR, 668 pp.

Kahn, S., O. Arakawa, and Y. Onoue. 1996. Neurotoxin production by a chloromonad *Fibrocapsa japonica* (Raphidophyceae). *Journal of the World Aquaculture Society* 27:254–263.

Kahn, S., O. Arakawa, and Y. Onoue. 1997. Neurotoxins in a toxic red tide of Heterosigma akashiwo (Raphidophyceae) in Kagoshima Bay, Japan. *Aquaculture Research* 28:9–14.

Kalbe, L., and D. Tiess. 1964. Entenmassensterben durch *Nodularia*-Wasserblüte am kleinen Jasmunder Bodden auf Rügen. Archiv für Experimentelle Veterinarmedizin (Leipzig) 18:535–555.

Kao, C.Y. 1993. Paralytic shellfish poisoning. In *Algal Toxins in Seafood and Drinking Water,* I. Falconer (ed.). Academic Press, London, U.K., pp. 75–86.

Koch, R. 1891. Über bakteriologische forschung verhandlung des X Internationalen Medizinischen Congresses, Berlin, 1890. In *Xth International Congress of Medicine.* August Hirschwald, Berlin, DEU, pp. 35–47.

Kodama, M., T. Ogata, and S. Sato. 1988. Bacterial production of saxitoxin. Agricultural and Biological Chemistry 52:1075–1077.

Kodama, M. 2000. Paralytic shellfish poisoning. Ecobiology, classification, and origin. In *Seafood and Freshwater Toxins: Pharmacology, Physiology, and Detection,* L.M. Botana (ed.). Marcel Dekker, New York, NY, U.S.A., pp. 125–149.

Konovalova, G.V. 1989. Phytoplankton blooms and red tides in the far east coastal waters of the USSR. In *Red Tides, Biology, Environmental Science and Toxicology,* T. Okaichi, D.M. Anderson, and T. Nemoto (eds.). Elsevier Press, New York, NY, U.S.A., pp. 97–100.

Konovalova, G.V. 1993. Toxic and potentially toxic dinoflagellates from the Far east coastal waters of Russia. In *Toxic Phytoplankton Blooms in the Sea,* T.J. Smayda and Y. Shimuzu (eds.). Elsevier Press, Amsterdam, NLD, pp. 275–279.

Kreuder, C., J.A.K. Mazet, G.D. Bossart, T.E. Carpenter, M. Holyoak, M.S. Elie, and S.D. Wright. 2002. Clinicopathologic features of suspected brevetoxicosis in double-crested cormorants (*Phalacrocorax auritus*) along the Florida Gulf coast. *Journal of Zoo and Wildlife Medicine* 33:8–15.

Krienitz L., A. Ballot, K. Kotut, C. Wiegand, S. Pütz, J.S. Metcalf, G.A. Codd, and S. Pflügmacher. 2003. Contribution of hot spring cyanobacteria to the mysterious deaths of lesser flamingos at Lake Bogoria, Kenya. *Federation of European Microbiology Societies Microbiology Ecology* 43:141–148.

Kvitek, R.G. 1991. Sequestered paralytic shellfish poisoning toxins mediate glaucous-winged gull predation on bivalve prey. *The Auk* 108:381–392.

Kvitek, R.G., and C. Bretz. 2005. Shorebird foraging behavior, diet, and abundance vary with harmful algal bloom toxin concentrations in invertebrate prey. *Marine Ecology Progress Series* 293:303–309.

Lam, A.K.Y., Prepas, E.E., Spink, D., and Hrudey, S.E. 1995. Chemical control of hepatotoxic phytoplankton blooms: implications for human health. *Water Research* 29:1845–1854.

Landsberg, J.H. 2002. The effects of harmful algal blooms on aquatic organisms. *Reviews in Fisheries Science* 10:113–390.

Landsberg, J.H., F. Van Dolah, and G. Doucette. 2005. Marine and estuarine harmful algal blooms: impacts on human and animal health. In *Oceans and Health: Pathogens in the Marine Environment,* S. Belkin and R. Colwell (eds.). Springer, New York, NY, U.S.A., pp. 165–215.

Larsen, R.S., F.B. Nutter, T. Augspurger, T.E. Rocke, L. Tomlinson, N.J. Thomas, and M.K. Stoskopf. 2002. Clinical features of avian vacuolar myelinopathy in American coots. *Journal of the American Veterinary Medical Association* 221:80–85.

Larsen, R.S., F.B. Nutter, T. Augspurger, T.E. Rocke, N.J. Thomas, and M.K. Stoskopf. 2003. Failure to transmit avian vacuolar myelinopathy to mallard ducks. *Journal of Wildlife Diseases* 39:707–711.

Lewis-Weis, L.A., R.W. Gerhold, and J.R. Fischer. 2004. Attempts to reproduce vacuolar myelinopathy in domestic swine and chickens. *Journal of Wildlife Diseases* 40:476–484.

Llewellyn, L., A. Negri, and M. Quilliam. 2004. High affinity for the rat brain sodium channel of newly discovered hydroxybenzoate saxitoxin analogues from the dinoflagellate *Gymnodinium catenatum. Toxicon* 43:101–104.

Luukkainen, R., K. Sivonen, M. Namikoshi, M. Färdig, K.L. Rinehart, and S.I. Niemelä 1993. Isolation and identification of eight microcystins from thirteen *Oscillatoria agardhii* strains and structure of a new microcystin. *Applied and Environmental Microbiology* 59:2204–2209.

Matsunaga, H., K. Harada, M. Senma, Y. Ito, N. Yasuda, S. Ushida, and Y. Kimura. 1999. Possible cause of unnatural mass death of wild birds in a pond in Nishinomiya, Japan: sudden appearance of toxic cyanobacteria. *Natural Toxins* 7:81–84.

Matsushima, R., S. Yoshizawa, M.F. Watanabe, K.-I. Harada, M. Furusawa, W.W. Carmichael, and H. Fujiki. 1990. *In vitro* and *in vivo* effects of protein phosphatase inhibitors, microcystins and nodularin, on mouse skin and fibroblasts. *Biochemical and Biophysical Research Communications* 171:867–874.

McKernan, D.L., and V.B. Scheffer. 1942. Unusual numbers of dead birds on the Washington Coast. *The Condor* 44:264–266.

Moore, M.A. 1882. Fish mortality in the Gulf of Mexico. *Proceedings of the United States National Museum* 4:125–126.

Moustaka-Gouni, M., C.M. Cook, S. Gkelis, E. Michaloudi, K. Pantlelidakis, M. Pyrovetsi, and T. Lanaras. 2004. The coincidence of a *Prymnesium parvum* bloom and the mass kill of birds and fish in Lake Koronia. *Harmful Algae News* 26:1–2.

Mur, L.R., O. Skulberg, and H. Utkilen. 1999. Cyanobacteria in the environment. In *Toxic Cyanobacteria in Water: A Guide to Their Public Health Consequences, Monitoring and Management,* I. Chorus, and J. Bartram (eds.). E. and F.N. Spon, London, U.K., pp. 15–40.

Murphy, T., A. Lawson, C. Nalewajiko, H. Murkin, L. Ross, K. Oguma, and T. McIntyre. 2000. Algal toxins—initiators of avian botulism? *Environmental Toxicology* 15:558–567.

Murphy, T.P., K. Irvine, J. Guo, J. Davies, H. Murkin, M. Charlton, and S.B. Watson. 2003. New microcystin concerns in the lower Great Lakes. *Water Quality Research Journal of Canada* 38:127–140.

Negri, A.P., G.J. Jones, and M. Hindmarsh. 1995. Sheep mortality associated with paralytic shellfish poisons from the cyanobacterium *Anabaena circinalis. Toxicon* 33:1321–1329.

Nisbet, I.C. 1983. Paralytic shellfish poisoning: effects on breeding terns. *The Condor* 85:338–345.

Novelli, A., J. Kispert, A. Reilly and V. Zitko. 1990. Excitatory amino acids toxicity in cerebellar granule cells in primary culture. *Canada Diseases Weekly Report 16 Supplement* 1E:83–88; discussion pp. 88–89.

Ogata, T., S. Sato, and M. Kodama. 1989. Paralytic shellfish toxins in bivalves which are not associated with dinoflagellates. *Toxicon* 27:1241–1244.

Ogata, T., M. Kodama, K. Komaru, S. Sakamoto, S. Sato, and U. Simidu. 1990. Production of paralytic shellfish toxins by bacteria isolated from toxic dinoflagellates. In *Toxic Marine Phytoplankton,* E. Granéli, B. Sundström, L. Edler, and D. M. Anderson (eds.). Elsevier, New York, NY, U.S.A., pp. 311–315.

Ohta, T., E. Sueoka, N. Iida, A. Komori, M. Suganuma, R. Nishiwaki, M. Tatematsu, S.J. Kim, W.W. Carmichael, and H. Fujiki. 1994. Nodularin, a potent inhibitor of protein phosphatases 1 and 2A, is a new environmental carcinogen in male F344 rat liver. *Cancer Research* 54:6402–6406.

Onodera, H., M. Satake, Y. Oshima, T. Yasumoto, and W.W. Carmichael. 1997a. New saxitoxin analogues from the freshwater filamentous cyanobacterium *Lyngbya wollei. Natural Toxins* 5:146–151.

Onodera, H., Y. Oshima, P. Henriksen, and T. Yasumoto. 1997b. Confirmation of anatoxin-a(s), in the cyanobacterium *Anabaena lemmermannii,* as the cause of bird kills in the Danish lakes. *Toxicon* 35:1645–1648.

O'Shea, T.J., G.B. Rathbun, R.K. Bonde, C.D. Buergelt, and D.K. Odell. 1991. An epizootic of Florida manatees associated with a dinoflagellate bloom. *Marine Mammal Science* 7:165–179.

Oshima, Y., T. Sugino, and T. Yasumoto. 1989. Latest advances in HPLC analysis of paralytic shellfish toxins. In *Mycotoxins and Phycotoxins '88,* S. Natori, K. Hashimoto, and Y. Ueno (eds.). Elsevier, Amsterdam, NLD, pp. 319–326.

Oshima, Y. 1995. Chemical and enzymatic transformation of shellfish toxins in marine organisms. In *Harmful Marine Algal Blooms,* P. Lassus, G. Arzul, E. Erard-LeDenn, P. Gentien, and C. Marcaillou-LeBaut (eds.). Lavoisier, Paris, FR, pp. 475–480.

Pierce, R.H. 1986. Red tide (*Ptychodiscus brevis*) toxin aerosols: a review. *Toxicon* 24:955–965.

Pierce, R.H., M.S. Henry, L.S. Proffitt, and P.A. Hasbrouck. 1990. Red tide toxin (brevetoxin) enrichment in marine aerosol. In *Toxic Marine Phytoplankton,* E. Graneli, B. Sundstrom, L. Edler, and D. Anderson (eds.). Elsevier, Amsterdam, NLD, pp. 128–131.

Poli, M.A., T.J. Mende, and D.G. Baden. 1986. Brevetoxins, unique activators of voltage-sensitive sodium channels, bind to specific sites in rat brain synaptosomes. *Molecular Pharmacology* 30:129–135.

Popkiss, M.E.E., D.A. Horstman, and D. Harpur. 1979. Paralytic shellfish poisoning: a report of 17 cases in Cape Town. *South African Medical Journal* 55: 1017–1023.

Pütz, K., A.P. Clausen, N. Huin, and J.P. Croxall. 2003. Evaluation of historical Rockhopper Penguin population data in the Falkland Islands. *Waterbirds* 26: 169–175.

Pybus, M., D. Hobson, and D.K. Onderka.1986. Mass mortality of bats due to probable blue-green algae toxicity. *Journal of Wildlife Diseases* 22:449–450.

Quick, J.A., and G.E. Henderson. 1974. Effects of *Gymnodinium breve* red tide on fishes and birds: a preliminary report on behavior, anatomy, hematology and histopathology. In *Proceedings of the Gulf Coast Regional Symposium on Diseases of Aquatic Animals,* R.L. Amborski, M.A. Hood, and R.R. Miller (eds.). Louisiana State University: Louisiana Sea Grant, Louisiana, U.S.A., pp. 85–113.

Reynolds, C.S. 1997. Vegetation processes in the pelagic: A model for ecosystem theory. In *Excellence in Ecology,* Vol. 9, O. Kinne (ed.). Ecology Institute, Oldendorf-Luhe, GER, 371 pp.

Rinehart, K.L., M. Namikoshi, and B. Choi. 1994. Structure and biosynthesis of toxins from blue-green algae (cyanobacteria). *Journal of Applied Phycology* 6:159–176.

Rocke, T.E., N.J. Thomas, T. Augspurger, and K. Miller. 2002. Epizootiologic studies of avian vacuolar myelinopathy in waterbirds. *Journal of Wildlife Diseases* 38:678–684.

Rocke, T.E., N.J. Thomas, C.U. Meteyer, C.F. Quist, J.R. Fischer, T. Augspurger, and S.E. Ward. 2005. Attempts to identify the source of avian vacuolar myelinopathy for waterbirds. *Journal of Wildlife Diseases* 41: 163–170.

Runnegar, M.T., A.R.B. Jackson, and I.R. Falconer. 1988. Toxicity of the cyanobacterium, *Nodularia spumigens* Mertens. *Toxicon* 26:143–151.

Sasner, J.J., M. Ikawa, and B.E. Barrett. 1975. The 1972 red tide in New Hampshire. In *Proceedings of the First International Conference on Toxic Dinoflagellate Blooms,* V. R. LoCicero (ed.). Massachusetts Science and Technology Foundation, Wakefield, Massachusetts, U.S.A., pp. 517–523.

Scholin, C.A., F. Gulland, G.J. Doucette, S. Benson, M. Busman, F.P. Chavez, J. Cordaro, R. Delong, A. De Vogelaera, J. Harvey, M. Haulena, K. Lefebvre, T. Lipscomb, S. Loscutoff, L.J. Lowenstine, R. Marin III, P.E. Miller, W.A. McLellan, P.D.R. Moeller, C.L. Powell, T. Rowles, P. Silvagni, M. Silver, T. Spraker, V. Trainer, and F.M. Van Dolah. 2000. Mortality of sea lions along the central California coast linked to a toxic diatom bloom. *Nature* 403:80–84.

Schwimmer, D., and M. Schwimmer. 1968. Medical aspects of phycology. In *Algae, Man and the Environment,* D. Jackson (ed.). Syracuse University Press, Syracuse, New York, U.S.A., pp. 279–358.

SEANET. 2005. Red tide in MA to ME has potential to affect birds. Seabird Ecological Assessment Network (SEANET), Tufts University, North Grafton, MA. [Online.] Retrieved from the World Wide Web: www.tufts.edu/vet/seanet/seanet_news.shtml.

Short, S.B., and W.C. Edwards. 1990. Blue-green algae toxicoses in Oklahoma. *Veterinary and Human Toxicology* 32:558–560.

Shumway, S.E. 1990. A review of the effects of algal blooms on shellfish and aquaculture. *Journal of the World Aquaculture Society* 21: 65–104.

Shumway, S.E., S.M. Allen, and P.D. Boersma. 2003. Marine birds and harmful algal blooms: sporadic victims or under-reported events? *Harmful Algae* 2:1–17.

Sierra Beltran, A., M. Palafox-Uribe, J. Grajales-Montiel, A. Cruz-Villacorta, and J.L. Ochoa. 1997. Sea bird mortality at Cabo San Lucas, Mexico: evidence that toxic diatom blooms are spreading. *Toxicon* 35:447–453.

Sipia, V.O., K.A. Karlsson, J.A.O. Meriluoto, and H.T. Kankaanpaa. 2004. Eiders (*Somateria mollissima*) obtain nodularin, a cyanobacterial hepatotoxin, in Baltic Sea food web. *Environmental Toxicology and Chemistry* 23:1256–1260.

Sivonen, K., and G. Jones. 1999. Cyanobacterial toxins. In *Toxic Cyanobacteria in Water,* I. Chorus, and J. Bartram (eds.). Routledge, London, UK, pp. 41–111.

Smayda, T.J. 1990. Novel and nuisance phytoplankton blooms in the sea: evidence for a global epidemic. In *Toxic Marine Phytoplankton,* E. Granéli, B. Sundstrom, L. Edler, and D.M. Anderson (eds.). Academic Press: New York, U.S.A., pp. 29–40.

Smayda, T.J. 1992. Global epidemic of noxious phytoplankton blooms and food chain consequences in large ecosystems. In *Food Chains, Models, and Management of Large Marine Ecosystems,* K. Sherman, L.M. Alexander, and B.D. Gold (eds.). Westview Press, San Francisco, CA, U.S.A., pp.275–307.

Smith, G.B. 1975. The 1971 red tide and its impact on certain reef communities in the mideastern Gulf of Mexico. *Environmental Letters* 9:141–152.

Smith, J.C., P. Odense, R. Angus, S. Bates, C.J. Bird, R. Cormier, A.S.W. deFreitas, C. Leger, D.O'Neil, K. Pauley, and J. Worms. 1990. Variation in domoic acid levels in *Nitzschia* species: implications for monitoring programs. *Bulletin of the Aquaculture Association of Canada* 90:27–31.

Smith, P.T. 2000. Freshwater neurotoxins: mechanisms of action, pharmacology, toxicology, and impacts on aquaculture. In *Seafood and Freshwater Toxins: Pharmacology, Physiology, and Detection,* L.M. Botana (ed.). Marcel Dekker, New York, NY, U.S.A., pp. 583–602.

Steidinger, K.A. 1993. Some taxonomic and biologic aspects of toxic dinoflagellates. In *Algal Toxins in Seafood and Drinking Water,* I. Falconer (ed.). Academic Press, London, U.K., pp. 1–28.

Steidinger, K.A., and D.G. Baden. 1984. Toxic marine dinoflagellates. In *Dinoflagellates,* D.C. Spector (ed.). Academic Press, New York, NY, U.S.A., pp. 201–261.

Steidinger, K.A. and K. Tangen. 1996. Dinoflagellates. In *Identifying Marine Diatoms and Dinoflagellates,* C.R. Tomas (ed.). Academic Press, New York, NY, U.S.A., pp. 387–584.

Steidinger, K.A., M. Burklew, and R. M. Ingle. 1973. The effects of *Gymnodinium breve* toxin on estuarine animals. In *Marine Pharmacognosy: Action of Marine Toxins at the Cellular level,* D.F. Martin, and G.M. Padilla (eds.). Academic Press, New York, NY, U.S.A., pp. 179–202.

Steidinger, K.A., L.S. Tester, and F.J.R. Taylor. 1980. A redescription of *Pyrodinium bahamense* var. *compressa* (Böhm) stat. nov. from Pacific red tides. *Phycologia* 19:329–334.

Stephens, E.L. 1948. *Microcystis toxica* sp. nov., a poisonous alga from the Transvaal and Orange Free State. *Transactions of the Royal Society of South Africa* 32:105–112.

Steyn, D.G. 1945. Poisoning of animals and human beings by algae. *South African Journal of Science* 41:243–244.

Subba Rao, D.V., M.A. Quilliam, and R. Pocklington. 1988. Domoic acid—a neurotoxic amino acid produced by the marine diatom *Nitzschia pungens* in culture. *Canadian Journal of Fisheries and Aquatic Sciences* 45:2076–2079.

Sudaranam, S., G. Duke-Virca, D.J. March, and S. Srinivasan. 1992. An approach to computer aided inhibitor design: application to cathepsin I. *Journal of Computer-Aided Molecular Design* 6:223–233.

Suter, G.W. III, R.A. Efroymson, B.E. Sample, and D.S. Jones (eds.). 1993. Ecological risk assessment. Lewis Publishers, Boca Raton, FL, U.S.A., 438 pp.

Takahashi, S., and K. Kaya. 1993. Quail spleen is enlarged by microcystin RR as a blue-green algal hepatotoxin. *Natural Toxins* 1:283–285.

Takemoto, T., and K. Daigo. 1958. Constituents of *Chondria armata. Chemical and Pharmaceutical Bulletin* 6:578–580.

Tangen, K., U. Winther, and E. Dragsund. 1992. Adverse effects of an *Alexandrium excavatum* bloom in Norwegian waters. *Red Tide Newsletter* 5:2.

Taylor, F. J. R., Y. Fukuyo, J. Larsen, and G. M. Hallegraeff. 2003. Taxonomy of harmful dinoflagellates. In *Manual on Harmful Marine Microalgae,* G.M. Hallegraeff, D.M. Anderson, and A.D. Cembella (eds.), United Nations Educational, Scientific and Cultural Organization Publishers (UNESCO Press), Paris, FR, pp. 389–432.

Tester, P.A., R.P. Stumpf, and K. Steidinger. 1998. Ocean color imagery: What is the minimum detection level for *Gymnodinium brevis* blooms? In *Harmful Algae,* B. Reguera, J. Blanco, M. L. Fernández, and T. Wyatt (eds.). Intergovernmental Oceanographic Commission of the United Nations Educational, Scientific and Cultural Organization, Xunta de Galicia and Paris, pp. 149–151.

Thomas, N.J., C.U. Meteyer, and L. Sileo. 1998. Epizootic vacuolar myelinopathy of the central nervous system of bald eagles (*Haliaeetus leucocephalus*) and American coots (*Fulica americana*). *Veterinary Pathology* 35:479–487.

Throndsen, J. 1996. The planktonic marine flagellates. In *Identifying Marine Diatoms and Dinoflagellates,* C.R Tomas (ed.). Academic Press, New York, NY, U.S.A., pp. 591–729.

Tomas, C.R., and D.G. Baden. 1993. The influence of phosphorus source on the growth and cellular toxin content of the benthic dinoflagellate *Prorocentrum lima.* In *Toxic Phytoplankton in the Sea,* T.J. Smayda and Y. Shimizu (eds.). Elsevier Science Publishers, Amsterdam, NLD, pp. 565–570.

Van Dolah, F.M. 2000. Diversity of marine and freshwater algal toxins. In *Seafood and Freshwater Toxins: Pharmacology, Physiology, and Detection,* L.M. Botana (ed.). Marcel Dekker, New York, NY, U.S.A., pp. 19–43.

Vargo, G.A., K. Atwood, M. van Deventer, and R. Harris. 2006. Beached bird surveys on Shell Key, Pinellas County, Florida. *Florida Field Naturalist* 34:21–27.

Vollenweider, R., and Kerekes, J. 1982. *Eutrophication of Waters, Monitoring, Assessment, Control.* Organisation for Economic Co-operation and Development, Paris, FR, 154 pp.

Walker, S. T. 1884. Fish mortality in the Gulf of Mexico. In *Proceedings of the United States National Museum* 6:105–109.

Wilde, S.B., T.M. Murphy, C.P. Hope, S.K. Habrun, J. Kempton, A. Birrenkott, F. Wiley, W. W. Bowerman, and A. J. Lewitus. 2005. Avian vacuolar myelinopathy linked to exotic aquatic plants and a novel cyanobacterial species. *Environmental Toxicology* 20:348–353.

Wirsing, B., L. Hoffman, R. Heinze, D. Klein, D. Daloze, J.C. Braekman, and J. Weckesser. 1998. First report on the identification of microcystin in a water bloom collected in Belgium. *Systematic and Applied Microbiology* 21:23–27.

Woodman, J.N., and E.B. Cowling. 1987. Airborne chemicals and forest health. *Environmental Science and Technology* 21:120–126.

Work, T.M., B. Bar, A.M. Beale, L. Fritz, M.A. Quilliam, and J.L.C. Wright. 1992. Epidemiology of domoic acid poisoning in brown pelicans (*Pelecanus occidentalis*) and Brandt's cormorants (*Phalacrocorax penicillatus*) in California. *Journal of Zoology and Wildlife Medicine* 24:54–62.

Work, T.M., A.M. Beale, L. Fritz, M.A. Quilliam, M. Silver, K. Buck, and J.L.C. Wright. 1993. Domoic acid intoxication of brown pelicans and cormorants in Santa Cruz, California. In *Toxic Phytoplankton Blooms in the Sea,* T.J. Smayda, and Y. Shimizu (eds.). Elsevier, Amsterdam, NLD, pp. 643–649.

Yoshizawa, S., R. Matsushima, M. Watanabe, K.-I. Harada, A. Ichihara, W.W. Carmichael, and H. Fujiki. 1990. Inhibition of protein phosphatases by microcystins and nodularin associated with hepatoxicity. *Journal of Cancer Research and Clinical Oncology* 116:609–614.

Index

Printed and bound by CPI Group (UK) Ltd, Croydon, CR0 4YY

16/04/2025

14658458-0005